# The SAGES Manual of Strategic Decision Making

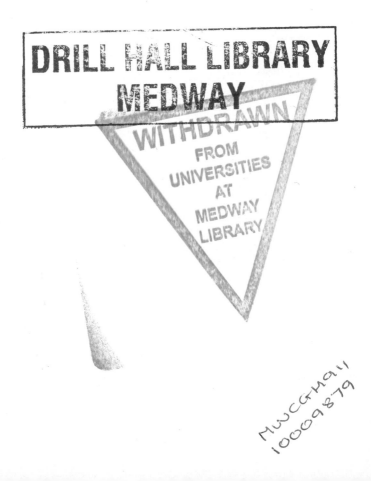

# The SAGES Manual of Strategic Decision Making

## Case Studies in Minimal Access Surgery

Carol E.H. Scott-Conner, MD, PhD
University of Iowa Hospitals and Clinics, Iowa City, IA, USA.

Editor

José E. Torres, MD
University of Iowa, Iowa City, IA, USA.

and

Nate Thepjatri, MD
University of Iowa, Iowa City, IA, USA.

Case Editors

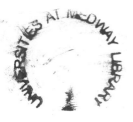

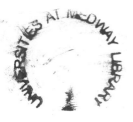

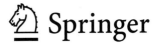 Springer

*Editor*
Carol E.H. Scott-Conner, MD, PhD
Professor
Department of Surgery
University of Iowa Hospitals and Clinics
Iowa City, IA
USA

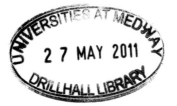

ISBN: 978-0-387-76670-6     e-ISBN: 978-0-387-76671-3
DOI: 10.1007/978-0-387-76671-3

Library of Congress Control Number: 2007940439

Printed on acid-free paper

9  8  7  6  5  4  3  2  1

springer.com

# Foreword

Minimal access, whenever feasible, in the performance of most general surgical procedures is now well established. However, many areas still need clarification. They range from indications and contraindications to the optimal route of access, as well as to choices to be made among the various procedures possible for any single surgical problem. This *Manual* is unique in that unlike most manuals it is not so much a "how to" but more a "when to," the "how to" having been covered to a significant extent in the two previous SAGES manuals. This work takes a series of common clinical scenarios and offers various, detailed, often contrasting approaches, commonly but not exclusively minimal access, discussing indications, limitations, and potential complications.

In this age of evidence-based surgical practice, the reader will find it refreshing to have abundant data and references to support or reject a particular approach or technique. With a cadre of surgeon authors skilled in open as well as minimal access surgery, including flexible endoscopy, the student and practitioner of surgery is exposed to not only varying approaches to many common surgical conditions but also comes to appreciate how flexibility and integration of various approaches can improve the outcome for the patient.

The forty-six chapters can each constitute a stand-alone discussion. The format of each chapter is uniformly an introduction of the problem to be considered or question to be answered. This is followed by a case history, after which, in almost every instance two authors each declare his or her preference of approach and management, giving reasons and offering evidence, if it exists, and acknowledging lack of data if they are insufficient. Each chapter concludes with a summary discussion, bringing the reader up to date on the state of the art and making recommendations based on available data. Integration of ultrasound, MRI, PET scanning, and computed tomography is detailed when these modalities are employed for diagnosis or therapy as is the use of endoscopically deployed stenting for biliary tract and colonic obstructions.

Some topics, such as gastroesophageal reflux, complicated as they are and controversial as their management often is, require more than one chapter for adequate discussion, and the editor, Dr. Carol E.H. Scott-Conner, is to be congratulated for her orchestration of these subjects, addressed as they are by multiple authors with minimal repetition evident to the reader. The inclusion of chapters on enteral access and nutrition, the discussions of management of complications of minimal access surgery, such bleeding and cystic duct stump leakage after laparoscopic cholecystectomy, opinions on when to convert to open operation are well treated. There is even detailed discussion of medical therapy when it is considered an appropriate alternative approach to a problem.

The contributing authors not only discuss differences in minimal access approaches but also address the integration of various methods of access (for example, flexible endoscopic combined with laparoscopic), various tools of dissection (hand, ultrasound, thermal) as well as varying techniques of specimen retrieval and extraction.

The surgeon involved in advanced laparoscopic surgery will find of special value the treatment of conditions that have been more recently managed by surgeons in specialties other than general surgery but, with overlapping training and practice, are increasingly performed by surgeons skilled in minimal access techniques.

While this work is labeled a "manual," it is a veritable textbook, albeit not covering every imaginable aspect of minimal access surgery. It will provide guidance for those who are interested in putting into logical context the role of minimal access procedures in the management of diseases managed by surgeons rather than the sometimes unfortunate perception that the new and the old are in competition. While it does provide clear and detailed descriptions of some procedures, open, endoscopic, and combined, its greatest strength is in the new knowledge it summarizes and the results it shares.

These are changing times in the world of surgery. The face of surgery is changing and the face of those who perform surgery is changing. Many of these chapters may need revision as time passes, as instruments are retooled, new modalities introduced, and more results accumulated, but this work serves for the present as a practical guide and logical basis for which approach today's surgeon should consider and why. Since minimal access will be the common practice of surgery when they graduate, this work should be read by all surgical residents. It will obviously appeal to fellows in advanced laparoscopic training programs, to teachers as well as practitioners of minimal access surgery and, hopefully, to surgical program directors and their faculty at large. It should also be of special interest to those surgeons who received their instruction in a previous generation and wish to know more of the substance and less of the hyperbole of minimal access surgery.

*Kenneth A. Forde, MD*
New York, NY
January 2008

# Preface

This book is all about choices and alternatives. Its purpose is to explore different approaches in minimal access surgery. The order of the chapters follows that of *The SAGES Manual: Fundamentals of Laparoscopy, Thoracoscopy, and GI Endoscopy*, beginning with the basic question of how to access the abdomen for laparoscopy and culminating with thoracoscopic sympathectomy. Trainees will find balanced presentations of two or more approaches, followed by concluding sections that weigh the evidence and give both references and selected readings. Practicing surgeons will find alternatives to their preferred approach in a situation— alternatives that we hope will expand their repertoire of techniques. Experts have been generous in sharing technical tips and pearls.

Readers of the SAGES Manual series gave us the idea for this book. They requested a "case studies" book that would explore the concepts of minimal access surgery through a series of actual clinical cases. SAGES responded by appointing an editorial advisory board, and together the members hammered out a list of topics that we felt, exemplified some of the issues on which experts disagree. Topics were chosen to span the spectrum of laparoscopic and endoscopic topics. For each topic, two viewpoints were identified. We did not attempt to cover every procedure in the SAGES manual, but rather selected clinical scenarios where we felt expert opinion diverged on management.

Then the fun began!

I was given the privilege of editing the book. Two Case Studies editors, Dr. Jose Torres and Dr. Nate Thepjatri, accumulated actual cases from the rich clinical material at the University of Iowa Hospitals and Clinics. Experts were recruited. I was rapidly reminded of the speed with which this field is developing and changing. In some areas, we identified more than two alternatives. In others, there was one overwhelmingly popular choice, and one that no one wanted to champion. I wrote a few of those orphan sections myself.

Many individuals deserve my profound thanks. I will name just a few here. A long list of authors were endlessly patient during a long editing process. Our residents and students, who contributed most of the cases, continue to inspire and teach all of us. Thanks go also to our editor, Paula Callaghan, who was endlessly patient with a highly fluid table of contents (reflecting changes in the field) through the process. The SAGES Editorial Advisory

Board consisted of Frederick Greene MD, Mark Talamini MD, and Tracey Arnell MD. My husband provided unswerving support. Finally, I wish to give thanks to SAGES, an organization that epitomizes surgeons working together to share and increase surgical knowledge.

*Carol E.H. Scott-Conner MD PhD*
Iowa City, Iowa
January 25, 2008

# Contents

# Contributors

*Prasad S. Adusumilli, MD*
General Surgeon, Memorial Sloan-Kettering Cancer Center,
New York, NY, USA

*Mohammad Allam, MD*
Cardiovascular Surgeon, Cardiovascular Clinic, Lafayette, LA, USA

*Basil J. Ammori, MD*
General Surgeon, Manchester Royal Infirmary, Manchester, UK

*Jared L. Antevil, MD*
General Surgeon, Naval Medical Center San Diego, San Diego,
CA, USA

*Muzaffar A. Anwar, MBBS*
General Surgeon, Whiston Hospital, Prescot, Merseyside, UK

*Evgeny V. Arshava, MD*
Resident, Department of Surgery, University of Iowa, Iowa City,
IA, USA

*Tracey D. Arnell, MD*
Assistant Attending Surgeon, NewYork-Presbyterian
Hospital/Columbia, New York, NY, USA

*Howard A. Aubert, MD*
Department of Urology, University of Iowa Hospitals and Clinics, Iowa
City, IA, USA

*Amanda Ayers, MD*
Resident, Department of General Surgery, University of Connecticut,
Integrated General Surgery Residency, Farmington, CT, USA

*Desmond Birkett, MB, BS, FACS*
Chairman, Department of General Surgery, Lahey Clinic Medical
Center, Burlington, MA, USA

*Samuel E. Bledsoe, MD*
Resident, Department of Surgery, Physicians Medical Center Carraway, Birmingham, AL, USA

*Fred Brody, MD, MBA*
Associate, Professor of Surgery, The George Washington University Medical Center, Washington, DC, USA

*Christoph E. Broelsch, MD*
General Surgeon, University of Chicago Medical Center, Chicago, IL, USA

*Carlos V. R. Brown, MD, FACS*
Chief of Trauma, Brackenridge Hospital, Associate, Professor of Surgery, University of Texas Medical Branch, Austin, TX, USA

*L. Michael Brunt, MD*
Professor, Department of Surgery, Washington University School of Medicine, St. Louis, MO, USA

*Sathyaprasad C. Burjonrappa, MD, FRCS(Ed)*
Fellow in Pediatric Surgery, University of Montreal, Montreal, Quebec, Canada

*Jo Buyske, MD*
General Surgeon, Presbyterian Medical Center, Philadelphia, PA, USA

*Marco Casaccia, MD*
Assistant Professor, Department of Surgery, General and Transplant Surgery Department, University of Genoa, Italy

*Edward H. Chin, MD*
Department of Surgery, Mount Sinai School of Medicine, New York, NY, USA

*Kent Choi, MD*
General Surgeon, University of Iowa Hospitals and Clinics, Iowa City, IA, USA

*Hui Sen Chong, MD*
Resident, Department of Surgery, University of Iowa, Iowa City, IA, USA

*Joseph Y. Chung, MD*
Department of Surgery, University of Iowa Hospitals and Clinics, Iowa City, IA, USA

*Ronald H. Clements, MD, FACS*
Associate, Professor of Surgery, University of Alabama-Birmingham, AL, USA

*Jeffrey L. Cohen, MD, FACS, FASCRS*
President, Connecticut Surgical Group, Professor of Clinical Surgery, University of Connecticut, Hartford, CT, USA

*Michael Cook, DO*
Radiologist, Beth Israel Medical Center, Brooklyn, NY, USA

*John Morgan Cosgrove, MD, FACS*
Director, American College of Surgeons, Chairman, Department of Surgery, Bronx Lebanon Hospital Center/Albert Einstein College, Bronx, NY, USA

*Jorge Cueto, MD, FACS*
Professor, Department of Minimally Invasive Surgery, Universidad Anahuac, Mexico City, Department of Surgery. American British Cowdray Hospital of Mexico City, Mexico

*Myriam J. Curet, MD, FACS*
Professor, Department of Surgery, Senior Associate Dean for Graduate and Continuing Medical Education, Stanford University School of Medicine, Stanford, CA, USA

*S. Scott Davis, Jr., MD*
Clinical Assistant Professor, Emory Endosurgery Unit, Atlanta, GA, USA

*Daniel J. Deziel, MD*
General Surgeon, Rush University Hospital, Chicago, IL , USA

*Francis D'Souza, FRCS*
General Surgeon, Whiston Hospital, Prescot, Merseyside, UK

*Quan-Yang Duh, MD*
Professor, Department of Surgery, Universisty of California,
San Francisco, San Francisco, CA, USA

*David Duppler, MD, FACS*
Fox Valley Surgical Associatess, Appleton Medical Center, Appleton,
WI, USA

*David Easter, MD, FACS*
Professor, Department of Clinical Surgery, University of California at
San Diego, San Diego, CA, USA

*Michael A. Edwards, MD*
Assistant Professor, Department of Surgery, Director, Virtual Education
and Surgical Skills Lab, Medical College of Georgia, Augusta, GA, USA

*George M. Eid, MD*
Assistant Professor, Department of Surgery, University of Pittsburgh
College of Medicine, Pittsburgh, PA, USA

*Farshad Elmi, MD*
Department of Internal Medicine, University of Iowa Hospitals
and Clinics, Iowa City, IA, USA

*Randy D. Ernst, MD*
Associate Professor, Department of Diagnostic Radiology,
The University of Texas M. D. Anderson Cancer Center, Houston,
TX, USA

*Sandy M. Fang, MD*
Department of Surgery, University of Iowa Hospitals and Clinics,
Iowa City, IA, USA

*Daniel L. Feingold, MD*
Assisting Attending Surgeon, NewYork-Presbyterian Hospital/
Columbia, New York, NY, USA

*Robert Fitzgibbons Jr., MD, FACS*
Harry E. Stuckenhoff Professor, Department of Surgery, Chief of the
Division of General Surgery, Associate Chairman, Department of
Surgery, Creighton University School of Medicine, Omaha, NE, USA

*Kenneth A. Forde, MD, FACS, FASCRS*
Jose M. Ferrer Professor Emeritus, Department of Surgery, College of
Physicians and Surgeons, Columbia University, New York, NY, USA

*James K. Fullerton, MD*
General Surgeon, Springfield Clinic, Springfield, IL, USA

*Henning Gerke, MD*
Gastroenterologist, University of Iowa Hospitals and Clinics, Iowa City,
IA, USA

*Frederick L. Greene, MD, FACS*
Chairman and Residency Program Director, Department of Surgery,
Carolinas Medical Center, Charlotte, NC, USA

*Susan S. Hagen, PhD*
Associate Director, Department of Surgical Research, Associate
Professor, Department of Surgery, Beth Israel Deaconess Medical
Center, Boston, MA, USA

*Daniel M. Hallam, MD*
Department of Surgery, University of Iowa Hospitals and Clinics,
Iowa City, IA, USA

*Zane T. Hammoud, MD*
Assistant Professor, Department of Surgery, Indianapolis, IN, USA

*Robert Hanfland, MD*
Department of Surgery, University of Iowa Hospitals and Clinics,
Iowa City, IA, USA

*Jeffrey Hannon, MD, FACS*
Assistant Professor, Department of Surgery, University of South
Alabama, School of Medicine, Mobile, AL, USA

*Samad Hashimi, MD*
Department of Surgery, University of Iowa Hospitals and Clinics,
Iowa City, IA, USA

*David Hazzan. MD*
Department of Surgery, Carmel Medical Center, Haifa, Israel

*Junko Honda, MD*
Outpatient Medical Master, Department of Digestive and Pediatric
Surgery, Institute of Health Biosciences, The University of Tokushima
Graduate School, Tokushima, Japan

*Tzu-Chi Hsu, MD, FACS*
Attending Surgeon, Mackay Memorial Hospital, Associate Professor,
Department of Surgery, Taipei Medical University, Taipei, Taiwan

*John G. Hunter, MD*
Chairman of Surgery, Oregon Health & Science University, Portland,
OR, USA

*Sayeed Ikramuddin, MD*
Director of Bariatric Surgery, Associate Professor, Department of
Surgery, University of Minnesota, Minneapolis, MN, USA

*Mohammad Jamal, MD*
Clinical Assistant Professor, Department of Surgery, Division of
Gasrointestinal, Minimally Invasive and Bariatric Surgery, University
of Iowa Hospitals and Clinics, Iowa City, IA, USA

*Jason T. Jankowski, MD*
Chief Resident, Department of Urology, Director, Pancreas Transplant
Program, University Hospitals - Case Medical Center, Case Western
Reserve University, Cleveland, OH, USA

*Louis O. Jeansonne IV, MD*
Emory Endosurgery Unit, Emory University School of Medicine,
Atlanta, GA, USA

*Manjula Jeyapalan, MD*
Department of Surgery, Good Samaritan Hospital, San Jose, CA, USA

*Jason M. Johnson, DO, MAJ, MC*
Adjunct Assistant Professor, Department of Surgery, Uniformed
Services University of the Health Sciences, William Beaumont Army
Medical Center, El Paso, TX, USA

*Mark Johnston, MD, FACP, FACG*
Lancaster Gastroenterology Inc., Lancaster, PA, USA

*Namir Katkhouda, MD, FACS*
Professor, Department of Surgery, Chief, Minimally Invasive Surgery,
University of Southern California, USC School of Medicine,
Los Angeles, CA, USA

*Katsunobu Kawahara, MD*
Second, Department of Surgery, Fukuoka University School of
Medicine, Fukuoka, Japan

*John J. Kelly, MD, FACS*
Associate Professor, Department of Surgery, University
of Massachusetts Medical School, Chief of General Surgery, Director
of Bariatric and Minimally Invasive Surgery, University
of Massachusetts Memorial Medical Center, Worcester, MA, USA

*Tony Kelly, MBChB*
Resident, SHO, Department of Surgery, Whiston Hospital, Prescot, UK

*Michael Kent, MD*
Instructor in Surgery, Harvard Medical School, Attending Surgeon,
Division of Thoracic Surgery, Beth Israel Deaconess Medical Center,
Boston, MA, USA

*Kent W. Kercher, MD, FACS*
Chief, Minimal Access Surgery, Division of Gastrointestinal and
Minimally Invasive Surgery, Carolinas Medical Center, Charlotte,
NC, USA

*Kenneth A. Kesler, MD*
Professor, Department of Surgery, Cardiothoracic Division, Indiana
University, Indianapolis, IN, USA

*Iftikhar M. Khan, FRCS, MD*
Associate, Department of Surgery/Liver Transplant, Mount Sinai
Medical Center, New York, NY, USA

*Geeta Lal, MD*
Assistant Professor, Department of Surgery, Division of Surgical
Oncology and Endocrine Surgery, University of Iowa Hospitals
and Clinics, Iowa City, IA, USA

*Teresa L. LaMasters, MD*
General Surgeon, Stanford University Medical Center, Stanford,
CA, USA

*Barbara A. Latenser, MD, FACS*
Clara L. Smith Professor, Department of Burn Surgery, University of
Iowa Carver College of Medicine, Iowa City, IA, USA

*James N. Lau, MD*
Assistant Professor, Department of Surgery, University of Nevada
School of Medicine, Las Vegas, NY, USA

*Chad R. Laurich, MD*
Department of Surgery, University of Iowa Hospitals and Clinics,
Iowa City, IA, USA

*James A. Lee, MD*
Assistant Professor, Department of Surgery, Columbia University,
New York, NY, USA

*Steve A. Lee-Kong, MD*
Resident, Department of Surgery, Columbia University College
of Physicians and Surgeons, New York, NY, USA

*John Leung, MD*
Emergency Medicine, Yale-New Haven Hospital, New Haven, CT,
USA

*Anne Lidor, MD, MPH*
Assistant Professor, Johns Hopkins Center for Bariatric Surgery,
Johns Hopkins Bayview Medical Center, Baltimore, MD, USA

*Edward Lin, DO, FACS, CNSP*
Director, Emory Endosurgery Unit, Emory University School of
Medicine, Atlanta, GA, USA

*Ingrid Lizarraga, MD*
General Surgeon, University of Iowa Hospitals and Clinics, Iowa City,
IA, USA

*James Luketich, MD*
Chief, Professor of Surgery, Division of Thoracic and Foregut
Surgery, UPMC Presbyterian, Digestive Disorders Center, Pittsburgh,
PA, USA

*Bruce MacFadyen, Jr., MD*
Moretz/Mansberger Distinguished Chair, Professor of Surgery, Medical
College of Georgia, Augusta, GA, USA

*Shishir K. Maithel, MD*
Fellow, Department of Surgical Oncology, Memorial Sloan-Kettering
Cancer Center, New York, NY, USA

*Anne T. Mancino, MD, FACS*
Associate Professor, Department of Surgery, University of Arkansas for
Medical Sciences, Chief, General Surgery, Central Arkansas Veterans
Healthcare System, Little Rock, AK, USA

*John H. Marks, MD*
General Surgeon, Colon and Rectal Surgeon, Lankenau Hospital,
Wynnewood, PA, USA

*Michael Marohn, MD*
Associate Professor, Department of Surgery, The Johns Hopkins School
of Medicine, Baltimore, MD, USA

*Samuel M. Maurice, MD*
Department of Surgery, University of Iowa Hospitals and Clinics,
Iowa City, IA, USA

*Carol McCloskey, MD*
Assistant Professor, Department of Surgery, University of Pittsburgh
School of Medicine, Pittsburgh, PA, USA

*Michele McElroy, MD*
General Surgery Resident, University of California, San Diego,
San Diego, CA, USA

*Gill McHattie, MSc, BSc, RGN*
Clinical Nurse Specialist, Nutrition, Southern General Hospital, NHS
Greater Glasgow & Clyde, Glasgow, UK

*John Meehan, MD*
Assistant Professor, Department of Surgery, Division of Pediatric
Surgery, University of Iowa Hospitals and Clinics, Iowa City, IA, USA

*Ross Meidinger, MD*
Gastroenterology-Hepatology Fellow, University of Iowa Hospitals
and Clinics, Iowa City, IA, USA

*Muhammed Ashraf Memon, MBBS, DCH, FRCSI, FRCSEd, FRCSEng,
PGD Clin* Edu
Consultant Surgeon, Department of Surgery, Ipswich Hospital,
Queensland, Australia, Associate Professor, Department of Surgery,
The University of Queensland, Herston, Queensland, Australia,
Associate Professor, Faculty of Health Sciences and Medicine, Bond
University, Gold Coast, Queensland, Australia

*Eiichi Miyasaka, MD*
Department of Surgery, University of Iowa Hospitals and Clinics,
Iowa City, IA, USA

*Kamran Mohiuddin, MD*
Department of Surgery, Aga Khan University Hospital, Karachi,
Pakistan

*Gamal Mostafa, MD*
Director, Acute Care Surgical Service, Department of Surgery,
Carolinas Medical Center, Charlotte, NC, USA

*Jonathan A. Myers, MD*
Assistant Professor, Department of Surgery, Director, Undergraduate
Surgical Education, Rush Medical College, Rush University Medical
Center, Chicago, IL, USA

*Satish N. Nadig, MD*
Research Fellow, Transplant Immunology, University of Oxford,
Oxford, UK, Resident in General Surgery, Harvard Medical School,
Beth-Israel Deaconess Medical Center, Boston, MA, USA

*Kenneth G. Nepple, MD*
Department of Urology, University of Iowa, Iowa City, IA, USA

*Richard Nguyen, MD*
Head Physician, Buena Vista Family Medical Center, Oxnard, CA, USA

*Rachael Nicholson, MD*
Department of Surgery, University of Iowa, Iowa City, IA, USA

*Saira Nizami FCPS, MRCS*
Department of Surgery, Aga Khan University Hospital, Karachi, Pakistan

*Andrew Nowell, MD*
Senior Resident, University of Iowa, Iowa City, IA, USA

*Kerri Maiers Nowell, MD*
Department of Surgery, University of Iowa, Iowa City, IA, USA

*Robert W. O'Rourke, MD*
Assistant Professor, Department of Surgery, Oregon Health and Science
University, Portland, OR, USA

*James W. Ostroff, MD*
Professor, Department of Clinical Medicine, Pediatrics and Radiology,
Lynne and Marc Benioff Endowed Chair in Gastroenterology, Director,
Endoscopy Unit and GI Consultation Service, University of California,
San Francisco, CA, USA

*Aytekin Oto, M.D.*
Associate Professor, Director, Body Imaging, Vice Chairman
for Research, The University of Texas Medical Branch, Galveston,
TX, USA

*Kalpaj R. Parekh, MD*
Assistant Professor, Division of General Thoracic Surgery, University
of Iowa, Iowa City, IA, USA

*Amit N. Patel, MD, MS*
Cardiothoracic Surgery, University of Pittsburgh, Pittsburgh, PA, USA

*Anand Patel, MD*
Instructor of Pediatrics, School of Medicine, Washington University
in St. Louis, St. Louis, MO, USA

*Marco G. Patti, MD*
Professor, Department of Surgery, Director, Center for Esophageal
Disorders, University of Chicago School of Medicine, Chicago, IL, USA

*Eric Pham, MD*
Bariatric Surgery Care Center of Orange County, Orange, CA, USA

*Todd A. Ponsky, MD*
Professor, Department of Surgery, Children's National Medical Center,
George Washington University Medical Center, Washington, DC

*Eric Pontey, MD*
Division of General Surgery, University of Iowa, Iowa City, IA, USA

*Bruce Ramshaw, MD*
Chief, Division of General Surgery, University of Missouri Health
Care, Columbia, MO, USA

*Beate Rau, MD*
Charité Medical School, Humboldt University, Department of Surgery
and Surgical Oncology, Robert-Roessle Klinik, Berlin, Germany

*William Richards, MD, FACS*
Ingram Professor, Department of Surgical Sciences, Director of
Laparoendoscopic Surgery, Medical Director of the Center for Surgical
Weight Loss, Vanderbilt University School of Medicine, New Orleans,
LA, USA

*Heidi H. Richardson, MD*
Surgical Oncology Fellow, Department of Surgery, University of Iowa,
Iowa City, IA, USA

*William Richardson, MD*
Division Chief of General Surgery, Ochsner Clinic, New Orleans, LA

*Maged Rizk, MD*
Department of Internal Medicine, Gastroenterology-Hepatology Fellow,
University of Iowa Health Care, Iowa City, IA, USA

*Nora A. Royer, MD*
Department of Surgery, University of Iowa Hospitals and Clinics,
Iowa City, IA, USA

*Bashar Safar, MD*
Department of Colorectal Surgery, Cleveland Clinic Florida, Weston,
FL, USA

*Barry A. Salky, MD*
Professor, Department of Surgery, Mount Sinai Medical Center,
New York, NY, USA

*Anthony Sandler, MD*
Pediatric Surgeon, Childrens National Medical Center, Washington,
DC, USA

*Juan R. Sanabria, MD, MSc, FRCSC, FACS*
Assistant Professor, Department of Surgery, Nutrition and Metabolism,
Case Western Reserve University, Director Pancreas Transplant Program,
University Hospitals, Case Medical Center, Cleveland, OH, USA

*Andras Sandor, MD, FACS*
Attending Surgeon, Commonwealth Surgical Associates, Stoneham,
MA, USA

*Sharfi Sarker, MD, MPH, FACS*
Assistant Professor, Department of Surgery, Director, Virtual Surgical
Training, Loyola University Health System, Maywood, IL, USA

*Leopoldo Sarli, MD*
Associate Professor, Department of General Surgery, Parma University
School of Medicine, Parma, Italy

*David Scheeres, MD, FACS*
Associate Professor, Department of Surgery, Michigan State University,
College of Human Medicine, Grand Rapids, MI, USA

*Janet Schlechte, MD*
Professor, Departments of Endocrine-Metabolism and Internal
Medicine, University of Iowa Health Care, Iowa City, IA, USA

*Benjamin E. Schneider, MD, FACS*
Instructor in Surgery, Harvard Medical School, Beth Israel Deaconess
Medical Center, Boston, MA, USA

*Rob Schuster, MD*
Banner Gateway Medical Center, Gilbert, AZ, USA

*Carol E.H. Scott-Conner, MD, PhD*
Professor, Department of Surgery, University of Iowa Hospitals and
Clinics, Iowa City, IA, USA

*Junichi Seike, MD*
Oncological and Regenerative Surgery, University of Tokushima
School of Medicine, Shikoku, Japan

*Matthew D. Shane, MD*
House Staff, Emory University, Atlanta, GA, USA

*Melhem Sharafuddin, MD*
Assistant Professor, Department of Surgery, University of Iowa
Hospitals and Clinics, Iowa City, IA, USA

*Vafa Shayani, MD*
Department of Surgery, Loyola University Medical Center, Maywood,
IL, USA

*Amal Shibli-Rahhal, M.D.*
Clinical Assistant Professor, Department of Internal Medicine,
University of Iowa Health Care, Iowa City, IA, USA

*Takayuki Shirakusa, MD*
Advisory Editorial Board, Japanese Association for Thoracic Surgery,
Department of Surgery, Fukuoka University, Fukuoka, Japan

*Kristen C. Sihler, MD, MS*
Assistant Professor, Department of Surgery, University of Michigan,
Ann Arbor, MI, USA

*William B. Silverman, MD*
Department of Internal Medicine, University of Iowa Health Care,
Iowa City, IA, USA

*Christopher M. Simons, MD*
Resident, Department of Urology, University of Iowa, Iowa City,
IA, USA

*Dionne Skeete, MD*
Assistant Professor, Department of Surgery, University of Iowa Health
Care, Iowa City, IA, USA

*Georgios C. Sotiropoulos, MD*
Department of General Surgery and Transplantation, University
Hospital Essen, Essen, Germany

*Steven C. Stain, MD*
Neil Lempert Professor and Chair, Department of Surgery,
Albany Medical College, Albany, NY, USA

*Kimberly Steele, MD*
Department of Surgery, The Johns Hopkins Medical Institutions,
Baltimore, MD, USA

*Gregory Van Stiegmann, MD*
Professor and Head, Department of Gastrointestinal, Tumor and
Endocrine Surgery, University of Colorado, Denver School of
Medicine, Denver, CO, USA

*Choichi Sugawa, MD*
Professor, Department of Surgery, Wayne State University School
of Medicine, Director of Endoscopy, Detroit Medical Center, Detroit,
MI, USA

*Ronald M. Summers, MD, Ph.D.*
Senior Investigator, Staff Radiologist, National Institutes of Health
Clinical Center, Bethesda, MD, USA

*Lee Swanström, MD*
Clinical Professor, Department of Surgery, Oregon Health Sciences
University, Director, Division of Minimally Invasive Surgery, Legacy
Health System, Portland, OR, USA

*Akira Tangoku, MD*
Professor and Chairman, Department of Oncological and
Regenerative Surgery, University of Tokushima Graduate School,
Tokushima, Japan

*Paul B. Tessmann, MD*
Surgery Resident, University of Iowa Health Care, Iowa City,
IA, USA

*Rahul Tevar, MD*
Resident, Department of General Surgery, The George Washington
University Medical Center, Washington, DC, USA

*Nate Thepjatri, MD*
Department of Surgery, University of Iowa Hospitals and Clinics,
Iowa City, IA, USA

*Rebecca Thoreson, MD*
Surgery Resident, University of Iowa Health Care, Iowa City, IA, USA

*José E. Torres, MD*
Department of Surgery, University of Iowa Hospitals and Clinics,
Iowa City, IA, USA

*Atsushi Umemoto, MD*
Department of Surgery, Graduate School of Medicine, The University
of Tokushima, Tokushima, Japan

*Brian T. Valerian, MD*
Assistant Professor, Department of Surgery, Albany Medical College,
Albany, NY, USA

*José A. Vazquez-Frias, MD*
Department of Surgery, American British Cowdray Hospital of Mexico
City, Districto Federal (Mexico City), Mexico

*Gary C. Vitale, MD*
Professor, Department of Surgery, University of Louisville School of
Medicine, Louisville, KY, USA

*David A. Vivas, MD*
Department of Colorectal Surgery, Cleveland Clinic Florida, Weston, FL, USA

*Erik Wallace, MD*
Associate Program Director, Department of Internal Medicine, Oklahoma University-Tulsa, Tulsa, OK, USA

*Steven D. Wexner, MD, FACS, FRCS, FRCS Ed, FASCRS, FACG*
Editorial Board Chairman, Department of Colorectal Surgery, Cleveland Clinic Florida Weston, FL, USA

*Sherry M. Wren, MD*
Chief, Department of General Surgery, Associate Professor, Stanford University Medical Center, Palo Alto, CA, USA

*Satoshi Yamamoto, MD*
Department of Surgery, Osaka City University, Graduate School of Medicine, Osaka, Japan

*Srinath C. Yeshwant, BS*
Postbaccalaureate Intramural Research Trainee Award Fellow, National Institutes of Health Clinical Center, Bethesda, MD, USA

*Takahiro Yoshida, MD*
Oncological and Regenerative Surgery, University of Tokushima School of Medicine, Shikoku, Japan

# 1. Access to the Abdomen

## A. Introduction

Initial access to the abdomen may be achieved percutaneously with a Veress needle (closed technique), or by a small cutdown and direct placement of a blunt-tipped Hassan cannula into the peritoneum under visual control (open technique). A variety of optical access trocars are also available, but most are used after pneumoperitoneum is first established percutaneously. Laparoscopic surgeons need to be facile in both the open and closed techniques, but most have a strong preference for one or the other method and will use that method preferentially, modifying the technique if unusual circumstances exist. This chapter uses the case of a healthy young woman with no previous abdominal surgery to explore these choices and preferences. Both techniques are thoroughly described in the SAGES manuals.

## B. Case

*Daniel M. Hallam*

A 26-year-old woman came to the emergency department complaining of severe, nonradiating right lower quadrant abdominal pain. The pain began approximately 12 hours earlier as a dull, generalized abdominal pain. It then localized to the periumbilical region, and then the right lower quadrant. The pain intensified with any movement. She rated it as a 9 out of 10.

She had not eaten since the pain began. She was nauseated, and vomited twice. She was taking oral contraceptives. Her last menstrual period was approximately 18 days ago. She had no previous abdominal surgery, and was healthy except for asthma and seasonal allergies. She was married, with a 2-year-old son (vaginal delivery). She did not smoke, and had about one glass of wine per week.

On physical examination, her temperature was 38.1 °C, respiratory rate 18, blood pressure 120/70, and pulse 90. Her height was 5 feet 6 inches, and she weighed 65 kg. Her abdomen was not distended, without scars or hernias. It was moderately tender, with decreased bowel sounds and voluntary guarding. Rovsing's sign was positive, and the psoas and obturator signs were negative.

Laboratory examination was significant, with a white cell count of 15.5. Hematocrit and hemoglobin were normal. Urinalysis was negative.

Computed tomography (CT) abdomen and pelvis revealed a thickened appendix with periappendiceal inflammation consistent with acute appendicitis. No fluid was seen.

**Laparoscopic appendectomy was planned. Would you prefer a Veress needle or a Hassan cannula for abdominal access in this patient?**

# C. Veress Needle

*Muzaffar A. Anwar, Iftikhar M. Khan, Muhammed Ashraf Memon*

Our preference would be to use a Veress needle for creating pneumoperitoneum. Veress needle access is rapid and safe in experienced hands. Our personal experience has been confirmed by several studies.

Merlin et al. published a systematic review examining the safety and effectiveness of various access techniques for the creation of pneumoperitoneum. The authors (1) wanted to test the hypothesis that open (Hasson) access is safer than closed (needle/trocar) technique, and (2) examined the differences in the safety and effectiveness of the outcomes based on patient age, sex, weight, previous abdominal surgery, indication for surgery, and surgical experience. They found no statistical difference in major complications between open and closed methods (0–2% vs. 0–4%). Separate subanalysis for bowel and vascular injury once again failed to reveal any significant difference. Other major complications such as hematoma and access-site herniation seem to be more common with the open access method compared to the closed methods. Once again, these differences were small and of no significance. Conversion to laparotomy in nonobese patients was on a lesser magnitude, with the open access method compared to the closed access methods. When the authors analyzed the effectiveness of establishing pneumoperitoneum between the two methods, the open access method was faster to some extent, but of no clinical significance. The authors concluded that although there is a trend toward a reduced risk of major complications with the open access method, the evidence on the comparative safety and effectiveness of the different access methods was not definite.

Van der Voort et al. performed a systematic review addressing the incidence of bowel injury as a complication of laparoscopy. The incidence of bowel injury in 28 studies (329,935 laparoscopies) was 0.13% (430 patients). These injuries occurred most frequently during the access phase of laparoscopy. Surprisingly, only 19 were caused by insertion of a trocar and eight by the insertion of a Veress needle. Most of these were discovered during the procedure and appropriately dealt with.

Gunenc et al., in a recent randomized prospective trial, studied the efficacy of two closed methods, namely direct trocar insertion and Veress needle, for the creation of pneumoperitoneum in almost 500 patients. Neither technique was associated with any major vascular or bowel injury. Two further comparative studies (Agresta et al., Inan et al.) evaluating direct trocar and Veress needle insertion described only four major complications with Veress needle and no deaths (in 872 patients). However, the incidence of minor complications such as subcutaneous emphysema or extraperitoneal insufflation was slightly higher with the Veress needle. These minor complications, although a nuisance, did not lead to any major problems for the patients. These two studies further consolidate the evidence that Veress needle when performed carefully is a safe and effective method of creating pneumoperitoneum.

The following steps, we feel, will minimize the risk of any major injury when inserting the Veress needle for the creation of pneumoperitoneum:

- Elevate the skin on either side of the umbilicus using two Littlewoods or similar fine-toothed tissue forceps.
- Make an infraumbilical transverse skin incision and replace one of the forceps to grasp the umbilical tube, thereby lifting the rectus sheath upwards. Use the second forceps to retract the lower edge of the skin incision.
- While continuing to elevate the rectus sheath, under direct vision insert the Veress needle where the umbilical tube joins the rectus sheath.
- Insert the Veress needle, angling it toward the pelvis.

- Once the Veress needle is satisfactorily introduced into the abdominal cavity, do the saline drop test, ascertaining that the negative intraabdominal pressure sucks the saline drop when the Veress needle valve is opened.
- Start insufflation with $CO_2$ on a low setting while observing good flow and low intraabdominal pressure readings. Once satisfied, increase the flow to a maximum, but continue to observe both the flow and pressure gauge readings. Do not remove the Littlewoods tissue forceps from the umbilicus tube until you have inserted the first trocar.
- Once sufficient insufflation has been achieved, remove the Veress needle and insert the first trocar angling it toward the pelvis while continuing to maintain the upward lift on the umbilical tube with the Littlewoods forceps.
- Once satisfied with the trocar entry, open the gas valve to release some gas to confirm its position in the peritoneal cavity.

Laparoscopists should consider alternatives to the closed technique of creating pneumoperitoneum such as the Hasson method and optical-access design trocars for patients in the following situations:

- Multiple previous abdominal surgeries
- Severe abdominal adhesions
- Enterocutaneous fistula(s)
- Small or large bowel dilatation
- Endometriosis
- Active inflammatory bowel disease
- Carcinomatosis
- Morbid obesity (may require an extra-long Veress needle)
- Lower abdomen skin that cannot be adequately stabilized (women after multiple pregnancies, patients with atrophic abdominal musculature, thin patients)

An alternative access method would also be recommended in the following patients:

- Children
- Small, thin adults
- Pregnant women

Again, most of the above contraindications are relative, and an experienced laparoscopic surgeon may still decide to start with a Veress needle. However, it is extremely important that pride should not come in the way of patient safety.

# D. Hasson Canula

*Kimberly Steele and Anne Lidor*

We would access the abdomen using an Hasson cannula. We favor this technique because it is derived from the same safe general surgical principles used to enter the abdomen during a traditional laparotomy. Furthermore, we believe that the risk of serious vascular complications is less than with a blind percutaneous approach.

Although laparoscopic surgical techniques have been in widespread use for decades and are supplanting open laparotomies for many indications, the optimal method for gaining initial entry into the peritoneum remains a source of controversy. Two methods, the Veress needle approach and the Hasson technique, are most commonly debated.

Although the first descriptions of laparoscopy date back to Kelling's experiments in dogs at the turn of the 20th century, routine use of laparoscopy in humans did not become common until the 1970s. The initial approach to creating a pneumoperitoneum involved the use of the Veress needle, a large-bore hollow needle containing a spring-loaded blunt probe. This was invented in 1938 by the Hungarian physician Janos Veress, who noted that "it is without any doubt a very important moment when the needle goes through the pleura or the peritoneum, because it is at this time that the lung or intestine can be easily injured with the tip of the instrument." He used his device to drain fluid or air from the pleural space or the peritoneum, and treated almost 2000 pneumothoraces without incident. Although the needle was widely adopted by gynecologic laparoscopists, concerns arose regarding the safety of a blind entry into the peritoneum. In 1971, H.M. Hasson, a gynecologist, described an open technique involving direct visualization and dissection of the preperitoneal tissues followed by incision of the peritoneum and insertion of a blunt trocar. Variations on the Hassan technique and newer methods employing optical trocars (e.g., Visiport™ or Optiview™ [US Surgical Division of Tyco International, Ltd., Princeton, NJ]) have subsequently been developed in an attempt to improve safety. However, the Veress and Hasson techniques remain the most widely used. Regardless of the method used, gaining access to the abdomen and initiating pneumoperitoneum remains a source of morbidity or mortality, with the most common complications being visceral and vascular injuries. The individual surgeon's choice of technique is typically guided by considerations of safety, speed, and familiarity.

The Veress needle or closed technique involves making a tiny incision to allow for the insertion of the Veress needle. As the device is pushed through the subcutaneous fat and fascia, the spring-loaded blunt tip retracts into the needle. Upon penetration of the parietal peritoneum, the blunt tip springs out, theoretically protecting the abdominal viscera and vessels from injury. Once inserted, location of the needle tip in the peritoneal cavity is confirmed, and a pneumoperitoneum is created. The needle is then removed, and initial trocar inserted blindly at the same site.

In contrast, the Hasson or open technique resembles that of a mini-laparotomy. A small incision is made, usually just above or below the umbilicus, where the abdominal wall is thinnest. Using direct visualization, the subcutaneous tissues are dissected, the fascia is grasped and divided, and anchoring sutures are secured. The peritoneum is grasped and entered sharply, and the blunt Hasson trocar is inserted into the peritoneal under direct visualization.

In 2005, Larobina and Nottle published a combined prospective and retrospective review, consisting of a single surgeon series of 5900 open laparoscopic cases, along with a meta-analysis of all reported open and closed laparoscopic cases, utilizing Medline and PubMed. They discovered over 700 major vascular injuries that were in some way related to the use of the closed technique. In comparison, no major vascular injuries were reported when reviewing the literature from 1975 to 2002 using the open technique. While the Hasson technique is not without risk of complications, two major advantages favor its use: major abdominal vessel injury is much less frequent; and visceral injuries, should they occur, are immediately apparent, facilitating repair in most circumstances.

Since the introduction of Hasson's technique many articles have been written that have attempted to prove that one method is superior to the other. While most of these have been retrospective series, literature reviews, and surveys, at least one randomized controlled trial has been published, supporting the superiority of the Hassan approach in laparoscopic cholecystectomy. However, a recent systematic review of the safety and effectiveness of the different methods was unable to reach a definitive conclusion, and the authors wrote that "a multicenter randomized controlled trial with over 10,000 patients in each study arm" would be needed to settle the issue. To date, no one has stepped forward to undertake this monumental task.

In conclusion, the evidence comparing the Hassan and Veress techniques is not definitive. The largest studies to date are retrospective in nature. While it is probably impossible to adequately account for all of the potential confounding factors affecting outcomes, it does seem apparent that the use of the Veress needle is associated with a higher risk of intraabdominal vascular injury, and that the open and closed techniques are approximately equally risky with respect to visceral injuries. Regardless of the technique that is chosen, one must abide by the safe general principles of surgery: be meticulous, take your time, and be highly alert for the appearance of signs of injury.

# E. Conclusions

*Daniel M. Hallam*

Laparoscopic procedures use pneumoperitoneum in order to create a working space and examine the abdominal cavity and its contents. Significant complications of peritoneal access include bleeding from the abdominal wall, injury to the great vessels, and damage to intraperitoneal viscera. Delayed complications of trocar insertion include metastatic seeding from malignant neoplasms, dehiscence, and incisional hernia.

Although the closed and open techniques have been in clinical practice for many years, there is still no true "gold standard" with regard to relative safety and effectiveness. Studies comparing the closed (Veress needle) and open (Hasson cannula) techniques have primarily focused on immediate rather than delayed complications. Individual studies have generally been statistically underpowered and thus unable to detect differences in these rare life-threatening complications. Bonjer et al., in a retrospective review of the literature, concluded that open techniques were less apt to result in visceral or vascular injury than closed methods, but found no difference in mortality rates. Jansen et al., using a combination of a questionnaire and literature search, reported that the number of complications was not necessarily reduced when open-entry techniques were performed. They concluded that there was no evidence to abandon the closed-entry techniques, but the selection of an open- or alternative-entry method was recommended for special indications. Likewise, two recent meta-analyses demonstrated no definitive evidence of the safety and effectiveness of closed versus open access methods (Merlin et al., Molloy et al.). Therefore, there still remain no true clear evidence-based "gold standard" in regard to the relative safety and effectiveness of introducing and maintaining pneumoperitoneum. There have been some trends in the data and literature, and with further research and development an optimal form of laparoscopic entry should be discovered. Surgeons should be familiar with both techniques, and adapt their entry technique to individual patient circumstances.

# References

Agresta F, De Simone P, Ciardo LF, Bedin N. Direct trocar insertion vs Veress needle in nonobese patients undergoing laparoscopic procedures: a randomized prospective single-center study. Surg Endosc 2004;18:1778–1781.

Bonjer HJ, Hazebroek EJ, Kazemier G, et al. Open versus closed establishment of pneumoperitoneum in laparoscopic surgery. Br J Surg 1997;84:599–602.

Gunenc MZ, Yesildaglar N, Bingol B, Onalan G, Tabak S, Gokmen B. The safety and efficacy of direct trocar insertion with elevation of the rectus sheath instead of the skin for pneumoperitoneum. Surg Laparosc Endosc Percutan Tech 2005;15:80–81.

Inan A, Sen M, Dener C, Bozer M. Comparison of direct trocar and Veress needle insertion in the performance of pneumoperitoneum in laparoscopic cholecystectomy. Acta Chir Belg 2005;105:515–518.

Jansen FW, Kolkman W, Bakkum EA, et al. Complications of laparoscopy: an inquiry about closed- versus open entry technique. Am J Obstet Gynecol 2004;190:634–638.

Larobina M, Nottle P. Complete evidence regarding major vascular injuries during laparoscopic access. Surg Laparosc Endosc Percutan Tech 2005;15(3):119–123.

Merlin TL, Hiller JE, Maddern GJ, Jamieson GG, Brown AR, Kolbe A. Systematic review of the safety and effectiveness of methods used to establish pneumoperitoneum in laparoscopic surgery. Br J Surg 2003;90:668–679.

Molloy D, Kaloo PD, Cooper M, Nguyen TV. Laparoscopic entry: a literature review and analysis of techniques and complications of primary port entry. Aust N Z J Obstet Gynaecol 2002;42:246–254.

Van der Voort M, Heijnsdijk EAM, Gouma DJ. Bowel injury as a complication of laparoscopy. Br J Surg 2004;91:1253–1258.

Veress J. Neus Instrument Zur Ausfuhrung von brustoder Bachpunktionen und Pneumothoraybehundlung. Dtsch Med Wochenschr 1938;64:1480–1481.

# Suggested Reading

Catarci M, Carlini M, Gentlieschi P, Santoro E. Major and minor injuries during the creation of pneumoperitoneum. A multicenter study on 12,919 cases. Surg Endosc 2001;15(6):566–569.

Chandrakanth A, Talamini MA. Port site closure methods and hernia prevention. In: Whelan RL, Fleshman JW, Fowler DL, eds. The SAGES Manual: Perioperative Care in Minimally Invasive Surgery. New York: Springer-Verlag, 2006.

Cogliandolo A, Manganaro T, Saitta FP, Micali B. Blind versus open approach to laparoscopic cholecystectomy: a randomized study. Surg Laparosc Endosc 1998;8(5):353–355.

Hasson H. Open laparoscopy: a report of 150 cases. J Reprod Med 1974;12:234–238.

Lafullarde T, Van Hee R, Gys T. A safe and simple method for routine open access in laparoscopic procedures. Surg Endosc 1999;13(8):769–772.

Munro M. Laparoscopic access: complications, technologies, and techniques. Curr Opin Obstet Gynecol 2002;14:365–374.

Soper NJ. Access to abdomen. In: CEH Scott-Conner, ed. The SAGES Manual: Fundamentals of Laparoscopy, Thoracoscopy, and GI Endoscopy, 2nd ed. New York: Springer-Verlag, 2006:16–30.

String A, Berber E, Foroutani A, Macho JR, Pearl JM, Siperstein AE. Use of the optical access trocar for safe and rapid entry in various laparoscopic procedures. Surg Endosc 2001;15(6):570–573.

# 2. Appendicitis During Pregnancy

## A. Introduction

As laparoscopic surgery has evolved, the number of conditions once thought to present contraindications to laparoscopic (as opposed to open) surgery has gradually decreased. Obesity, previous abdominal surgery, and acute infectious processes are examples of comorbid conditions that are no longer thought to preclude laparoscopy. Clinicians have gradually become comfortable performing laparoscopic cholecystectomies during pregnancy. This chapter explores choice of operative approach for treatment of acute appendicitis during pregnancy.

## B. Case

*Rachael Nicholson*

A 30-year-old woman came to the emergency department complaining of abdominal pain. The pain began in the epigastrium approximately 12 hours earlier and then moved to the right lower quadrant, gradually becoming more severe. She was nauseated and anorexic. She had also had chills and sweats over the past 12 hours. Her last bowel movement, the day before, was normal in nature. She had dysuria, urinary frequency, and urgency.

She was a married homemaker, 8 weeks pregnant with her fourth child. Her previous deliveries had all been normal, spontaneous, vaginal deliveries. She had no prior surgery. Her past medical history was negative. She did not smoke or use alcohol.

Physical examination was significant for a temperature of 38.7 °C and pulse 110. She was not jaundiced. Abdominal exam revealed tenderness in the right lower quadrant with guarding and rebound tenderness. Rovsing's and psoas signs were positive. Digital rectal exam was negative.

Laboratory tests were significant for a white cell count of 16.2 with a left shift. Hematocrit was 46. Urinalysis was negative.

Ultrasound of the right lower quadrant revealed an enlarged appendix with a thickened hyperechoic wall, measuring 1.2 cm in diameter at the tip. The adjacent fat showed hyperechoic changes consistent with inflammation.

**What approach is the most appropriate way to remove the appendix in a pregnant woman?**

# C.  Laparoscopic Appendectomy

*Myriam J. Curet*

The decision as to whether a pregnant patient with appendicitis should undergo a laparoscopic or open appendectomy is still an unsettled one. Part of the issue is that the role of laparoscopic appendectomy in the general population is still debated. Given the short lengths of stay for patients with open appendectomy, and the higher operative costs for a laparoscopic appendectomy, many authors have found the minimally invasive approach not to be cost-effective. In addition, there have been concerns that in the pregnant patient, increased intraabdominal pressure and a carbon dioxide pneumoperitoneum may have deleterious effects on the fetus.

The first issue to address is whether the pregnant patient needs an operation at all. It is well known that there is an inherent risk of fetal loss with any surgery, even during the second trimester, which has traditionally been considered the safest period. It is important to remember, though, that delays in diagnosis and treatment in pregnant patients with appendicitis result in greater morbidity to the fetus, with mortality rates nearing 60%. Although the diagnosis of appendicitis in a pregnant patient can be difficult to make, especially later in the pregnancy, this patient is in her first trimester, which is when appendicitis most closely mimics its presentation in the nonpregnant patient. Despite the higher rate of spontaneous abortion during surgery in the first trimester, this patient should undergo an appendectomy.

In this case, the benefits of a laparoscopic approach are similar to those seen in the nonpregnant patient. Many authors have found less narcotic usage, quicker ambulation, quicker return of gastrointestinal function, shorter hospital stays, and more rapid return to normal activity after laparoscopic appendectomy. These benefits should apply in this patient as well. In addition, less narcotic usage may decrease problems with fetal depression secondary to narcotics. Also, patients undergoing a minimally invasive appendectomy generally have fewer wound-related problems, including infections and hernias. In a pregnant patient, where the abdominal wall is going to stretch significantly, smaller incisions, which have less chance of developing hernias, would be extremely beneficial.

In a pregnant patient with appendicitis who is further along in her pregnancy, laparoscopy may offer additional benefits compared to an open approach. It has been suggested that there is less uterine manipulation with a laparoscopic approach, so patients may experience less uterine irritability and fetal distress. In the late second trimester and in the third trimester, exploration of the abdomen during an open appendectomy is limited because of the size of the uterus. A laparoscopic approach enables the surgeon to better explore the abdomen, which will be particularly important if the appendix appears grossly normal. Finally, as the appendix moves in a cephalad direction with advancing gestational age, it can be difficult to know where to place the appropriate open incision. Placement of the operating ports in the best position is facilitated with the laparoscope.

Prior to a laparoscopic appendectomy, this patient should be well hydrated and should receive prophylactic antibiotics. Even though she is in only the first trimester and the uterus is not particularly enlarged, it is best to place either the patient or the bed in such a way that she is on her left side so the uterus is displaced off the vena cava. This position should be maintained throughout the operation. Because of the high risk of thromboembolic events during laparoscopy and pregnancy, the patient should have sequential compression devices placed preoperatively and maintained in place until she is fully ambulatory postoperatively. Precautions to prevent aspiration should be in place when intubating a pregnant patient. Intraoperative monitoring should include measurement of end-tidal $CO_2$ to prevent maternal or fetal acidosis. The reverse Trendelenburg position should be minimized while still maintaining adequate visualization. Intraabdominal pressure should be kept as low as possible while still allowing for adequate visualization, but should not be higher than 15 mm Hg. Finally, the operation should be done in an expeditious manner to minimize operative time.

With this patient, determination of fundal height is important. If the uterus is well below the umbilicus, the camera port can be placed safely just above the umbilicus. It would be important to use a Hassan trocar to avoid uterine puncture. The abdominal cavity can be explored visually with the laparoscope, and the two operating ports can be placed in the appropriate locations based on the visual survey while carefully avoiding injury to the uterus. A fourth trocar can be placed if necessary to more fully explore the abdomen if the appendix appears normal.

The question of fetal monitoring always arises when considering operation during pregnancy. In this case, since the fetus is not of a viable gestational age, intraoperative monitoring is not necessary. However, the presence of fetal heart tone and the fetal heart rate should be documented pre- and postoperatively. Tocolytics should not be administered prophylactically but should be used for preterm labor.

In conclusion, if the surgeon uses proper precautions when operating on a pregnant patient, there are numerous advantages to performing the appendectomy laparoscopically.

## D. Open Appendectomy

### Carol E.H. Scott-Conner

I would perform an open appendectomy. Although I am an enthusiastic advocate of laparoscopic appendectomy for acute appendicitis, I continue to prefer open appendectomy when the patient is pregnant. Two lives, not one, are at stake, and despite increasing numbers of case series documenting safe outcomes, I remain concerned about the scattered reports of uterine perforations or fetal loss in this situation. Indeed, fetal loss may occur after an episode of acute appendicitis even with optimum surgical care.

As pregnancy advances, the gravid uterus pushes the cecum and appendix up out of the pelvis. The incision for open appendectomy must be made correspondingly higher. I prefer a relatively high transverse muscle-splitting incision, lateral to the rectus sheath. It is better to err on the side of making the incision too high, as it is far easier to lift the cecum and appendix up into the wound than it is to reach up and pull the appendix down (if the incision is too low). Generally the cecum will be quite mobile and the appendix easily delivered. Such an incision allows easy access with minimal manipulation of the gravid uterus.

## E. Conclusions

### Rachael Nicholson

Acute appendicitis in the gravid patient demands urgent surgical intervention. In the past, pregnancy was considered an absolute contraindication for laparoscopy. However, the potential advantages of a minimally invasive approach have driven the use of laparoscopy in pregnancy.

Acute appendicitis is the most common acute general surgery condition encountered during pregnancy. It occurs with the same frequency in pregnant and nonpregnant females. Therefore, approximately one of every 1000 to 2000 pregnant patients requires an appendectomy.

A high index of suspicion and a low threshold for operative exploration must be held when the diagnosis of appendicitis is entertained in a gravid patient because of the dire consequences related to appendiceal perforation. The rate of fetal loss for uncomplicated appendicitis is approximately 1.5%. However, in the face of appendiceal rupture, fetal demise can be as high as 35% and maternal mortality has been reported at 0.9%. In addition, rupture is also associated with a 33% to 40% chance of preterm labor and premature delivery.

Some publications raise concern over the use of laparoscopy in pregnancy. Amos et al. reported four fetal deaths in seven patients who underwent laparoscopic surgery. In that small series it is unclear whether or not the fetal deaths were related to laparoscopy or to the disease process that prompted the surgery. Other reports demonstrate a more direct relationship between laparoscopy and adverse events, such as with uterine trocar or Veress needle injuries. Some of these injuries had no adverse consequences. However, Friedman et al. reported pneumoamnion from a Veress needle injury, resulting in the spontaneous labor and delivery of a stillborn fetus at 21 weeks estimated gestational age. Alternative trocar entry sites for the Veress needle or insufflation via a Hassan trocar have been suggested.

The effect of pneumoperitoneum on maternal-fetal acid-base status is another area of concern. Carbon dioxide pneumoperitoneum has been shown in animal models to result in fetal acidosis. In a ewe model, Hunter et al. demonstrated fetal acidosis with insufflation of $CO_2$, which was not seen when nitrous oxide was used instead. In their study, end-tidal $CO_2$ did not correlate to maternal $PaCO_2$. Curet et al. also published the results of $CO_2$ insufflation in a ewe model and also demonstrated significant fetal acidosis. However, in their report, end-tidal $CO_2$ did parallel maternal $PaCO_2$, and acidosis did not appear to affect the outcome of the pregnancy. Recommendations were made for end-tidal $CO_2$ monitoring. In a human study, Conron et al. reported 12 laparoscopic and nine open cases in 21 pregnant women with no difference in end-tidal $CO_2$ between the groups.

In addition to acidosis, pneumoperitoneum can also reduce venous return, potentially compromising uterine blood flow. However, Barnard et al. demonstrated that the ewe fetal placenta has sufficient flow reserves or compensatory mechanisms to maintain adequate gas exchange despite decreases in maternal placental blood flow caused by pneumoperitoneum.

Laparoscopy offers many potential advantages over conventional open surgery. These include a faster recovery and earlier return to normal physical activity, which could possibly reduce the risk of thromboembolism. There is less potential for wound infections and incisional hernias. Postoperative narcotic requirements are less due to decreased amounts of pain, thus resulting in less fetal depression related to narcotic exposure and maternal hypoventilation. Less uterine manipulation during surgery might theoretically lead to a lower incidence of preterm labor. Smaller incisions provide better cosmesis. Alterations in anatomy and physiology can make the diagnosis of common acute intraabdominal pathology difficult. Laparoscopy offers a way to define that pathology better than can some open approaches.

There are several small series that support the use of laparoscopic surgery for appendicitis. Affleck et al. published an 8-year retrospective review of pregnancies that required either open or laparoscopic appendectomies or cholecystectomies. Of the 98 laparoscopic and open cases, there were no incidents of birth defects, fetal loss, or uterine injuries. Furthermore, there were no significant differences in birth weights, Apgar scores, and preterm delivery rates between the open and laparoscopic groups.

Rollins et al. described 59 pregnant patients undergoing laparoscopy with minimal complications with recommendations of intraoperative monitoring of maternal end-tidal $CO_2$, fetal heart tone monitoring pre- and postoperatively, and maternal acid-base status monitoring.

Lyass et al. prospectively studied 11 pregnant patients who underwent laparoscopic appendectomies and compared these with 11 other pregnant patients who underwent open appendectomies during the same time period. There were no operative complications. Both groups delivered at term. Both groups had one patient each who had postoperative uterine contractions successfully treated with tocolytic therapy. The laparoscopic group had a significantly shorter length of hospital stay. At 30-month follow-up there were no abnormalities in infant development in either group.

In a large retrospective review of the Swedish Health Registry, Reedy et al. observed no difference between pregnant patients undergoing laparoscopy versus laparotomy. No significant differences were found between laparoscopy and laparotomy. However, when compared to pregnancies not requiring surgery at all, both surgical groups were found to have an increased risk of low birth weight ($<2500\,g$), premature delivery, and growth restriction. These conclusions were consistent with previous data from the Swedish Health Registry reported by Mazze and Kallen.

Laparoscopic appendectomy appears to be a safe alternative to open appendectomy in pregnant patients. Concerns about fetal acidosis and diminished blood flow have been demonstrated in animal models only. There have been reported injuries directly related to the use of laparoscopic techniques, which have pushed some authors to advocate for the use of the Hasson trocar for insufflation. In contrast, there have been a number of series that demonstrate safe outcomes with laparoscopy. Others have compared open appendectomy to laparoscopic appendectomy without a demonstration of significant difference in outcomes between the two groups. Therefore, a laparoscopic approach to appendectomy appears to be an acceptable alternative to the pregnant patient with acute appendicitis.

# References

Affleck DG, Hanrahan DL, Egger MJ, Price RR. The laparoscopic management of appendicitis and cholelithiasis during pregnancy. Am J Surg 1999;178:523–529.

Amos JD, Schoor SJ, Norman PF, et al. Laparoscopic surgery during pregnancy. Am J Surg 1996;171:435–437.

Barnard JM, Chaffin D, Droste S, Tierney A, Phernetton T. Fetal response to carbon dioxide pneumoperitoneum in the pregnant ewe. Obstet Gynecol 1995;5(5, pt 1):669–674.

Conron RW Jr, Abbruzzi K, Cochrane SO, Sarno AJ, Cochrane PJ. Laparoscopic procedures in pregnancy. Am Surg 1999;65(3):259.

Curet MJ, Vogt DA, Schob O, Qualls C, Izquierdo LA, Zucker KA. Effects of $CO_2$ pneumoperitoneum in pregnant ewes. J Surg Res 1995;63:339–344.

Friedman JD, Ramsey PS, Ramin KD, Berry C. Pneumoamnion and pregnancy loss after second-trimester laparoscopic surgery. Obstet Gynecol 2002;99:512–513.

Hunter JG, Swanstrom L, Thornburg K. Carbon dioxide pneumoperitoneum induces fetal acidosis in a pregnant ewe model. Surg Endosc 1995;9:272–279.

Lyass S, Pikarshy A, Eisenberg VH, Elchalal U, Schenker JG, Reissman P. Is laparoscopic appendectomy safe in pregnant women? Surg Endosc 2001;15:377–379.

Mazze RI, Kallen B. Appendectomy during pregnancy: a Swedish Registry Study of 778 cases. Obstet Gynecol 1991;77(6):835–840.

Reedy MB, Kallen B, Kuehl TJ. Laparoscopy during pregnancy: a study of five fetal outcome parameters with use of the Swedish Health Registry. Am J Obstet Gynecol 1997;177:673–679.

Rollins MD, Chan KJ, Price RR. Laparoscopy for appendicitis and cholelithiasis during pregnancy: a new standard of care. Surg Endosc 2004;18:237–241.

# Suggested Readings

Bisharah M, Tulandi T. Laparoscopic surgery in pregnancy. Clin Obstet Gynecol 2003;46:92–97.

Curet MJ, Allen D, Josloff RK, et al. Laparoscopy during pregnancy. Arch Surg 1996;131:546–551.

Horowitz MD, Gomez GA, Santiesteban R. Acute appendicitis in pregnancy. Arch Surg 1995:120:1362–1367.

Lemaire BMD, van Erp WFM. Laparoscopic surgery during pregnancy. Surg Endosc 1997;11:15–18.

Mazze RI, Kallen B. Reproductive outcome after anesthesia and operation during pregnancy: a registry study of 5405 cases. Am J Obstet Gynecol 1989;161:1178–1185.

Rizzo AG. Laparoscopic surgery in pregnancy: long term follow-up. J Laparoendosc Adv Surg Tech A 2003;13:11–15.

Schwartzberg BS, Conyers JA, Moore JA. First trimester of pregnancy laparoscopic procedures. Surg Endosc 1997;11:1216–1217.

Society of American Gastrointestinal Endoscopic Surgeons (SAGES). Guidelines for laparoscopic surgery during pregnancy. Surg Endosc 1998;12:189–190.

Weingold AB. Appendicitis in pregnancy. Clin Obstet Gynecol 1983;26:801–809.

# 3. Stab Wound to the Abdomen

## A. Introduction

One of the earliest applications of laparoscopy was abdominal exploration. Indeed, laparoscopy was applied to the evaluation of stable trauma patients before diagnostic peritoneal lavage, ultrasound, and computed tomographic scanning were accepted modalities. The role of laparoscopy in the evaluation of the stable trauma patient is explored in this chapter.

## B. Case

### Kristen C. Sihler

A 25-year-old woman was brought to the emergency department approximately 20 minutes after an altercation in which she was stabbed with a pocket knife. She denied loss of consciousness or other injuries. She stated that she had had about four beers but no illicit drugs. Paramedics report that her pulse was 90 and her blood pressure 130/80 at the scene of the incident and that she remained stable through transport.

Her past medical history was negative. Her only prior surgery was an intramedullary nail of the right femur after a motor vehicle accident (MVA) at age 17. She had no known allergies and was on no medications. Her family history was significant for a mother with diabetes. The patient has not had any contact with her father. Her brother died at age 19 in an MVA.

The patient was single with two children, only the youngest of which resided with her. She has smoked a pack of cigarettes per day for the past 12 years and drinks five to seven beers on weekend nights. She reports marijuana use and no intravenous drug use.

The review of symptoms was otherwise negative. Her last menstrual period started 3 days earlier, and her last meal was 1 hour before the altercation.

On physical examination, her temperature was 36.8 °C, pulse 90, respiratory rate 22, blood pressure 126/69. Her height was 5 feet 3 inches and she weighed 140 pounds. There were no lacerations, ecchymosis, or abrasions to face or neck. She did not have periorbital ecchymosis, Battle's sign, or hemotympanum. Her neck was supple and nontender. Her trachea was midline and there were no step-offs on the cervical spine. She did not have jugular venous distention. Her cardiac rate and rhythm were regular. Breath sounds were equal and normal bilaterally. There was no chest wall instability, no flail segments, no tenderness, and no lacerations.

There was a laceration of the skin of the abdomen at the level of the umbilicus, over the rectus muscle, approximately 5 cm in length. It was bleeding moderately but was easily tamponaded with direct pressure. It was not obviously contaminated. Muscle was visible, but no omentum or bowel contents were seen. Her abdomen was nontender except immediately around the laceration, and she had no peritoneal signs. Bowel sounds were normoactive. There were no scars, no other lacerations, abrasions, or ecchymosis, other than the surgical scar from her prior femur surgery.

Digital rectal examination revealed normal sphincter tone, no masses, and guaiac-negative brown stool. Examination of her back was normal. A superficial laceration approximately 8 cm long was noted on the left arm. Exposed fat but no muscle was visible. Neurologic examination was normal.

Laboratory examination included a hematocrit of 34%, normal amylase and lipase, normal electrolytes, and a negative urine drug screen. Chest x-ray showed no pneumothorax or rib fractures. Computed tomography (CT) of abdomen and pelvis showed no solid organ injury and a small amount of free fluid in the pelvis.

**In addition to irrigating and suturing the arm laceration, how would you manage the stab wound to the abdomen? Wound you perform laparoscopy or formal laparotomy? Is there a role for diagnostic peritoneal lavage in this situation?**

# C. Laparoscopic Exploration

*Samuel E. Bledsoe and Ronald H. Clements*

We would perform a laparoscopy. Over the past two decades, the treatment of abdominal stab wounds has changed significantly. Traditionally, an exploratory laparotomy (EL) was required whenever peritoneal violation was suspected based on clinical presentation or local wound exploration.

This approach resulted in a high rate of nontherapeutic laparotomies with the consequent morbidity and mortality. As diagnostic imaging has improved, CT and bedside ultrasound have been used with success to predict patients who can be managed nonoperatively. While these tests have been proven to be adequately sensitive and specific, it is still difficult to definitively evaluate the patient for certain intraabdominal injuries, with small bowel, diaphragmatic, and pancreatic injuries being the most notorious.

Diagnostic peritoneal lavage (DPL) has also been employed as a diagnostic and screening tool in determining which patients would benefit from EL. However, DPL is an invasive procedure with its own discrete morbidity, and it results in a high rate of nontherapeutic laparotomy because of its high sensitivity but low specificity. In this particular case, the small amount of fluid may be blood related to the patient's menstrual cycle, rather than to an intraabdominal injury. This unrelated finding of such a small amount of blood could easily be detected on DPL, leading to an unnecessary surgical procedure.

Laparoscopy has emerged as a tool in the armamentarium of the trauma surgeon for diagnosing and treating intraabdominal injuries due to stab wounds. Gazzaniga et al. in 1976 published the first manuscript describing a series of trauma patients to be evaluated by laparoscopy. However, at that time, there were few options for laparoscopic intervention if an intraabdominal injury was identified. Since that time, two things have changed that have caused a resurgence in the interest of using laparoscopy penetrating trauma. The first factor is the technologic breakthroughs. High-resolution laparoscopes connected to high-definition plasma-screen monitors have replaced the old scopes with the cumbersome eyepieces. Technically advanced instruments and equipment are popular and widely available. This has allowed surgeons to expose previously inaccessible areas and intervene in injuries previously thought to be amenable only to laparotomy. Second, surgeons have gained a great deal of experience with laparoscopy. Laparoscopic Roux-en-Y gastric bypasses, laparoscopic splenectomy, laparoscopic colon resections, and other advanced procedures are performed daily at many hospitals across the United States. This increased experience in advanced laparoscopy has given surgeons the confidence and ability to diagnose and treat most intraabdominal injuries.

The literature demonstrates tremendous advantages to using laparoscopy in the evaluation of select trauma patients. Laparoscopy decreases nontherapeutic laparotomies, shortens the length of hospital stay, and diminishes the cost of hospital admission. An impressive number of injuries have been amenable to laparoscopy. All of this can be accomplished with a low rate of missed injuries, few conversions to open procedures, low morbidity, and low mortality.

As with any technique, there are disadvantages to using laparoscopy. There is a need for the hospital to make a significant financial investment in the technology, and the surgeon should be skilled at both laparoscopic and open techniques for trauma intervention. Peritoneal insufflation can induce a tension pneumothorax when there is a diaphragmatic laceration present. For those patients with closed head injuries, intracranial hypertension has been shown to worsen with pneumoperitoneum and the Trendelenburg position. The concerns for air embolism seem to be more theoretical than real at this point, with no documented instances in the literature to our knowledge.

Proper patient selection is of the utmost importance when employing laparoscopy in the setting of abdominal trauma. The only absolute contraindication for laparoscopy is the hemodynamically unstable patient who does not respond appropriately to proper fluid resuscitation. In this instance, emergent laparotomy and rapid control of hemorrhage is indicated. Relative contraindications include uncorrectable coagulopathy, diminished cardiopulmonary reserves from preexisting conditions, and extremely distended bowel. Care should also be used in extremes of age, pregnancy, and previous operations. Our current algorithm for management is given in Figure 3.1.

In preparing the patient for surgery, it is important to apply the usual rules of trauma care, including adequate intravenous access, Foley catheterization, and stomach decompression with a nasogastric tube. Preoperative chest x-ray should be carefully examined to rule out pneumothorax. Positive-pressure ventilation can convert an occult pneumothorax into a tension pneumothorax, and pneumoperitoneum can also cause tension pneumothorax when a diaphragmatic injury is present. The patient should be prepped in the supine position from chin to thighs in anticipation of a possible conversion to an open procedure. The entrance sites of the penetrating injury can be closed or covered with an occlusive dressing to allow for abdominal insufflation.

The placement of the first port should be at a site remote from the location of the penetrating injury. After the abdomen is entered, the peritoneum should be carefully examined for violation. An angled laparoscope is helpful in inspecting the anterior abdominal wall as the stab wound site is depressed with a finger to direct attention to the location of interest. If there is no penetration into the abdominal cavity, the operation can be safely terminated and the laceration irrigated and closed in the usual fashion.

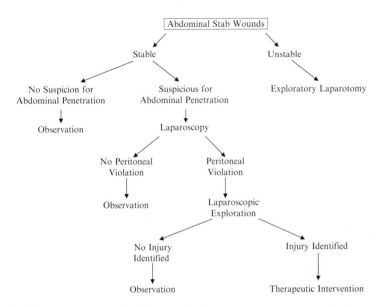

Fig. 3.1. Our preferred algorithm for the laparoscopic management of abdominal stab wounds. (Adapted from Choi and Lim.)

When there is definite penetration of the abdomen, a systematic evaluation of the abdominal organs should be conducted. Many surgeons may choose to convert to an open procedure at this point; others, with sufficient advanced laparoscopic skills, will proceed if conditions are favorable. The bowel is run from the ligament of Treitz to the rectum. The liver, spleen, stomach, and omentum must be carefully examined as well as the diaphragm. The retroperitoneum should also be visually examined for hematoma or violation.

If a small bowel injury is found, there are several options. Laparoscopic primary repair with suture is possible when there is a small enterotomy without devitalization of surrounding intestine. When there is significant injury or contamination, the bowel can be resected and anastomosed laparoscopically, if the surgeon is experienced with this technique. Another option is to lengthen the incision, exteriorize, resect, and anastomose the bowel and then return it to the peritoneal cavity.

Injuries to the liver or spleen can also be treated laparoscopically. There are a number of hemostatic treatments that have been documented as effective: thrombostat, fibrin glue, Gelfoam, diathermy coagulation, and absorbable meshes, to name a few. Laparoscopic splenectomy is considered in cases where the hemorrhage cannot be controlled with more conservative intervention. If hemorrhage from solid organs cannot be controlled by laparoscopic techniques, the operation should be immediately converted to an open procedure.

Diaphragmatic injuries are well suited for diagnosis by laparoscopy and are frequently missed by diagnostic imaging studies. If a laceration is identified in the diaphragm during exploration, the need for a chest tube must be repeatedly assessed during the laparoscopic operation. A chest tube may not be necessary since the lungs are being inflated with positive pressure. This fact may force any pleural gas back below the diaphragm, thus preventing pneumothorax and tension pneumothorax. The repair of a diaphragmatic laceration is best accomplished with large, nonabsorbable monofilament suture. Similarly, a stab wound to the lower chest with question of diaphragmatic injury may be explored laparoscopically, after placement of a chest tube.

The anterior stomach can be checked without great difficulty. If necessary, the omental sac can be entered to inspect the posterior surface of the stomach and the pancreas. Suture or staples can be used when repairing the stomach. Distal pancreatectomy is appropriate for significant injuries to the pancreatic tail, and fibrin glue can be applied to accomplish hemostasis of the pancreas.

The retroperitoneum should be carefully inspected. If an expanding hematoma is found, that is an indication to convert to an open procedure for further exploration and control of hemorrhage. Additionally, if a major vascular injury is suspected or discovered, immediate conversion should be accomplished.

It is advisable to be aware of indications for conversion to an open procedure. In addition to the previously described indications, if the patient becomes unstable during the procedure or if there is any concern about inadequate exploration, the laparoscopic operation should be abandoned and a laparotomy performed without hesitation.

# D. Laparotomy

## *Barbara Latenser*

Stab wounds to the anterior abdomen present a diagnostic and management dilemma. The days of mandatory laparotomy for all penetrating abdominal wounds are over. The attentive surgeon must balance the patient's clinical situation with the best choices for diagnosis that carry the least likelihood for complications or missed injury. In today's medical climate, the cost-effectiveness of interventions must always be considered. Thus, a selective approach to anterior abdominal stab wounds first popularized by Shaftan in the 1960s remains a rational management method.

The first issue to determine is patient stability. In a stable patient, there is time for diagnostic evaluation. The most aggressive option is selective conservatism: admit the patient for observation, keeping in mind that the patient must undergo diligent serial abdominal examinations over the next 24 hours. The optimal way to perform this process is to have the same staff person evaluate the patient over time, something that cannot be done with either shift work or in an institution where there are not personnel to evaluate the person over time. Coupled with serial abdominal examination is the process of monitoring the wound for bleeding, evisceration of omentum, or abdominal contents, and continued overall evaluation of the patient's hemodynamic status. A change in the patients' status warrants moving the patients' evaluation to the next level.

As for deciding on a diagnostic course of action for this patient, who has a mid-abdominal stab wound that is 5 cm in length, the viscoelastic properties of skin mean that the actual wound size beneath the skin will undoubtedly be greater than this dimension, increasing my concern that there may be intraabdominal injury. Patients who have sustained stab wounds are not always reliable historians. They may not have seen the stabbing instrument, may have been distracted, or may have been impaired by alcohol or other drugs during the event/altercation. I have found that descriptions of the size of the wounding implement are often inaccurate. Although stab wounds are low-velocity injuries with damage confined to the missile tract, the mobility of the intestinal contents, depending on the patient's size, position when she was stabbed, and size of the knife, means the entire intraabdominal contents could be at risk for injury.

The next assessment maneuver is to perform a local wound exploration to evaluate for peritoneal penetration. Since there is no thoracic component to this patient's injury, local wound exploration is a safe process. It can be quite challenging in a patient whose mentation is clouded by drugs, alcohol, or other reasons. Lack of fascial penetration is not ruled out with digital or instrumental wound probing, and I discourage either of these two methods of wound assessment. Inability to visualize the end of the stab wound with local wound exploration means you cannot evaluate the abdominal fascia. Abdominal fascial violation will eventually require surgical repair to prevent a future ventral hernia.

Although not all injuries providing fascial violation result in injury requiring repair, those injuries must be identified and treated to prevent serious complications or even death. A diagnostic peritoneal lavage (DPL), popularized in the 1970s as a method to determine peritoneal penetration and injury, may be used to determine the presence of abdominal injury. Red cell and white blood cell counts as well as aspiration of food particles indicate the need for immediate laparotomy, but the absolute cell count levels indicating a positive DPL vary in the literature. Even a transmural small bowel injury may produce little bleeding, making the DPL less than the ideal test. Peritoneal lavage is a nonspecific test and does not provide preoperative diagnostic information regarding the specific location of injury. Performing a DPL makes interpretation of a later computed tomography (CT) scan more difficult, as there will be some residual free fluid in the pelvis and lateral gutters.

Although abdominal ultrasound (FAST, focused abdominal sonography for trauma) has largely replaced DPL in the evaluation of the trauma patient, it shows significant amounts of peritoneal fluid due to large enteric lacerations or vascular injury, rather than small amounts of fluid due to a small penetrating bowel injury and is probably not helpful in this patient. A CT scan of the abdomen and pelvis with triple contrast (e.g. IV, oral, and rectal), will show large defects and fluid collections but may be insufficient to demonstrate small holes that will eventually develop infections and serious sepsis for the patient.

The next most invasive procedure is laparoscopy. This procedure requires general anesthesia, and carries the risks of pneumothorax and gas embolism. Although laparoscopy may be considered for patients with stab wounds to the flank or thoracoabdominal areas, not all injuries are easily found. A missed injury may be catastrophic. And laparoscopy is not a benign procedure. The time taken for therapeutic laparoscopy in penetrating trauma in one study was nearly 2 hours (111 minutes), and in that same study, several patients had additional bowel injuries diagnosed and repaired during subsequent laparotomy. If you are certain that laparoscopy is indicated, laparotomy should be the next step.

Hence, we are left with the least aggressive, and most definitive option for diagnosing and treating a 5-cm stab wound to the abdomen: exploratory laparotomy. Although there are certainly negative laparotomies, the risk of missing a significant injury may outweigh the risk of not doing a laparotomy. Mandatory laparotomy in such cases will detect some unexpected organ injuries earlier and more accurately but result in a higher nontherapeutic laparotomy rate. Although a negative laparotomy carries a small but definable risk of complications, a missed enteric injury could be needlessly life-threatening.

The safest algorithm for anterior abdominal wall stab wounds is a selective, individualized approach to evaluation and intervention. First, determine patient stability, followed by signs of peritoneal irritation. If the patient is stable without peritoneal signs, determine whether or not there is evidence of peritoneal penetration by local wound exploration. If there is no evidence of peritoneal penetration, the patient may be safely discharged. If there is evidence of peritoneal penetration on local wound exploration, the stable patient who has no peritoneal signs may be safely observed. If the patient has or develops peritoneal signs or any change in hemodynamic status, exploratory laparotomy is indicated. Avoid unnecessary operative exploration as well as diagnostic delays. The thoughtful approach to the patient will minimize complications while providing the most appropriate diagnostic and treatment options for the patient.

# E. Conclusions

*Kristen C. Sihler*

Stab wounds are a low-energy form of penetrating injury. Many do not penetrate the peritoneum and those that do may not result in injury to intraabdominal organs. Because of this, mandatory laparotomy results in a high nontherapeutic operation rate with all the attendant morbidities and costs. Local wound exploration at the bedside with local anesthesia is done for anterior abdominal wounds to determine if the anterior fascia has been penetrated. If the anterior fascia has not been violated, then no further explorations are needed. However, determining if peritoneal penetration has occurred is quite difficult at the bedside. Diagnostic peritoneal lavage was first advocated by Thal in 1977. The advantages are that it is sensitive for bowel injuries and solid organ injuries, especially if the lower threshold of 1000 red blood cells/mL is used as the threshold for operation. However, it is not sensitive for diaphragmatic injury. White blood cell counts of greater than 500/mm$^3$ are often used as indicators for hollow visceral injury, but even that may be unreliable.

In the year before Thal described using DPL for stab wounds, Gazzaniga et al. first described laparoscopy for stab wounds. In their series, 14 of 37 patients avoided laparotomy by undergoing laparoscopy. There was one missed injury in the group that did not have a laparotomy.

Because of this concern for missed injuries, a common current practice is to use laparoscopy for diagnosis of peritoneal penetration only. If peritoneal penetration is found, laparotomy is performed. Centers with an expertise in advanced laparoscopic techniques have reported evaluation of the abdomen and even repair of injuries laparoscopically, but reports of missed injuries suggest that these more advanced maneuvers should remain confined to these centers.

The technique for diagnostic laparoscopy is straightforward. Candidates for laparoscopy must be hemodynamically stable and have an anterior wound, as the retroperitoneum is not accessible laparoscopically. Patients with a stab wound between the nipples and the costal margin has their chest prepped. This way an unrecognized diaphragmatic injury leading to a tension pneumothorax at the time of insufflation can be quickly treated with a chest tube. Alternatively, for those familiar with it, a gasless technique can be used. A 30-degree scope is place through a periumbilical port site and the peritoneum is inspected. If no penetration is seen and there is no concern for diaphragmatic injury, then the procedure is terminated. If the wound is above the level of the costal margin, the diaphragm can be inspected laparoscopically if the surgeon is comfortable with this (Friese et al., Murray et al.). A series of 34 patients whose diaphragms were evaluated laparoscopically and who then underwent confirmatory laparotomy showed a sensitivity of 87.5% and a negative predictive value of 96.8%.

The advantages of diagnostic laparoscopy include fewer negative or nontherapeutic laparotomies, with resultant reductions in morbidity and possibly costs. The disadvantages include the risk of tension pneumothorax with insufflation and missed diaphragmatic injuries if the patient is at risk.

An accepted algorithm for anterior wall abdominal stab wounds is shown in Figure 3.2. Readers should be aware that there are multiple algorithms for managing anterior abdominal stab wounds and myriad small studies supporting one method over another. For instance, Demetriades and Rabinowitz performed a prospective study of observation of abdominal stab wounds in 306 patients. The only indications for immediate operation were signs of acute abdomen. Patients with other signs such as shock, evisceration, positive DPL, and air under the diaphragm on radiographic studies, as well as asymptomatic patients, were observed. Only 3.6% of these patients required subsequent operation, and there were no deaths in any of the patients who underwent observation with or without subsequent operation. Of note, this was done in a high-volume trauma center, and patients were examined every 2 to 4 hours for the first day.

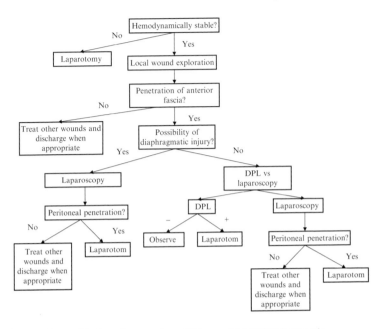

*Centers with advanced laparoscopic capabilities may wish to perform laparoscopic exploration with or without laparoscopic repair of injuries.

Fig. 3.2. Algorithm for management of abdominal stab wound.

Triple-contrast (oral, rectal, and intravenous) CT is often used for the evaluation of stab wounds. Soto et al. reported on 32 patients who underwent CT scan and were observed after stab wounds to the abdomen with peritoneal penetration as diagnosed by local wound exploration. Several patients had abnormalities on CT scan including free fluid, hepatic laceration, renal laceration, and mesenteric hematoma. Only one patient required subsequent operation for increasing abdominal pain and peritoneal signs with hypotension. A hepatic laceration was found at laparotomy, which had been seen on CT scan, but which did not have active contrast extravasation. Patients had to be hemodynamically stable after initial fluid resuscitation, and have no peritoneal signs, gastrointestinal bleeding, or evisceration. The authors indicate that active contrast extravasation or "definite" bowel perforation would have been indications for immediate operation, but no patients had these findings. In another study triple contrast CT was examined to evaluate peritoneal violation in penetrating thoracic trauma; 60% of patients with a positive

CT scan received an operation, and the remainder were observed. Computed tomography scan was judged to have 100% sensitivity, 96% specificity, 100% negative predictive value, and 97% accuracy in predicting the need for laparotomy.

# References

Choi YB, Lim KS. Therapeutic laparoscopy for abdominal trauma. Surg Endosc 2003;17:421–427.

Demetriades D, Rabinowitz B. Indications for operation in abdominal stab wounds. A prospective study of 651 patients. Ann Surg 1987;205(2):129–132.

Friese RS, Coln CE, Gentilello LM. Laparoscopy is sufficient to exclude occult diaphragm injury after penetrating abdominal injury. J Trauma 2005;58:789–792.

Gazzaniga AB, Stanton WW, Barlett RH. Laparoscopy in the diagnosis of blunt and penetrating injuries to the abdomen. Am J Surg 1976;131:315–318.

Murray JA, Demetriades D, Asensio JA, et al. Occult injuries to the diaphragm: prospective evaluation of laparoscopy in penetrating injuries to the left chest. J Am Coll Surg 1998;187:626–630.

Soto JA, Morales C, Munera F, Sanabria A, Guevara JM, Suarez T. Penetrating stab wounds to the abdomen: use of serial US and contrast-enhanced CT in stable patients. Radiology 2001;220:365–371.

Thal ER. Evaluation of peritoneal lavage and local exploration in lower chest and abdominal stab wounds. J Trauma 1977;17:642–648.

# Suggested Readings

Ahmed N, Whalen J, Brownlee J, et al. The contribution of laparoscopy in evaluation of penetrating abdominal wounds. J Am Coll Surg 2005;201(2):213–216.

Burnweit CA, Thal ER. Significance of omental evisceration in abdominal stab wounds. Am J Surg 1986;152(6):670–673.

D'Amelio LF, Rhodes M. A reassessment of the peritoneal lavage leukocyte count in blunt abdominal trauma. J Trauma 1990;30:1291–1293.

De Lacy AM, Pera M, Garcia-Valdecasas JC, et al. Management of penetrating abdominal stab wounds. Br J Surg 1988;75(3):231–233.

Fabiani P, Iannelli A, Mazza D, et al. Diagnostic and therapeutic laparoscopy for stab wounds of the anterior abdomen. J Laparoendosc Adv Surg Tech 2003;13(5):309–312.

Ivatury RR, Simon RJ, Stahl WM. A critical evaluation of laparoscopy in penetrating abdominal trauma. J Trauma 1993;34:822–827.

Lee WC, Uddo JF Jr, Nance FC. Surgical judgment in the management of abdominal stab wounds: utilizing clinical criteria from a 10-year experience. Ann Surg 1984;199(5):549–554.

Leppaniemi A, Salo J, Haapianen R. Complications of negative laparotomy for truncal stab wounds. J Trauma Injury Infect Crit Care 1995;38(1):54–58.

Leppäniemi AK, Haapiainen RK. Selective nonoperative management of abdominal stab wounds: prospective, randomized study. World J Surg 1996;20(8):1101–1106.

Leppäniemi AK, Voutilainen PR, Haapiainen RK. Indications for early mandatory laparotomy in abdominal stab wounds. Br J Surg 2003;86(1):76–80.

Liu M, Lee CH, P'eng FK. Prospective comparison of diagnostic peritoneal lavage, computed tomographic scanning, and ultrasonography for the diagnosis of blunt abdominal trauma. J Trauma 1993;35(2):267–270.

Livingston DH, Tortella BJ, Blackwood J, Machiedo GW, Rush BF. The role of laparoscopy in abdominal trauma. J Trauma 1992;33:471–475.

Marks JM, Youngelman DF, Berk T. Cost analysis of diagnostic laparoscopy vs laparotomy in the evaluation of penetrating abdominal trauma. Surg Endosc 1997;11:272–276.

Nagy K, Roberts R, Joseph K, Barrett J. Evisceration after abdominal stab wounds: is laparotomy required? J Trauma Injury Infect Crit Care 1999;47(4):622.

Rehm CG, Sherman R, Hinz TW. The role of CT scan in evaluation for laparotomy in patients with stab wounds of the abdomen. J Trauma 1989;29(4):446–450.

Robin AP, Andrews JR, Lange DA, Roberts RR, Moska M, Barrett JA. Selective management of anterior abdominal stab wounds. J Trauma 1989;29(12):1684–1689.

Rosemurgy AS 2nd, Albrink MH, Olson SM, et al. Abdominal stab wound protocol: prospective study documents applicability for widespread use. Am Surg 1995;61(2):112–116.

Salvino CK, Esposito TJ, Marshall WJ, Dries DJ, Morris RC, Gamelli RL. The role of diagnostic laparoscopy in the management of trauma patients: a preliminary assessment. J Trauma 1993;34:506–513.

Shanmuganathan K, Mirvis SE, Chiu WC, Killeen KL, Scalea TM. Triple-contrast helical CT in penetrating torso trauma: a prospective study to determine peritoneal violation and the need for laparotomy. AJR 2001;177;1247–1256.

Shorr RM, Gottlieb MM, Webb K, Ishiguro L, Berne TV. Selective management of abdominal stab wounds: importance of the physical examination. Arch Surg 1988;123(9):1141–1145.

Taviloglu K, Günay K, Ertekin C, Calis A, Türel Ö. Abdominal stab wounds: the role of selective management. Eur J Surg 1998;164(1):17–21.

Thomsen JS, Moore EE, Van Duzer-Moore S, Moore JB, Galloway AC. The evolution of abdominal stab wound management. J Trauma 1980;20(6):478–484.

Zantut LF, Ivatury RR, Smith RS, et al. Diagnostic and therapeutic laparoscopy for penetrating abdominal trauma: a multicenter experience. J Trauma 1997;42:825–831.

# 4. Elective Laparoscopic Cholecystectomy

## A. Introduction

In the early days of laparoscopic cholecystectomy, cholangiography was advocated as a way to avoid common duct injury by delineating the anatomy, as well as a method of detecting or excluding the presence of unsuspected common duct stones. This chapter explores whether routine cholangiography is needed in the routine case of a patient with no evidence of common duct stones, and explores alternatives, including the use of intraoperative ultrasound.

## B. Case

*Nate Thepjatri*

A 42-year-old woman presented for surgical evaluation with a 1-year history of intermittent right upper quadrant pain. The pain occurred approximately 20 minutes after eating, especially after she ate fatty foods. She described it as sharp, radiating to the right shoulder, and lasting about 1 to 3 hours. She had approximately three attacks per week. These episodes were not associated with nausea, vomiting, chills, or fever. She had never noted the whites of her eyes to become yellow, dark urine, or light stools. She had been seen in her local emergency department twice over the past month, told she had gallstones, and given oral pain medication.

Her past medical history was negative as was her past surgical history. Her father was alive at age 65, with diabetes. Her mother was alive and hypertensive at age 65.

The patient was employed as a schoolteacher. She smoked one pack of cigarettes per day for 20 years and drank two to three beers per week.

Her only medications were Tylenol as needed for headaches. She had no allergies.

On physical examination, she was afebrile and not visibly icteric. Her pulse was 95 and her blood pressure was 140/84. Her abdomen was soft without masses. She was mildly tender to direct palpation of the right upper quadrant. Bowel sounds were present. Murphy's sign was absent. Rectal examination was negative.

Her laboratory results were as follows: complete blood count (CBC), normal; serum bilirubin, 0.9; direct bilirubin, 0.5; alkaline phosphatase, 101; aspartate aminotransferase (AST), 23; alanine aminotransferase (ALT), 34; amylase, 55; and lipase, 55.

Ultrasound of the right upper quadrant showed a gallbladder containing multiple gallstones. The gallbladder wall was not thickened. There was no pericholecystic fluid. The common duct and the intrahepatic ducts were not dilated.

The impression was symptomatic cholelithiasis and the plan was for an elective laparoscopic cholecystectomy. **Would you do a cholangiogram during cholecystectomy?**

# C. Intraoperative Cholangiogram

## Carol E.H. Scott-Conner

Operative fluorocholangiography (intraoperative cholangiogram, IOC) remains the most accurate means to detect unexpected findings at cholecystectomy, whether open or laparoscopic. These findings may include small calculi in the common duct not seen on preoperative ultrasound, or significant anomalies of the biliary tract. While it has been difficult to prove an advantage in prospective trials, surgeons who routinely perform cholangiography strongly believe that it improves safety. Performance using fluoroscopy allows immediate interpretation of results in the operating room, assures quality of images by allowing immediate correction of patient position or overlying trocar shadows, and facilitates clearance of small calculi or bubbles from the distal duct by flushing. The technique is very well described by Berci in the SAGES manual.

Although it has been difficult to demonstrate any difference in common duct injury rates between patients who did and did not undergo cholangiography, there is a general consensus that injuries due to cholangiography (most commonly, a nick in the common duct when the common duct was cannulated) are less severe than the complete transactions noted without cholangiography. In addition, routine cholangiography facilitates recognition and management of any common duct injury, a key factor for successful repair.

Subtle biliary anomalies, such as an anomalous entrance of the right hepatic duct into the cystic duct, may be detected during cholangiography. This may help the surgeon to avoid injury, although the routine practice of keeping the dissection high at the gallbladder–cystic duct junction may help avoid this as well.

There are other advantages to routine use of IOC. Amott et al. noted no difference in complications or operative time with IOC in a small prospective cohort study. However, they commented that "IOC was easier to perform when the staff were expecting it. Thus a policy of routine IOC has been adopted." Surgeons who routinely perform operative cholangiography are more apt to be facile in laparoscopic techniques for common duct clearance as well (see Chapter 7), allowing confident management of the entire spectrum of biliary tract disorders with less reliance on endoscopic retrograde cholangiopancreatography (ERCP).

Nickkholgh et al. reported on 2130 consecutive laparoscopic cholecystectomies with a follow-up period of 9 years. They used an evolving policy, which began with the selective use of IOC but then switched to routine IOC. Sensitivity and specificity for routine IOC were extremely high, and their only two common duct injuries occurred during the selective phase of their consecutive series.

In summary, routine fluoroscopic performance of IOC allows the surgeon and the operating room team to become facile in this important method of detecting ductal anomalies and stones. It does not require specialized equipment or training (like laparoscopic ultrasound). When performed by an experienced team, it does not significantly extend operating room time.

# D.  No Cholangiogram

## *Jeffrey Hannon*

As originally presented by Mirizzi, IOC is an excellent adjunct to delineate anatomy and to demonstrate common duct stones. It should be a familiar procedure for all laparoscopic surgeons, but we do not advocate using it routinely. There is no indication for IOC in the case presented, and the decision not to perform IOC in this case should be based on a number of important factors.

The routine performance of IOC yields little information that cannot be obtained by simpler and more direct means in this patient. When used in cases with potential for retained common duct stones, or those at real risk of injury to the common duct, IOC complements the preoperative workup and meticulous dissection. Workup and dissection are more important factors in selecting the patients in whom the IOC is most likely to yield clinically significant results.

Since 1997, our group has used a selective approach to IOC. This protocol was validated in 2043 patients, and we have continued to use it in another 2400 patients since that time. We have shown that when the likelihood of the presence of common duct stones is suggested through historical, physical, laboratory, or radiologic data, then IOC is indicated. We perform IOC with real-time C-arm fluoroscopy and radiologist review. In our practice, selective IOC based on historical indications, physical findings, the elevation of any liver function test (i.e., total bilirubin, alkaline phosphatase, AST, ALT) or elevation of pancreatic enzymes (i.e., amylase or lipase), or suggestion of stones in the common bile duct on radiologic imaging, has led to a 21% IOC rate with one-third positive common duct exploration, for an overall common duct stone rate of 7% in our most recent series of 2400 patients.

Even with high-quality radiologic equipment and professional review, routine IOC is not perfect and does not always show every stone in the common duct, in our experience. One of the interesting findings in our subgroup of patients with common duct stones is that only 87% of the IOCs performed showed stones in the duct at surgery. This means that in 13% of patients with common duct stones recovered at surgery, IOCs were either falsely negative or indeterminate at the time of surgery. Therefore, in these patients, the only clear proof of a common duct stone was a positive common duct exploration. Because of the preoperative workup or the intraoperative dissection findings, the apparently negative or indeterminate intraoperative IOC did not keep the surgeon from proceeding with the common duct exploration that revealed stones in the common duct in these cases.

By avoiding IOC in 79% of all of our patients, the overall cost of cholecystectomy is lowered, and risks to the patient decreased with shortened operative time and reduced use of radiologic equipment. Intraoperative cholangiogram has been reported to take an average of 10 to 15 minutes, although this varies among hospitals and surgeons. Even if it takes 5 minutes, the risk of exposure to unnecessary radiation, dye allergy, longer anesthesia, and operative costs are higher than if the IOC was not performed.

During the course of dissection of the gallbladder and delineation of the anatomy, the ductal anatomy can be examined, and indications for IOC can be found if the common duct is unusually enlarged (a fact most often seen on preoperative radiographs) or if stones are seen in the common duct or at the junction of the common duct and cystic duct. An IOC can then be obtained in the case of any unexpected intraoperative findings.

Routine IOC is said to show anatomy and thereby to reduce the incidence of common duct injury. The risk of common duct injury in one recent large retrospective series varied from 0.39% with IOC to 0.58% without IOC. The study was touted to encourage routine IOC. However, in the discussion of this large multicenter Medicare retrospective series, the authors acknowledged that "the relationship among a surgeon's experience, frequency of IOC use, and incidence of common duct injury is not clear.... Even with the routine use of IOC, common duct injuries will, unfortunately continue to occur." It is not clear that routine IOC will prevent common duct injury any better than good surgical technique and meticulous dissection.

No common duct injury was seen in our group's series of selective IOC patients. The complete dissection of the junction of the neck of the gallbladder with the cystic duct seems critical to us in avoiding common duct injury. Through inferolateral retraction of the fundus of the gallbladder, the junction of the cystic duct with the gallbladder can be dissected for clear visualization. During the course of this maneuver, the small cystic duct branch of the cystic artery is usually seen laparoscopically so as to confirm the anatomy. Meticulous dissection of the triangle of Calot in this manner will decrease the risk of common duct injury. This dissection, in my experience, is necessary whether the IOC is to be performed or not, and, when properly done, obviates the need for IOC for anatomic delineation in most cases.

The detection of clinically insignificant stones in the common bile duct is another point in consideration of routine IOC and has many implications. The most important of these is to make sure that the treatment is no worse than the disease. That is to say that many of these small stones in small ducts will supposedly pass uneventfully, whereas surgical or ERCP efforts to retrieve them have real risks of damage or complications.

The incidence of major pancreatitis, perforation, and hemorrhage with ERCP ranges from 0.1% to over 1.0% in several studies. These numbers may be misleading in reference to our patient, as the incidence of problems with ERCP spincterotomy can be higher in patients with small common ducts, similar to this patient with no indication for selective IOC. A routine IOC could show a small clinically insignificant stone in a small common duct. The decision to "chase" this stone could lead to problems. Most of these stones that do not cause enzyme elevation or other clinical signs may pass spontaneously, in which case surgical or ERCP manipulation would be unnecessary.

Table 4.1. Indications for selective intraoperative cholangiogram.

**Preoperative Indications**

**History**

*Relative*
Choledochalgia
Acholic stools
Dark urine
*Absolute*
Jaundice
Pancreatitis
Cholangitis

**Physical examination**
Jaundice

**Ultrasound**
Defect in common duct
Dilated common duct

**Radionuclide hepatobiliary scan**
Obstructed common duct
Dilated common duct

**Abnormal lab values**
Bilirubin
Alanine aminotransferase (ALT)
Aspartate aminotransferase (AST)
Lactate dehydrogenase (LDH)
Alkaline phosphatase
Amylase
Lipase

**Intraoperative Indications**

**Dilated bile ducts**

Cystic duct > 5 mm
Common duct > 10 mm

**Proximal obstruction of the cystic duct**

**Stones or sludge in the cystic or common duct**

**Questionable anatomy**

**Questionable ductal injury**

We did not have any patients that needed postoperative ERCP for missed common duct stones in our series of patients with selective IOC. The incidence of clinically significant missed stones in other series of selective IOC ranges from 0.4% to 0.6%. These stones are usually handled by postoperative ERCP.

Some selective IOC advocates use preoperative ERCP to clear the duct prior to laparoscopic cholecystectomy. We have not used this route because, as noted, most preoperative criteria would still result in negative ERCP, and an unnecessary ERCP carries higher risk than IOC.

One other potential danger of IOC is the real risk of anaphylaxis to the contrast. Few instances of dye anaphylaxis in IOC exist in the literature, but the reported episodes were severe. Most instances of anaphylaxis are totally unexpected, and the results can be devastating. The only way to lower this risk is to avoid unnecessary IOC.

In summary, the patient as presented has no indication for IOC outside of a dogged routine to perform IOC on all patients. As discussed, the routine performance of IOC, in my experience, increases risks to the patient, with very little benefit. An IOC will not stop common duct injury, cannot completely obviate further invasive procedures, increases costs, and without clear indications can even be misleading and falsely negative. The best course of action for this patient is thorough preoperative workup with a focused history and physical exam, good radiologic imaging, and appropriate laboratory studies. This should be followed by a careful laparoscopic cholecystectomy with meticulous dissection of the triangle of Calot and the junction of the cystic duct and the gallbladder neck. We recommend the selective use of IOC based only on the criteria as outlined in Table 4.1.

# E. Intraoperative Ultrasound

*Daniel J. Deziel*

Surgeons have long debated the necessity of routine intraoperative imaging of the common bile duct during an elective cholecystectomy. Routine imaging can be defined as the use of imaging in nearly all cases, regardless of the presence or absence of factors that may be predictive for choledocholithiasis. Proponents of routine imaging argue that such an approach detects unexpected stones in a small, but finite, proportion of patients, and that these stones may be clinically relevant. Implicit in this philosophy is the concept that it is generally better to treat bile duct stones at the time of operation than to wait until afterward. When bile duct stones are not present, routine imaging may still be valuable for defining the anatomy of the bile ducts. This may occasionally facilitate the detection of other pathology and, in particular, may be useful to prevent, to minimize, or to diagnose bile duct injury in that unfortunate circumstance. Routine imaging has been established to be safe, rapid, and inexpensive. In surgical training programs it is considered a necessary tool for the development of requisite technical skills by the resident trainees.

Selective intraoperative imaging can be defined as limiting use to patients who have a statistically greater probability of having concomitant choledocholithiasis based on clinical, laboratory, or preoperative imaging criteria. This approach contends that occult bile duct stones are infrequent and are even less frequently likely to require any intervention. The data that routine imaging prevents bile duct injury are not considered compelling. Moreover, imaging unnecessarily adds some operative time and expense and occasionally can even be harmful. The proportion of cases in which selective surgeons actually image the bile ducts varies tremendously in clinical practice. Although "routine" may not literally mean always, "selective" should not mean rarely or never.

Compounding the debate is the issue of which method of intraoperative imaging is better: digital fluorocholangiography or ultrasonography or both (static cholangiography is clearly inferior). For the patient undergoing elective laparoscopic cholecystectomy with a low probability of bile duct stones, routine laparoscopic ultrasound is a logical first choice for evaluating the bile duct. The rationale for routine imaging has been outlined. The recommendation for laparoscopic ultrasound is based on the body of peer-reviewed literature that has accrued for more than a decade now and is supported by my own clinical practice during that time.

There are a number of advantages to laparoscopic ultrasound of the bile duct. First, it is highly accurate for the detection of choledocholithiasis. Common bile duct stones can be identified in up to 5% of patients with absolutely no preoperative risk factors, that is, normal liver enzymes, normal-caliber bile duct by transabdominal ultrasound, and no clinical history of jaundice, cholangitis, or pancreatitis. Figure 4.1 shows a stone in the distal common bile duct diagnosed in just such a patient. The consensus of the published data demonstrates that the sensitivity and specificity of intraoperative ultrasound are excellent, equaling and often exceeding those of intraoperative cholangiography. The positive

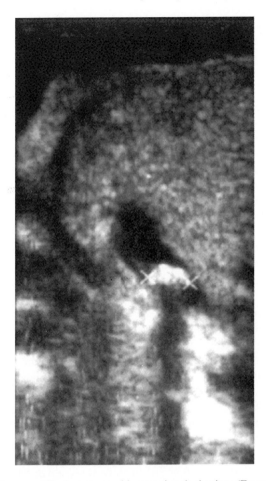

Fig. 4.1. Common bile duct stone with posterior shadowing. (From Scott-Conner CEH, ed. The SAGES Manual: Fundamentals of Laparoscopy, Thoracoscopy, and GI Endoscopy, 2nd ed. New York: Springer-Verlag, 2006, with permission.)

predictive value of intraoperative ultrasound has been significantly better than that of intraoperative cholangiography. In other words, ultrasound has resulted in a lower rate of negative common bile duct explorations. Wu et al. showed that laparoscopic ultrasound is more sensitive than cholangiography for the detection of small stones or sludge found in 6% of patients. Although these may not necessarily be clinically important, they can usually be cleared out of the duct by simple flushing.

Laparoscopic ultrasound can be useful for identifying the location of the common bile duct and common hepatic duct in difficult cases. The cystic duct–common duct junction can usually be visualized sonographically, thus allowing the surgeon to determine whether the dissection can be accomplished safely away from the common duct. Biffl et al. observed that the use of laparoscopic ultrasound has been associated with lower rates of conversion to open cholecystectomy during operations for acute cholecystitis and also lower rates of bile duct injury. While laparoscopic ultrasound may be helpful for locating the common bile duct, it is inferior to cholangiography for complete definition of the bile duct anatomy. The branching pattern of the proximal bile ducts cannot be reliably determined, and the distal intrapancreatic portion of the duct and ampulla are not always well visualized. Other pertinent anatomy can be identified by laparoscopic ultrasound during routine cases as well, particularly variations in the origination of the hepatic arteries from the celiac or superior mesenteric vessels. Unexpected liver or pancreatic masses or lymphadenopathy will also sometimes be discovered.

There are other practical advantages to using laparoscopic ultrasound as the first method for imaging the bile duct. Laparoscopic ultrasonography has been shown in several series to require significantly less time to complete than does an intraoperative cholangiogram: 5 to 10 minutes versus 15 to 18 minutes. Ultrasound examination does not require opening the ductal system for direct access. Sonographic imaging can easily be repeated as necessary during the procedure. This is useful for assessing stone clearance in situations when stones have been unexpectedly encountered and manipulated. In special circumstances, such as with a pregnant patient, ultrasound is obviously preferable since there is no exposure to ionizing radiation.

Inherent to any technique are the limitations and disadvantages that must be recognized. Laparoscopic ultrasound requires special transducers, and in many institutions the equipment may not be available. The surgeon must be familiar with the operation of the ultrasound machine settings and handling of the transducer to acquire optimal sonographic images of the duct. Halpin et al. have shown that with experience, technically adequate visualization can be achieved in more than 95% of cases. Intraoperative ultrasound should never be considered a replacement for intraoperative cholangiography. The techniques are complementary, and it is advantageous to have a surgeon capable of utilizing both. In the elective scenario when the anticipation of bile duct stones is low, routine laparoscopic ultrasound evaluation is sensible and well supported.

# F. Conclusions

*Nate Thepjatri*

The decision as to whether or not to perform intraoperative imaging, and which imaging modality to use, is a difficult one when there is a low suspicion that the patient has choledocholithiasis, as in the present case. This is implied with normal liver function tests, no history of jaundice, no history of pancreatitis, and preoperative ultrasound showing no evidence of biliary tree calculi or dilatation.

Metcalfe et al. performed a Medline search in 2004 to identify laparoscopic cholecystectomy series in which either routine or selective intraoperative cholangiograms were performed. They identified eight laparoscopic cholecystectomy series from 1991 to 2001 with a routine cholangiogram policy. A total of 4209 laparoscopic cholecystectomies were performed, with 170 (4%) having unsuspected retained common bile duct stones. The false positive rate was 0.8% (34/4209). They further identified nine series from 1989 to 2001 with a selective cholangiogram policy. None of the patients had a history of pancreatitis, jaundice, or common bile stones by ultrasound. Of a total of 5179 cases, 32 patients (0.06%) developed symptoms from residual stones. They concluded that the true incidence of common bile duct stones in an asymptomatic patient was 4%, and 0.6% actually become symptomatic. Thus only 15% of retained common bile stones go on to develop problems.

It is often stated that routine cholangiogram helps define the biliary anatomy and thus reduces injury during laparoscopic cholecystectomy. Metcalf et al. looked at 11 series from 1987 to 2001. The rate of common bile duct transaction with routine (1/6024 = 0.02%) and selective (3/3268 = 0.09%) cholangiogram was not statically different (*p* = .13). Overall, Metcalf et al. advocated a selective policy for intraoperative cholangiogram.

Collins et al. performed a prospective trial to study common bile duct calculi in patients undergoing laparoscopic cholecystectomy. Over an 11-year period from 1990 to 2001, 997 patients underwent laparoscopic cholecystectomy. Intraoperative cholangiogram was attempted in all patients, with a success rate of 96% (962 patients). In total, 46 patients had a filling defect for a rate of 4.6%. In those with a filling defect, the cholangiogram catheter was left in place, and a cholangiogram was repeated in 48 hours and at 6 weeks. Twelve had a normal cholangiogram at 48 hours for a false-positive rate of 26%. An additional 12 had a normal cholangiogram at 6 weeks. The remaining 22 with an abnormal cholangiogram at 6 weeks underwent ERCP.

Collins et al. concluded that choledocholithiasis occurs in 3.4%, but almost a third pass the stone at 6 weeks. Based on these data, treatment based on an IOC finding would have resulted in unnecessary intervention in 50% of the patients.

Birth et al. performed a prospective randomized trail in 1998 to compare laparoscopic ultrasonography and intraoperative cholangiography. From June 1994 to April 1996, a total of 518 consecutive patients were randomized to either ultrasound or cholangiogram. Ultrasound failed in two patients (0.4%) and cholangiogram failed in 41 patients (7.9%). The results of ultrasound versus cholangiogram in terms of identifying unsuspected common bile duct stones were (1) sensitivity 83.3% versus 100%, (2) specificity 100% versus 98.9%, and (3) accuracy 99.2% versus 98.9%. The authors concluded that laparoscopic ultrasound in the hands of experienced surgeons is good and effective in assessing the common bile duct. It has the advantage of unlimited ability to repeat the study, lack of adverse effects, shorter examination time, and lower costs.

Ohtani et al. performed a prospective study in 1997 to compare intraoperative ultrasound with cholangiography. They wanted to compare the effectiveness in identifying gallstones, detecting hepatobiliary structures, and demonstrating congenital anomalies. In 65 patients, intraoperative ultrasound was performed first, followed by cholangiography. Ultrasound was successful in 65 patients, and IOC was successful in 54 patients. Less time was needed for intraoperative ultrasound than for IOC ($p < .001$). Intraoperative ultrasound imaged the hepatic ducts and their confluence, the common hepatic duct, the common bile duct, and the ampulla of Vater in 97%, 100%, 97%, and 51%. Intraoperative ultrasound imaged these structures in 85%, 89%, 100%, and 94%. In terms of sensitivity, specificity, positive predictive value, negative predictive value, and accuracy in identifying bile duct stones, intraoperative ultrasound was 80%, 98%, 80%, 98%, and 97%, and IOC was 80%, 97%, 67%, 98%, and 95%, respectively. The authors concluded that intraoperative ultrasound is superior to intraoperative cholangiography in regard to safety, shorter exam time, and ease of administration to patients.

Machi et al. performed a review of 12 prospective studies comparing laparoscopic ultrasound and intraoperative cholangiography. There were a total of 2059 patients. The success rate was comparable for both tests: 88% to 100%. The average time needed for laparoscopic ultrasound was

7 minutes, or one-half the time needed for IOC. Laparoscopic ultrasound had fewer false positives (4 versus 23), better positive predictive value, and better specificity. Sensitivity and negative predictive value were comparable. Intraoperative cholangiogram detected ductal variations more distinctly than laparoscopic ultrasound.

In conclusion, the true incidence of common bile duct stones in an asymptomatic patient was 4%, and 0.6% actually become symptomatic. Thus only 15% of retained common bile stones will go on to develop problems. Because of this, a routine policy of IOC is not advocated.

Laparoscopic ultrasound has many advantages. It is quick, can be used repeatedly, and has a lower cost. Some disadvantages are surgeon inexperience and need for a special probe. It takes a surgeon about 30 to 40 laparoscopic ultrasound exams to become more proficient. Because of this learning curve, IOC and laparoscopic ultrasound should be used in a complementary manner. Once one becomes more accustomed to the laparoscopic ultrasound, it can be used as the primary screening tool for bile duct stones. If the laparoscopic ultrasound is definitely negative or positive for stones, IOC is not necessary.

When bile duct stones are suspected, laparoscopic ultrasound is emerging as an important diagnostic tool. When the learning curve is surpassed, it is as accurate as IOC in identifying bile duct stones. Because of its ease, speed, and fewer side effects, ultrasound should be used as the initial screening tool. If the ultrasound results are not conclusive, then proceed with a cholangiogram. At this time, ultrasound and cholangiogram should be used in a complementary manner.

# References

Amott D, Webb A, Tulloh B. Prospective comparison of routine and selective operative cholangiography. ANZ J Surg 2005;75:378–382.

Berci G. Laparoscopic cholecystectomy: cholangiography. In: Scott-Conner CEH, ed. The SAGES Manual: Fundamentals of Laparoscopy, Endoscopy, and Thoracoscopy, 2nd ed. New York: Springer-Verlag, 2006:145–164.

Biffl WL, Moore EE, Offner PJ, Franciose RJ, Burch JM. Routine intraoperative laparoscopic ultrasonography with selective cholangiography reduces bile duct complications during laparoscopic cholecystectomy. J Am Coll Surg 2001;193(3):272–280.

Birth M, Ehlers KU, Delinikolas K, et al. Prospective randomized comparison of laparoscopic ultrasonography using a flexible-tip ultrasound probe and intraoperative dynamic cholangiography during laparoscopic cholecystectomy. Surg Endosc 1998;12:30–36.

Collins C, Maguire D, Ireland A, et al. A prospective study of common bile duct calculi in patients undergoing laparoscopic cholecystectomy. Ann Surg 2004;239:28–33.

Halpin VJ, Dunnegan D, Soper NJ. Laparoscopic intracorporeal ultrasound versus fluoroscopic intraoperative cholangiography: after the learning curve. Surg Endosc 2002; 16(2): 336–41.

Machi J, Tateishi T, Oishi AJ, et al. Laparoscopic ultrasonography versus operative cholangiography during laparoscopic cholecystectomy: review of the literature and a comparison with open intraoperative ultrasonography. J Am Coll Surg 1999;188(4):360–367.

Metcalfe MS, Chir MBB, Ong T, et al. Is laparoscopic intraoperative cholangiogram a matter of routine. Am J Surg 2004;187:475–481.

Mirizzi, PL. Operative cholangiography. Surg Gynecol Obstet 1937;65:702–710.

Nickkholgh A, Soltaniyekta S, Kalbasi H. Routine versus selective cholangiography during laparoscopic cholecystectomy: a survey of 2,130 patients undergoing laparoscopic cholecystectomy. Surg Endosc 2006;20:868–874.

Ohtani T, Kawai C, Shirai Y, et al. Intraoperative ultrasonography versus cholangiography during laparoscopic cholecystectomy: a prospective comparative study. J Am Coll Surg 1997;185:286–295.

Wu JS, Dunnegan DL, Soper NJ. The utility of intracorporeal ultrasonography for screening the bile duct during laparoscopic cholecystectomy. J Gastrointest Surg 1998;2(1):50–60.

# Suggested Readings

Catheline J, Rizk N, Champault G. A comparison of laparoscopic ultrasound versus cholangiography in the evaluation of the biliary tree during laparoscopic cholecystectomy. Eur J Ultrasound 1999;10(1):1–9.

Chi-Liang Cheng MD, et al. Risk factors for post-ERCP pancreatitis: a prospective multicenter study. Am J Gastroenterol 2006;101(1):139–147.

Cotton PB, Leung JWC. ERCP: risks, prevention, and management. Advanced Digestive Endoscopy, ERCP Section http://www.ddc.musc.edu/ddc_pro/pro_development/reading_list/articles/ERCP_risks_082004.pdf

Flum DR, et al. Intraoperative cholangiography and risk of common bile duct injury during cholecystectomy. JAMA 2003;289:1639–1644.

Livingston EH, et al. Indications for selective intraoperative cholangiography. J Gastrointest Surg 2005;9(9):1371–1377.

McLean TR. Risk management observations from litigation involving laparoscopic cholecystectomy. Arch Surg 2006;141:643–648.

Moskovitz AH, et al. Anaphylactoid reaction to intraoperative cholangiogram. Report of a case, review of literature, and guidelines for prevention. Surg Endosc 2001;15(10):1227.

Snow LL, Weinstein LS, Hannon JK, Lane DR. Evaluation of operative cholangiography in 2043 patients undergoing laparoscopic cholecystectomy. Surg Endosc 2001;15:14–20.

Tranter SE, Thompson MH. A prospective single-blinded controlled study comparing laparoscopic ultrasound of the common bile duct with operative cholangiography. Surg Endosc 2003;17(2):216–219.

# 5. Gallstone Pancreatitis

## A. Introduction

Gallstones and alcohol use are the two most common causes of acute pancreatitis in most developed countries. For many patients, an episode of pancreatitis is the first clue that they have calculous biliary tract disease. Cholecystectomy is required to prevent recurrence, but the optimum management of the common duct—specifically, how to determine whether or not stones are still present and, if so, how to clear those stones—is a matter of debate. This chapter explores those issues. Chapter 6 expands upon these themes by considering management of the patient with *known* choledocholithiasis.

## B. Case

*Farshad Elmi and William B. Silverman*

A 51-year-old woman presented to the emergency department complaining of upper abdominal pain and nausea. The pain began 4 hours earlier, while she was grocery shopping. The pain was described as constant, sharp, and rated as 10/10. She had not had any fever or chills. She reported that she had had some indigestion over the past 3 to 4 months and had been using antacids, with partial relief. She described these attacks as intermittent abdominal pain and nausea, usually after fatty meals, lasting for just a few hours. The pain that brought her to the emergency department this time was more severe and radiated to the back. She was otherwise healthy and walked 1 to 2 miles per day without difficulty.

Her past medical history was significant only for three normal vaginal deliveries of term infants. She had not had any prior surgery. She was married and lived with her husband. She worked as an English teacher. She was a nonsmoker. She did not drink. Her only medications were multivitamins and calcium. She used antacids periodically, as noted above. Her review of symptoms was negative except as noted above.

On physical examination, she was awake, alert, oriented, and in moderate distress due to abdominal pain. She was not visibly jaundiced. Her pulse was 95, temperature 37.5 °C, blood pressure 140/85. Her mucous membranes were moist, and her jugular veins were nondistended. Her cardiovascular examination was normal.

Abdominal examination was significant for a soft abdomen with moderate tenderness over the epigastric region. There was no rebound tenderness, no Murphy's sign. Bowel sounds were present. Rectal examination revealed normal sphincter tone, no masses or gross blood, and stool was guaiac negative.

Laboratory examinations were significant for a white cell count of 12,500 cells. Total bilirubin was 1.2 mg/dL, aspartate aminotransferase was elevated at 95 U/L, alanine aminotransferase was elevated at 84 U/L, alkaline phosphatase normal at 95 U/L, $\gamma$-glutamyltransferase normal at 35 U/L. Amylase was 1400 U/L and lipase 730 U/L, both significantly elevated.

Ultrasound of the right upper quadrant showed a normal liver, several stones within the gallbladder, and dilatation of intra- and extrahepatic biliary ducts with maximum diameter of common bile duct 10 mm. The sonographic Murphy's sign was negative.

**The impression was biliary pancreatitis. Which would you recommend: endoscopic retrograde cholangiopancreatography (ERCP) followed by laparoscopic cholecystectomy, or laparoscopic cholecystectomy with intraoperative cholangiogram (and laparoscopic common bile duct exploration, if cholangiogram positive)?**

# C. Endoscopic Retrograde Cholangiopancreatography with Laparoscopic Cholecystectomy

*Farshad Elmi and William B. Silverman*

Alcoholism and biliary stones (also known as biliary pancreatitis) are the two most common causes of acute pancreatitis in the United States; each accounts for 35% of cases. Although gallstones are common etiology of acute pancreatitis, acute pancreatitis develops only in 3% to 7% of patients with gallstone disease. Smaller stones (<5 mm in size) carry more risk of acute pancreatitis, as the small size favors the migration of stones into the common bile ducts.

It is estimated that up to 50% of gallstones are asymptomatic, 30% present as biliary colic, and 20% present as complications such as acute cholecystitis, cholangitis, and acute pancreatitis. However, once an episode of biliary colic has occurred, there is a high risk of repeated attacks of pain. More than 90% of the complications have been preceded by biliary colic.

Biliary pancreatitis is precipitated by the transient or persistent obstruction of the ampulla of Vater by a stone. This is usually accompanied by passage of a stone from the common bile duct into the lumen of the intestinal tract. In most patients this process occurs on the day of the attack, and by the time they reach the emergency department the stone may have already passed into the intestinal tract.

In terms of laboratory findings, amylase and lipase rise quickly during the pancreatitis, but amylase has a shorter half-life and may be normalized by the second or third day, while lipase could remain elevated for a longer period of time. Liver transaminase levels also increase and then fluctuate. Alkaline phosphatase and bilirubin levels go up only with persistent biliary obstruction.

This patient has had biliary colic for a few months, which has been treated as indigestion with antacid medications. She has been intermittently experiencing these bouts of postprandial abdominal pain until one of the stones has passed into the common bile duct and caused obstruction of the papilla leading to pancreatitis. Her abdominal pain on the day of presentation to the emergency department has been different compared to the usual biliary colic. It was more severe and also radiating to the back, suggestive of a pancreatic process. The clinical picture along with elevation of amylase/lipase and liver transaminases prompts the physicians to obtain the liver ultrasound and perform ERCP followed by laparoscopic cholecystectomy.

An ERCP allows careful examination of the biliary tree under ideal conditions. Any stones still present in the distal duct can be removed, and a spincterotomy performed to allow free drainage of bile and prevent recurrence. It allows the most expedient resolution of the immediate problem. Laparoscopic cholecystectomy should be done during the same hospitalization to prevent recurrence.

# D. Laparoscopic Cholecystectomy with Cholangiogram, Laparoscopic Common Duct Exploration if Needed

*Shishir K. Maithel and Benjamin E. Schneider*

Since its advent in 1987, laparoscopic cholecystectomy has become the treatment of choice for symptomatic cholelithiasis. The incidence of concomitant choledocholithiasis has been reported to be as high as

15% to 20%, thus causing some to advocate performing routine intraoperative cholangiography. When symptoms suggest choledocholithiasis, whether pain, sepsis, pancreatitis, or simply a rise in liver enzymes, the treatment algorithm becomes slightly more complex. Many options exist for management of this problem, including performing ERCP either pre-, intra-, or postoperatively, or performing a common bile duct exploration at the time of laparoscopic cholecystectomy. We advocate the latter. The advantages of performing a laparoscopic common bile duct exploration (LCBDE) over the other options listed above are mainly twofold: (1) direct benefits to the patient, and (2) efficient utilization of hospital resources.

In terms of direct patient benefits, an LCBDE is performed at the same time as the laparoscopic cholecystectomy. Thus, in contrast with pre- or postoperative ERCP, the patient is spared a second intervention that requires conscious sedation, and occasionally requires general anesthesia. Furthermore, the patient is not subjected to the inherent risks that accompany ERCP, such as bowel perforation, post-ERCP pancreatitis, cholangitis, bleeding after sphincterotomy, and bacteremia or septicemia.

If a surgeon is skilled in LCBDE, the definitive diagnosis of choledocholithiasis can be made in the operating room and can be managed in the same setting. This also potentially reduces patients' hospital stay and allows them to return to their daily activities and occupation in a timely manner.

Furthermore, in today's era of limited resources, rising health care costs, and a growing number of patients without health care insurance, we must inevitably consider these factors when deciding on treatment options for our patients. Laparoscopic common bile duct exploration and ERCP have been compared in terms of resource utilization in numerous studies. Poulose et al. recently reported on nearly 41,000 patients who were identified in the 2002 U.S. National Inpatient Sample and who underwent laparoscopic cholecystectomy but who also had choledocholithiasis. Ninety-three percent of these patients underwent ERCP to clear their common bile duct, while only 7% underwent LCBDE at the time of cholecystectomy. The total in-hospital charges and length of hospital stay were significantly lower for the LCBDE group. Mean hospital charges and length of stay were almost $5000 and one full day less, respectively, for the LCBDE group.

Similar findings are reported by Urbach et al. after conducting an extensive decision analysis of four treatment strategies for choledocholithiasis in terms of their cost-effectiveness and ability to avoid retained common bile duct stones. The four treatment options were (1) routine preoperative ERCP, (2) selective LCBDE, (3) selective postoperative ERCP, and (4) expectant management. Selective LCBDE was more cost-effective and slightly better at preventing residual choledocholithiasis compared to selective postoperative ERCP. Selective LCBDE added less than $500 to hospital costs compared to laparoscopic cholecystectomy alone. While routine preoperative ERCP is very effective in preventing residual common bile duct stones, its poor cost-effectiveness was prohibitive. Furthermore, this strategy would subject many patients to an unnecessary invasive procedure. Expectant management is not recommended due to the potential of highly morbid complications that may result from untreated choledocholithiasis.

One may rebut that *intraoperative* ERCP accomplishes common bile duct clearance at the time of cholecystectomy with the same success and cost-efficiency as LCBDE (see Chapter 6 for a detailed discussion of this modality). In fact, several studies have demonstrated that there is no difference between these two treatment strategies in terms of surgical time, success rate, number of stone extractions, postoperative complications, retained common bile duct stones, postoperative length of stay, and hospital charges. However, we firmly believe that difficulty with scheduling logistics would prohibit adoption of this treatment strategy as a routine practice. Intraoperative ERCP would require synchronization of the gastroenterologist and surgeon's schedules, a feat that we are sure would be nearly impossible to achieve on a regular basis.

The long-term effects of each treatment option must also be considered. There is a growing suspicion that patients who undergo ERCP with sphincterotomy may have more frequent complications with cholangitis over the long-term. Macadam and Goodall reported that nearly 20% of patients who had previously undergone sphincterotomy had symptoms suggestive of cholangitis. Furthermore, the potential consequences of free duodenobiliary reflux after sphincterotomy that results in bactibilia has been shown to lead to mild portal tract inflammation on liver biopsy.

Thus, it seems clear that LCBDE is the most viable option for treating choledocholithiasis, both in terms of direct patient benefits, as well as efficient utilization of limited health care resources. However, as with any invasive procedure, there is a technical learning curve that must be mastered in order to provide the best care to patients. Laparoscopic common bile duct exploration can be accomplished through a transcystic approach or directly via a choledochotomy, the latter of which is technically more challenging. The following are some technical pearls that may increase one's success in performing LCBDE.

## Transcystic Approach

1.  It is often best to incise the cystic duct via the same port through which the cholangiogram catheter will be introduced in order to facilitate a simpler introduction of the catheter by optimizing the angle of incision.
2.  Intravenous administration of 1.0 mg of glucagon can sometimes further facilitate stone clearance with simple saline flushes by relaxing the sphincter of Oddi.
3.  When using a Fogarty balloon catheter to retrieve stones, it is important to prevent stones from traveling proximally into the common hepatic duct, a situation that may require performing a choledochotomy or a postoperative ERCP.
4.  A larger 5-French (F) catheter should be used to perform a transcystic cholangiogram if transcystic choledochoscopy is planned to facilitate passage of the choledochoscope into the common bile duct. Furthermore, the cystic duct can be dilated by passing an 8F balloon angioplasty catheter over a guidewire and inflating the balloon to 6 atmospheres of pressure for 5 minutes.

## Choledochotomy

1.  Indications for doing a choledochotomy include an extremely short cystic duct, distal insertion of the cystic duct into the common bile duct, multiple large stones that cannot be extracted via the transcystic approach, and proximal stones in the common hepatic duct.
2.  Choledochotomy should be avoided in situations where the common bile duct measures less than 8 mm in diameter or is surrounded by significant inflammation. In this case, a postoperative ERCP may be the better treatment strategy.
3.  A choledochotomy incision is made along the right anterolateral surface, just distal to the insertion of the cystic duct, for a length of approximately 5 to 6 mm.
4.  Consider placing a T-tube in the common bile duct in order to minimize postoperative strictures, and a closed suction drain should be left in place in the operative field.

In summary, laparoscopic common bile duct exploration is definitely underutilized by surgeons, despite its clear benefits to patients and its more efficient use of hospital resources. One reason for this may be the lack of technical abilities or know-how of many general surgeons who routinely perform laparoscopic cholecystectomies. The widespread use of laparoscopic surgical simulation as a teaching tool may help to narrow this technical gap and make LCBDE a readily available treatment strategy to patients.

# E. Conclusions

## Susan S. Hagen

Acute pancreatitis is generally characterized by abdominal pain with elevated pancreatic enzymes. It is most commonly caused by gallstones and chronic alcohol abuse. The annual incidence of acute pancreatitis ranges from 5 to 80 per 100,000. Gallstone pancreatitis is a result of transient or persistent blockage of the ampulla of Vater by biliary calculi. Cholecystectomy and clearing of duct stone will prevent recurrence, and it is accepted practice to perform this once symptoms have resolved during the same hospitalization. Laparoscopic cholecystectomy is the gold standard for treatment of symptomatic cholelithiasis. Without treatment, the risk of recurrence of symptoms is high, occurring in one third to two thirds of patients. An additional 5% to 20% of patients can have necrotizing pancreatitis and systemic organ failure.

## Preoperative Endoscopic Retrograde Cholangiopancreatography

The change from open cholecystectomy to laparoscopic cholecystectomy has increased surgeon's reliance on endoscopists to perform ERCP, as many surgeons are not comfortable performing laparoscopic duct exploration.

The current literature supports preoperative ERCP only in select patients. If patients meet criteria such as high serum bilirubin value, severe cholangitis, and a common bile duct dilatation, a preoperative ERCP is performed. Even following the above criteria, Enochsson et al. noted that 10% of preoperative ERCP will be negative.

According to the Japanese (JPN) Guidelines, "an emergency endoscopy approach is beneficial in patients with acute pancreatitis in whom bile duct obstruction is suspected or there are complications from cholangitis." The endoscopic approach can include sphincterotomy, papillary balloon dilation, nasobiliary drainage, and stenting. The end result of draining the bile duct and removing the stone relieves the obstruction of the pancreatic duct. After the stones are cleared via endoscopy, laparoscopic cholecystectomy should be performed during the same hospital stay. The National Institutes of Health has a similar stance. An ERCP and sphincterotomy with stone removal is therapeutic for those with choledocholithiasis with jaundice, dilated common bile duct, acute pancreatitis, or cholangitis. In those with severe biliary pancreatitis, early intervention with ERCP reduces morbidity and mortality compared with delayed ERCP. If there is low probability of choledocholithiasis, then preoperative ERCP is not warranted. ERCP should be avoided if there is a low likelihood of biliary stone or structure. Complications of ERCP include pancreatitis, sepsis, hemorrhage, and retroperitoneal duodenal perforation. Sekimoto et al. cite an incidence of acute pancreatitis following ERCP of 0.4% to 1.5%, increasing to 1.6% to 5.4% if endoscopic sphincterotomy is performed.

## Intraoperative Cholangiogram

Those who do not meet criteria for preoperative ERCP often have an intraoperative cholangiogram (IOC). In 2000, Chang and colleagues performed a prospective randomized controlled trial to assess if ERCP and common bile duct stone extraction should be performed prior to surgery or selectively after surgery in patients who demonstrated a stone on intraoperative cholangiogram. All patients with mild to moderate gallstone pancreatitis were randomized ($n = 59$). In the postoperative ERCP group, in only seven of 29 patients (24%) was a postoperative ERCP necessary. This study demonstrates that routine preoperative ERCP is not warranted in the case of mild to moderate gallstone pancreatitis and that routine post operative ERCP is not necessary.

## Methods for Clearing Common Bile Duct Stones if Intraoperative Cholangiogram Is Positive

According to Petelin, percutaneous intraoperative cholangiograms were performed and abnormal cholangiograms were identified in 10% of patients. In most cases, laparoscopic common bile duct exploration successfully treated the patients usually via the cystic duct (82.5%) or through a choledochotomy (17.5%). In the remaining patients, ERCP and open common bile duct exploration treated the disease. According to the National Institutes of Health, laparoscopic common bile duct exploration and postoperative ERCP are both safe and reliable in clearing common bile duct stones.

Nathanson et al., in a randomized trial across seven metropolitan hospitals in Australia, evaluated whether retained stones, failing extraction transcystically, should be extracted via laparoscopic choledochotomy or postoperative ERCP. Over a nearly 5-year period, 372 patients had bile duct stones, with successful clearance performed through the cystic duct in 286 patients (77%). The remaining patients ($n = 86$) were randomized to either choledochotomy ($n = 41$) or ERCP clearance ($n = 45$). There were five bile leaks in the choledochotomy group, and two eventually required ERCP and one patient required reoperation and cystic stump relegation ($p = .01$). There were no differences in postoperative pancreatitis, morbidity, or hospital length of stay. In the ERCP group, two patients required re-operation and 2 patients required transfusion due to gastrointestinal (GI) bleeding. This study demonstrates that the majority of stones that are identified can be extracted transcystically, and those patients failing extraction can have either choledochotomy or postoperative ERCP.

Rhodes et al. assessed retention of common bile duct stones over a 2-year period. Preoperative ERCP was avoided unless the patient had acute cholangitis or severe pancreatitis. A total of 480 patients with symptomatic gallstones were treated, and 427 (89%) had a preoperative cholangiogram where 80 (17% of the total number of patients) were found to have stones in the common bile duct. Patients were randomized to either have laparoscopic exploration of the common bile duct or postoperative ERCP. In the group randomized to the laparoscopic exploration ($n = 40$) with stones less than 9 mm the transcystic approach was attempted first ($n = 28$) and five patients required additional intervention such as a postoperative ERCP. In stones greater than 9 mm, choledochotomy was performed ($n = 12$). In the ERCP group ($n = 40$) ERCP cleared the stone after the first attempt in 30 patients, an additional five cleared after the second attempt, and two more after the third attempt. Although the results are similar, the authors note that the hospital stay was much shorter for those in the laparoscopic exploration of the common bile duct group.

Enochsson et al. assessed the effectiveness of intraoperative ERCP for those with positive IOC. These authors have developed a strong working relationship with the endoscopists, and have developed a system to ensure the endoscopists are available during the surgery. Intraoperative cholangiograms were performed in 87.8% of patients, and in 5.7% it was immediately followed by an intraoperative ERCP. When a common bile duct stone was identified, most were treated by sphincterotomy (91.1%) with stone removal or a stent was placed. There was no difference in length of hospitalization versus cholecystectomy alone.

## Evidence Against Routine Intraoperative Cholangiogram

More recently, even the IOC has been criticized as a routine tool because of the relative infrequency of common bile duct stones being found along with a high false-positive rate, resulting in unnecessary treatment and risk from the common bile duct exploration.

Bennion et al. retrospectively analyzed the medical records of 200 patients who were diagnosed and treated for acute gallstone pancreatitis; 163 patients had a laparoscopic cholecystectomy and 59 (29.5%) had IOC, with abnormalities detected only in nine (15.5%) of these patients (one was ultimately found to be a false positive). The other 141 (70.5%) patients did not have IOC, 30 of which had a preoperative ERCP. Of the remaining 111 patients, only three underwent ERCP for retained stones. Following discharge, seven patients in the no-IOC group returned for persistent symptoms, all receiving postoperative ERCP, and stones were found in only one patient. Of those who had IOC, five patients had a postoperative ERCP with known stones found in two patients and retained stones in one patient. One patient in the IOC group returned postoperatively for persistent symptoms, had an ERCP with no stones found. In short, only 11 (6.6%) of patients who did not have a preoperative ERCP were found to have common bile duct stones. In this study, IOC did not alter the likelihood of retained stones.

Korman et al. reviewed records of 343 patients who had a laparoscopic cholecystectomy; 42 patients had a preoperative ERCP (based on common bile duct dilatation on ultrasound and enzyme abnormalities), with 27 patients (64%) having common bile duct stones. Intraoperative cholangiogram was performed for 101 patients; 95 were negative, and six were positive, yet three of the six were actually found to be false positives on postoperative ERCP. These studies similarly suggest that routine IOC may not be necessary.

A final option for patients who do not show high serum bilirubin value, severe cholangitis, and a common bile duct dilatation yet the practitioner has a high index of suspicion that the patient may have a retained common bile duct stone is to perform noninvasive biliary imaging such as magnetic resonance cholangiopancreatography (MRCP) or endoscopic ultrasound. These modalities can help determine which patients would be most likely to benefit from ERCP. An MRCP can be highly accurate for the diagnosis of choledocholithiasis, but may not be when detecting small stones. Endoscopic ultrasound (EUS) has a positive predictive value of 91% to 100% and a negative predictive value of 93% to 100% with a sensitivity and specificity of 95%. Both modalities are accurate and can help guide conversion to ERCP. According to the National Institutes of Health, ERCP, MRCP, and endoscopic ultrasonography have comparable sensitivity and specificity in the diagnosis of choledocholithiasis.

In summary, preoperative ERCP is warranted in the case of abnormal liver enzymes such as high serum bilirubin, severe cholangitis, and common bile duct dilatation on ultrasound. Intraoperative cholangiogram can be performed on the remaining patients with the understanding that very few common bile duct stones will be found. If common bile duct stones are found, they can be treated by clearance via the transcystic duct if less than 9 mm, choledochotomy for larger stones, intraoperative ERCP, or postoperative ERCP. If the patient is monitored carefully, one can choose not to do the IOP and only selectively perform ERCP in patients who return with persistent symptoms. Health care practitioners can also utilize other noninvasive imaging modalities such as MRCP and EUS to determine who would benefit from ERCP.

# References

Bennion RS, Wyatt LE, Thompson JJE. Effect of intraoperative cholangiography during cholecystectomy on outcome after gallstone pancreatitis. J Gastrointest Surg 2002;6:575–581.

Chang L, et al. Preoperative versus postoperative endoscopic retrograde cholangiopancreatography in mild to moderate gallstone pancreatitis. A prospective randomized trial. Ann Surg 2000;231(1):82–87.

Enochsson L, Lindberg B, Swahn F, Arnelo U. Intraoperative endoscopic retrograde cholangiopancreatography (ERCP) to remove common bile duct stones during routine laparoscopic cholecystectomy does not prolong hospitalization: a 2-year experience. Surg Endosc 2004;18(3):367–371.

Korman J, et al. The role of endoscopic retrograde cholangiopancreatography and cholangiography in the laparoscopic era. Ann Surg 1996;223(2):212–216.

Macadam RCA, Goodall RJR. Long-term symptoms following endoscopic sphincterotomy for common bile duct stones. Surg Endosc 2004;18(3):363–366.

Mayumi T, Takada T, Kawarada Y, et al. Management strategy for acute pancreatitis in the JPN Guidelines. J Hepatobiliary Pancreat Surg 2006;13:1–67.

Nathanson LK, et al. Postoperative ERCP versus laparoscopic choledochotomy for clearance of selected bile duct calculi. Ann Surg 2005;242(2):188–192.

Petelin JB. Laparoscopic common bile duct exploration. Surg Endosc 2003;17:1705–1715.

Poulose BK, Arbogast PG, Holzman MD. National analysis of in-hospital resource utilization in choledocholithiasis management using propensity scores. Surg Endosc 2006;20(2):186–190.

Rhodes M, et al. Randomised trial of laparoscopic exploration of common bile duct versus postoperative endoscopic retrograde cholangiography for common bile duct stones. Lancet 1998;351:159–161.

Sekimoto M, et al. JPN guidelines for the management of acute pancreatitis: epidemiology, etiology, natural history, and outcome predictors in acute pancreatitis. J Hepatobiliary Pancreat Surg 2006;13:10–24.

# Suggested Readings

Heider TR, et al. Endoscopic sphincterotomy permits interval laparoscopic cholecystectomy in patients with moderately severe gallstone pancreatitis. J Gastrointest Surg 2006;10:1–5.

Hong DF, Xin Y, Chen DW. Comparison of laparoscopic cholecystectomy combined with intraoperative endoscopic sphincterotomy and laparoscopic exploration of the common bile duct for cholecystocholedocholithiasis. Surg Endosc 2006;20:424–427.

Jones DB, Maithel SK, Schneider BE. Atlas of Minimally Invasive Surgery. Woodbury, CT: Cine-Med, 2006.

Kimura Y, et al. JPN guidelines for the management of acute pancreatitis: treatment of gallstone-induced acute pancreatitis. J Hepatobiliary Pancreat Surg 2006;13:p. 56–60.

Lee S, Ko C. Gallstones. In: Yamada T, et al. Textbook of Gastroenterology, 4th ed. Lippincott, Williams & Wilkins; Philadelphia, PA. 2003:2177–2200.

NIH state-of-the-science statement on endoscopic retrograde cholangiopancreatography (ERCP) for diagnosis and therapy. NIH Consens State Sci Statements 2002;19(1):1–26.

Riela A, Zinsmeister AR, Melton LJ, DiMagno EP. Etiology, incidence, and survival of acute pancreatitis in Olmsted County, Minnesota. Gastroenterology 1991;100:A296.

Romagnuolo J, Currie G. Noninvasive vs. selective invasive biliary imaging for acute biliary pancreatitis: an economic evaluation by using decision tree analysis. Gastrointest Endosc 2005;61:86–97.

Tenner S, Dubner H, Steinberg W. Predicting gallstone pancreatitis with laboratory parameters: a meta-analysis. Am J Gastroenterol 1994;89(10):1863–1866.

Topazian M, Gorelick F. Acute pancreatitis. In: Yamada T, et al. Textbook of Gastroenterology, 4th ed. Lippincott, Williams & Wilkins; Philadelphia, PA. 2003:2026–2061.

UK Guidelines for the management of acute pancreatitis. Gut 2005;54:1–9.

Urbach DR, Khajanchee YS, Jobe BA, Standage BA, Hansen PD, Swanstrom LL. Cost-effective management of common bile duct stones: A decision analysis of the use of endoscopic retrograde cholangiopancreatography (ERCP), intraoperative cholangiography, and laparoscopic common bile duct exploration. Surg Endosc 2001;15(1):4–13.

West DM, Adrales GL, Schwartz RW. Current diagnosis and management of gallstone pancreatitis. Curr Surg 2002;59(3):296–298.

# 6. Cholelithiasis with Choledocholithiasis

## A. Introduction

Stones in the common duct complicate minimal access management of cholelithiasis. Before the laparoscopic era, open common duct exploration at the time of cholecystectomy was the procedure of choice. In the current era, common duct stones may be managed endoscopically (by endoscopic retrograde cholangiopancreatography [ERCP]) or laparoscopically; ERCP management can occur before, after, or even during laparoscopic cholecystectomy. This chapter explores several alternatives and preferences. A slightly different scenario was discussed in Chapter 5, which discussed gallstone pancreatitis.

## B. Case

*Samuel M. Maurice*

A 50-year-old woman came to the emergency department with severe right upper quadrant pain of 10 hours' duration. She characterized the pain as dull and nonradiating. It awakened her from sleep and had steadily increased in intensity. There were no alleviating or aggravating factors. She had not had any fever, chills, nausea, or vomiting. She had not had any change in her bowel habits.

Her past medical history was significant for bipolar disorder, hypertension, and hypothyroidism, all well controlled with medication. She had not had any previous surgery. She has smoked half a pack of cigarettes per day for 30 years. She does not consume alcoholic beverages.

On physical examination, her temperature was 36.2 °C, respiratory rate 22, blood pressure 167/92, and pulse 94. Her height was 5 feet 5 inches, and she weighed 96 kg. She was not visibly jaundiced. Her abdomen was soft without scars or masses. She had tenderness to deep palpation in the right upper quadrant, with mild voluntary guarding. Bowel sounds were normal. She did not have a Murphy's sign. Rectal examination was normal.

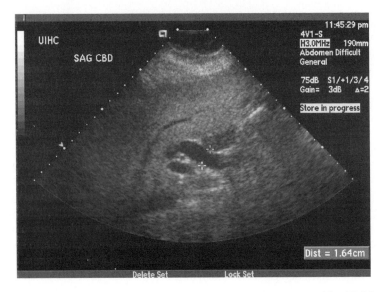

Fig. 6.1. Ultrasound showing dilated common duct. A stone was identified in the distal common duct.

Laboratory examination was significant for a white cell count of 10.2. Total bilirubin was 2.1 with direct bilirubin of 0.9. Alkaline phosphatase was 141, aspartate aminotransferase (AST) 38, alanine aminotransferase (ALT) 66, and γ-glutamyltransferase (GGT) 418. Her amylase and lipase were normal.

Ultrasound of the right upper quadrant revealed four mobile gallstones in the gallbladder without evidence of acute cholecystitis. The gallbladder wall was not thickened. There was no pericholecystic fluid. Negative sonographic Murphy's sign. A stone was identified in a grossly dilated common duct, measuring 16 mm (Fig. 6.1).

**How would you proceed in this patient with both cholelithiasis and choledocholithiasis?**

# C. Laparoscopic Cholecystectomy and Common Duct Exploration

*Shishir K. Maithel and Benjamin E. Schneider*

We advocate combined laparoscopic cholecystectomy with laparoscopic common bile duct exploration (LCBDE) over other options for two primary reasons: (1) direct benefits to the patient, and (2) efficient utilization of hospital resources.

In terms of direct patient benefits, an LCBDE is performed under the same anesthesia as laparoscopic cholecystectomy. Thus, in contrast to pre- or postoperative ERCP, the patient is spared a second intervention that requires conscious sedation, and occasionally requires general anesthesia. Furthermore, the patient is not subjected to the inherent risks that accompany ERCP, such as bowel perforation, post-ERCP pancreatitis, cholangitis, bleeding after sphincterotomy, and bacteremia or septicemia. If a surgeon is skilled in LCBDE, the definitive diagnosis of choledocholithiasis can be made in the operating room and managed in the same setting. This potentially reduces the hospital stay and allows the patient to return to daily activities and occupation faster.

Laparoscopic common bile duct exploration and ERCP have been compared in terms of resource utilization in numerous studies. Poulose et al. recently reported on nearly 41,000 patients who were identified in the 2002 U.S. National Inpatient Sample who underwent laparoscopic cholecystectomy but who also had choledocholithiasis. Ninety-three percent of these patients underwent ERCP to clear their common bile duct, while only 7% underwent LCBDE at the time of cholecystectomy. The total in-hospital charges and length of stay were significantly lower for the LCBDE group. Mean hospital charges and length of stay were almost $5000 and one full day less, respectively, for the LCBDE group.

Similar findings are reported by Urbach et al. after conducting an extensive decision analysis of four treatment strategies for choledocholithiasis in terms of their cost-effectiveness and ability to avoid retained common bile duct stones: (1) routine preoperative ERCP, (2) selective LCBDE, (3) selective postoperative ERCP, and (4) expectant management. Selective LCBDE was more cost-effective and slightly better at preventing residual choledocholithiasis compared to selective postoperative ERCP. Selective LCBDE added less than $500 to hospital costs compared to laparoscopic cholecystectomy alone. While routine preoperative ERCP is very effective in preventing residual common bile duct stones, its poor cost-effectiveness was prohibitive. Furthermore, this strategy would subject many patients to an unnecessary invasive procedure. Expectant management is not recommended due to the potential of highly morbid complications that may result from untreated choledocholithiasis.

One may argue that intraoperative ERCP accomplishes common bile duct clearance at the time of cholecystectomy with the same success and cost-efficiency as LCBDE. In fact, several studies have demonstrated that there is no difference between these two treatment strategies in terms of surgical time, success rate, number of stone extractions, postoperative complications, retained common bile duct stones, postoperative length of stay, and hospital charges. We firmly believe that difficulty with scheduling logistics would prohibit adoption of this treatment strategy as a routine practice. Lacking significant numbers of surgeons skilled in both laparoscopy and ERCP, intraoperative ERCP would require synchronization of the gastroenterologist and surgeon's schedules, a feat that we are sure would be nearly impossible to achieve on a regular basis.

The long-term effects of each treatment option must also be considered. There is a growing suspicion that patients who undergo ERCP with sphincterotomy may have more frequent complications with cholangitis over the long-term. Macadam and Goodall reported that nearly 20% of patients who had previously undergone sphincterotomy had symptoms suggestive of cholangitis. Furthermore, the potential consequences of free duodenobiliary reflux after sphincterotomy that results in bactibilia has been shown to lead to mild portal tract inflammation on liver biopsy.

Thus, it seems clear that LCBDE is the most viable option for treating choledocholithiasis, both in terms of direct patient benefits, as well as efficient utilization of limited health care resources. However, as with any invasive procedure, there is a technical learning curve that must be mastered in order to provide the best care to patients. Laparoscopic common bile duct exploration can be accomplished through a transcystic approach or directly via a choledochotomy, the latter of which is technically more challenging. The following are some technical pearls that may increase one's success in performing LCBDE. Additional information on these techniques in found in the SAGES manuals.

## Transcystic Approach

1. It is often best to incise the cystic duct via the same port through which the cholangiogram catheter will be introduced in order to facilitate a simpler introduction of the catheter by optimizing the angle of incision.
2. Intravenous administration of 1.0 mg of glucagon can sometimes further facilitate stone clearance with simple saline flushes by relaxing the sphincter of Oddi.
3. When using a Fogarty balloon catheter to retrieve stones, it is important to prevent stones from traveling proximally into the common hepatic duct, a situation that may require performing a choledochotomy or a postoperative ERCP.
4. A larger 5-French catheter should be used to perform a transcystic cholangiogram if transcystic choledochoscopy is planned to facilitate passage of the choledochoscope into the common

bile duct. Furthermore, the cystic duct can be dilated by passing an 8F balloon angioplasty catheter over a guidewire and inflating the balloon to 6 atmospheres of pressure for 5 minutes.

## *Choledochotomy*

1. Indications for making a choledochotomy include an extremely short cystic duct, distal insertion of the cystic duct into the common bile duct, multiple large stones that cannot be extracted via the transcystic approach, and proximal stones in the common hepatic duct.
2. Avoid choledochotomy in situations where the common bile duct measures less than 8 mm in diameter or is surrounded by significant inflammation. In this case, a postoperative ERCP may be the better treatment strategy.
3. Make the choledochotomy incision along the right anterolateral surface, just distal to the insertion of the cystic duct, for a length of approximately 5 to 6 mm.
4. Consider placing a T-tube in the common bile duct in order to minimize postoperative strictures.
5. Place a closed suction drain in the operative field.

Laparoscopic common bile duct exploration is definitely underutilized by surgeons, despite its clear benefits to patients and its more efficient use of hospital resources. One reason for this may be the lack of technical abilities or know-how of many general surgeons who routinely perform laparoscopic cholecystectomies. The widespread use of laparoscopic surgical simulation as a teaching tool may help to narrow this technical gap and make LCBDE a readily available treatment strategy to patients.

# D. Laparoscopic Cholecystectomy with Intraoperative Endoscopic Retrograde Cholangiopancreatography

## *John Morgan Cosgrove*

The time for combined laparoscopic cholecystectomy (LC) and intraoperative ERCP and endoscopic sphincterotomy (IERCP + ES) has arrived. The advantages are many and the disadvantages are few. The most tangible benefit is that the patient has "one-stop shopping." Any of us who have had to deal with hospitalization and all the attendant problems can appreciate that. The patient avoids the extra anesthesia induction with its own risks and disadvantages. Often the hospital stay is consolidated. Most importantly, the added intraoperative procedure, performed by a skilled endoscopist, adds minimal or no morbidity.

Kalimi, Cosgrove et al. reported on their experience with combined LC and IERCP + ES in 29 patients. Stones were successfully retrieved in 20 of 21 patients (95%). There was no mortality and minimal morbidity. The mean time for combined procedure was 173 minutes. In our last 10 patients the average time has been 126 minutes. The one "failure" was a patient with a past history of Billroth II gastrojejunostomy. The unsuccessful IERCP was followed by conversion to an open common bile duct exploration (CBDE) with successful stone extraction.

The options for management of choledocholithiasis in the minimally invasive era are preoperative ERCP + ES followed by LC, laparoscopic transcystic with common bile duct cannulation, laparoscopic CBDE, or postoperative ERCP + ES. Postoperative ERCP + ES carries the risk, albeit low, of failure and need for return to the operating room. Nakajima et al. report a 5% failure rate of postoperative endoscopic therapy. The problem with a liberal preoperative ERCP policy is a high rate of negative procedures. Liu, Lai, et al. reported that 10% of patients with elevated liver function tests (LFTs) had no common bile duct stones. The attendant complications of bleeding, pancreatitis and stricture invariably multiply.

Due to the poor predictive value of LFTs we recommend performance of a transcystic cholangiogram in questionable cases before making the decision to perform IERCP. The performance of "routine" ERCP for elevated LFTs would result in an unnecessary complication rate estimated at 4% and a 0.58% mortality.

Saccomani et al. report on IERCP + ES with a rendezvous technique. This is based on passing a guidewire transcystically through the ampulla of Vater so that the endoscopist can be guided in performance of a sphincterotomy. We feel this is an unnecessary step and have not had to resort to it. Having a "seasoned" endoscopist has made the rendezvous technique unnecessary in our institution. The rendezvous technique is proposed to avoid papillary edema and pancreatitis. However, we have not experienced any clinical pancreatitis in our series. Transient hyperamylasemia was seen in only two patients.

In our system of combining LC and IERCP we simply complete our cholecystectomy, close the trocar incisions, and "scrub out" (Table 6.1). The gastroenterologist then sets up his equipment and performs an ERCP

Table 6.1. Algorithms for suspected choledocholithiasis.

Cholelithiasis (normal LFTs) → Laparoscopic cholecystectomy (LC)
Cholelithiasis (abnormal LFTs) → LC with intraoperative cholangiogram
    (IOC), followed by IERCP + ES if IOC is positive
Cholelithiasis (jaundice/cholangitis) → LC with IERCP + ES (no IOC)

ES, endoscopic sphincterotomy; IERCP, intraoperative endoscopic retrograde cholangio-pancreatography; LFT, liver function test.

+ ES. We remove the operative field equipment and our video tower to prevent clutter. Furthermore, we avoid the distorted laparoscopic view that results from endoscopic air insufflation. Our first case was done after ERCP and we found that the pneumoperitoneum was compromised due to small bowel distention. Since then we have always performed the LC first. In our opinion ERCP insufflates the gastrointestinal tract too much to perform safe laparoscopic surgery.

The literature describes transcystic common bile duct clearance with a biliary Fogarty catheter. Large stones (>1 cm) cannot be removed or cleared from the common bile duct this way. We have shown that large stones can be cleared safely with IERCP + ES. Also, direct laparoscopic common bile duct exploration (essentially a "cutdown") is more a theoretic than real possibility. Inflammation and distorted anatomy conspire against keeping the procedure simple and safe.

Preoperative ERCP + ES followed by LC has a couple of limitations. It requires two anesthetic inductions and the added inconvenience of a second procedure. Also, a negative ERCP does not guarantee the absence of stone migration in the interval between ERCP and LC. Aliperti et al. recommends the performance of laparoscopic cholecystectomy within 1 day of preoperative ERCP. Anecdotally, in our limited experience with this approach we have performed LC after ERCP on the same day and have not seen any pancreatitis or "retained" stones.

Patients with a resolving gallstone pancreatitis may benefit from magnetic resonance cholangiopancreatography (MRCP). Hallal et al. proposed its use in moderate/mild resolving gallstone pancreatitis. However, in two of 29 cases the MRCP was falsely positive. There were no false- negative results.

Our approach has been to do routine intraoperative cholangiogram (IOC) in all patients with gallstone pancreatitis. We feel that MRCP may miss some small stones (Table 6.2). However, it may help delineate anatomy as well as providing reassurance in backing out of difficult transcystic cannulations. We have the endoscopist on standby, and if

Table 6.2. Algorithm for gallstone pancreatitis.

| |
|---|
| Gallstone pancreatitis with resolution of LFTs → LC + IOC if IOC, then IERCP + ES |

Table 6.3. Algorithm for prior foregut reconstruction and abnormal LFTs.

| |
|---|
| Magnetic resonance cholangiopancreatography (MRCP) negative → LC ± IOC MRCP positive → LC with IOC; if IOC positive, transcystic cannulation/ manipulation, possible open common bile duct exploration (CBDE) |

the IOC is positive, an IERCP + ES will be performed. Even in cases of cholangitis we have found that fluid resuscitation and intravenous antibiotics followed by LC and IERCP + ES is the most rewarding. Finally in cases where there has been foregut reconstruction, MRCP may be helpful (Table 6.3). The caveat is that small stones may be missed.

In summary, our experience with combined laparoscopic cholecystectomy and intraoperative ERCP has been favorable, and we would advocate its use in this situation.

# E. Endoscopic Retrograde Cholangiopancreatography Followed by Laparoscopic Cholecystectomy

## James K. Fullerton and Gary C. Vitale

This is a common clinical scenario faced by most general surgeons. In patients with symptomatic cholelithiasis the incidence of common bile duct stones is estimated to be between 10% and 20%. Open cholecystectomy and CBDE had been the treatment of choice for symptomatic cholelithiasis and choledocholithiasis with little debate since the first gallstone was surgically removed by way of the common bile duct in 1890. With the advancement of minimally invasive approaches such as ERCP, ES, and LC, management has changed dramatically over the last few decades. An ERCP with ES became the main treatment option for suspected choledocholithiasis, once laparoscopic cholecystectomy was accepted as the standard for treating symptomatic cholelithiasis. Very few patients now require an open common bile duct exploration. More recently surgeons have described laparoscopic CBDE in the treatment of choledocholithiasis at the time of cholecystectomy. This technique has some potential advantages but has only been mastered in a few medical centers. Although these advanced minimally invasive approaches have provided more options in the treatment of bile duct stones, they have provoked much controversy on what is the optimal perioperative management of choledocholithiasis.

## Management

There are now many ways to address the clinical scenario of choledocholithiasis. The options are pre/postoperative ERCP with cholecystectomy (laparoscopic or open), laparoscopic cholecystectomy with laparoscopic CBDE, open cholecystectomy with CBDE, ERCP and no cholecystectomy, and percutaneous transhepatic cholangiography. The optimal treatment approach likely varies from patient to patient, depending on the local availability of certain modalities and the expertise of the endoscopist, radiologist, and surgeon.

In the presented case scenario, the 50-year-old woman has symptoms consistent with symptomatic cholelithiasis and suspected choledocholithiasis. The ultrasound revealed multiple gallstones, a 16-mm dilated common bile duct, and a stone visible in the distal bile duct. Preoperative variables that predict common bile duct stones include an imaging study demonstrating a stone within the common bile duct, a dilated common bile duct, increasing liver enzymes, and severe acute biliary pancreatitis. When there is a high likelihood of a therapeutic ERCP, we feel ERCP preoperatively provides a safe and established management strategy in a busy endoscopy center. If the ERCP is successful, it eliminates a potential need for common bile duct exploration or a second trip to the operating room in the case of a failed postcholecystectomy ERCP.

## Endoscopic Retrograde Cholangiopancreatography Technique and Interventions

The patient with suspected choledocholithiasis is first hydrated, a coagulation profile documented, and antibiotics started. A dedicated ERCP suite with fluoroscopy is beneficial, along with an experienced endoscopy team to increase the success rate of therapeutic ERCP. The patient is placed in the prone position and sedation is administered. A side-viewing duodenoscope is used and passed down the oropharynx into the stomach. The scope is then passed through the pylorus and the ampulla is identified.

The common bile is selectively cannulated with either an opacifying cannula or guidewire technique. The bile duct is opacified after deep cannulation, and any filling defects or strictures are noted. If an ES is likely, we often cannulate initially with a sphincterotome and guidewire. Once the bile duct stone is identified on cholangiography, a sphincterotomy is performed. The sphincterotome is deeply cannulated and a wire is advanced up into the bile duct. The cutting wire of the sphincterotome is positioned in contact with the papilla at the 11 o'clock to 12 o'clock position and the wire is tightened slightly. Blended current is used to slowly cut through the sphincter. The sphincterotomy length is individualized but is usually 1 cm in length. Rarely, a precut sphincterotomy or percutaneous transhepatic cholangiography rendezvous sphincterotomy is needed to gain access to the bile duct for stone extraction. Endoscopic balloon dilatation prior to stone extraction is another alternative to ES especially in patients who are coagulopathic or have small stones.

Bile duct stones can be removed with multiple accessories. We typically use the Dormia wire basket first to retrieve stones (Figs. 6.2 and 6.3). The wire basket is advanced into the bile duct up past the stone under fluoroscopic guidance. It is best to start with the most distal bile duct stone encountered and remove stones separately. The basket is opened and then moved up and down near the stone to trap it between the wires. Once the stone is engaged, the basket is closed and pulled back through the ampulla. Sometimes the endoscope has to be angled with downward tip deflection and rotation to remove the stone. Stone extraction balloon catheters (8-, 12-, 15-mm diameters) can also be used to remove small stones. The balloon is advanced past the stone, inflated, and then withdrawn into the duodenum. After all the stones are thought to have been removed, a balloon occlusion cholangiogram is performed to document no residual stones. The balloon is inflated at the hepatic duct bifurcation, contrast is injected, and the balloon is slowly withdrawn. For larger stones (>15mm), mechanical lithotripsy is often needed to fracture and facilitate safe removal of large stones. We typically use the preassembled through-the-scope lithotripsy basket. After the stone is engaged in the wire basket, a metal sheath is advanced up to the basket. The wheel on the mechanical lithotripter is cranked until the stone is crushed by the wire basket. In cases were there are suspected retained stones, intrahepatic stones, or a difficult cannulation with an edematous ampulla, we have found it beneficial to place plastic biliary stents. This facilitates a repeat ERCP when the patient's condition has improved

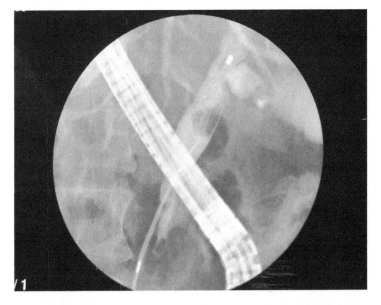

Fig. 6.2. Endoscopic retrograde cholangiopancreatography (ERCP) image showing Dormia basket engaging stone.

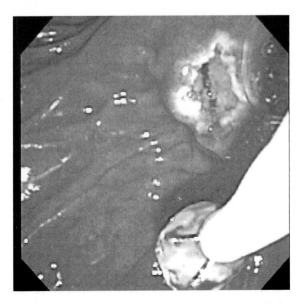

Fig. 6.3. Endoscopic photograph showing stone being extracted through papillotomy incision.

and the edema resolved. Also placing the patient on ursodeoxycholic acid during the period of stenting sometimes reduces the size of residual stones and increases the success rate of stone extraction. We have found that adjunct devices such as intraductal laser lithotripsy and extracorporeal shock-wave lithotripsy are rarely necessary, and their availability is limited. Laparoscopic or open common bile duct exploration should be utilized for definitive treatment if preoperative ERCP is unsuccessful in an experienced endoscopy center.

## Selection Criteria for Endoscopic Retrograde Cholangiopancreatography

Endoscopic retrograde cholangiopancreatography, with ES and stone extraction, has been shown to be highly effective in clearing the common bile duct of stones in >90% of cases. However, the rate of negative ERCPs in many studies has been high, exposing the patient to the risks of ERCP. In the study by Vitale et al., bile duct clearance by ERCP was successful in all cases. Elevated liver function tests and a dilated common bile duct visualized by ultrasound were the most accurate predictors of stones. The limitation of this study was that only 33% of preoperative ERCPs detected bile duct stones. Other studies have demonstrated approximately a 50% negative ERCP rate when different positive predictors are used for suspected choledocholithiasis. In the randomized trial by Cuschieri et al. comparing preoperative ERCP to laparoscopic CBDE, only 23% of patients had a normal cholangiogram on preoperative ERCP. In a more recent study by Hamy et al., bile duct stones were found in 86% of patients (268/310), with a duct clearance rate of 99% (256/258). The criteria used to select patients for preoperative ERCP were persistent jaundice, common bile duct larger than 8 mm on ultrasound, cholestasis (elevated alkaline phosphatase and glutamyl transpeptidase), or severe acute pancreatitis. There were five cases of mild pancreatitis caused by ES. This study demonstrates that with strict criteria, negative ERCP rates can be reduced.

Magnetic resonance cholangiopancreatography (MRCP) has emerged has a useful noninvasive diagnostic tool in reducing the rate of negative ERCPs and optimizing its therapeutic potential. Liu, Consorti, et al. categorized patients into groups based on their risk of harboring bile duct stones. Group 1 patients (cholelithiasis, common bile duct [CBD] >5 mm, elevated liver enzymes, and no evidence of cholecystitis or pancreatitis) underwent preoperative ERCP. Group 2 patients (cholelithiasis,

CBD >5 mm, elevated liver enzymes, with cholecystitis, pancreatitis, or apparent resolving choledocholithiasis) underwent MRCP prior to any intervention. When the MRCP demonstrated common bile duct stones, the patients underwent preoperative ERCP. However, if the MRCP was negative, laparoscopic cholecystectomy with cholangiogram was performed. In the very high risk group (group 1), 92.6% (25/27) were identified with CBD stones with an 88% clearance rate by ERCP. Group 2 had MRCP performed in all patients, with 32% (12/37) of patients having CBD stones on MRCP. Of the 12 patients with a positive MRCP, 11 had a positive ERCP. Only one of the patients with a negative MRCP had a bile duct stone on intraoperative cholangiogram. This algorithm resulted in the identification of CBD stones during preoperative ERCP in 92% of patients and unsuspected stones in only 1.4%. MRCP can be a very helpful diagnostic tool in patients with probable resolving choledocholithiasis (decreasing liver enzymes and improving pain) and can improve the rate of therapeutic ERCPs.

## Potential Complications

The most common complications from ERCP and ES include bleeding, perforation, pancreatitis, and cholangitis. The overall complication rate is approximately 10%, with a mortality of 0% to 1%. In the study by Freeman et al., the complication rate was lowest (4.9%) in patients undergoing bile duct stone removal within 30 days of laparoscopic cholecystectomy. In 1921 sphincterotomies reported by Cotton et al., the overall complication rate was 5.8%. There was no demonstrated increased risk in younger patients or in those with small bile ducts. Cuschieri et al. demonstrated no difference in the complication rates when comparing the ERCP/ES (12.8%) and laparoscopic CBDE (15.8%) groups. These studies demonstrate that ERCP with ES can be performed with minimal morbidity when performed for choledocholithiasis in experienced centers.

## Other Indications for Preoperative Endoscopic Retrograde Cholangiopancreatography

Cuschieri et al. demonstrated that preoperative ERCP with laparoscopic cholecystectomy and laparoscopic CBDE have similar success rates and morbidity in the treatment of choledocholithiasis. We believe the best management strategy for choledocholithiasis should rely on the local expertise and will vary between institutions. There are certain indications, however, when ERCP preoperatively has been shown to be advantageous. Urgent ERCP with ES decreases the morbidity and mortality associated with worsening gallstone pancreatitis. Cholangitis with increasing jaundice, fever, elevated white blood cell count (WBC), and worsening abdominal pain should also have prompt preoperative ERCP. Intrahepatic and very large common bile duct stones can be difficult to remove laparoscopically. If intrahepatic or large (>1.5 cm) stones are suspected by preoperative imaging, endoscopic clearance may be the best treatment choice.

The treatment of elderly patients who present with obstructive jaundice can raise further questions on what the appropriate management should be. If the patient is unfit for general anesthesia and considered a high surgical risk, then ERCP with ES is the best treatment option for suspected symptomatic choledocholithiasis. Leaving the gallbladder in situ after clearing the bile duct of stones is also a reasonable option, especially for patients with severe comorbidities. The elevation of liver enzymes in the elderly patient should also raise the suspicion for malignancy. Diagnostic evaluation with an MRCP, computed tomography (CT), and possible ERCP should be sought before surgery if there is any question of malignancy.

# F. Conclusions

*Samuel M. Maurice*

Prior to the advent of minimally invasive approaches, the treatment of choice for common bile duct stones was an open cholecystectomy with open common bile duct exploration. When ERCP was developed, it assumed a role in managing patients with a significant operative risk, such as those with multiple comorbidities, cholangitis, or pancreatitis. As laparoscopic cholecystectomy became standard management of symptomatic cholelithiasis, ERCP took on a greater role in managing common bile duct stones, even in the young and healthy, in hopes of avoiding laparotomy and open common bile duct explorations. With increasing advances and experience in laparoscopic techniques, laparoscopic approaches to managing choledocholithiasis have emerged. Numerous management approaches to choledocholithiasis have been validated in the literature, but there still is no consensus regarding optimal treatment.

In comparing laparoscopic and endoscopic management, four questions must be answered: (1) How high should one's suspicion of common bile duct stones be before one would consider preoperative ERCP? (2) How do endoscopic and laparoscopic approaches compare in terms of effectiveness, morbidity, and mortality? (3) Which method is most cost-effective? (4) Are the studies comparing these approaches applicable to all practices given the differing resources and experiences of local surgeons/endoscopists?

Both prospective (Nehaus et al.) and retrospective (Miller et al.) studies have shown that ERCP may be normal in up to 50% of patients with clinical or biochemical signs of choledocholithiasis. In hopes of avoiding negative ERCPs on the one hand and retained CBD stones on the other hand, attempts have been made to refine predictors of common bile duct stones. Miller et al. found that besides the presence of a CBD stone on ultrasound (which was 100% predictive), the next factor most predictive of CBD stones was a conjunction of abnormal LFTs and a dilated CBD (>8 mm), which predicted 82% of stones. Barr et al., in a model based on GGT and CBD diameter as positive predictors and amylase as a negative predictor, correctly classified 78% of patients with common bile duct stones. Hamy et al., using jaundice for >72 hours, CBD >8 mm on ultrasound, cholestasis, and acute biliary pancreatitis as selection criteria, increased the yield of ERCPs to 86%. All these strategies, however, lead to a rate of negative ERCPS that exceeds the 8% false-negative rate when ERCPs are performed after laparoscopic cholecystectomy with intraoperative cholangiogram.

An analysis of the efficacy, morbidity, and mortality of laparoscopic and endoscopic approaches is important in comparing the two techniques. Tranter and Thompson, in their review of the literature, reported similar rates of duct clearance with 75% to 96% success with ES and 75% to 98% with LCBDE. The morbidity of LC with ES, 3% to 16% (median 13%), was comparable to the 2% to 17% (median 8%) morbidity of LCBDE. The mortality rates of ES and LCBDE were also similar, 0% to 6% (median 1%) for ES and 0% to 5% (median 1%) for LCBDE.

Two randomized controlled trials compared endoscopic and laparoscopic techniques. The European Association of Endoscopic Surgery (EAES) study, a multicenter prospective randomized controlled trial restricted to American Society of Anesthesiologists (ASA) class I and II patients compared preoperative endoscopic retrograde cholangiography (ERC) and LC to LC with LCBDE. It found equivalent success rates (85% for LCBDE and 84% for ERC and ESE [endoscopic stone extraction]) and patient morbidity (15.8% for LCBDE vs. 12.8% for ERC and ESE) for the two management options. However, it also showed a significantly shorter hospital stay with the one-stage laparoscopic technique (9 days vs. 6 days). A randomized controlled trial by Rhodes compared LCBDE with LC and postoperative ERCP. It also found similar efficacy, with 75% clearance rates in both groups after the first intervention with comparable subsequent success rates of 100% in the laparoscopic group and 93% in the ERCP group. Subsequent treatments after initial failed attempts were predominantly ERCPs. Morbidity was similar, 17.5% for LCBDE and 15% for ERCP. The length of hospital stay, including readmissions, was significantly shorter in the laparoscopic group with a median stay of 1 day in the laparoscopic group and 3.5 days in the ERCP group.

Although there are many reports on early and intermediate results of ERCP/ES and LCBDE, there is little data on long-term complications. Uncontrolled retrospective and prospective reviews with mean follow-up times of 36 to 60 months have suggested no increased risk of stricture or late biliary complications after LCBDE. With ES, there is considerable concern over possible consequences of sphincter destruction with potential for recurrent stones and biliary cancer. Investigators have suggested that the reflux of digestive enzymes, pancreatic juices, and bacterial flora following destruction of the sphincter of Oddi could potentially promote carcinogenesis or recurrent bilirubinate stone formation. Tranter and Thompson reported recurrent bile duct stones following ERCP with ES in 2% to 16% of patients. These stones are almost universally of the bilirubinate type, making the reflux of bacterial flora through an incompetent sphincter a compelling explanation. Indeed, investigators who have cultured the biliary system after ES have found enteric organisms present.

Hakamada et al., in a retrospective review of 108 patients following transduodenal sphincteroplasty, found a 7.4% incidence of bile duct cancer a median of 18 years after the operation. This and other studies, however, are without controls. Karlson et al., in a population-based cohort study of 992 patients, found no increased risk of biliary cancer 9 to 10 years following ES compared to population controls. Until long-term prospective randomized controlled trials are conducted, this issue will remain a subject of debate.

Time and efficiency are also important. Many have criticized LCBDE for being an inefficient use of operative time. Certainly, the amount of time is operator- and institution-dependent. Berber et al., in a retrospective review, found that LCBDE added an average of only 17.5 minutes to a laparoscopic cholecystectomy but prolonged the anesthesia and setup time by approximately 62 minutes. As pointed out by Petelin in his review of more than 12 years of experience with LCBDE, efficient use of operating room time requires attention to operating room setup and readily available and appropriate equipment.

Heili et al., in a retrospective review of 913 patients, found that LCBDE was associated with a significantly shorter length of stay and a trend toward lower cost compared to ERCP/ES. Similarly, Liberman et al., in a smaller retrospective review of 76 patients, found that LCBDE resulted in a significantly shorter length of stay and lower cost. Urbach et al., using a decision-making model, found LCBDE more cost-effective than pre- or postoperative ERCP. Selective postoperative ERCP was more cost-effective than preoperative ERCP, unless the probability of CBD stones was greater than 80%.

Ultimately, the resources available and the experience of the practitioner dictate practice. The importance of experience with LCBDE was highlighted by Hawasli et al.'s retrospective study of LCBDEs. Success with LCBDE increased from 59% in the first 38 months of the study to 96% in the last 6 years of the study. Lack of an institutional commitment to purchasing and maintaining adequate equipment, inadequate laparoscopic training, and unavailability of a dedicated operating room team represent potential obstacles to performing LCBDE.

Laparoscopic common bile duct exploration exhibits comparable effectiveness, morbidity, and mortality to ERCP in the management of choledocholithiasis. In some centers, LCBDE appears to be more cost-effective than endoscopic means, but differing levels of experience, local resources, and institutional dedication to setup and maintenance of equipment presents obstacles to use in some settings. Preoperative ERCP may have a place when the probability of choledocholithiasis is high, but LCBDE or postoperative ERCP is preferential for most other cases.

# References

Aliperti G, Edmundowicz S, et al. Combined endoscopic sphincterotomy and laparoscopic cholecystectomy in patients with choledocholithiasis and cholecystolithiasis. Ann Intern Med 1991;15(10):783–784.

Barr LL, Frame BC, Coulanjon A. Proposed criteria for preoperative endoscopic retrograde cholangiography in candidates for laparoscopic cholecystectomy. Surg Endosc 1999;13:778–781.

Berber E, Engle KL, Garland A, et al. A critical analysis of intraoperative time utilization in laparoscopic cholecystectomy. Surg Endosc 2001;15:161–165.

Cotton PB, Geenan JE, Sherman S, et al. Endoscopic Sphincterotomy for stones by experts is safe, even in younger patients with normal ducts. Ann Surg 1998;227:201–204.

Cuschieri A, Lezoche E, Morino M, et al. E.A.E.S. multicenter prospective randomized trial comparing two-stage vs. single-stage management of patients with gallstone disease and ductal calculi. Surg Endosc 1999;13:952–957.

Freeman ML, Nelson DB, Sherman S, et al. Complications of endoscopic biliary sphincterotomy. N Engl J Med 1996;335:909–918.

Hakamada K, Sasaki M, Endoh M, Itoh T, Morita T, Konn M. Late development of bile duct cancer after sphincteroplasty: a ten- to twenty-two year follow-up study. Surgery 1997;121:488–492.

Hallal A, Amortegui J, Jeroukhimov I, et al. Magnetic resonance cholangiopancreatography accurately detects common bile duct stones in resolving gallstone pancreatitis. J Am Coll Surg 2005;200(6):869–875.

Hamy A, Hennekinne S, Pessaux P, et al. Endoscopic sphincterotomy prior to laparoscopic cholecystectomy for the treatment of cholelithiasis. Surg Endosc 2003;17:872–875.

Hawasli A, Lloyd L, Cacucci B, Management of choledocholithiasis in the era of laparoscopic surgery. Am Surg 2000;66(5):425–430.

Heili MJ, Wintz NK, Fowler DL. Choledocholithiasis: endoscopic versus laparoscopic management. Ann Surg 1999;65(2):135–138.

Hong DF, Xin Y, Chen DW. Comparison of laparoscopic cholecystectomy combined with intraoperative endoscopic sphincterotomy and laparoscopic exploration of the common bile duct for cholecystocholedocholithiasis. Surg Endosc 2006;20:424–427.

Jones DB, Maithel SK, Schneider BE. Atlas of Minimally Invasive Surgery. Woodbury, CT: Cine-Med, 2006.

Kalimi R, Cosgrove JM, Marini M, Gecelter G, Stark B, Cohen JR. Combined intraoperative and laparoscopic cholecystectomy and ERCP: Lessons learned from 29 cases. Surg Endosc 2000;14(3):232–234.

Karlson BM, Ekbom A, Arvidsson D, Yuen J, Krusemo UB. Population-based study of cancer risk and relative survival following sphincterotomy for stones in the common bile duct. Br J Surg 1997;84:1235–1238.

Liberman MA, Phillips EH, Carroll BL, Fallas MJ, Rosenthal R, Hiatt J. Cost-effective management of complicated choledocholithiasis: laparoscopic transcystic duct exploration or endoscopic sphincterotomy. J Am Coll Surg 1996;182:488–494.

Liu C, Lai E, et al. Combined laparoscopic and endoscopic approach in patients with cholelithiasis and choledocholithiasis. Surgery 1996;119(5):534–537.

Liu TH, Consorti ET, Kawashima A, et al. Patient evaluation and management with selective use of magnetic resonance cholangiography and endoscopic retrograde cholangiopancreatography before laparoscopic cholecystectomy. Ann Surg 2001;234:33–40.

Loperfido S, Angelini G, et al. Major early complications from diagnostic and therapeutic ERCP: a prospective multicenter trial. Gastrointest Endosc 1988;48(1):1–10.

Macadam RCA, Goodall RJR. Long-term symptoms following endoscopic sphincterotomy for common bile duct stones. Surg Endosc 2004;18(3):363–366.

Miller RE, Kimmelstiel FM, Winkler WP. Management of common bile duct stones in the era of laparoscopic cholecystectomy. Am J Surg 1995;169:273–276.

Nakajima H, Okubo H, Masuko Y. Intraoperative endoscopic sphincterotomy during laparoscopic cholecystectomy. Endoscopy 1996;28(2):264.

Nehaus H, Feussner H, Ungeheuer A, Hoffmann W, Siewert JR, Classen M. Prospective evaluation of the use of endoscopic retrograde cholangiography prior to laparoscopic cholecystectomy. Endoscopy 1992;24:745–749.

Petelin JB. Laparoscopic common bile duct exploration. Surg Endosc 2003;17:1705–1715.

Poulose BK, Arbogast PG, Holzman MD. National analysis of in-hospital resource utilization in choledocholithiasis management using propensity scores. Surg Endosc 2006;20(2):186–190.

Rhodes M, Sussman L, Cohen L, Lewis MP. Randomised trial of laparoscopic exploration of common bile duct versus postoperative endoscopic retrograde cholangiography for common bile duct stones. Lancet. 1998;351(9097):159–161.

Saccomani G, Durante V, Magnolia M, et al. Combined endoscopic treatment for cholelithiasis associated with choledocholithiasis. Surg Endosc 2005;19(7):910–914.

Tranter SE, Thompson MH. Comparison of endoscopic sphincterotomy and laparoscopic exploration of the common bile duct. Br J Surg 2002;89:1495–1504.

Urbach DR, Khajanchee YS, Jobe BA, Standage BA, Hansen PD, Swanstrom LL. Cost-effective management of common bile duct stones: a decision analysis of the use of endoscopic retrograde cholangiopancreatography (ERCP), intraoperative cholangiography, and laparoscopic common bile duct exploration. Surg Endosc 2001;15(1):4–13.

Vitale GC, Larson GM, Wieman TJ, Cheadle WG, Miller FB. The use of ERCP in the management of common bile duct stones in patients undergoing laparoscopic cholecystectomy. Surg Endosc 1993;7:9–11.

# Suggested Readings

Enochsson L, Lindberg B, Swahn F, Arnelo U. Intraoperative endoscopic retrograde cholangiopancreatography (ERCP) to remove common bile duct stones during routine laparoscopic cholecystectomy does not prolong hospitalization: a 2-year experience. Surg Endosc 2004;18(3):367–371.

Harris HW, Davis BR, Vitale GC. Cholecystectomy after endoscopic cholecystectomy for common bile duct stones: Is surgery necessary? Surg Innov 2005;12:187–194.

Lella F, Bagnolo F, Rebuffat C, et al. Use of the laparoscopic-endoscopic approach, the so-called "rendezvous" technique in cholecystocholedocholithiasis. Surg Endosc 2006;20:419–423.

Vitale GC, Rangnekar NJ, Hewlett SC. Advanced interventional endoscopy. Curr Probl Surg 2002;39:968–1053.

# 7. Choice of Approach for Laparoscopic Common Duct Exploration

## A. Introduction

When laparoscopic cholecystectomy is undertaken in the presence of known common duct stones, laparoscopic common duct exploration is generally part of the planned procedure. Chapters 5 and 6 explored alternatives in the management of choledocholithiasis, including the role of endoscopic retrograde cholangiopancreatography (ERCP). This chapter deals specifically with the relative merits of the transcystic duct approach versus laparoscopic choledochotomy (a procedure that more nearly mimics what was done during open surgery for this problem).

## B. Case

### Rachael Nicholson

A 35-year-old woman complained of pain in the epigastric region and right upper quadrant of the abdomen. The pain radiated to her back. It began 2 to 3 hours after eating a fatty meal. She had nausea, but no vomiting. She did not have diarrhea, constipation, fever, or chills. She had had several previous episodes, but none was as severe as the present one.

Her past medical and surgical history was remarkable only for three spontaneous vaginal deliveries of healthy term infants, and a laparoscopic bilateral tubal ligation. She was on no medications and had no known allergies. Her mother and sister had required surgery for gallbladder disease.

She was a married homemaker. She was a nonsmoker and drank one to two glasses of wine per month. The review of systems was negative, except as noted above.

Physical examination revealed a moderately obese woman, alert and oriented, in no acute distress. She was not visibly jaundiced. Her pulse was 85, temperature 36.5 °C, blood pressure 128/70, and body mass index (BMI) 30. Her mucosa were pink and dry. Her cardiopulmonary examination was normal.

Her abdomen was soft to palpation and not distended. There was tenderness to palpation in the right upper quadrant. There was no Murphy's sign, and no rebound tenderness. Bowel sounds were normal. Rectal examination was negative and stool was guaiac negative.

Laboratory examination was significant for a white cell count of 9500. Her total bilirubin was 2.2, direct bilirubin 1.8, γ-glutamyltransaminase was elevated at 260, lactic dehydrogenase elevated at 450, alkaline phosphatase was elevated at 146, aspartate aminotransferase (AST) and alanine aminotransferase (ALT) were normal, and amylase and lipase were normal.

Ultrasound of the right upper quadrant showed a gallbladder with normal wall thickness containing multiple stones, all mobile. There was no pericholecystic fluid. The common bile duct measured within normal limits and no filling defects were found in the common duct.

She was taken to the operating room for laparoscopic cholecystectomy and intraoperative cholangiogram (IOC). The IOC revealed a 5-mm stone within the common bile duct. The cystic duct measured 5 mm, and the common duct 6 mm. **How would you approach this stone? Via a transcystic duct approach, or by performing a laparoscopic choledochotomy?**

# C. Laparoscopic Common Bile Duct Exploration Via Transcystic Approach

*Teresa L. LaMasters and Sherry M. Wren*

Choledocholithiasis may be encountered at the time of laparoscopic cholecystectomy in up to 10% of younger patients and increases to over 25% in patients age 65 and older. Stones are often identified during intraoperative cholangiogram or ultrasonography of the common bile duct. Once a stone is identified, it can become a therapeutic dilemma. In the early years of laparoscopic cholecystectomy, most algorithms advocated preoperative ERCP for suspected common bile duct (CBD) stones or postoperative ERCP if stones were encountered unexpectedly intraoperatively (see also Chapter 6). The ERCP was not a risk-free solution since it has an 11% to 14% failure rate in CBD stone removal, a morbidity of 5% to 10%, and a mortality of 0.02% to 0.5%. Overall, 5% of patients get pancreatitis postprocedure. In addition, the economic cost of routine preoperative ERCP for suspected cases of CBD stones was excessive, since only one in four to five studies required intervention. Multiple investigators have demonstrated the safety and effectiveness of laparoscopic CBD exploration, which allows for the treatment of choledocholithiasis in one stage, avoiding the potential morbidity of ERCP, and reduces the inpatient length of stay.

Options for management of choledocholithiasis discovered intraoperatively include laparoscopic transcystic common bile duct exploration (TCBDE), laparoscopic common bile duct exploration via choledochotomy (LCBDE-C), open choledochotomy, and postoperative ERCP with or without sphincterotomy. The choice of a TCBDE versus LCBDE-C is based on patient and stone characteristics, ductal anatomy, and surgeon's expertise. In general, indications for an attempt at TCBDE are fewer than nine stones, stones located distal to the cystic duct–CBD junction, and stones <6mm in size. In contrast, those patients with intrahepatic stones, stones above the cystic duct–CBD junction, and CBD larger than 7mm may be better served by an LCBDE-C.

Overall, approximately 85% to 95% of patients can be managed successfully with a laparoscopic transcystic approach. The outcomes of these patients are similar to those undergoing simple laparoscopic cholecystectomy without a bile duct exploration. Multiple techniques may be utilized depending on patient characteristics, availability of equipment, and the surgeon's expertise. The techniques of transcystic stone extraction include lavage with saline, Fogarty balloon catheters or biliary baskets, and choledochoscopy with stone removal using wire baskets under direct vision. Antegrade sphincterotomy and lithotripsy techniques have been described and utilized successfully; however, these techniques are not widely used. The following are several common techniques of TCBDE, all of which are best performed using fluorocholangiography to guide therapy.

Once a filling defect consistent with a stone is identified, the operating room personnel should ready the additional needed equipment required to perform TCBDE. Ideally, this equipment would be packaged together and ready for immediate utilization (Table 7.1).

For CBD stones less than 4mm in diameter, one should first attempt to mechanically flush the stones from the duct using saline after administration of 1mg of glucagon intravenously. This relaxes the sphincter of Oddi to allow small stones to pass more easily. After waiting 3 to 4 minutes, the cystic duct catheter should be flushed with saline, and the fluorocholangiography repeated. If small stones remain in the duct

Table 7.1. Equipment required.

---

Flexible choledochoscope or ureteroscope with 1.2-mm working channel
Laparoscopic padded graspers for manipulation of choledochoscope
Second camera and light source for choledochoscope
Second video monitor or video mixer for picture in picture
Pressurized saline connection for working port of choledochoscope
5-French cholangiogram or ureteral catheter
0.035-inch flexible tipped hydrophilic guidewire (long >90 cm)
5-French angioplasty catheter with 8-mm balloon (optional)
12-French abdominal wall introducer sheath (optional)
Additional 5-mm port with 3-mm inner cannula
Fluoroscope (C-arm)
Glucagon, 1 to 2 mg to be given by anesthetist
Fogarty catheters 4-French
Dormia or Segura type wire baskets for stone retrieval
Absorbable suture 4–0 or 5–0 size for closure of common duct if needed
T-tube 14-French

---

(<3 mm in size), but there is free flow of contrast into the duodenum, a decision to observe these stones may be considered, as the majority of small stones will pass spontaneously into the duodenum (Tranter and Thompson, Watson et al.).

For stones that are too large to clear by simple flushing, the next step may then be removal utilizing a Fogarty balloon catheter. A 4-French Fogarty can be inserted transcystically beyond the stones, inflated, and withdrawn. Stones can then be retrieved from the abdomen after falling out of the cystic duct. Alternatively, a stone retrieval basket may be inserted under fluoroscopic guidance and used to retrieve or crush the stone. This basket can be slowly closed and withdrawn with the stone, and any fragments can be flushed through the duct. Completion cholangiogram must be performed following either method.

Another approach is to introduce the choledochoscope through the cystic duct. This approach allows for stone removal with a basket under direct vision and can be very successful. It does, however, require additional equipment including a second light source, camera, and monitor or preferably a video splitter to view both the choledochoscope and laparoscope images on the same monitor (Table 7.1). Placement of a fifth port along the right subcostal margin can facilitate the exploration and passage of the choledochoscope while the other ports may continue to be utilized for retraction and manipulation. If a standard 5-mm port is used, a 3-mm inner cannula also should be used to protect the choledocho-scope from breaking while being passed though the valve. Alternatively, a 12F sheath may be inserted percutaneously for this purpose. It can be necessary at times to dilate the cystic duct to allow the choledochoscope to be placed. This can be done with an 8-mm angioplasty balloon or a biliary Fogarty as a less expensive alternative.

A 3-mm choledochoscope or ureteroscope can then be introduced over a guidewire placed through the cholangiogram catheter or directly into the cystic duct. Extra care should be taken in the manipulation of the scope to prevent damage to the fragile optic fibers, and padded graspers should be utilized if possible. Pressurized saline is then connected to the working side port of the choledochoscope to allow adequate visualiza-tion of the stones. A watertight valve is required on the working port to prevent leakage of saline during passage of guidewires and baskets.

When a stone is encountered, a wire retrieval basket is passed through the working port. Under direct vision the stone is grasped and pulled back against the scope. The entire assembly is then removed as one unit. The stone is released into the abdomen in a convenient location in order to retrieve at the end of the procedure. If a stone is impacted at the ampulla or cannot be removed with a basket, attempts may be made to gently push the stone into the duodenum using the tip of the choledochoscope. A completion cholangiogram should then be performed with subsequent ligation of the cystic duct. If stones are encountered in the hepatic ducts or proximal to the cystic–common duct junction, retrieval may be more difficult. Occasionally the endoscope can be angled into the upper tract, which may be facilitated by extending the dissection of the cystic duct near the common duct junction; however, this is often difficult. This sce-nario usually requires choledochotomy for further exploration or referral for postoperative ERCP.

For the patient presented in this case, with a small single stone, transcystic exploration would be the simplest alternative and does not require incision onto the duct or closure over a T-tube. Table 7.2 outlines general characteristics of clinical scenarios appropriate for each of the two techniques.

Situations in which an LCBDE-C should be considered include mul-tiple stones (more than nine), stones >10 mm, small cystic duct, CBD larger than 6 mm, and proximally located stones. This approach is safe and highly successful. It allows treatment of the stones without an additional procedure and decreased hospital stay in comparison with ERCP. This approach does, however, require advanced endoscopic and laparoscopic skills including intracorporeal laparoscopic suturing. A T-tube

Table 7.2. Characteristics of transcystic common bile duct exploration (TCBDE) versus laparoscopic common bile duct exploration via choledochotomy (LCBDE-C).

| |
|---|
| Transcystic approach—appropriate for the majority of patients and surgeons |
|     Fewer than 9 stones |
|     Stone diameter <6 mm |
|     Cystic duct >4 mm |
|     Diameter of CBD <6 mm |
|     Marked inflammation |
|     Surgeon with little experience in laparoscopic suturing |
| Choledochotomy approach |
|     Multiple stone >9 |
|     Stone diameter >6 mm |
|     Intrahepatic stones |
|     Cystic duct <4 mm diameter |
|     Distal or posterior cystic duct entrance |
|     Surgeon with expertise in laparoscopic suturing |

for biliary drainage with its inherent morbidity is also required in the majority of cases.

Treatment of choledocholithiasis via a transcystic approach is successful when combined with laparoscopic choledochotomy in the appropriate clinical scenario as a one-stage treatment in 95% of patients. A one-stage technique also contributes to a decreased hospital stay compared with cholecystectomy and staged ERCP. When laparoscopic techniques are unsuccessful in clearing the duct of stones, a transcystic catheter may be left in place to facilitate postoperative ERCP, improving the probability that the ampulla will be able to be cannulated. Postoperative ERCP remains an important adjunct in the small percentage of patients unable to be treated with laparoscopic techniques. The use of ERCP selectively avoids subjecting the vast majority of patients to the potentially long-term risks incurred with this procedure.

In summary, the laparoscopic transcystic CBD exploration should be the preferred approach to treatment of choledocholithiasis discovered intraoperatively. It is safe and effective, sparing the patient the risk of incision directly on the CBD with a need for T-tube drainage or an endoscopic procedure that could lead to morbidities such as pancreatitis, recurrent stones, or stricture. The skills required should be a part of every laparoscopic surgeon's armamentarium.

# D. Laparoscopic Common Bile Duct Exploration Via Choledochotomy

*Tony Kelly and Muhammed Ashraf Memon*

Our preference would be to perform one-stage laparoscopic chole-cystectomy (LC) and LCBDE. This can be achieved safely and expeditiously if the surgeon is experienced in advanced laparoscopic surgery and specialized equipment is available.

Surgical exploration of the CBD for ductal stones (CBDS) dates back to 1889, first performed by the famous Swiss surgeon Ludwig Courvoisier. From an early, yet still valuable, open approach, the next major shift in technique was endoscopic management of CBDS by ERCP and endoscopic sphincterotomy (ES) in the 1970s. With the increasing popularity, safety, and success of LC in the 1990s, the LCBDE technique was a logical extension. However, the benefits of LCBDE over endoscopic management are still controversial.

Three approaches have been popularized for LCBDE, namely transcystic-CBD exploration (TC-CBDE), laparoscopic choledochotomy (LCD), and lastly laparoscopic antegrade sphincterotomy (LAS).

## Laparoscopic Common Bile Duct Exploration for Suspected or Proven Common Bile Duct Stones

The incidence of choledocholothiasis is reported to range between 3% and 20% for patients undergoing cholecystectomy. In the early LC era, patients with the slightest suspicion of CBDS were submitted for preoperative ERCP under the assumption that CBDS could be removed by ES. Failing that, an open common bile duct exploration (OCBDE) was undertaken. The endoscopic approach, however, has been increasingly questioned, as the patients often do not have CBDS and there is a significant risk of complications such as bleeding (3%), pancreatitis (2%), duodenal perforation (1%), late papillotomy stenosis (10% to 33%), and a failure rate that ultimately leads to operative management.

The medical literature is supportive of LCBDE, as a number of randomized controlled trials have shown this approach to be a safe alternative to ES or OCBDE. Rhodes et al., in their randomized clinical trial comparing LCBDE vs. postoperative ERCP for proven stones on intraoperative cholangiography, showed that both techniques had equal clearance rates at first intervention of about 75%. However, the procedure time required for LC + LCBDE was relatively shorter compared to LC + postoperative ERCP. The most significant result noted in this trial was shorter hospital stay in the group treated by LCBDE. Later a European multicenter randomized clinical trial by Cuschieri et al. confirmed Rhodes et al.'s findings of reduced hospital stay and equal clearance rates of CBDS with laparoscopic approach.

Nathanson et al. looked at the management of failed TC-CBDE either by ERCP or choledochotomy. The study found comparable results for CBDS clearance by either procedure. However, the authors felt that there is a role for each technique in different clinical scenarios. The ERCP was felt to be beneficial for stones smaller than 7 mm, and choledochotomy was a good choice for CBDS greater than 8 mm, failed ERCP, institutions with poor availability of ERCP, and patients after Billroth II gastrectomy.

Long-term results from LCBDE are presently limited due to the relative short history of this technique, but a number of retrospective studies have shown encouraging results. Riciardi et al., in a large retrospective 11-year follow-up study of over 346 LCBDE procedures, did show a low incidence of retained stones and no long-term stricture or other biliary complications over a mean follow-up period of 43 months. These promising data were further supported by another retrospective study of 175 consecutive LCBDE (Waage et al.). Over a median period of 36 months, the authors of this study did not find any evidence of CBD stricture in their patients. However, data from ES is now in its fourth decade and many centers are showing disappointing rates of recurrent CBDS after ES. For example, Peppelenbosch et al. found that only 2% of patients with OCBDE had CBDS compared to 19% after ES. The mechanism responsible for such high recurrence is believed to be the loss of the function in the sphincter of Oddi and the effects of bacterobilia (infection of bile) from duodenobiliary reflux, which leads to stone formation with time. Interestingly, there is a laboratory-based theory of reactive change to the biliary epithelium from such duodenobiliary reflux, leading to hyperplasia, metaplasia, and thus a theoretical risk of neoplastic change over time.

In summary, on the basis of the above evidence, LCBDE is a safe and effective procedure that carries a lower morbidity and mortality compared to ERCP, most notably pancreatitis. While initial setup costs of LCBDE are high, this cost can be recouped by cost savings in other areas such as inpatient stay and total length of procedure time (LC + LCBDE vs. LC + postoperative ERCP). Benefits to both the surgeon and patient are the principles of one-stage management and full control over CBD pathology. Definite algorithms are yet to be established and agreed upon but international data continues to refine the indications of ERCP over LCBDE and vice versa. We present our algorithm for laparoscopic management of CBDS (Fig. 7.1).

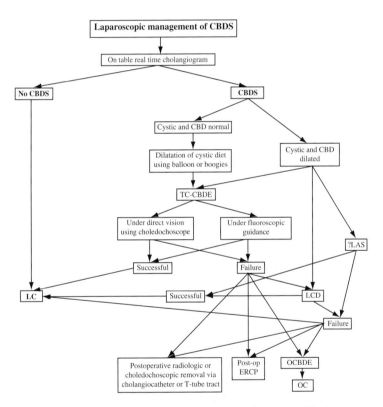

Fig. 7.1. Algorithm for laparoscopic management of common bile duct stones (CBDS). CBD, common bile duct; ERCP, endoscopic retrograde cholangiopan-creatography; LAS, laparoscopic antegrade sphincterotomy; LC, laparoscopic cholecystectomy LCD, laparoscopic choledochotomy; OC, open cholangiogram; OCBDE, open common bile duct exploration; TC-CBDE, transcystic-CBD exploration (Reprinted from American Journal of Surgeons, 179:309–315, Memon MA, ©2000, with permission from Excerpta Medica, Inc.)

# E.  Conclusions

## *Carol E.H. Scott-Conner*

The laparoscopic biliary surgeon who is unable to provide laparoscopic clearance of common duct stones dooms the patient to a separate procedure, usually ERCP, for clearance. Preparation is everything, whether the transcystic approach or approach via choledochotomy is selected. Assembling all needed materials together on a cart (see Table 7.1) as advocated by Petelin, will facilitate the procedure. Positioning the patient on a table that allows fluorocholangiography is essential. Finally, allowing sufficient time and energy to patiently complete the procedure is essential.

The procedures are mutually complementary, not exclusionary. By its nature, choledochotomy is best for large stones in a large duct. Small stones may easily be retrieved or flushed from the common duct by utilizing a transcystic approach.

Both procedures have potential complications, including incomplete clearance, pancreatitis, bile leak, and—particularly when a choledochotomy is performed—stricture. Both have their place in the management of calculous biliary tract disease.

# References

Cuschieri A, Lezoche E, Morino M, et al. E.A.E.S. multicenter prospective randomized trial comparing two-stage vs single-stage management of patients with gallstone disease and ductal calculi. Surg Endosc 1999;13:952–957.

Memon MA, Hassaballa H, Memon MI. Laparoscopic common bile duct exploration: the past, the present, and the future. Am J Surg 2000;179:309–315.

Nathanson LK, O'Rourke NA, Martin IJ, et al. Postoperative ERCP versus laparoscopic choledochotomy for clearance of selected bile duct calculi: a randomized trial. Ann Surg 2005;242:188–192.

Peppelenbosch AG, Naber AHJ, van Goor H. Recurrence rate of common bile duct stones is higher after endoscopic sphincterotomy than after common bile duct exploration in patients below 60 years of age: a long–term follow-up study. Br J Surg 1998;85:54(abstr).

Petelin JB. Tools of the trade: the common bile duct stone cart. J Gastrointest Surg 2000;4:336–337.

Rhodes M, Sussman L, Cohen L, et al. Randomized trial of laparoscopic exploration of common bile duct versus postoperative endoscopic retrograde cholangiography for common bile duct stones. Lancet 1998;351:159–161.

Riciardi R, Islam S, Canete JJ, Arcand PL, Stoker ME. Effectiveness and long-term results of laparoscopic common bile duct exploration. Surg Endosc 2003;17:19–22.

Tranter SE, Thompson MH. Comparison of endoscopic sphincterotomy and laparoscopic exploration of the common bile duct. Br J Surg 2002;89:1495–1504.

Waage A, Stromberg C, Leijonmarck CE, Arvidsson D. Long-term results from laparoscopic common bile duct exploration. Surg Endosc 2003;17:1181–1185.

Watson MJ, Hamilton EC, Jones DB, Laparoscopic common bile duct exploration. Oper Tech Gen Surg 2005;7(1):23–38.

# Suggested Readings

Akopian G, Blitz J, Vander Laan T. Positive intraoperative cholangiography during laparoscopic cholecystectomy: is laparoscopic common bile duct exploration necessary? Am Surg 2005;71:750–753.

Dorman JP, Franklin ME, Glass JL. Laparoscopic common bile duct exploration by choledochotomy. Surg Endosc 1998;12:926–928.

Lyass S, Phillips EH. Laparoscopic transcystic duct common bile duct exploration. Surg Endosc 2006;20:441–445.

Paganini AM, Guerrieri M, Sarnari J, et al. Thirteen years' experience with laparoscopic transcystic common bile duct exploration for stones. Surg Endosc 2007;21:34–40.

Petelin JB. Laparoscopic common bile duct exploration. Surg Endosc 2003;17:1705–1715.

# 8. Bleeding After Laparoscopic Cholecystectomy

## A. Introduction

Bleeding can occur after any surgical procedure. Prompt management and efficient treatment minimize the sequelae. This chapter explores the options when postoperative hemorrhage complicates laparoscopic cholecystectomy.

## B. Case

*Kerri Maiers Nowell*

A 20-year-old woman presented to the emergency department after 3 days of right upper quadrant (RUQ) pain, nausea, and vomiting. The pain began shortly after finishing supper at a fast-food restaurant. The pain was a sharp, crampy pressure in the RUQ that radiated straight through to her back and was rated at 9/10. The pain was not relieved by either Tylenol or ibuprofen. Overnight, the pain subsided slightly, but she was still nauseated and unable to eat or drink over the next 48 hours. She denied fevers or chills. When she was unable to attend classes because of the pain, she sought medical attention. She is a student studying education, smokes one pack of cigarettes per day, drinks socially, and denies drug use. She is recently single and no longer sexually active.

Her past medical history was unremarkable except for migraine headaches. She had not had any prior surgery. Medications were Imitrex and birth control pills. She had no known allergies.

On physical exam, she was a well-developed, well-nourished young woman in no acute distress. She was not visibly jaundiced. Her temperature was 36.6 °C, pulse was 82, and blood pressure was 120/70. The cardiopulmonary examination was benign.

Her abdomen was soft and nondistended, with active bowel sounds. She had mild tenderness to palpation in the epigastrium and RUQ. There was no guarding or rebound tenderness. Extremities were free of edema with palpable pulses.

Laboratory studies were significant for a white blood cell count (WBC) of 8100, and hemoglobin/hematocrit (Hgb/Hct) of 14.0/41. Total and direct bilirubin were 1.4 and 0.8. Alkaline phosphatase was 102, γ-glutamyltransferase (GGT) 194, aspartate aminotransferase (AST) 154, and alanine aminotransferase (ALT) 176.

Abdominal ultrasound showed a normal-sized liver without intrahepatic or extrahepatic ductal dilatation. The gallbladder was distended with sludge. At least three nonmobile stones were seen in the fundus. The gallbladder wall was not thickened (3 mm). No pericholecystic fluid was noted. The pancreas and spleen were normal.

The patient was taken to the operating room the following morning for a laparoscopic cholecystectomy. Pneumoperitoneum was attained with a Veress needle through an infraumbilical incision. There were no apparent complications during the case. The cystic duct and artery were dissected circumferentially and clipped twice proximally and once distally. After hemostasis was attained, the pneumoperitoneum was released. The patient was extubated and transported to the recovery room. Over the next 2 hours, the patient became tachycardic, with beats per minute in the 120 s, and her blood pressure dropped with systolic pressures in the 80 s to 90 s. Postoperative Hgb/Hct were 8.3 and 24. Two units of packed red blood cells (PRBCs) were transfused and the patient was taken back to the operating room emergently.

The obvious concern is postoperative hemorrhage following this uncomplicated laparoscopic cholecystectomy. **What is the best and safest way to approach this case—through an open or laparoscopic exploration?**

# C. Open Exploration

*Rahul Tevar and Fred Brody*

Intraabdominal bleeding after a laparoscopic cholecystectomy is a rare but potentially serious complication. Historically, the rate of postoperative bleeding ranges from 0.08% to 0.1%, with a mortality rate of 8% to 17%. Deziel et al. noted that the gallbladder fossa is the most common source of bleeding, followed by port sites, the cystic artery, and other intraabdominal vasculature. Minor postoperative bleeding presents with tachycardia, decreased hematocrit, increased abdominal discomfort, or an abdominal wall hematoma. As in the present case, major postoperative bleeding usually presents with hemorrhagic shock. The choice of laparoscopy versus laparotomy for postoperative hemorrhage is based on the bleeding source and the hemodynamic stability of the patient.

As noted earlier, the gallbladder fossa is the most common source of postoperative blood loss. Usually, simple venous oozing from inadequate hemostasis of the liver bed can be controlled laparoscopically with electrocautery, argon beam coagulation, or hemostatic agents such as Surgicel, Avitene, or fibrin glue. Arterial bleeding from the gallbladder fossa may originate from small branches of the cystic artery that run superficially through the parenchyma of the liver bed, as noted by Schafer et al. Coagulopathic bleeding from the liver bed is extremely difficult to manage laparoscopically, let alone through an open laparotomy. If hemorrhage from the liver induces hypotension, a laparotomy is necessary to pack the RUQ. Once the abdomen is packed, resuscitation continues with blood products and fluids until the patient is stabilized. Subsequently, blood and old clot are evacuated quickly and the bleeding source is visualized and secured. In the case of coagulopathic bleeding from the liver, the fossa is packed with laparotomy pads and the patient is closed with a silo. Depending on the nature and severity of the patient's hematologic studies and core temperature, a second-look operation is scheduled to remove the packs and ensure hemostasis.

Bleeding from trocar sites is also an uncommon complication of laparoscopic cholecystectomy. Damage to the inferior epigastric arteries and veins may present as external or internal bleeding. External bleeding from the abdominal wall is treated with pressure or a simple stitch. Bleeding *into* the abdominal wall can present with massive bruising of the abdominal wall or rectus sheath and is usually managed nonoperatively. It is exceedingly rare for a patient to develop hemodynamic instability from external bleeding. The patient may exhibit mild tachycardia, but a significant blood pressure change with hemodynamic instability is rare. Internal bleeding can be detected intraoperatively as blood drips down trocars, instruments, or the abdominal wall. This is managed with endoscopic suturing or fascial closure devices. However, internal bleeding from port sites may go undetected intraoperatively. In addition, the pneumoperitoneum may tamponade lacerated veins that ultimately bleed once the pressure is released. Furthermore, small arteries may spasm during surgery, only to bleed postoperatively. If conservative management fails and the patient's hemoglobin continues to decrease, repeat laparoscopy affords an excellent view of the abdominal wall. Bleeding vessels can be controlled with port site closure devices, or a Foley catheter can be inserted to tamponade the bleeding. On the other hand, brisk bleeding that presents with hemorrhagic shock would necessitate a laparotomy.

Hemorrhage from the cystic artery can occur postoperatively if clips are improperly placed or dislodged. Also, an injury to an unrecognized aberrant or accessory artery can present with postoperative hemorrhage. Laparoscopic management of postoperative cystic artery bleeding may be attempted in a stable patient. But vigorous irrigation and suctioning of clots may dislodge clips from the cystic duct or induce more bleeding from the hepatic bed. Blind electrocautery or clips may injure the cystic duct stump, the common bile duct, or the hepatic vessels. The cystic artery can be avulsed with an exponential increase in bleeding. An open exploration of the abdomen minimizes these risks and affords definitive control of bleeding in an unstable postoperative patient.

Major vascular injury during laparoscopic cholecystectomy occurs very rarely but can be catastrophic, especially with a delay in recognition. Wherry et al. reviewed 9130 laparoscopic cholecystectomies performed at 94 military hospitals between 1993 and 1994 and found a 0.11% rate of major vascular injury. The most common site of injury was the hepatic artery (40%), followed by the portal vein (30%), common iliac artery (20%), and mesenteric arteries (10%). Of these injuries, 90% were identified intraoperatively and 10% postoperatively. Also, the aortic bifurcation lies directly beneath the umbilicus and is susceptible to injuries from a Veress needle or a blind trocar. Other vascular structures including the iliac arteries and veins and the vena cava are susceptible as well. Commonly, these injuries demand an emergent laparotomy. Rarely, a major vascular injury may escape unnoticed only to present in the early postoperative period as a pseudoaneurysm. Again, this scenario necessitates a laparotomy, not a laparoscopy, for proximal and distal control of the bleeding vessel.

Finally, in the setting of hypotension and poor tissue perfusion, a repeat laparoscopy with a pneumoperitoneum increases intraabdominal pressure and impedes venous return to the heart. This exacerbates an already inadequate preload created by acute hypovolemia. Animal models of hemorrhagic shock demonstrate that a pneumoperitoneum of just 5 mm Hg decreases mean arterial pressure and cardiac output, worsens acidosis, and decreases renal perfusion. An emergent laparotomy does not induce these pathophysiologic alterations.

The source of postoperative hemorrhage after a laparoscopic cholecystectomy dictates the management algorithm. However, if operative intervention is required, the choice of access is influenced by the hemodynamic stability of the patient. As demonstrated in the present case, postoperative bleeding after a laparoscopic cholecystectomy can present as severe, life-threatening hemorrhage. There are multiple possible sources of bleeding, but safe and rapid control in the emergent setting requires a laparotomy. In addition, a pneumoperitoneum is potentially harmful in the setting of hemorrhagic shock. An open exploration provides the best and safest approach to control postoperative bleeding associated with hemorrhagic shock following a laparoscopic cholecystectomy.

# D.  Repeat Laparoscopy, with Preparation to Convert to Open Laparotomy

*Carol E.H. Scott-Conner*

In the case presented, bleeding is recognized in the recovery room. Immediate preparation for return to surgery must be made, while the patient is resuscitated and coagulation studies sent to the laboratory. If the patient stabilizes after administration of two units of packed cells, as evidenced by return of pulse and blood pressure to normal levels, then a case can be made for a quick laparoscopic exploration. Preparations for immediate conversion to full laparotomy must be available if laparoscopy fails, and the surgeon attempting the repeat laparoscopy must be an experienced laparoscopist, ideally one with experience in laparoscopy for trauma.

At all times, the experience of the laparoscopist, the likely nature of the injury, and the safety of the patient must determine the extent to which this minimal access route is attempted or how long it is pursued. Failure to identify a bleeding site or hemodynamic instability provoked by pneumoperitoneum mandate immediate conversion to formal laparotomy.

If these precautions are followed, success may follow a repeat laparoscopy. Dexter et al. reported a small series of patients who underwent repeat laparoscopy for complications of laparoscopy cholecystectomy, including two patients with postoperative bleeding. Duca et al. reported results from a slightly larger series.

Of the potential bleeding sites, those most likely to be amenable to laparoscopic management include the trocar site (managed by suture closure of the trocar site), the cystic artery (management by grasping the stump of the artery gently with a forceps and securing it with a clip or pre-tied loop ligature), and the gallbladder fossa (management by electrocautery, argon beam coagulator, or hemostatic agents). Even if laparoscopic management is unsuccessful, localization of the site to the RUQ (as opposed to a retroperitoneal vascular injury) allows a mini-laparotomy incision to be made right over the bleeding site.

It is helpful to review the trauma literature in this context. Laparoscopy is a recognized modality for diagnosis and even management of abdominal injuries. Several caveats must be observed. First, the patient must be hemodynamically stable. Thus, in the case presented, hemodynamic stability would need to have been achieved with the two-unit transfusion. Second, the laparoscopic team must be experienced. Chol and Lim reported that in 78 hemodynamically stable trauma patients, diagnostic or therapeutic laparoscopy was successful in all cases.

Clearly, any previously undiagnosed coagulopathy must be corrected. While in most cases the problem is surgical in nature (inadequate surgical hemostasis at the initial surgery), occasionally a previously undiagnosed patient with mild von Willebrand's disease or other congenital abnormality of coagulation presents with surgical bleeding. Similarly, patients may be taking over-the-counter medications that interfere with coagulation, such as nonsteroidal antiinflammatory agents. Some herbal medications can affect the coagulation system as well. It is always worthwhile to speak with the patient and family to determine if there is any family history of abnormal bleeding or bruising.

If a retroperitoneal vascular injury is suspected, then prompt midline laparotomy with the assistance of an experienced vascular surgeon is the best option.

Finally, if the laparoscopic surgeon is at all uncomfortable with the concept of laparoscopy for hemoperitoneum, then open laparotomy is the best and safest course.

# E. Conclusions

*Kerri Maiers Nowell*

Laparoscopic cholecystectomy is widely accepted as the treatment of choice for patients with gallstone disease and cholecystitis. However, this has introduced a new set of complications, including access injuries and procedure-related problems. Major retroperitoneal vascular injuries were extremely rare before the days of laparoscopy. Catarci et al. found a 0.05% incidence of major vascular injuries in a retrospective study of

12,919 patients. Geers and Holden found a 0.14% incidence. Although the majority of these injuries were recognized in the operating room, a few were diagnosed within 24 hours, similar to the patient in the case presented here.

The most dangerous step during laparoscopy is believed to be establishment of the pneumoperitoneum. Mayol et al. demonstrated a 5% complication rate specifically related to accessing the abdominal cavity, including abdominal wall hematoma (2.0%), umbilical hernia (1.5%), and umbilical wound infection (1.2%). Of these, 75% were related to the umbilical insertion site.

The Swiss Association for Laparoscopic and Thoracoscopic Surgery (SALTS) collected data on 14,243 patients undergoing various standard laparoscopic procedures between 1995 and 1997. Laparoscopic cholecystectomy comprised 60% of the surgical cases. The database looked at injuries occurring during establishing the pneumoperitoneum. There were 22 trocar and four Veress needle injuries. This corresponded to an incidence of 0.18%. Nineteen involved visceral organs (0.133%) and seven (0.049%) were vessel injuries. The majority of the vascular lesions (six of seven) were venous bleeding of either the greater omentum or mesentery. The one remaining was an injury to the right iliac vessel. Of all the injuries, 21.7% were repaired laparoscopically and 78.3% had conversion to an open procedure. Laparoscopic repair of the vascular injuries included using monopolar current, clips, or sutures. The authors believe that injuries in the retroperitoneum require rapid conversion to open technique to achieve hemostasis and avoid further complications. It is also noted that small lesions restricted to the surface of parenchymatous organs can be managed laparoscopically.

Bove et al. reported the results of a study of 1100 laparoscopic cholecystectomies in which there were four hemoperitoneums, all treated with a minimally invasive approach. These authors believe that, with early diagnosis, it is possible to treat the majority of complications arising after laparoscopic cholecystectomy with minimally invasive methods.

It is not surprising that laparoscopy is associated with some new and unique complications. The complications range from simple abdominal wall hematomas to devastating retroperitoneal vascular injuries that require emergent reexploration. What is the best way to approach a reexploration when bleeding is diagnosed in the postoperative period? After reviewing the published data, it appears the answer depends partly on the stability of the patient. If the patient is relatively stable, one should opt for laparoscopy, as many complications may be amended in such a manner. However, there are certain instances in which a conversion to an open procedure is appropriate. One would start with a laparotomy if the patient was hemodynamically unstable, or convert to an open procedure if a vascular lesion is diagnosed that is not amenable to laparoscopic maneuvers, such as an expanding retroperitoneal hematoma. Another reason for conversion would be if the necessary repair was not within the comfort levels of the operating surgeon.

It appears that a reexploration may proceed in a laparoscopic manner in many cases of bleeding diagnosed after a laparoscopic cholecystectomy. A laparoscopic repair may proceed as long as two crucial criteria are met: (1) the safety of the patient is never compromised, and (2) the operating surgeon is competent at a minimally invasive repair.

# References

Bove A, Bongarzoni G, Palone G, Chiarini S, Corbellini L. Minimally invasive approach of the most common complications after laparoscopic cholecystectomy. Ann Ital Chir 2005;76(3):235–238.

Catarci M, Carlini M, Gentileschi P, Santoro E. Major and minor injuries during the creation of pneumoperitoneum, a multicenter study on 12,919 cases. Surg Endosc 2001;15:566–569.

Chol YB, Lim KS. Therapeutic laparoscopy for abdominal trauma. Surg Endosc 2003;17:421–427.

Dexter SP, Miller GV, Davides D, et al. Relaparoscopy for the detection and treatment of complications of laparoscopic cholecystectomy. Am J Surg 2000;179(4):316–319.

Deziel DJ, Millikan KW, Economou SG, et al. Complications of laparoscopic cholecystectomy: a national survey of 4,292 hospitals and an analysis of 77,604 cases. Am J Surg 1993;165:9–14.

Duca S, Iancu C, Bălă O, et al. Mini-invasive treatment of complications following laparoscopic cholecystectomy. Acta Chir Belg 2004;104(3):309–312.

Geers J, Holden C. Major vascular injury as a complication of laparoscopic surgery: a report of three cases and review of the literature. Am Surg 1996;62(5):377.

Mayol J, Garcia-Aguilar J, et al. Risks of the minimal access approach for laparoscopic surgery: multivariate analysis of morbidity related to umbilical trocar insertion. World J Surg 1997;21:529–533.

Schafer M, Lauper M, Krahenbuhl L. Trocar and Veress needle injuries during laparoscopy. Surg Endosc 2001;15:275–280.

Wherry DC, et al. An external audit of laparoscopic cholecystectomy in the steady state performed in medical treatment facilities of the department of defense. Ann Surg 1996;22(2):145–154.

# Suggested Readings

Bailey RW, Flowers JL, eds. Complications of Laparoscopic Surgery. St. Louis: Quality Medical Publishing, 1995.

Bergamaschi R, Ignjatovic D. Anatomic rationale for arterial bleeding from the liver bed during and/or after laparoscopic cholecystectomy: a postmortem study. Surg Laparosc Endosc 1999;9(4):267.

Bulut F, et al. Is pneumoperitoneum harmful during intra-abdominal hemorrhage in rats? J Laparoendosc 2005;15:112–120.

Demetriades D, Hadjizacharia P, Constantinou C, et al. Selective nonoperative management of penetrating abdominal solid organ injuries. Ann Surg 2006;2444:620–628.

Kheirabadi BS, et al. Metabolic and hemodynamic effects of $CO_2$ pneumoperitoneum in a controlled hemorrhage model. J Trauma 2001;50:1031–1043.

Soper NJ, Swanstrom LL, Eubanks WS, eds. Mastery of Endoscopic and Laparoscopic Surgery. Philadelphia: Lippincott, 2005.

Steinman M, et al. Hemodynamic and metabolic effects of $CO_2$ pneumoperitoneum in an experimental model of hemorrhagic shock due to retroperitoneal hematoma. Surg Endosc 1998;12:416–420.

Usal H, et al. Major vascular injuries during laparoscopic cholecystectomy: an institutional review of experience with 2589 procedures and literature review. Surg Endosc 1998;12:960–962.

# 9. Cystic Duct Stump Leak After Cholecystectomy

## A. Introduction

Things do not always go smoothly after a laparoscopic cholecystectomy. One of the more common complications is bile leak. Common bile duct injury must always be ruled in or out in this circumstance. Other causes of leak include aberrant bile ducts, which drain from the liver into the gallbladder fossa, or failure of the cystic duct stump closure. This chapter explores options for management of cystic duct stump leak.

## B. Case

### Mohammad Allam

A 45-year-old man underwent uncomplicated laparoscopic cholecystectomy for symptomatic cholelithiasis. He was discharged less than 24 hours after the procedure, but returned to the emergency department 2 days later complaining of increasing abdominal pain and distention. His family thought that he was starting to appear slightly yellow.

His past medical history was negative. He had not had any other previous surgery. His family history was significant for gallstones in his mother and in one sister. His medications were only the usual postoperative medications of Tylenol No. 3 and Colace. He had no known drug allergies. He was married, worked as a car salesman, and did not smoke or drink alcoholic beverages. The review of symptoms was negative except as noted above.

On physical examination, he appeared slightly jaundiced. He was well developed and well nourished, and appeared anxious. His vital signs were significant for a temperature of 38.3 °C, pulse 122, and blood pressure 128/64. The head and neck examination was negative, except for slight jaundice. Cardiopulmonary examination revealed decreased breath sounds at the right base.

His abdomen was slightly distended and diffusely tender to palpation. There were no masses. Bowel sounds were hypoactive. His trocar sites were clean without ecchymosis or erythema. No hernias were detected. Rectal examination was negative and stool was guaiac negative.

Laboratory examination was significant for white cell count of 20,200. Hematocrit was 44. Blood urea nitrogen (BUN) and creatinine were normal, as were electrolytes. Total bilirubin was 5.2 with a direct bilirubin of 3.2, aspartate aminotransferase (AST) was 67, alanine aminotransferase (ALT) 93, γ-glutamyltransferase (GGT) 288, alkaline phosphatase 124, amylase 34, and lipase 13.

Ultrasound examination of the right upper quadrant revealed fluid around the liver. The bile ducts could not be visualized due to bowel gas. A hepatobiliary iminodiacetic acid (HIDA) scan showed prompt flow of contrast into the common duct, which was well delineated. There was free flow into the duodenum. Leakage of contrast was noted from the medial aspect of the gallbladder fossa.

The assessment was a cystic duct leak after laparoscopic cholecystectomy. **How would you address this— endoscopic retrograde cholangiopancreatography (ERCP) with percutaneous drainage, or repeat laparoscopy?**

# C. Endoscopic Retrograde Cholangiopancreatography and Percutaneous Drainage of the Biloma

*David Scheeres*

A cystic duct stump leak after a laparoscopic cholecystectomy usually presents with a bile leak. In this situation, the patient develops abdominal pain, mild to moderate jaundice, mild to moderate leukocytosis, occasional fever, and shoulder pain. The next step in the workup of the patient is often either an ultrasound or computed tomography (CT) to evaluate the diameter of the bile ducts and determine if a fluid collection is present. If such a fluid collection is found, further interventions are needed to determine what the fluid is composed of.

Percutaneous drainage allows identification of what type of fluid is present, differentiating among an abscess, biloma, or hematoma. However, while this intervention alone is curative for an abscess and hematoma, it has been shown not to be definitive therapy for a biloma. Drainage as sole therapy of a biloma has been shown to result in failure and sepsis.

The etiology of a biloma can be from numerous causes, including a leak from the closure of the cystic duct, as in this case, or from the ducts of Luschka, associated biliary obstruction whether from a stone or stricture, or biliary injury with an associated bile leak. The management of such a bile leak differs based on the cause of the biloma. Once the biloma has been drained, resolution of the cause of the bile leak requires accurate imaging. A bile leak can be confirmed with a HIDA nuclear scan, although the exact location of the leak and the fact that this is only a diagnostic test limit its usefulness. Noninvasive magnetic resonance cholangiopancreatography (MRCP) gives greater definition of the biliary tree, helping exclude a biliary tract injury, but still is only diagnostic and often does not demonstrate the site of the bile leak. The distinction between a test that is only diagnostic versus one that can be both diagnostic and therapeutic is important. Many times a bile leak can be large enough to cause problems, but small enough to defy definition. Therefore, proceeding with therapy during the ERCP will resolve the problem, even if the exact site of leakage cannot be seen.

Attempts at finding the leak with surgical exploration, open or laparoscopic, and reapplication of a clip to the cystic duct may not always resolve the cause of the bile leak, and may still leak because the cystic duct is inflammatory and may not hold the clip or tie. There have not been reports of clip application succeeding as routine therapy for a cystic duct leak, especially when done after several days or a week have passed. In addition, case series of patients with bile leaks have found that a significant number of patients do not have a cystic duct stump leak as the source of the bile leak. This leads to a significant nontherapeutic laparotomy rate in those cases where the cystic duct stump is not the problem.

Endoscopic retrograde cholangiopancreatography allows definitive evaluation of the biliary tree to ensure that an injury has not resulted from the prior laparoscopic cholecystectomy. If an injury has resulted from the surgery, it can be identified and described, allowing the surgeon to plan an operative strategy for repair of the biliary tract injury. The ability to do this without a laparotomy is important, especially in light of the current literature, which recommends a delayed repair of biliary tract injuries rather than an immediate repair.

Endoscopic retrograde cholangiopancreatography also allows correction of biliary obstruction that may have caused ductal hypertension, leading to the leak and biloma. Removal of obstructing common bile duct (CBD) stones or debris, sphincterotomy, or dilation of ampullary strictures all can resolve the cause of the leak and ductal hypertension that contributed to the leak in the first place.

Treatment of the biliary leak and fistula, which is what the biloma is converted to if drained externally, is performed using established principles of fistula management for gastrointestinal (GI) tract fistulas. One of these principles is removal of distal obstruction, and it can be applied to the biliary tree easily with ERCP, sphincterotomy, and transampullary stenting. Normally, the ampullary sphincters are in a contracted state at rest, slowing drainage of bile through the ampulla into the duodenum. When an endoscopic sphincterotomy is performed and a stent is placed, this removes the resistance to flow out of the biliary system, and encourages bile to drain through the ampulla, rather than through the leak and fistula. An ERCP with sphincterotomy and stenting can accomplish this and resolve the problem, even if the bile leak is small and cannot be visualized during the cholangiogram (Fig. 9.1). Prospective, randomized series have not been performed to determine the best management method for a bile leak; however, there have been many case series published that establish endoscopic drainage as a successful treatment modality in most cases.

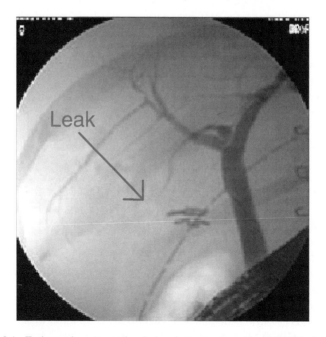

Fig. 9.1. Endoscopic retrograde cholangiopancreatography (ERCP) showing leak from cystic duct stump.

Drainage can also be accomplished with a nasobiliary tube, where a 5-French pigtail catheter is placed in the bile duct and exited through the nose. This decompresses the bile duct sufficiently to allow resolution of the bile leak. However, most patients do not tolerate a tube in their nose for the 7 to 14 days it requires to treat the problem, making this method an imperfect solution. The advantage of such a tube is that it can be removed simply by withdrawing it, without performing another endoscopy.

Drainage can also be accomplished by placement of a biliary endo-prosthesis across the ampulla, with one end in the bile duct and the other end in the duodenum (Fig. 9.2). This theoretically should work better, since the resistance to flow through the ampulla is lower than a nasobiliary tube, because the length is shorter, and a larger, 8.5F to 11F stent, can be placed, further decreasing the resistance to flow and therefore better decompressing the biliary tree and stopping the leak. Barkun et al. noted a better success rate with stenting over that of nasobiliary drainage. Series have reported a high success rate with biliary stenting. Endoscopic sphinc-terotomy alone has also been shown to be helpful in stopping the biliary leak; however, it has less success than when stenting is added to it.

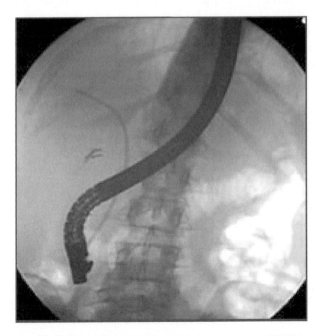

Fig. 9.2. Endoscopic retrograde cholangiopancreatography (ERCP) showing stent in common duct.

Therefore, ERCP with endoscopic sphincterotomy and stenting, is the preferred method of diagnosis and then immediate management of a bile leak. It allows management of most causes of bile leak that are not caused by a bile duct injury requiring surgical correction. It also allows resolution of any distal CBD obstruction that may have caused the leak to occur.

## D.  Repeat Laparoscopy

*Carol E.H. Scott-Conner*

I would perform repeat laparoscopy in this patient. This single procedure allows the surgeon to identify and close the bile leak, perform a cholangiogram if necessary, and irrigate and drain any intra-abdominal bile collections.

The first concern when a patient returns with a bile leak must be to exclude the presence of a bile duct injury. In this particular case, a HIDA scan demonstrated prompt flow into the duodenum (hence an intact bile duct) and leakage of contrast from the medial aspect of the gallbladder fossa. These findings suggest that the source of the leak is either a cystic duct stump blowout (in which case the cystic duct simply needs to be identified and secured) or a duct of Luschka (in which case, a well-placed laparoscopic suture should suffice). Less common causes include injury to an accessory duct or to the right hepatic duct.

The second concern is whether or not distal bile duct obstruction, most likely from previously-undiagnosed bile duct stones, have caused the leak. The HIDA scan is reassuring, but not totally diagnostic, on this point. A cholangiogram should be done if there is any question. If necessary, laparoscopic common duct exploration, can be performed.

The advantage of this approach is that it does not require the special skills or expertise needed for ERCP with stenting (which may not be available at all hospitals), and that it allows the problem to be treated during a single procedure rather than two procedures.

Several points are important for success: first, the index of suspicion for a bile duct injury must be low. In this situation, an operative cholangiogram from the initial operation is literally "worth is weight in gold". This does not, of course, exclude the possibility of bile duct injury, but does give important anatomic information such as the length of cystic duct remaining. It may even, in retrospect, show a tiny duct of Luschka leak. Second, repeat laparoscopy is most successful when performed within a few days of the initial procedure. Third, it may be difficult to identify the site of leakage, especially if the leak is small. Copious irrigation and even cholangiography may be needed. Fourth, if the leak appears to originate from the cystic duct, a catheter should be passed into the site of injury and a cholangiogram done to confirm the anatomy and exclude right hepatic duct injury or common duct stones. Generally a catheter can be gently inserted over a guidewire to obtain the cholangiogram. Additional cystic duct length will need to be obtained by gentle dissection prior to attempt at closure. Doubly-ligating the cystic duct is probably more secure than clipping it – especially since it is likely that it was clipped at the first operation. Finally, a leak coming directly from the gallbladder fossa itself may be a duct of Luschka, and can be suture-ligated.

Copiously suction-irrigating the subhepatic space and any areas of contamination concludes the procedure. I would place a closed suction drain in the subhepatic space.

If a major duct injury is identified, a drain should be placed and the procedure should be terminated. The patient should then be referred to a center with expertise in complex biliary reconstructions. Endoscopic stenting may be used as part of the preoperative preparation, but should be done at the discretion of the surgeon who will perform the reconstruction.

# E. Conclusions

## *Carol E.H. Scott-Conner*

For many surgeons who routinely perform laparoscopic cholecystectomy, in-house ERCP capability is a luxury. Facility with techniques of laparoscopic cholangiography and trans-cystic duct exploration (see chapters 4, 5, and 6) tremendously extend the surgeon's capability to prevent, diagnose, and manage some of the problems associated with the procedure.

One such problem is postoperative bile duct leakage. Wills et al. reported an incidence of 15 patients in 1779 sequential laparoscopic cholecystectomies. Two of these patients resolved spontaneously. Ten patients with leakage from the gallbladder bed responded to repeat laparoscopy (although one subsequently required laparotomy for drainage of a pelvic abscess). Of the three patients with cystic duct stump leak, one was managed laparoscopically and the other two endoscopically. They recommended the use of HIDA scan, as was done in this case, to assist in identification of patients in whom this approach might be useful.

Barkun et al. reported on the diagnosis and management of post-laparoscopic cholecystectomy (LC) bile leaks in 64 patients. Biliary obstruction was demonstrated in 31%, and the majority of these had stones. Most patients had leakage from the cystic duct stump, and were managed by endoscopic decompression and/or percutaneous drainage. They noted that occurrence of a complication at LC increased the probability of a postoperative leak.

Many groups begin with placement of a percutaneous drain and reserve more intervention for failure of the drainage to subside. This is very similar to the approach familiar to older surgeons (such as myself) from the open cholecystectomy days. Routine drain placement was part of open cholecystectomy for several decades, and appearance of bile in the drains was occasionally observed, and generally subsided spontaneously.

The increased risk of common duct injury during LC changed the algorithm, because early diagnosis and treatment of a bile duct injury gives the best chance of a good outcome. Thus many surgeon combine percutaneous drainage with ERCP and/or placement of a stent. This excludes major bile duct injury and helps to seal the leak. Numerous subsequent reports (see Selected Readings) attest to the efficacy of ERCP in this setting. Ahmad et al. advocated the use of laparoscopy when ERCP and percutaneous drainage failed.

Because the complication is so rare, prospective randomized trials are unlikely to be performed. And, indeed, the preference of one modality over another may well depend upon local expertise and availability. The key points are a low index of suspicion for a bile duct injury (which requires prompt diagnosis and expert repair), and a selective minimally-invasive approach to duct of Luschka injuries or cystic duct stump leaks.

# References

Ahmad F, Saunders RN, Lloyd GM, Lloyd DM, Robertson GS. An algorithm for the management of bile leak following laparoscopic cholecystectomy. Ann R Coll Surg Engl 2007;89(1):51–6.

Barkun AN, Rezieg M, Mehta SN, et al. Postcholecystectomy biliary leaks in the laparoscopic era: risk factors, presentation, and management. McGill Gallstone Treatment Group. Gastrointest Endosc 1997;45(3):277–282.

Christoforidid E, Vasiliadis K, Goulimaris I, Tsalis K, Kanellos I, Papachilea T, Tsorlini E, Betsis D. A single center experience in minimally invasive treatment of postcholecystectomy bile leak, complicated with biloma formation. J Surg Res 2007;141(2):171–175.

Sefr R, Ochmann J, Kozumplik L, Vrastyak J, Penka I. The role of relaparoscopy in the management of bile leaks after laparoscopic cholecystectomy. Int Surg 1995;80(4):356–357.

Wills VL, Jorgensen JO, Hunt DR. Role of relaparoscopy in the management of minor bile leakage after laparoscopic cholecystectomy. Br J Surg 2000;87(2):176–180.

# Suggested Readings

Bose SM, Mazumdar A, Singh V. The role of endoscopic procedures in the management of postcholecystectomy and posttraumatic biliary leak. Surg Today 2001;31(1):45–50.

Chow S, Bosco JJ, Heiss FW, Shea JA, Qaseem T, Howell D. Successful treatment of postcholecystectomy bile leaks using nasobiliary tube drainage and sphincterotomy. Am J Gastroenterol 1997;92(10):1839–1843.

Hanazaki K, Igarashi J, Sodeyama H, Matsuda Y. Bile leakage resulting from clip displacement of the cystic duct stump: a potential pitfall of laparoscopic cholecystectomy. Surg Endosc 1999;13(2):168–171.

Himal HS. The role of ERCP in laparoscopic cholecystectomy-related cystic duct stump leaks. Surg Endosc 1996;10(6):653–655.

Katsinelos P, Paroutoglou G, Beltsis A, et al. Endobiliary endoprosthesis without sphincterotomy for the treatment of biliary leakage. Surg Endosc 2004;18(1):165–166.

Khalid TR, Casillas VJ, Montalvo BM, Centeno R, Levi JU. Using MR cholangiopancreatography to evaluate iatrogenic bile duct injury. AJR Am J Roentgenol 2001;177(6):1347–1352.

Mergener K, Strobel JC, Suhocki P, et al. The role of ERCP in diagnosis and management of accessory bile duct leaks after cholecystectomy. Gastrointest Endosc 1999;50(4):527–531.

Neidich R, Soper N, Edmundowicz S, Chokshi H, Aliperti G. Endoscopic management of bile duct leaks after attempted laparoscopic cholecystectomy. Surg Laparosc Endosc 1996;6(5):348–354.

Ponsky JL. Endoscopic approaches to common bile duct injuries. Surg Clin North Am 1996;76(3):505–513.

Sandoval BA, Goettler CE, Robinson AV, O'Donnell JK, Adler LP, Stellato TA. Cholescintigraphy in the diagnosis of bile leak after laparoscopic cholecystectomy. Am Surg 1997;63(7):611–616.

# 10. Medical Versus Surgical Management of Uncomplicated Gastroesophageal Reflux Disease

## A. Introduction

Significant advances have occurred in both medical and surgical management of gastroesophageal reflux disease (GERD), an extremely common condition in the United States and other industrialized nations. This chapter explores the pros and cons of medical versus surgical management of uncomplicated GERD. Subsequent chapters deal with other related issues, and a chapter introducing endoscopic options for management is included later in Chapter 42. The importance of this topic is underscored by development of a protocol for systematic review of the topic (Wileman et al.), the results of which have not yet been published.

## B. Case

### Eric Wallace

A 42-year-old man had symptoms of "heartburn" for about 3 years. At first, the symptoms occurred sporadically, usually after meals consisting of spicy foods. Initially this happened about once a month. Over the past 3 years the symptoms had become more frequent, but not necessarily more severe, until they occurred about three to four times a week. There was no longer any correlation with the type of food that was eaten. The patient still described the symptoms as "heartburn." He had not noticed any regurgitation. The discomfort was not severe and was usually relieved with over-the-counter antacids.

He had recently started a new job, and with his new health insurance he had started seeing a new primary care provider (PCP). Because of the duration of symptoms his new PCP requested an esophagogastroduodenoscopy (EGD) and placed him on a proton-pump inhibitor. The EGD demonstrated mild gastroesophageal reflux without esophagitis or Barrett's metaplasia.

After just 3 weeks on the proton-pump inhibitor, the patient's symptoms had resolved. However, a coworker at his new job told him about an operation his sister just had to control her GERD. He said it was great because she no longer had to take any medication and she could eat and drink whatever she wanted without problems. Also, because it was laparoscopic surgery she had minimal pain and a quick recovery. The patient requested referral for evaluation for possible surgical therapy for his GERD.

His past medical history was significant only for hypertension and GERD. He had had an inguinal hernia repaired as a child. His family history was significant for adult-onset diabetes in his father. His mother died of a heart attack at age 68.

His medications included hydrochlorothiazide and a multivitamin, in addition to his proton-pump inhibitor. He had no known drug allergies. He was a nonsmoker, and he drank two to four beers per month.

The review of symptoms was positive only for heartburn (now resolved), occasional headaches, and an ingrown left great toenail.

On physical examination, he was a well-appearing male in no acute distress. Vital signs included a temperature of 37.4 °C, pulse 78, blood pressure 128/82. He was 185 cm tall and weighed 98 kilograms. The body mass index (BMI) was 28.6. The head and neck examination was negative, as was the cardiopulmonary examination.

Abdominal examination revealed a soft, mildly obese abdomen without masses or tenderness. Bowel sounds were normal. There was a well-healed right inguinal hernia scar. There were no hernias. Rectal examination revealed normal sphincter tone and a smooth prostate. Stool was guaiac negative.

All laboratory tests, including a complete blood count, electrolytes, blood urea nitrogen (BUN), creatinine, and liver function studies were normal. Chest x-ray was normal.

**Which would you recommend—laparoscopic fundoplication or continued medical management?**

# C. Laparoscopic Fundoplication

*Carol E.H. Scott-Conner*

It is difficult to make a strong case for surgical intervention in this man, and I would not offer it at this point in his history. However, it is instructive to discuss the procedure and potential complications and pitfalls. I would, in fact, have such a discussion with the patient to stress to him that this was not a procedure to be entertained lightly. SAGES provides a patient information Web site, www.GERDSurgery.info, that is useful in educating patients about these issues.

If this patient failed medical management, he would need additional tests before surgery intervention could be contemplated. Before fundoplication, he would need a more comprehensive workup, including 24-hour pH monitoring to document reflux and esophageal motility studies to exclude motility disorders.

Laparoscopic fundoplication is considered an advanced procedure. Considerable facility in manipulation and suturing is required. This procedure, like other minimal access adaptations of standard open surgical procedures, has gone through an evolution and become standardized. Several trade-offs have become apparent. For example, is a complete (360-degree wrap) or a partial fundoplication desirable (see Chapter 11)?

I prefer to do a full, 360-degree wrap, a procedure with 50 years of experience behind it. I use the technique described by Peters et al. The crucial elements are exposure and dissection of the hiatus, full mobilization of the esophagus with identification and protection of both vagal trunks, division of the short gastric vessels, and construction of a complete but floppy wrap. The wrap must be anchored to the esophagus to avoid slippage. The hiatus must be closed after dissection to avoid herniation of viscera (this is a point of difference with the corresponding open technique).

The patient is positioned with legs spread so that the surgeon can stand comfortably between the legs and look directly up at the hiatus. Port placement depends on the habitus. It is easy to underestimate the distance to the hiatus and find that one's instruments do not reach. The camera port should be above the umbilicus, generally about two thirds of the distance down from the umbilicus to the xiphoid. Subsequent port placement can be informed by the initial view. Generally four more ports are required for retraction and dissection.

In contrast to the exposure used during open Nissen fundoplication, exposure of the hiatus is achieved by lifting the left lobe of the liver with a liver retractor. The peritoneum overlying the hiatus is divided and the esophagus mobilized. Dissection concentrates on working on both sides of the esophagus, avoiding the two vagal trunks, and progresses well up into the mediastinum. The esophagus is gently encircled and elevated. This maneuver must be done with care to avoid injury to the back wall of the esophagus (Fig. 10.1). Dissection proceeds until a generous length of esophagus has been mobilized into the abdomen. This also provides

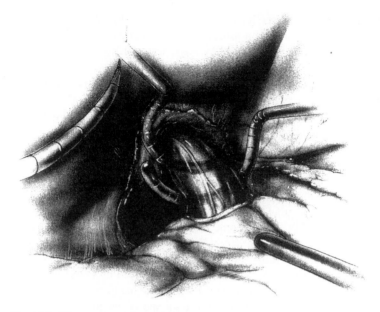

Fig. 10.1. The esophagus is gently retracted after adequate mobilization has been performed. Note the anterior vagal trunk visible on the surface. (From Scott-Conner CEH. Chassin's Operative Strategy in General Surgery: An Expositive Atlas, 3rd ed. New York: Springer-Verlag, 2001, with permission.)

a wide posterior window to admit the wrap. The esophageal hiatus is closed by approximating the crura behind the esophagus (Fig. 10.2).

The short gastric vessels are then divided. Generally the ultrasonic shears provide sufficient control. The stomach must be mobilized adequately to provide a floppy wrap. Passage of a 60-French mercury-weighted bougie assures that the wrap will not constrict the esophagus. I prefer to break scrub and pass the bougie myself. It is crucial that the esophagus be allowed to return to its normal position during this maneuver. If the esophagus is "tented up" by retraction, the bougie may perforate the back wall of the esophagus.

The stomach is then passed gently behind the esophagus and tested to see if the wrap will come together without tension. This wrap should encircle the vagal trunks. If it is difficult to pass the stomach behind the esophagus despite adequate division of the short gastric vessels, the posterior window must be enlarged.

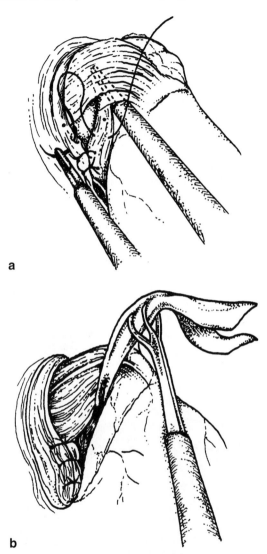

Fig. 10.2. (A) The hiatus is closed by approximating the crura behind the esophagus. (B) Generally three to six interrupted sutures of 0 silk are required. (From Scott-Conner CEH, ed. The SAGES Manual: Fundamentals of Laparoscopy, Thoracoscopy, and GI Endoscopy, 2nd ed. New York: Springer-Verlag, 2006, with permission.)

The wrap is secured with three or four interrupted sutures (Fig. 10.3). Pledgets may be used. The suture line generally comes to lie naturally facing the right side of the abdomen.

Life-threatening complications may occur. Esophageal perforation, if not immediately recognized and treated by suture and coverage with the wrap, is perhaps the most concerning. Insufflation of air into the distal esophagus with observation under saline for bubbles is an easy way to exclude full-thickness injury and should be part of the routine. Failure to adequately close the hiatus may allow small bowel or other viscera to herniate into the chest.

In summary, if this patient were referred to me, I would discuss laparoscopic fundoplication as an option but stress that an initial trial of medical management is preferable, and then review the situation in 6 months. If he failed medical management, additional workup including 24-hour pH

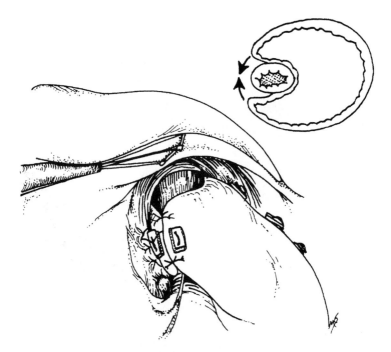

Fig. 10.3. Completed fundoplication. Inset shows proper orientation of the wrap. (From Scott-Conner CEH, ed. The SAGES Manual: Fundamentals of Laparoscopy, Thoracoscopy, and GI Endoscopy, 2nd ed. New York: Springer-Verlag, 2006, with permission.)

monitoring and esophageal motility studies would be required. Patient education materials, such as those produced by SAGES and accessible over the Web, are helpful in this discussion.

# D. Continued Medical Management

*Ross Meidinger*

Because this patient is being treated for the first time for GERD, has had an EGD that shows no esophagitis or metaplasia, and has had resolution of symptoms with proton pump inhibitor (PPI) treatment, there is no indication for surgical intervention at this time. Typical indications for surgical intervention include persistent or recurrent symptoms despite medical therapy, inability to tolerate medication, noncompliance with medication, severe esophagitis on endoscopy, Barrett's metaplasia, stricture development, or recurrent pulmonary symptoms such as asthma or aspiration pneumonia associated with GERD.

In this case as in most cases, GERD can be diagnosed on a clinical basis as heartburn and acid regurgitation, and treated empirically. Initiation of medical treatment usually involves a step-up or step-down approach along with lifestyle modifications. The step-up approach dictates starting a standard daily dose of a histamine-$H_2$ receptor antagonist ($H_2$ blocker) for an 8-week trial, and if symptoms do not resolve, progressing to twice-a-day dosing. If this is not effective, starting a daily PPI is indicated. If symptoms persist, twice-a-day PPI dosing should be tried. Proton pump inhibitors are typically taken 30 to 60 minutes before the first meal of the day (and 30 to 60 minutes before the evening meal for twice-a-day dosing) to allow absorption before stimulating gastric proton pumps with food. The step-down approach involves initiating treatment with a PPI for 8 weeks, and if symptoms are controlled, downgrading to an $H_2$ blocker. The goal is to find the lowest effective dose and type of medication to achieve symptom relief. The patient should continue this treatment for 8 weeks with a subsequent trial off of the treatment.

If symptoms recur in more than 3 months after stopping treatment, a repeat course of the previously effective treatment should be reinstituted, and another trial off of treatment should be attempted. If the patient continues to have recurrent symptoms, maintenance therapy should be initiated. If the patient has infrequent relapses, as-needed treatment is reasonable.

If symptoms recur in less than 3 months after stopping treatment, EGD should be considered for evaluation and maintenance therapy, with the previously effective treatment resumed and continued indefinitely. If recurrent symptoms of GERD persist despite maximum therapy, manometry and pH studies while on treatment should be considered for diagnosis confirmation. If studies show refractory GERD, the patient should be considered for antireflux surgery.

Along with medical treatment, the patient should always be educated about lifestyle modifications to reduce factors that may precipitate acid reflux. These include avoiding foods known to induce acid reflux by causing decreasing lower esophageal sphincter tone or spasm, such as fatty foods, spicy foods, chocolate, peppermint, alcohol, onion, garlic, and caffeinated beverages, and avoiding foods with an acidic pH that can exacerbate symptoms, such as citrus or tomato-based products, colas, and red wine. Patients are also encouraged to keep track of other foods that give them heartburn symptoms, and then avoid them. In addition, if patients complain of nocturnal symptoms, they should be instructed not to eat meals within 3 to 4 hours of bedtime and to elevate the head of their bed by placing 6- to 8-inch blocks under the legs at the head of the bed or by placing a Styrofoam wedge under the mattress. Increasing salivation by gum chewing and smoking cessation will help neutralize refluxed acid as well. Patients should be encouraged to avoid large meals, not to wear tight-fitting clothing around the waist, and to lose weight, as large meals, tight-fitting clothing, and being overweight can cause increased intraabdominal or intragastric pressure and increase reflux. Finally, patients should be cautioned about medications that can potentiate GERD symptoms due to their muscle relaxation effect on the lower esophagus and lower esophageal sphincter, such as calcium channel blockers, β-agonists, α-agonists, theophylline, and nitrates.

If the patient has had long-term symptoms (usually several years, as in the case presented here) with or without patient-directed therapy using antacids or over-the-counter acid suppressants, initial endoscopic assessment is indicated to exclude complications of GERD (Barrett's esophagus, stricture, esophagitis). When heartburn is uncontrolled by measures described above or is at any time accompanied by warning signs of more complicated disease such as dysphagia, odynophagia, bleeding, weight loss, or anemia, endoscopic evaluation is indicated.

Efficacy of the different classes of GERD treatment has been established in several studies. Antacids have been shown in two long-term trials to result in effective symptom relief in approximately 20% of patients using over-the-counter agents. However, they may be considered less effective than $H_2$ blockers in chronic GERD since their duration of action is much shorter. $H_2$ blockers have been shown to be effective for less severe cases of GERD, but even in divided doses are inferior to PPIs. DeVault and Castell reviewed the results of 33 randomized trials totaling over 3000 patients with erosive esophagitis, and found symptomatic relief in 27% of placebo-treated patients, 60% of $H_2$-blocker–treated patients, and 83% of PPI-treated patients. Esophagitis healed in 24% of the placebo treated, 50% of the $H_2$-blocker treated, and 78% of the PPI treated. These results suggest that initial treatment with a PPI may be indicated if esophagitis is present on EGD. Promotility agents may be considered as an adjunct in treating GERD, but currently are not recommended as monotherapy due to potential side effects and insufficient data to support their use.

Questions have been raised about the potential long-term consequences of PPIs for treatment of GERD. Concern has been raised about an increased incidence of pneumonia due to reduction in gastric acid, allowing pathogens to more easily colonize the upper gastrointestinal tract; however, this increased incidence has not been convincingly demonstrated in studies. It has been suggested that hypergastrinemia resulting from chronic acid suppression contributes to gastrocolic carcinomas, but the relationship has not been established since the introduction of this class of medications (omeprazole was approved by the Food and Drug Administration [FDA] in 1989). Similarly, the propensity of inducing chronic atrophic gastritis has been shown in long-term PPI use, but has not been shown to increase the risk of gastric cancer. Other data have suggested that PPIs can interfere with the absorption of vitamin $B_{12}$, but no clinical evidence has been established showing such nutritional deficiencies.

Because of high rates of recurrence, lifelong treatment may be needed if symptom relapse occurs within the first 3 months off of treatment, unless the patient opts for antireflux surgery after a thorough discussion of the associated risks and benefits.

It is unknown if surveillance endoscopy is indicated in patients treated for GERD with long-term maintenance therapy. It has been suggested that in patients without Barrett's esophagus on initial examination, the cancer risk may be too low to justify a follow-up endoscopy. Exceptions are patients who develop bleeding, dysphagia, or a significant change in symptoms while on effective therapy. Once-in-a-lifetime screening for Barrett's esophagus has been proposed for patients with GERD, but data supporting cost-effectiveness are lacking.

In summary, this patient with recently diagnosed GERD has responded well to medical therapy. The EGD did not show complications of GERD. Surgery intervention would not be warranted at this time.

# E. Conclusions

## Eric Wallace

Gastroesophageal reflux disease is one of the most common chronic disorders of the gastrointestinal tract, affecting an estimated 10% of the U.S. population. Most often, patients with GERD present with a long-standing history of heartburn, and perhaps a shorter history of regurgitation or dysphagia. Approximately 40% of patients with symptomatic GERD go on to develop reflux esophagitis. This can be complicated by bleeding, stricture, and Barrett's esophagus. The latter is a strong risk factor for esophageal adenocarcinoma (see also Chapter 12).

The diagnosis and treatment of GERD has advanced tremendously over the past several decades. Advances in the understanding of the pathophysiology of reflux as well as esophageal and gastric motility helped lay the foundation for today's management strategies. The introduction of new diagnostic modalities along with new pharmacologic agents ($H_2$ blockers, PPIs) and options for endoscopic (Stretta; see chapter 42) and surgical (fundoplication, open, or laparoscopic) treatment brings us to an exciting and sometimes confusing place when considering options for treatment of GERD.

Gastroesophageal reflux disease can be treated with medication or surgery. The medications available for management of GERD include antacids, motility agents, $H_2$ blockers, and PPIs. There is little doubt that the development of PPIs has been a revolution in the pharmacologic treatment of GERD. These drugs act by irreversibly binding the proton pump in the parietal cells in the stomach, thus effectively stopping gastric acid production. Compared with $H_2$ blockers, PPIs are more effective at healing esophageal ulceration secondary to acid exposure. They are relatively well tolerated, but are expensive. On the whole, patients with GERD consume over-the counter (OTC) therapies costing more than $1 billion per year , and among physician-prescribed medications the drugs used to treat GERD rank among the highest in sales. Figures vary, but Spelcher et al. (1992) estimated that the total cost for antacids and antisecretory medications probably tops $5 billion per year in the United States.

The mainstay of surgical therapy for GERD is the fundoplication. Although other options for endoscopic intervention exist (Stretta; see Chapter 42), this discussion focuses on fundoplication. Open fundoplication was first performed for GERD with reflux esophagitis in 1955 by Rudolph Nissen, and rapidly proved to be a reproducible and durable operation. Laparoscopic fundoplication was introduced in 1991, and performed by analogy with the open procedure. As with other minimally invasive techniques, laparoscopic fundoplication has been shown to provide lower wound-related morbidity, better cosmesis, a shorter hospital stay, and an earlier return to normal activity when compared to the open approach. These benefits, together with improvement in quality of life and possible elimination of the need for continuous pharmacologic treatment, demand that surgical treatment be considered in carefully selected patients with GERD.

In practice, once the diagnosis of GERD is suspected by history and physical examination, physicians may initiate a 4- to 8-week trial of empiric acid-suppressive therapy. The relief of symptoms with therapy and their return when therapy is discontinued are highly suggestive of GERD. There is no gold standard for diagnosing GERD, but 24-hour pH monitoring is considered by most to be the accepted standard for establishing or excluding its presence. Esophagogastroduodenoscopy is successful at identifying the esophageal complications of reflux, but lacks sensitivity for identifying pathologic reflux itself. Empiric treatment for GERD is usually performed using a step-up or step-down approach with the goal of complete, cost-effective symptom relief with the lowest effective dosage and type of medication. Diagnostic testing should be reserved for patients who present with early warning signs and symptoms (e.g., gastrointestinal bleeding), have not responded to PPI therapy, or have disease duration greater than 5 years.

A number of randomized controlled trials have shown that $H_2$ blockers are more effective at relieving heartburn than placebo in patients with GERD, with up to 70% of patients reported symptomatic relief within several weeks in most series. Chiba et al. performed a meta-analysis of 43 randomized controlled trials and confirmed that there was a larger rate of healing of erosive esophagitis in patients treated with $H_2$ blockers compared to placebo.

Similarly, Chiba et al. also demonstrated that evidence from several randomized controlled trials revealed that symptomatic relief of GERD is higher with PPIs (83%) compared to $H_2$ blockers (60%) or placebo (27%). In the treatment of erosive esophagitis, faster healing rates were achieved in patients who received PPI therapy (78%) than in patients who were given H$_2$ blockers (50%) or placebo (24%). In patients with chronic or complicated GERD, the potential benefit of long-term therapy with PPIs generally outweighs the risk of adverse events.

Consideration of antireflux surgery must be individualized. Indications for surgery include failed medical management, patient preference for surgery despite successful medical management, complications of GERD, medical complications attributable to a large hiatal hernia, or atypical symptoms with reflux documented on 24-hour pH monitoring. Several studies have shown that surgical treatment of GERD is superior to medical treatment in controlling GERD symptoms. One potential advantage of antireflux surgery is the elimination of the need for expensive, lifelong pharmacologic therapy. However, Spelcher et al. (2001) noted that a modest percentage of patients continue pharmacologic treatment for GERD postoperatively. Should the antireflux surgery be viewed as a failure if a patient's symptoms require resumption of medical treatment? Laparoscopic fundoplication has been successful in abolishing GERD symptoms in the vast majority of patients. Over 80% of patients can expect symptomatic relief.

Of course, laparoscopic antireflux surgery is not without complication, reportedly as high as 20% in some series. Dysphagia, gas bloat, and slippage of the wrap are all potential pitfalls of the surgical approach. More serious complications of perforation and death are extremely rare but must also be considered. Even with these potential complications, patient satisfaction is high when the symptoms of GERD are controlled.

As stated above, the indications for surgery for uncomplicated GERD are still controversial. However, a reasonable approach seems to be to limit surgical therapy to those patients with evidence of pathologic GERD, who are highly motivated to have surgery and have a realistic understanding of its benefits and potential risks. A patient with classic GERD symptoms who responds well to PPIs should continue medical therapy unless there is a compelling reason to discontinue it (e.g., medication cost or the persistence of disabling symptoms, such as severe regurgitation, which do not respond as well to PPIs as heartburn).

# References

Chiba N, De Gara CJ, Wilkinson JM, Hunt RH. Speed of healing and symptom relief in grade II to IV gastroesophageal reflux disease: a meta-analysis. Gastroenterology 1997;112:1798–1810.

DeVault KR, Castell DO. Updated guidelines for the diagnosis and treatment of gastro-esophageal reflux disease. The Practice Parameters Committee of the American College of Gastroenterology. Am J Gastroenterol 1999;94:1434–1442.

Peters JH, et al. The treatment of gastroesophageal reflux disease with Nissen fundoplication. Ann Surg 1998;228:40–50.

Spechler SJ, et al. Comparison of medical and surgical therapy for complicated gastro-esophageal reflux disease in veterans. N Engl J Med 1992;326:786–792.

Spelcher SJ, et al. Long-term outcome of medical and surgical therapies for gastroesopha-geal reflux disease. JAMA 2001;285:2331–2338.

Wileman SM, McLeer SK, Campbell MK, Mowat NAG, Krukowski ZH, Grant AM. Laparoscopic fundoplication versus medical management for gastro-oesphageal reflux disease in adults (Protocol). Cochrane Database of Systematic Reviews 2001;CD003243.

# Suggested Readings

Arguedas MR, Heudebert GR, Spechler SJ, et al. Re-examination of the cost-effectiveness of surgical versus medical therapy in patients with gastroesophageal reflux disease: the value of long-term data collection. Am J Gastroenterol 2004;99:1023–1028.

Behar J, et al. Medical and surgical reflux esophagitis. N Engl J Med 1975;293:263–268.

Bell RW, et al. Laparoscopic fundoplication for symptomatic but physiologic gastro-esophageal reflux. J Gastrointestinal Endosc 2001;5:462–467.

Catarci M, Gentileschi P, Papi C, et al. Evidence-based appraisal of antireflux fundoplica-tion. Ann Surg 2004;239:325–337.

Donnelan C, Sharma N, Preston C, Moayyedi P. Medical treatments for the maintenance therapy of reflux oesophagitis and endoscopic negative reflux disease. Cochrane Database of Systematic Reviews 2004;4:CD003245.

GERDsurgery.info. Information about GERD surgery (surgery for heartburn, antireflux surgery) brought to you by the Society of American Gastrointestinal and Endoscopic Surgeons (SAGES). http://www.gerdsurgery.info/.

Gregor J. Acid suppression and pneumonia. A clinical indication for rational prescribing. JAMA 2004;292(16):2012–2013.

Heidelbaugh JJ, Nostrant TT, Kim C, van Harrison R. Management of gastroesophageal reflux disease. Am Fam Physician 2003;68:1311–1318,1321–1322.

Inadomi JM, Sampliner R, Lagergren J, et al. Screening and surveillance for Barrett esophagus in high-risk groups: a cost-utility analysis. Ann Intern Med 2003;138(3):176–186.

Lundell L, et al. Continued followup of a randomized clinical study comparing antire-flux surgery and omeprazole in gastroesophageal reflux disease. J Am Coll Surg 2001;192:1722–1729.

Mattioli S. Indications for anti-reflux surgery in gastro-oesophageal reflux disease. Ali-ment Pharmacol Ther 2003;2:60–67.

Papasavas PK, et al. Effectiveness of laparoscopic fundoplication in relieving the symptoms of gastroesophageal reflux disease and eliminating antireflux medical therapy. Surg Endosc 2003;17:1200–1205.

SAGES Guidelines for Surgical Treatment of Gastroesophageal Reflux Disease (GERD). http://www.sages.org/sagespublication.php?doc=22.

# 11. Partial or Complete Fundoplication for Gastroesophageal Reflux Disease

## A. Introduction

Laparoscopic fundoplication was initially patterned after the highly successful open Nissen fundoplication, which produces a complete 360-degree wrap. As experience with the operation progressed, several alternative partial fundoplications were devised. These included the Toupet (a posterior fundoplication very similar to the Nissen but only encompassing 270 degrees) and the Dor (an anterior fundoplication used primarily during surgery for achalasia) procedures. This chapter explores the issue of complete versus partial fundoplication in an otherwise uncomplicated case of gastroesophageal reflux disease (GERD).

## B. Case

*Christopher M. Simons*

A 44-year-old man was referred for surgical management of GERD. He had been experiencing burning retrosternal pain for about 1 year. This occurred after almost every meal. He also noted that he periodically could taste stomach contents in the back of his throat. He had lost 15 pounds, and tried lifestyle changes such as elevating the head of his bed and avoiding alcohol. Cardiac causes for his pain had been ruled out with an electrocardiogram (ECG) and exercise stress test. His physician put him on an $H_2$ blocker, and when that did not help, a proton pump inhibitor (PPI). The PPI provided relief for about 6 months, but then his symptoms recurred. A recent esophagogastroduodenoscopy demonstrated grade 2 (Savary-Miller) esophagitis. Esophageal manometry showed decreased lower esophageal sphincter pressure. A double-contrast barium study did not show any evidence of peptic stricture.

The patient's medical history was significant for hypertension and elevated serum lipids. He had had an appendectomy and a laparoscopic cholecystectomy. He was married, worked as a police officer, did not drink alcoholic beverages, and stopped smoking 5 years ago after a 23-pack-year smoking history.

The physical examination found the patient to be mildly hypertensive at 145/83. He was 6 feet 2 inches in height and weighed 90 kg. His abdomen was soft with a well-healed McBurney incision and trocar sites from his laparoscopic cholecystectomy. He had no masses or tenderness. The remainder of the examination, including rectal exam, was negative. Laboratory studies were unremarkable.

The impression was that he would benefit from laparoscopic fundoplication. **Would you suggest a complete or a partial fundoplication?**

# C. Complete (360-Degree) Fundoplication

## David Duppler

I would suggest a complete fundoplication. This procedure was first described by Rudolph Nissen in 1956. Although originally performed via the open approach, the technique has subsequently been adapted to the laparoscopic approach, first described by Dallemagne in 1991. It is the most commonly performed antireflux procedure, with multiple publications attesting to its effectiveness and durability.

The Nissen fundoplication, as originally described, sometimes causes dysphagia and gas bloat syndrome. In an effort to alleviate these problems partial fundoplications were developed, such as those described by Toupet, Guarner, and Belsey. Subsequent modifications to the Nissen fundoplication by Donahue and DeMeester, who described the construction of a short, floppy fundoplication, were also intended to alleviate these postoperative problems. There has continued to be controversy as to whether the total fundoplication as it is now performed or some type of partial fundoplication is the proper choice for patients undergoing antireflux surgery.

In close comparison to the Nissen fundoplication, the partial fundoplications have been proven to be less effective in controlling gastroesophageal reflux and do have similar side effects profiles. Farrell et al. compared 465 patients with normal esophageal motility who underwent Nissen fundoplication with 44 patients with abnormal motility who underwent Toupet fundoplication. Although heartburn rates were similar in both groups at 6 weeks, at 1 year the Toupet group had a higher incidence of both heartburn (18% to 8%, $p < .05$) and regurgitation (20% to 8%, $p = .06$) than the Nissen group. The dysphagia rates were similar in both groups. Fernando et al. followed cohorts of patients who underwent Nissen fundoplication ($n = 114$) and Toupet fundoplication ($n = 28$) for a mean of 19.7 months. The Toupet group had a higher incidence of dysphagia (34.5% vs. 15%, $p$ <.05) and postoperative PPI use (38% vs. 20%, $p$ <.05). When comparing the patients with impaired esophageal motility who had undergone the two procedures, they found no difference in quality of life indicators between the two groups. When comparing patients with normal esophageal motility, however, they found significantly worse quality of life scores in the Toupet group compared to the Nissen group. They also found no difference in postoperative bloating, early satiety, increased flatulence, and diarrhea between the two groups.

Patti and colleagues analyzed 357 patients who had undergone laparoscopic antireflux surgery. Group 1 was comprised of 94 patients with normal esophageal motility who had a Nissen fundoplication performed and 141 patients with decreased esophageal motility who underwent a 240-degree fundoplication. Group 2 was a later group of 122 patients who had a Nissen fundoplication performed irrespective of their preoperative motility findings. The average follow-up was 23 ± 10 months. In group 1, the partial fundoplication patients had a higher incidence of heartburn than the Nissen patients (33% vs. 15%, $p$ = .003). The incidence of dysphagia (partial 8% vs. Nissen 11%, nonsignificant [NS]), and the dysphagia score (partial 2.3 ± 1.1 vs. Nissen 2.2 ± 1.0, NS) were similar. In group 2, patients with weak peristalsis who underwent Nissen fundoplication had a similar incidence of heartburn (15% vs. 13%, NS), dysphagia (9% vs. 7%, NS), and dysphagia score (2.4 ± 1.1 vs. 2.0 ± 1.2, NS) when compared to those with normal preoperative peristalsis. In comparing the patients with weak peristalsis who had partial fundoplications in group 1 with patients with weak peristalsis who had Nissen fundoplications in group 2, the incidence of dysphagia (8% vs. 9%, NS) was similar, as was the dysphagia score (2.3 ± 1.1 vs. 2.4 ± 1.1, NS). However, the incidence of heartburn in the partial fundoplication group was significantly higher (33% vs. 13%, $p$ = .006). This led their group to conclude that total fundoplication is superior to partial fundoplication, even in patients with diminished esophageal peristalsis.

Chrysos et al. randomly assigned 33 consecutive patients with decreased esophageal peristalsis to either Nissen fundoplication (NF) or Toupet fundoplication (TF). Although the TF group had a lower incidence of gas bloat syndrome (21% vs. 50%) and dysphagia (16% vs. 57%) than the NF group at 3 months, by 12 months the differences had disappeared (gas bloat syndrome: NF 21% vs. TF 16%; dysphagia: NF 14% vs. TF 16%). All patients in both groups had control of reflux symptoms.

Ravi and colleagues studied 98 patients undergoing total fundoplication. Group 1 ($n$ = 60) had normal esophageal motility and group 2

($n = 38$) had dysmotility. At 6 months, the incidence of dysphagia, regurgitation, and heartburn were similar with 88% of the group 1 patients and 89% of the group 2 patients having no symptoms or minor symptoms not requiring medication; 89% of group 1 patients and 92% of group 2 patients consider their results good or excellent. Both group had similar improvement in their quality of life scores. pH studies showed improvement in both groups with the DeMeester score decreasing from 36 to 2.5 in group 1 and 53 to 4.2 in group 2. Of interest is the fact that motility reverted to normal in 53% of the group 2 patients. The authors concluded that good outcomes with improved quality of life after a Nissen fundoplication is equally achieved in patients with esophageal dysmotility and in patients with normal motility.

Jobe and colleagues studied 100 consecutive patients who underwent laparoscopic Toupet fundoplication for confirmed GERD. Seventy-four patients presented for follow-up at 22 months. Of these patients, 20% reported recurrence of heartburn. Ten patients with heartburn and 31 asymptomatic patients underwent postoperative pH studies. Nine of 10 symptomatic patients and 12 of 31 asymptomatic patients had positive pH studies and elevated DeMeester scores, for a total of 51% abnormal pH studies. This high failure rate led authors to conclude they could not recommend Toupet fundoplication in uncomplicated GERD.

In summary, the literature appears to support the idea that total fundoplication is superior to partial fundoplication in patients with uncomplicated GERD, even when esophageal dysmotility is present. Although partial fundoplication may play a role in patients with severe esophageal motility disorders, such as achalasia and scleroderma, the choice of Nissen fundoplication appears to be appropriate for most patients undergoing antireflux surgery.

# D.  Partial Fundoplication

## *Michael Cook and William Richardson*

This patient, like most patients referred for surgical correction of gastroesophageal reflux, has already failed maximal medical management, including medication (with $H_2$ blockers followed by PPIs), diet modification (bland diet, avoiding alcohol and caffeine), and behavioral modification (weight loss, elevation of head of bed). A thorough workup has been done and no further tests are necessary. For patients refractory to medical treatment, two common surgical options exist: a 360-degree, or complete fundoplication; and a partial fundoplication, of which the most commonly used is the Toupet fundoplication. As the argument for a complete fundoplication has already been made, this section discusses the reasoning behind performing a partial fundoplication in the selected patient. Although there is a trend in the recent literature toward the use of a 360-degree fundoplication for all patients with reflux, the data are inconclusive. This is also a dramatic change from the earlier dogma that the choice of fundoplication should be tailored to the individual patient. The argument in favor of a partial wrap centers on two issues: the adverse side effects of a full wrap, and the definition of treatment failure for a partial fundoplication.

The biggest drawbacks to complete fundoplication are the relatively high incidences of dysphagia, the inability to belch or vomit, and increased flatus for the first year after surgery. Several studies have even shown better control of heartburn with a partial wrap. Hagedorn et al. reported a randomized trial showing control of heartburn in 92% of partial fundoplication patients as compared to 88% of those undergoing full wraps. Five Nissen patients required reoperation in this study, whereas only two Toupet patients were taken back for revision. While all fundoplications generate some dysphagia related to swelling as a result of the surgery, this tends to be more severe with a total wrap. Furthermore, odynophagia, rectal flatus, and postprandial fullness were more common in the total fundoplication group. Several studies have noted increased dysphagia with Nissen fundoplication in comparison to partial fundoplication. Although most but not all clinically significant dysphagia does resolve or improve within the first year postoperatively, this is very disturbing for the patient and occasionally leads to the need for early reoperation for severe dysphagia.

Partial fundoplication has been advocated as a more physiologic antireflux procedure. While both types of fundoplication are similar in restoring the resting lower esophageal sphincter pressure (one of the dominant abnormalities in patients with GERD), Chrysos et al. note that only the Nissen fundoplication increases intragastric pressures in the postprandial state. This is likely the reason why patients often experience a sensation of bloating, inability to belch, and increased flatulence after complete fundoplication. In patients with normal peristalsis, Zornig et al. showed recurrent reflux in 8% of patients after Toupet fundoplication and 4% after Nissen (no statistically significant difference), while the dysphagia rates were 6% and 32% respectively ($p < .01$). More importantly patient satisfaction scores were similar in both groups.

Since a full wrap adds approximately 10 mm Hg to the lower esophageal sphincter (LES) pressure, it seems logical that at some point patients with low esophageal peristaltic pressure will not be able to push a bolus of food past the gastroesophageal (GE) junction. Randomized studies in patients with decreased peristalsis have shown increased rates of postoperative dysphagia at 3 months after Nissen fundoplication as compared to Toupet fundoplication (57% vs. 16%, respectively). However, the rates are equivalent at 1 year follow-up, suggesting that there is no need to tailor surgery based on manometric findings. Partial fundoplication has begun to fall out of favor for patients with weakened peristalsis, but most surgeons still feel that a partial wrap is the procedure of choice for the severe dysmotility disorders such as scleroderma or achalasia (in combination with esophageal myotomy).

The final argument in favor of partial fundoplication involves the need to reevaluate the definition of a treatment failure. In addition to the obvious failures such as slipped and herniated wraps, most documented failures of fundoplication include the need to restart medical therapy and the presence of abnormal postoperative pH studies. However, if our goal is patient satisfaction, prevention of long-term sequelae, or the ability to control patients' symptoms, many reported failures of partial wraps would no longer be considered as such. Lundell noted that some studies have documented recurrence of reflux in as many as 50% to 60% of patients after fundoplication of any type. With long-term patient satisfaction scores of 90% to 95% after total fundoplication and 85% to 90% after partial fundoplication, it is likely that not all recurrent reflux translates into significant symptoms. Allowing a patient who has severe reflux on maximal medical therapy preoperatively to be controlled with medication postoperatively should be considered a success, even if it is not the ideal scenario.

Taking only the European literature into account, there is a clear advantage to partial over complete fundoplication. While the long-term results of other studies show somewhat better control of reflux with a Nissen fundoplication, overall patient satisfaction is excellent for both types of wrap. Furthermore, Nissen fundoplication causes significantly higher rates of gas bloat, flatulence, and dysphagia during the first year after surgery as compared to Toupet fundoplication. This is important because some patients require revision for severe dysphagia. Therefore, partial fundoplication is at least a viable option for our patient (if not the preferred option), as he will likely have excellent long-term results with fewer adverse symptoms in the early postoperative period.

# E. Conclusions

## *Christopher M. Simons*

Gastroesophageal reflux disease is a common medical condition that affects about 30% of Western populations a minimum of once per month. The usual symptoms are chest pain, regurgitation, dysphagia, and heartburn; complications of long-standing GERD include Barrett's esophagus and stricture. The advent of medications such as $H_2$ blockers and PPIs has made it possible for many GERD patients to live symptom-free lives. Unfortunately, some GERD patients have disease that proves refractory to medical management that includes both lifestyle changes and pharmaceuticals. For these patients, surgery presents the best option for eliminating their symptoms.

In 1956, the Swiss surgeon Rudolf Nissen described a fundoplication, which consisted of a 360-degree wrap of the cardia of the stomach around the lower esophageal sphincter. The aim was to create a valve that would prevent acid reflux and alleviate symptoms. This operation was not without side effects, the most notable being what came to be known as gas bloat syndrome: postoperative dysphagia, bloating, and the inability to vomit or belch. Through the years, multiple modifications of Nissen's original procedure have been crafted in an attempt to alleviate these postoperative side effects. Many of these procedures centered on performing a partial wrap instead of the full 360-degree wrap. In 1991, antireflux surgery entered a new era as surgeons started to perform laparoscopic Nissen fundoplications, and now the laparoscopic approach to antireflux surgery has largely replaced the open operation in centers throughout the world.

Multiple studies have demonstrated both the safety and efficacy of laparoscopic antireflux surgery. These trials have typically included both functional and symptomatic outcomes. Functional outcomes are usually determined by comparing preoperative and postoperative esophageal manometry and 24-hour pH monitoring. Symptomatic outcomes typically include the evaluation of subjective complaints such as heartburn, regurgitation, and chest pain both before and after the operation.

While laparoscopic antireflux surgery has been proven both effective and safe, the subset of patients with diminished esophageal motility poses a conundrum. A hypothesis is that these patients are more prone to suffer postoperative obstructive complications after they undergo a total wrap. Therefore, the idea of tailoring antireflux surgery has gained favor. Currently, there are advocates for both laparoscopic total fundoplication and laparoscopic partial fundoplication in these patients. The main issue is whether or not a partial wrap lessens the likelihood of postoperative dysphagia and other obstructive difficulties in those with decreased esophageal motility.

Rydberg studied 106 patients, with 53 randomized to either a Nissen-Rossetti total fundic wrap or a Toupet partial, posterior fundic wrap. Patients with normal and impaired motility were included and motility was not used to determine what operation a particular patient received. The entire study population was evaluated postoperatively for a total of 3 years. The outcomes of heartburn, acid regurgitation, dysphagia, distention, flatulence, and 24-hour pH monitoring (% time pH <4) were similarly improved at 3 years in both arms of the study. For this reason, the authors questioned the utility of preoperative esophageal manometry for the purpose of tailoring antireflux surgery because both operations had similar results whether or not the patient had preoperative impaired esophageal motility.

Another prospective study that included 200 patients randomized to either a Nissen or Toupet fundoplication also discounted the necessity of tailoring antireflux surgery (Zornig et al.). This study was different in that each arm included 50 patients with normal esophageal motility and 50 with impaired motility. The study found that at 4 months 88% of the Nissen patients and 90% of the Toupet patients were pleased with the results from the operation, but swallowing difficulties were more common in the Nissen patients. While both operations proved equally effective for reflux control, the study found that postoperative complaints of dysphagia were just as frequent in the patients with normal motility as in those with impaired motility. This confuses the issue of whether or not there is a causal relationship between postoperative dysphagia and preoperative decreased esophageal motility.

An additional randomized study that compared Nissen and Toupet operations in 33 patients with impaired esophageal motility exclusively included 1 year of follow-up and showed that both operations were equally efficacious in the control of reflux (Chrysos et al.). At 3 months, dysphagia and gas-bloat syndrome were more common in the Nissen group, but at 1 year the incidence had fallen to where there was no difference between the Nissen and Toupet arms.

Hagedorn et al. reported another randomized, controlled clinical trial comparing the Nissen-Rossetti and the Toupet approaches with regard to the long-term management of GERD. This study differed from those mentioned previously in that the follow-up period spanned 11.5 years, and the procedures were done open rather than laparoscopically.

The study included 132 patients (65 randomized to Nissen and 67 to Toupet) and showed efficacy and decreased postoperative gas-bloat in the Toupet arm. This study did not look at patients with diminished preoperative esophageal motility exclusively.

In conclusion, GERD is a common disease with repercussions that can drastically affect the quality of life for the afflicted patients. Laparoscopic antireflux surgery has provided another avenue for those patients whose disease proves refractory to both lifestyle changes and medications. Studies have demonstrated the safety and efficacy of laparoscopic antireflux surgery. The prevailing thought has been that patients with preoperative diminished esophageal motility are more likely to suffer postoperative dysphagia and bloating after a Nissen. In an attempt to answer this question, head-to-head trials have been done to determine whether total or partial wraps have less postoperative complications with regard to dysphagia and bloating. The evidence is mixed as some studies show that total wraps are effective with minimal side effects in patients with impaired motility, while others have shown that these patients benefit from a partial wrap because of decreased postoperative obstruction symptoms. It appears that partial wrap patients may have less postoperative symptoms in the first few months after surgery, but by 1 year the incidence of these problems in the total wrap patients approaches those of the partial wrap. A definitive answer to this question remains elusive. At this time, either wrap may benefit a patient regardless of preoperative esophageal motility.

# References

Arguedas MR, Heudebert GR, Klapow JC, et al. Re-examination of the cost-effectiveness of surgical versus medical therapy in patients with gastroesophageal reflux disease: the value of long-term data collection. Am J Gastroenterol 2004;99(6):1023–1028.

Christian DJ, Buyske J. Current status of antireflux surgery. Surg Clin N Am 2005;85: 931–947.

Chrysos E, Tsiaoussis J, Zoras OJ, et al. Laparoscopic surgery for gastroesophageal reflux disease patients with impaired esophageal peristalsis: total or partial fundoplication? J Am Coll Surg 2003;197(1):8–15.

Dallemagne B, Weerts JM, Jehaes C. Laparoscopic Nissen fundoplication: preliminary report. Surg Laparosc Endosc 1991;1:138–143.

DeMeester TR, Bonavina L, Albertucci M. Nissen fundplication for gastroesophageal reflux disease. Evaluation of primary repair in 100 consecutive patients. Ann Surg 1986;204:9–20.

Donahue PE, Samelson S, Nyhus L, et al. The floppy Nissen fundoplication. Arch Surg 1985;120:663–667.

Farrell TM, Archer SB, Galloway KD. Heartburn is more frequent after Toupet fundoplication than Nissen fundoplication. Am Surg 2000;66:229–235.

Fernando HC, Luketich JD, Chritie NA, et al. Outcomes of laparoscopic Nissen fundoplication. Surg Endosc 2002;16:905–908.

Guarner V, Degollade JR, Tore NM. A new antireflux procedure at the esophagogastric junction: experimental and clinical evaluation. Arch Surg 1975;110:101–106.

Hagedorn C, et al. Long-term efficacy of total (Nissen-Rossetti) and posterior partial (Toupet) fundoplication: results of a randomized clinical trial. J Gastrointest Surg 2002;6(4):540–545.

Hinder RA, Filipi CJ, Wetscher G, et al. Laparoscopic Nissen fundoplication is an effective treatment for gastroesophageal reflux disease. Ann Surg 1994;220:472–483.

Hunter JG, Trus TL, Branum GD, et al. A physiologic approach to laparoscopic fundoplication for gastroesophageal reflux disease. Ann Surg 1996;223:673–687.

Jobe BA, Wallace J, Hansen PD, et al. Evaluation of laparscopic Toupet fundoplication as a primary repair for all patients with medically resistant gastroesophageal reflux. Surg Endosc 1997;11:1080–1083.

Limpert PA, Naunheim KS. Partial versus complete fundoplication: Is there a correct answer. Surg Clin N Am 399–410.

Lundell L. Continued (5–year) followup of a randomized clinical study comparing antireflux surgery and omeprazole in gastroesophageal reflux disease. J Am Coll Surg 2001;192:172–181.

Nissen R, Eine E, Einfat HE. Operation zur Beeinflussung der R drfluxochtitis [surgery to influence reflux esophagitis]. Schweiz Med Wochenschr 1956;86:590–592 (in German).

Patti MG, Robinson T, Galvani C, et al. Total fundoplication is superior to partial fundoplication even when esophageal peristalsis is weak. J Am Coll Surg 2004;198;6.

Ravi N, Al-Sarraf N, Morant, et al. Acid normalization and improved esophageal motility after Nissen fundoplication: equivalent outcomes in patients with normal and ineffective esophageal motility. Am J Surg 2005;190(3):445–450.

Ritter MP, Peters JH, DeMeester TR, et al. Outcome after laparoscopic fundoplication is not dependent on a structurally defective lower esophageal sphincter. J Gastrointest Surg 1998;6:567–571.

Rydberg L. Tailoring antireflux surgery: a randomized clinical trial. World J Surg 1999;23(6):612–18.

Toupet A. Technic of esophago-gastroplasty with phreno-gastropexy used in radical treatment of hiatal hernias as a supplement to Hellers operation in cardiospasms [in French]. Mem Acad Chir (Paris) 1963;89:384–389.

Zornig C, Strate U, Fibbe C, et al. Nissen vs. Toupet laparoscopic fundoplication: a prospective randomized study of 200 patients with and without preoperative esophageal motility disorders. Surg Endosc 2002;16:758–766.

# Suggested Readings

Chrysos E. The effect of total and anterior partial fundoplication on antireflux mechanisms of the gastroesophageal junction. Am J Surg 2004;188(1):39–44.

Granderath A, Kamolz T, Schweiger U, Pointner R. Laparoscopic antireflux surgery for gastroesophageal reflux disease: experience with 668 laparoscopic antireflux procedures. Int J Colorectal Dis 2003;18:73–77.

Hunter JG. Laparoscopic fundoplication failures: patterns of failure and response to fundoplication revision. Ann Surg 1999;230(4):595–604; discussion 604–606.

Kamolz T, Bammer T, Wykypiel H, et al. Quality of life and surgical outcome after laparoscopic Nissen and Toupet fundoplication: one-year follow-up. Endoscopy 2000;32(5):362–368.

Limpert PA. Partial versus complete fundoplication: is there a correct answer? Surg Clin North Am 2005;85(3):399–410.

Swanstrom L. Partial fundoplications for gastroesophageal reflux disease: indications and current status. J Clin Gastroenterol 1999;29(2):127–132.

Zornig C, Strate U, Fibbe C, et al. Nissen vs. Toupet laparoscopic fundoplication: a prospective randomized study of 200 patients with and without preoperative esophageal motility disorders. Surg Endosc 2002;16:758–766.

# 12. Barrett's Esophagus with High-Grade Dysplasia

## A. Introduction

When Barrett's esophagus (BE) complicates gastroesophageal reflux disease (GERD), is carcinoma far behind? The finding of high-grade dysplasia in this setting increases the stakes for adequate management of GERD and raises the possibility that a more definitive management strategy—surgical resection—might be required. This chapter explores options for the treatment of an older male patient with multiple comorbidities, in whom this condition is found.

## B. Case

*John Leung*

A 67-year-old man was referred for management of his BE. He has had GERD for more than 10 years, and his symptoms had been well controlled with omeprazole 40 mg PO qd until 2 years ago. At that time, he had persistent heartburn, sometimes accompanied by a bitter taste in the back of his throat, and regurgitation. His symptoms were worsened after larger meals or while he was lying in his bed at night. His primary care physician intensified his omeprazole to twice-a-day dosing and ordered a screening upper endoscopy to rule out complications of GERD. The upper endoscopy was negative for dysplasia. However, a recent repeat screening endoscopy did show focal high-grade dysplasia despite the patient's being symptom-free since he was switched to omeprazole b.i.d. 2 years ago.

The patient denied any heartburn, dysphagia, upper gastrointestinal (GI) bleeding, melena, hematochezia, weight loss, anorexia, chest pain, shortness of breath, or night sweats. He denied any change in his bowel habits. He had 30-degree orthopnea and could barely walk up two flights of stairs without shortness of breath or chest pain. He denied chest pain at rest.

His past medical history was significant for GERD, hypertension, myocardial infarction 5 years ago status post–five-vessel bypass, and mild congested heart failure. His family history was non-contributory.

His medications include aspirin 81 mg PO qd, metoprolol 50 mg PO b.i.d., lisinopril 10 mg PO qd, Lasix 20 mg PO qd, and omeprazole 40 mg PO b.i.d.

The patient is a retired accountant who lives independently. He had a 100-pack smoking history and denied any alcohol or illicit drug use.

On physical examination, he is an alert and obese Caucasian gentleman in no acute distress. His temperature is 36.7 °C, pulse 85, blood pressure 155/80, respiratory rate 14, and body mass index (BMI) 38. His head, ears, eyes, nose, and throat (HEENT) exam was unremarkable. There was no cervical or supraclavicular lymphadenopathy. Cardiac exam showed regular rate and rhythm without any murmur or gallops. His lungs were clear to auscultation without any wheezes, rales, or crackles. There was no tenderness on deep palpation of his abdomen, and no hepatosplenomegaly. He had good distal pulses and trace bilateral lower extremity edema. Rectal exam was normal and stool guaiac is negative. Complete blood count, liver function test, and electrolytes are within normal limits.

On review of his diagnostic studies, an initial screening esophagogastroduodenoscopy (EGD) 2 year ago was unremarkable. There was no evidence of dysplasia or malignancy on multiple biopsies. However, a recent EGD showed columnar epithelium lining a short segment of the distal esophagus, and biopsy revealed a focus of high-grade dysplasia.

**What would you recommend—surgical management, endoscopic mucosal ablation, or intensive medical management and surveillance?**

# C. Surgical Management

*Robert W. O'Rourke and John G. Hunter*

Treatment options for patients with GERD and BE have expanded greatly in the last decade, and now include medical, surgical, and endoscopic ablative and mucosal resection therapies. As underlying technologies advance, the roles of each of these treatment modalities in the management of BE will change, complicating choices for physicians and patients. The rapidity of technologic progress combined with the practical obstacles to designing large trials of BE treatment options makes rigorous prospective comparative study of optimal therapy difficult. Despite these challenges, medical, endoscopic, and surgical therapies play important and complementary roles in the treatment of BE. It is therefore important to define consensus roles for each in the management of specific subsets of patients with GERD and BE.

One of the challenges in achieving such a consensus is the clinical heterogeneity of this patient population. Barrett's esophagus may be a sole endoscopic finding, or occur along with esophagitis, stricture, ulcer, or dysplasia. Patients with dysplasia may have low-grade dysplasia (LGD) or high-grade dysplasia (HGD). Dysplasia may be focal or diffuse, and may occur on a background of short-segment or long-segment BE. Other important patient subsets to consider that are beyond the scope of this discussion include patients with localized invasive esophageal adenocarcinoma (T1a, T1b disease) and patients with intestinal metaplasia of the cardia.

The patient presented here has a long history of GERD. His symptoms worsened recently, requiring increased proton pump inhibitor (PPI) dosing. A recent endoscopy demonstrated BE and dysplasia. He has a history of coronary artery disease, has undergone coronary artery bypass, and has a long smoking history. Further management is dictated by the histology of the dysplasia. The preferred treatment in the case of HGD is laparoscopic transhiatal esophagectomy, and in the case of LGD, antireflux surgery.

It is well accepted that BE is a premalignant precursor of esophageal adenocarcinoma, and high-grade dysplasia is a final stage in the progression of BE to cancer. The diagnosis of HGD imparts a significant risk of harboring or developing adenocarcinoma of the esophagus. Accurate diagnosis of HGD is complicated by biopsy sampling error and pathologist concordance, such that anywhere from 15% to 65% of patients with HGD may harbor synchronous occult invasive cancer (Fernando et al., Sujendran et al., Tseng et al.). Of those who presumably do not have cancer at diagnosis, at least 50% of patients progress to invasive cancer within 3 years (Weston et al.). Longer follow-up is associated with even higher rates of disease progression, and as natural history data accumulate it is becoming clear that the majority of patients with HGD eventually develop cancer (Reid et al.).

Accurate clinical predictors of risk for cancer in patients with HGD have yet to be defined. Given the high risk of cancer and the current inability to risk-stratify patients, total esophagectomy is the treatment of choice and the only reliable means of cure for patients with HGD. In the past, this management strategy was well accepted. The recent introduction of high-dose PPI therapy with surveillance, as well as endoscopic ablative and resection techniques, has complicated management of these patients, however. The search for alternatives to surgical therapy is driven in a large part by the significant morbidity and mortality historically associated with esophagectomy. Centralization of care at high-volume centers and recent advances in surgical technique impact on these considerations.

High-dose PPI therapy with frequent surveillance is advocated for patients with BE and HGD by select groups with significant experience with this approach (Schnell et al.). Proponents argue that HGD may regress with PPI therapy (although regression in some cases may be attributable to biopsy sampling error or variability in histologic analysis), and that delayed esophageal resection in patients who are eventually given a diagnosis of invasive cancer has not been demonstrated to impact upon survival. Others, however, have reported significant rates of cancer development even with appropriate surveillance (Weston et al.), and have noted that little published data supports intensive surveillance for HGD (Spechler). Despite pioneering efforts by groups with experience with this approach, intensive surveillance is cumbersome, requires specific institutional expertise, and entails significant resource expenditure. Investigators have shown that compliance with surveillance may be quite poor (<50%) at centers without experience in this approach (Thomas et al.). In addition, the emotional stress associated with frequent surveillance may lead some patients to prefer esophagectomy despite its incumbent risk. For these reasons, this approach has yet to be embraced by the medical community as a whole, and therefore represents a preferred alternative to surgery only in patients who present excessive operative risk or who refuse surgery, and who have access to a center with expertise and resources in this area. These constraints have limited widespread application of this management strategy.

A variety of endoscopic ablative and resection techniques are currently being applied to patients with BE and HGD, and include photodynamic therapy (Hage et al.), argon plasma coagulation (Hage et al.), radiofrequency-based ablation (Salameh et al.), and endoscopic mucosal resection (May et al.). While such technologies likely represent the future of treatment for HGD, they have yet to meet this promise. Evaluation of the results of endoscopic therapies is difficult, as a complete posttreatment specimen is usually not available to determine the extent of disease and the success of ablation or resection. Recurrence rates and incomplete resection rates of endoscopic mucosal resection for patients with HGD may be as high as 25% (May et al.) and 80% (Lewis et al.), respectively, and the current lack of controlled, randomized, long-term follow-up data for all endoscopic treatments confounds analysis of efficacy (Faybush and Sampliner). The main concerns with all endoscopic techniques include failure to remove or ablate all affected mucosa, "buried BE," and the inability to accurately determine the presence of residual disease. In addition, patients with HGD who harbor occult nodal disease or invasive cancer are not effectively treated with endoscopic ablative or resection procedures. Patient selection therefore remains problematic. These problems limit the use of endoscopic procedures for HGD outside of the clinical trial setting. The primary questions that must be addressed before widespread application of these techniques in patients with HGD include the identification of accurate predictors of nodal disease and invasive cancer to allow proper patient selection, and verification of complete ablation or resection of all diseased tissue. Once these challenges are met, endoscopic techniques have the potential to be primary therapy for select patients with HGD.

The most commonly applied surgical therapy for HGD is total esophagectomy. Some investigators have suggested a role for limited surgical resection in such patients, however, including distal esophagectomy with either primary esophagoesophageal anastomosis or ileal interposition. These operations may be associated with less perioperative morbidity compared to total esophagectomy, and allow for preservation of the vagus nerves and the gastric reservoir, which may reduce long-term morbidity (Stein et al.). Few data exist that support these alternative surgical approaches to HGD, however, or definitively demonstrate lower morbidity. Partial esophageal resection also does not address concerns regarding a "field effect" for the development of dysplasia, and the natural history of such patients with respect to the development of dysplasia and cancer in the remnant esophagus remain poorly defined. Such approaches, therefore, while promising, require further study.

Total transhiatal esophagectomy represents the preferred treatment for HGD. The primary criticism lodged against esophagectomy as first-line therapy in such patients is that historically, associated morbidity and mortality are significant. Recent advances have led to improved results after esophagectomy, however. Results are significantly better at high-volume centers (Birkmeyer et al., Casson and van Lanschot), suggesting that centralization of these complex procedures at specialized centers will reduce postoperative morbidity and mortality. Advances in surgical technique have also resulted in improved outcomes. The introduction of laparoscopic transhiatal esophagectomy represents the most important recent technical advance. While prospective comparative data is lacking, data from centers with significant expertise suggest that a laparoscopic approach may be associated with lower morbidity and mortality than an open approach when compared to historical controls (Luketich et al.). As experience and prospective randomized data accumulate, the benefits of a laparoscopic approach to esophagectomy will be better delineated. Other pioneering efforts include the introduction of vagus-sparing esophagectomy, which may reduce long-term morbidity and improve quality of life (Banki et al.). These techniques are currently limited by a lack of long-term outcome data and concerns regarding oncologic soundness in the subset of patients who harbor invasive cancer and occult nodal disease. Improvement in preoperative determination of invasive and nodal disease, and accumulation of long-term outcome data, will define the role of such promising surgical modifications in reducing postoperative morbidity after esophagectomy. Finally, patients with HGD seem to enjoy a lower mortality, and possibly lower morbidity as well, after esophagectomy, than patients with invasive cancer (Thomas et al., Thomson and Cade, Tseng et al.), and long-term quality-of-life measures are also excellent in this subgroup (Headrick et al.). Taken together, these considerations suggest that morbidity and mortality data culled from previously published series of open esophagectomy for cancer may not apply to carefully selected patients with BE and HGD who are good operative candidates and who undergo laparoscopic transhiatal esophagectomy at a center with significant expertise. Such select patients likely enjoy significantly better outcomes than published benchmarks. Further study will better define specific morbidity and mortality of results of esophagectomy in this patient subgroup.

The high risk of cancer and lack of accurate clinical predictors of disease progression warrant an aggressive approach to patients with HGD. Despite continuing advances in the development of endoscopic techniques, and pioneering efforts in pharmacologic therapy and surveillance, total esophagectomy represents the most reliable means for definitive cure. Laparoscopic transhiatal esophagectomy performed at centers with expertise may be associated with lower morbidity and mortality than open esophagectomy, and is therefore the preferred treatment for HGD.

The natural history of LGD is less well understood than that of HGD. Data are conflicting regarding the risk of progression to HGD and cancer. Practical issues also complicate the diagnosis of LGD; even more so than in HGD, histologic diagnosis of LGD varies even among experienced pathologists, and the potential for biopsy sampling error exists. The primary initial task in the treatment of a patient with BE and a diagnosis of LGD is to eliminate the possibility that the patient in fact harbors occult HGD. Confirmation of histologic diagnosis by two experienced pathologists may increase diagnostic accuracy (Skacel et al.). Repeat biopsy after aggressive treatment and resolution of coexisting erosive esophagitis is usually performed to confirm a diagnosis of LGD (Sharma). If the patient presented here undergoes such diagnostic confirmation, then definitive management must be considered.

While the natural history of LGD remains poorly defined, the majority of reports demonstrate an increased risk of harboring or developing HGD or cancer in patients with LGD. While the exact incidence is unknown, various reports suggest that as many as 10% to 40% of patients with LGD may eventually progress to HGD or cancer (Oberg et al., Reid et al., Rossi et al., Skacel et al.).

Management choices in patients with BE and LGD include endoscopic surveillance alone, high-dose PPI therapy with surveillance, endoscopic ablative and resection techniques, antireflux surgery, or some combination of these therapies. Esophagectomy does not play a role in the treatment of LGD. Regardless of the treatment option chosen, accompanying surveillance endoscopy with biopsy is recommended, although data supporting its efficacy in detecting disease progression or improving survival are lacking (Sharma).

The role of endoscopic ablative and mucosal resection techniques in the management of LGD is currently unclear, but the same limitations mentioned above with respect to HGD apply to application of these techniques to LGD. Incomplete resection or ablation of diseased tissue, the risk of "buried" disease, current inability to identify patients with nodal or invasive cancer preoperatively, and the lack of long-term prospective outcome data currently limit application of these promising technologies in patients with LGD to the clinical trial setting.

Surveillance with or without high-dose PPI therapy has also been suggested as treatment for LGD. As outlined above, however, recent data suggest that LGD is in fact a significant risk factor for subsequent HGD. In addition, antireflux surgery has been shown to be more effective than medical therapy in preventing progression of BE to dysplasia (Oberg et al.) as well as promoting its regression (Rossi et al.). An obvious theoretical advantage of surgical therapy compared to medical therapy that may explain these differences in clinical outcome is the elimination of nonacid reflux, which has been shown to be important in the pathogenesis of dysplasia (Theisen et al.). Only antireflux surgery provides a mechanical barrier to both acid and nonacid refluxate. While debate persists, given the data demonstrating LGD to be a risk factor for HGD, and antireflux surgery to be effective treatment of BE and LGD, we recommend an aggressive approach, in which antireflux surgery is the preferred treatment for patients with LGD, except in cases in which operative risk is excessive or patients are unwilling to proceed with surgery.

It is important to consider the risks associated with antireflux surgery in defining optimal treatment for LGD. Perioperative mortality is approximately 0.1% to 0.2%, and major morbidity may be as high as 5% to 8% (Lundell). As in the case of esophagectomy, however, both short- and long-term results of antireflux surgery appear to be improved at centers of expertise, with experienced surgeons reporting excellent long-term results (Dallemagne et al.). These data again argue for performance of these complex procedures at centers with significant expertise. Other data suggest that BE itself may be an independent risk factor for failure after antireflux surgery (Csendes et al., Farrell et al., Hofstetter et al.). At least one recent study reports results in patients with BE comparable to those with simple GERD, however, casting doubt on this link (Parrilla et al.) Regardless, it is important to note that patients with BE are a subpopulation with a high incidence of severe GERD, and those who seek surgical therapy likely represent the "worst of the worst" of this subgroup and have already failed medical therapy. Analysis of surgical outcomes in such patients is therefore compromised by this selection bias.

The associated early and late morbidity of antireflux surgery must be considered individually in all patients with LGD, and such risks must be balanced with the benefits of maximizing the likelihood of halting progression of a premalignant process. Progression of LGD to HGD mandates esophagectomy in most cases, and antireflux surgery at the time of diagnosis of LGD currently provides the best chance for avoiding this outcome in patients who are good operative candidates.

Important related topics that are beyond the scope of this discussion include the cost-effectiveness of competing technologies, combination therapy, and the increasingly important role of endoscopic fundoplication methods as alternatives to antireflux surgery. These issues aside, current management of BE with dysplasia is primarily surgical. Total esophagectomy provides the best chance for cure and therefore remains the standard of care for patients with BE and HGD. Recent data demonstrate antireflux surgery to be the most effective current treatment to prevent progression and promote regression of LGD, and it is thus the preferred treatment for patients with BE and LGD. Surgical management of patients with BE and dysplasia should be performed at centers with significant expertise. A laparoscopic approach to such patients may result in improved outcomes. Despite an increasingly important role for endoscopic ablative and resection therapies in the management of BE with dysplasia, the lack of current prospective data limits their utility outside of the setting of clinical trials. Such alternative therapies, therefore, should be reserved for patients who are poor surgical candidates or who are unwilling to proceed to surgical therapy.

# D. Endoscopic Mucosal Ablation

*Mark Johnston*

Advocating mucosal ablation in this 67-year-old man with focal HGD and significant comorbidities must be assessed in relation to current practice guidelines and published literature. In the past it was argued that in the medically fit patient with HGD, esophagectomy was the treatment of choice. More recently, the risk of progression to cancer has been thought to be much lower, especially for focal HGD. Consequently, some experts argue that following such patients until cancer develops with serial endoscopy with four-quadrant biopsies every 1 cm, the length of the BE, in 3-month intervals is the management of choice. This approach is unsettling for many, and a more aggressive approach is often pursued. The latter is based on data such as the following: of 126 cases with HGD alone by endoscopic biopsy, 41% had cancer at the time of esophagectomy. Fortunately, a promising, less morbid, alternative exists—mucosal ablation. Because Barrett's esophagus does not spontaneously resolve with PPI treatment alone or after surgical antireflux procedure except on rare occasion, the concept of mucosal ablation entails the following steps:

1. Intentionally damage the BE mucosa in a controlled fashion.
2. Permit esophageal healing in a nonacid environment.
3. Create the ideal environment for esophageal healing with high-dose PPI or surgical antireflux procedure.
4. Maintain control of GERD to prevent return of BE through recurrent injury.

The armamentarium of ablative modalities available includes photodynamic therapy (PDT), laser, multipolar electrocoagulation (MPEC), argon plasma coagulation (APC), endoscopic mucosal resection (EMR), radiofrequency ablation, and cryoablation. These treatment options should be regarded as investigational for the treatment of HGD, with the exception of PDT. Photodynamic therapy is the only Food and Drug Administration (FDA)-approved technique for the specific indication of treating HGD in BE. Although I believe ablation is an excellent choice in this particular case, it is my opinion that it should be performed in the context of an approved research protocol because more data are needed to establish the long-term efficacy and safety of these modalities.

Why consider ablation therapy in comparison to watchful waiting or esophagectomy? First, it is relatively effective. Complete histologic remission, defined as the complete elimination of all specialized intestinal metaplasia (SIM), approaches 70%, although reported rates vary considerably. Additionally, surgery always remains an option after ablation, should it fail. It is also relatively safe. Although occurrences of esophageal perforation, stricture, and bleeding have been reported with virtually all of these modalities, the rates are very low and well below those of esophagectomy. Another concern is the presence of residual subsquamous SIM after ablation, which is reported to occur with all ablative techniques except with radio frequency ablation and cryoablation. However, these are the two newest modalities, and with additional publications, I suspect residual subsquamous SIM will be reported with them as well. Additionally, the cost of ablation is relatively low, with the exception of PDT, which can exceed that of esophagectomy when long-term follow-up is included. My recommendation is to pursue endoscopic ablation at a center that performs it under the guidance of an investigational review board (IRB)-approved protocol. The surgery option remains available should ablation fail, and ablation avoids the morbidity of esophagectomy and the anxiety of harboring a cancer.

# E. Intensive Medical Management and Surveillance

## John Leung

This patient should be managed with intensive medical management and endoscopic surveillance for the following reasons. First, the progression of HGD to cancer is not inevitable, and HGD may be present only intermittently or may regress to low-grade dysplasia spontaneously (Reid et al.). Second, surgical therapy, whether esophagectomy or laparoscopic fundoplication, is associated with significant risks, which may not be warranted in such a high-risk patient with a premalignant lesion. An effective endoscopic surveillance program coupled with intensive medical management is an attractive alternative in the predominately elderly population in which this problem occurs.

The American College of Gastroenterology (Sampliner et al.) recommend the following surveillance regimen. Patients without evidence of dysplasia on two endoscopies with biopsies should have followup endoscopy in three years. Patients with low grade dysplasia should have annual followup until dysplasia clears. Patients with high grade dysplasia need repeat biopsy to rule out carcinoma; followup endoscopy should be performed at intervals of three months. Review of the pathology by an expert may be necessary as the distinction between high grade dysplasia and carcinoma is not always clear cut. If such a regimen is carefully followed, surgery may be avoided unless progression of disease occurs.

# F. Conclusions

## John Leung

Clearly there are several alternatives to the management of a focus of HGD in this patient. Although this lesion is considered premalignant, it is important to note that surgical resection is not the only option. Intensive antireflux therapy, either medical or surgical (laparoscopic fundoplication), with or without mucosal ablation, is a very acceptable option provided that the patient is carefully followed.

Esophagectomy is associated with high rates of procedure-related mortality, postoperative complications, and long-term morbidity. In a U.S study, mortality rate was 3.0% in hospitals with high surgical volume and up to 12.2% in hospitals with low surgical volume (Levine et al.). Postoperative complications such as arrhythmia, myocardial infarction (MI), heart failure, pneumonia, urinary tract infection, and anastomotic leaks were reported in 30% to 50% of patients undergoing this procedure. Operative and hospital volume are significant predictors of outcome, and data support limiting this high-risk procedure to selected centers experienced in this therapeutic modality. Long-term morbidities such as weight loss, dysphagia, gastroesophageal reflux, and dumping syndromes have been documented in more than two thirds of patients who underwent esophagectomy.

Given the high-risk nature of resection, an effective surveillance program might potentially save thousands of patients who do not show definitive evidence of malignancy from exposure to the unnecessary mortality and morbidity inherent in esophagectomy. The efficacy of an endoscopic surveillance program was demonstrated by Reid and his colleagues. They reported that a surveillance program with an intensive biopsy protocol (four-quadrant biopsies every 1 cm with a jumbo biopsy forceps) is effective in detecting early mucosal and submucosal carcinoma at a time when the disease is still resectable and curative. Similar efficacy was demonstrated in a larger number of patients by Levine and coworkers. Despite its proven efficacy in these studies, one might still argue that sampling error can never be eliminated, and foci of invasive cancer might be missed. This argument is based on the observation that 41% of patients with only HGD confirmed by endoscopic biopsy had cancer at the time of esophagectomy. However, these studies did not follow a uniform and intensive endoscopic biopsy protocol, and the actual sampling error may be far less than what was suggested.

An additional consideration is that many patients who have Barrett's esophagus are elderly (the mean age at the time of diagnosis is approximately 60) and many die of unrelated causes (Levine et al., Reid et al.).

Less invasive alternative therapies are available even if early superficial adenocarcinoma develops. These include photodynamic therapy, argon plasma coagulation, laser treatment, and endoscopic mucosal resection. Technical improvement of the devices and accumulating experience with the techniques render them increasingly clinically attractive. Data from numerous small series are encouraging, but long-term clinical outcome data are lacking. As previously noted, these modalities are best applied in the context of a controlled clinical trial.

In conclusion, given the low risk of cancer progression in focal HGD, the high mortality and morbidity of esophagectomy, the effectiveness of intensive endoscopic surveillance program in detecting early resectable cancer, the patient's comorbidities, and potential alternative endoscopic therapy, it is reasonable to recommend against esophagectomy without proven evidence of malignancy. This recommendation is consistent with the guideline published by the Practice Parameters Committee of the American College of Gastroenterology (ACG) in 2002: "Patients with focal high-grade dysplasia (less than five crypts) may be followed with intensive endoscopic surveillance every 3 months." Surgical intervention can then be undertaken in a timely fashion.

# References

Banki F, Mason RJ, DeMeester SR, et al. Vagal sparing esophagectomy: a more physiologic alternative. Ann Surg 2002;236:324–336.

Birkmeyer JD, Stukel TA, Siewers AE, Goodney PP, Wennberg DE, Lucas FL. Surgeon volume and operative mortality in the United States. N Engl J Med 2003;349(22):2117–2127.

Casson AG, van Lanschot JJ. Improving outcomes after esophagectomy: the impact of operative volume. J Surg Oncol 2005;92(3):262–266.

Csendes A, Braghetto I, Burdiles P, et al. Long term results of classic antireflux surgery in 152 patients with Barrett's esophagus: clinical radiologic, endoscopic, manometric, and acid reflux test analysis before and late after operation. Surgery 1998;123:645–657.

Dallemagne B, Weerts J, Markiewicz S, et al. Clinical results of laparoscopic fundoplication at ten years after surgery. Surg Endosc 2006;20(1):159–165.

Farrell TM, Smith CD, Metreveli RE, et al. Fundoplication provides effective and durable symptom relief in patients with Barrett's esophagus. Am J Surg 1999;178:18–21.

Faybush EM, Sampliner RE. Randomized trails in the treatment of Barrett's esophagus. Dis Esoph 2005;18:291–297.

Fernando HC, Luketich JD, Buenaventura PO, Perry Y, Christie NA. Outcomes of minimally invasive esophagectomy (MIE) for high-grade dysplasia of the esophagus. Eur J Cardiothorac Surg 2002;22(1):1–6.

Hage M, Siersema PD, van Dekken H, et al. 5-aminolevulinic acid PDT vs. argon plasma coagulation of BE: a randomized trial. Gut 2004;53:785–790.

Headrick JR, Nichols FC 3rd, Miller DL, et al. High-grade esophageal dysplasia: long-term survival and quality of life after esophagectomy. Ann Thorac Surg 2002;73(6):1697–1702.

Hofstetter WA, Peters JH, DeMeester TR, et al. Long-term outcome of antireflux surgery in patients with Barrett's esophagus. Ann Surg 2001;234:532–539.

Levine DS, Haggitt RC, Blount PL, Rabinovitch PS, Rusch VW, Reid BJ. An endoscopic biopsy protocol can differentiate high-grade dysplasia from early adenocarcinoma in Barrett's esophagus. Gastroenterology 1993;105(1):40–50.

Lewis J, Lutzke L, Smyrk T, et al. The limitations of mucosal resection in Barrett's esophagus. Gastrointest Endosc 2004;59:AB101.

Luketich JD, Alvelo-Rivera M, Buenaventura PO, et al. Minimally invasive esophagectomy: outcomes in 222 patients. Ann Surg 2003;238(4):486–494.

Lundell L. Surgery of GERD: a competitive or complementary procedure. Dig Dis 2004;22:161–170.

May A, Gossner L, Pech O, et al. Local endoscopic therapy for intraepithelial high-grade neoplasia and early adenocarcinoma in Barrett's esophagus: acute-phase and intermediate results of a new treatment approach. Eur J Gastroentrol Hepatol 2002;14:1085–1091.

Oberg S, Wenner J, Johansson J, Walther B, Willen R. Barrett esophagus: risk factors for progression to dysplasia and adenocarcinoma. Ann Surg 2005;242(1):49–54.

Parrilla P, Martinez de Haro LF, Ortiz A, Munitiz V, Serrano A, Torres G. Barrett's esophagus without esophageal stricture does not increase the rate of failure of Nissen fundoplication. Ann Surg 2003;237(4):488–493.

Reid BJ, Levine DS, Longton G, Blount PL, Rabinovitch PS. Predictors of progression to cancer in Barrett's esophagus: baseline histology and flow cytometry identify low- and high-risk patient subsets. Am J Gastroenterol 2000;95(7):1669–1676.

Rossi M, Barreca M, de Bortoli N, et al. Efficacy of nissen fundoplication versus medical therapy in the regression of low-grade dysplasia in patients with Barrett esophagus: a prospective study. Ann Surg 2006;243(1):58–63.

Salameh F, Kudo T, Seidler H, Kawano T, Iwai T. An animal model study to clarify and investigate endoscopic tissue coagulation by using a new monopolar device. Gastrointest Endosc 2004;59(1):107–112.

Sampliner RE, and the Practice Parameters Committee of the American College of Gastroenterology. Updated guidelines for the diagnosis, surveillance, and therapy of Barrett's esophagus. Am J Gastroenterol 2002;97:1888–1895.

Schnell TG, Sontag SJ, Chejfec G, et al. Long-term nonsurgical management of Barrett's esophagus with high-grade dysplasia. Gastroenterology 2001;120(7):1607–1619.

Sharma P. Low grade dysplasia in Barrett's esophagus. Gastroenterology 2004; 127:1233–1238.

Skacel M, Petras RE, Gramlich TL, Sigel JE, Richter JE, Goldblum JR. The diagnosis of low-grade dysplasia in Barrett's esophagus and its implications for disease progression. Am J Gastroenterol 2000;95:3383–3387.

Spechler SJ. Dysplasia in Barrett's esophagus: limitations of current management strategies. Am J Gastroenterol 2005;100:927–935.

Stein HJ, Von Rahden BHA, Feith M. Surgery for Early-stage esophageal adenocarcinoma. J Surg Oncol 2005;92:210–217.

Sujendran V, Sica G, Warren B, Maynard N. Oesophagectomy remains the gold standard for treatment of high-grade dysplasia in Barrett's oesophagus. Eur J Cardiothorac Surg 2005;28(5):763–766.

Theisen J, Peters JH, Fein M, et al. The mutagenic potential of duodenoesophageal reflux. Ann Surg 2005;241(1):63–68.

Thomas T, Richards CJ, de Caestecker JS, Robinson RJ. High-grade dysplasia in Barrett's oesophagus: natural history and review of clinical practice. Aliment Pharmacol Ther 2005;21(6):747–755.

Thomson BN, Cade RJ. Oesophagectomy for early adenocarcinoma and dysplasia arising in Barrett's oesophagus. ANZ J Surg 2003;73(3):121–124.

Tseng EE, Wu TT, Yeo CJ, Heitmiller RF. Barrett's esophagus with high grade dysplasia: surgical results and long-term outcome—an update. J Gastrointest Surg 2003;7(2):164–170.

Weston AP, Sharma et al. Long-term follow-up of Barrett's high-grade dysplasia. Am J Gastroenterol 2000;95:1888–1093.

# Suggested Readings

Edwards MJ, Gable DR, Lentsch AB, et al. The rationale for esophagectomy as the optimal therapy for Barrett's esophagus with high grade dysplasia. Ann Surg 1996;223:585–591.

Heitmiller RF, Redmond M, Hamilton SR. Barrett's esophagus with high grade dysplasia. Ann Surg 1996;224:66–71.

Johnston MH. Technology insight: ablative techniques for Barrett's esophagus—current and emerging trends. Nat Clin Pract Gastroenterol Hepatol 2005;2(7):323–330.

# 13. Management of Gastroesophageal Reflux Disease in the Morbidly Obese

## A. Introduction

With the widespread acceptance of laparoscopic procedures for treatment of morbid obesity, has come the proposal that morbidly obese patients who suffer with gastroesophageal reflux disease (GERD) should be treated by laparoscopic Roux-en-Y gastric bypass rather than by an antireflux procedure. This chapter addresses this controversy. The procedures described, and the specific modifications in laparoscopic technique required in the morbidly obese patient, are described in both SAGES manuals.

## B. Case

### Rebecca Thoreson

A 43-year-old morbidly obese woman has failed therapy for GERD. Her symptoms included burning epigastric to retrosternal pain, with occasional regurgitation of acid-tasting material. She had tried proton pump inhibitors and histamine-2 antagonists without relief. She took antacids regularly with meals. She occasionally noted a sore throat after acid reflux episodes. She had a negative cardiac workup for this epigastric pain. She was referred for surgical management.

Her past medical history was significant for hypertension, obesity, glucose intolerance, and snoring (but no documented sleep apnea). She had a tonsillectomy as a child. She is married and works as a secretary in a high school. She previously smoked one pack per day for 10 years, but stopped when she was 29. She had never used alcohol.

Her physical examination was significant for a height of 65 inches, weight 235 pounds, and body mass index (BMI) 38. Her abdomen was soft without scars or masses. Physical examination was otherwise unremarkable.

Esophagogastroduodenoscopy showed esophagitis with an irregular Z-line. Biopsies showed inflammation, but no evidence of Barrett's esophagus. No hiatal hernia was noted. The stomach appeared normal. A 24-hour pH monitoring revealed multiple episodes of reflux.

**How would you treat this patient?**

# C. Fundoplication

*Lee Swanström*

I would offer this patient laparoscopic fundoplication. Obesity is frequently associated with GERD and may even be an etiologic factor in the rapid increase of this problem worldwide. Also, GERD is a frequent comorbidity of morbid obesity and much is made of the fact that a large percentage of gastric bypass patients have an improvement in their GERD symptoms after their surgery. I would argue that there is a large difference between the patient who seeks surgery for treatment of refractory reflux (and who happens to be obese) and the morbidly obese patient (with GERD as a comorbidity) who is seeking weight reduction surgery. The latter patient needs weight loss surgery to reduce *all* of the comorbid conditions and to improve one's quality of life by becoming thinner. To such a patient, the reflux problem most likely pales in comparison to comorbidities such as diabetes, congestive heart failure, joint dysfunction, sleep apnea, and social stigma. I believe that obese GERD patients deserve the best procedure for their specific complaint of reflux. Besides, the patient in question, with a BMI in the high 30s, has unfortunately become the "average" American and may even be insulted if the surgeon stresses her weight as the major issue. I believe that it is ethically incumbent on the surgeon to point out the dangers of obesity to such patients and to make sure that they know that (1) morbid obesity is a major health and anesthesia risk, (2) morbid obesity may compromise the longevity of an antireflux surgery, and (3) there is a surgery for obesity that is risky but successful and may also improve or correct their primary complaint of GERD. After that, if patients say that, while being thinner would be great, being reflux free is really their priority, I would have no qualms in offering a laparoscopic fundoplication if objective assessment confirms the diagnosis.

I base my opinion not only on the ethical considerations of patient choice but also on an assessment of the data regarding the relative success of fundoplication and bypass for the effective treatment of GERD. Roux-en-Y gastric bypass is an effective treatment for morbid obesity, although it is also associated with appreciable surgical morbidity and even a 1% to 4% mortality rate. It is also well known to improve the frequently associated comorbidity of GERD. Its effect on GERD is related both to the exclusion of large amounts of the acid-secreting oxyntic cells of the stomach and to the beneficial effects of losing intraabdominal fat. On the other hand, it is no better than laparoscopic Nissen in truly controlling pathologic reflux. We compared laparoscopic Nissen fundoplication with gastric bypass both symptomatically and objectively. At a follow-up of 12 months, we found no statistical difference between the outcomes of both groups. There was, in fact, a trend toward better GERD outcomes in the fundoplication group. In a study with the longest follow-up (3 years), which specifically looked at GERD symptoms following laparoscopic bypass, Schauer et al. reported only a 78% resolution in heartburn. There are also no long-term studies regarding the durability of the antireflux effect following bypass; it may be that its effectiveness fades with time as does the effect of its gastric restriction.

Overall success rates for laparoscopic fundoplication are 88% to 95% based on symptomatic improvement, and between 85% and 90% successful at correcting 24-hour pH. There is controversy regarding the impact of weight on the outcomes of antireflux surgery. Intuitively, morbid obesity would seem to compromise the results due to increased intraabdominal pressure and compulsive overeating. The vast majority of studies, however, which specifically looked at outcomes of laparoscopic fundoplication in the morbidly obese, found that results were the same as in the thin population.

I believe that extraordinary measures need to be taken when performing fundoplication in the morbidly obese population. Preoperative counseling should strongly encourage weight loss as part of the treatment of the patient's GERD. Patients should be warned about the risks of overeating and imbibing carbonated drinks after surgery. Even if they do not compromise the repair, it will make the patients' postsurgical course miserable for both the patients and the surgeon. During surgery extra care should be taken to avoid axial tension on the repair because, as with any laparoscopic fundoplication patient, wrap herniation is the most common reason for failure. This may require additional mediastinal dissection or even a Collis procedure to achieve 3 or 4 cm of intraabdominal esophageal length. In addition, a robust crural closure makes sense. I use heavy woven polyester sutures with Teflon pledgets placed as a horizontal mattress suture. It may eventually become standard to reinforce high-risk crural repairs with some sort of biological mesh, though the efficacy of this is still not fully documented. I also use extra fixation with all my laparoscopic wraps, including sutures from the back of the wrap to the closed crura, internal sutures between the inside of the wrap and the esophagus at the 3 o'clock and 9 o'clock positions, and each Nissen suture incorporating some anterior esophagus.

A final argument against performing a fundoplication in the morbidly obese is that it makes future bariatric surgery contraindicated or at least more dangerous. This has not been our experience in 11 patients with past fundoplications. In five cases we were able to create a small pouch (20 to 30 cc) by stapling below an intact fundoplication. In the other six, we took down the wrap either because it was not functioning or it was very floppy and we felt we could not tailor a small gastric pouch around it. There were no complications in this small series, and all patients experienced good to excellent weight loss. Raftopoulos et al. reported a similar experience.

In conclusion, I believe that obesity, even morbid obesity, is not a contraindication for an antireflux procedure. The literature supports equivalent outcomes in obese and thin patients, and with extra attention to the details of the technique the surgeon does not have to make gloomy predictions about the long-term success of the procedure. While patients should be informed of the higher risk but effective alternative of a bypass surgery, they should not be forced into that procedure, and if they decline bariatric referral, it is fine for the surgeon to perform a standard fundoplication.

# D. Roux-en-Y Gastric Bypass

*Sayeed Ikramuddin*

I would offer this patient laparoscopic Roux-en-Y gastric bypass. Clearly the patient has indications for an antireflux procedure. However, a much more appropriate answer would be a laparoscopic Roux-en-Y gastric bypass. Results are mixed in individual series of patients who are obese undergoing Nissen fundoplication. Perez et al., in a study originally designed to compare a thoracic Belsey Mark IV to an abdominal laparoscopic Nissen fundoplication, found the highest incidence of failure (23.7%) in patients with a BMI greater than 30 versus 5% in patients with a normal BMI. In a study of 257 patients from the University of South Florida, no significant difference was found in outcomes between normal weight and obese patients. No series truly dealt with the morbidly obese. Patterson et al. compared six morbidly obese patients undergoing gastric bypass with six undergoing the Nissen. Though the mean BMI of the two groups was significantly different at 55 versus 40 ($p$ <.05), the outcomes were not different.

Given the observations that obesity itself increases both mortality and the risk of comorbid illness, and that weight reduction decreases the relative risk of mortality by 89% over a 6-year period, the preferred approach in this patient, assuming that she is an appropriate candidate based on demonstrable willingness to modify her lifestyle, would be a gastric bypass.

# E.  Conclusions

## *Rebecca Thoreson*

Gastroesophageal reflux disease is a very common disorder, affecting up to 40% of the population. It is particularly common and has been noted to be more severe in the obese population. Control of GERD is extremely important, as it increases the risk of esophageal adenocarcinoma. In patients who continue to have symptoms of GERD despite maximal medical therapy, antireflux surgery is often the next step. The laparoscopic Nissen fundoplication (LNF) is a successful antireflux surgery in medically refractory GERD. However, recent studies based on the LNF procedure have shown conflicting evidence regarding its role in effectively reducing the symptoms of GERD in the obese patient. It has also been noted that obese patients who undergo a Roux-en-Y gastric bypass (RYGB) procedure have improved GERD symptoms. In fact, there is growing evidence supporting the benefits of the RYGB in relieving GERD symptoms. A review of the literature supports the idea that perhaps the next step for GERD refractory to pharmacologic therapy in the obese population should be the Roux-en-Y gastric bypass.

The Nissen fundoplication has been an accepted treatment for patients with GERD. The LNF is known to be a safe and effective treatment overall. Yet, in the obese population, there have been many studies completed with conflicting results. Anvari and Bamehriz prospectively compared two groups of patients with proven GERD who underwent a laparoscopic Nissen fundoplication, 70 patients with a BMI >35 and 70 patients with a BMI <30. Reflux symptom scores were significantly improved and esophageal acid exposure time was decreased to normal levels in the morbidly obese. However, Perez et al. reached different conclusions. They reviewed patients who underwent either the LNF or the Belsey Mark IV (BM4) and divided them into three categories: normal (BMI <25), overweight (BMI 25 to 29.9) and obese (BMI ≥30). There was a significantly higher failure rate in the obese group (31%) compared to the normal (4.5%) and overweight (8%) groups, independent of the type of surgery.

In comparison to the LNF done for antireflux treatment, it has been observed that GERD symptoms improve following a Roux-en-Y gastric bypass done for morbid obesity. Nelson et al. documented improved symptoms of GERD following this procedure in a prospective study. The sample population consisted of obese patients (mean BMI 51) undergoing a laparoscopic or open RYGB. Pre- and postoperative symptoms and antireflux medication use were studied. Results showed a significant decrease in the frequency of GERD symptoms at just 3 months postoperatively, with a decrease in medication usage as well. Improvement this early postoperatively is due to the operation itself and not to weight loss. Long-term (>9 months) follow-up continued to show significant improvement in symptoms. The authors concluded that gastric bypass relieves symptoms of GERD independent of weight loss. Patterson et al. compared the two surgeries, the LNF and laparoscopic gastric bypass (LGB), in the same-sized population. Morbidly obese patients with significant heartburn symptoms or objective evidence of acid reflux were included in the study. A total of 12 patients were studied: six underwent LNF (mean BMI 39.8) and 6 underwent LGB (mean BMI 55). Both groups had significant reduction in heartburn symptom scores as well as normalized lower esophageal sphincter resting pressures postoperatively, suggesting that both surgeries were effective.

Both the laparoscopic Nissen fundoplication and the Roux-en-Y gastric bypass are effective in relieving GERD symptoms. In an obese patient with GERD refractory to medical therapy who is seeking surgical treatment, it is important to offer both options. The LNF has been well established as an anti-reflux surgery in medically refractory GERD. However, patients should be made aware of the conflicting evidence regarding the LNF in the obese population. More recently, the RYGB has been shown to relieve the symptoms of GERD in morbidly obese patients. The RYGB also has the additional benefits that come with weight reduction, which may make it the more favorable choice for many patients. Long-term studies with larger numbers of patients are necessary to determine outcome and delineate which patients benefit from which procedure.

# References

Anvari M, Bamehriz F. Outcome of laparoscopic Nissen fundoplication in patients with body mass index ≥35. Surg Endosc 2006;20(2):230–234.

Nelson L, et al. Amelioration of gastroesophageal reflux symptoms following Roux-en-Y gastric bypass for clinically significant obesity. Am Surg 2005;71:950–954.

Patterson EJ, Davis DG, Khajanchee Y, Swanstrom LL. Comparison of objective outcomes following laparoscopic Nissen fundoplication versus laparoscopic gastric bypass in the morbidly obese with heartburn. Surg Endosc 2003;17(10):1561–1565.

Perez AR, Moncure AC, Rattner DW. Obesity adversely affects the outcome of antireflux operations. Surg Endosc 2001;15:986–989.

Raftopoulos I, Awais O, Courcoulas AP, Luketich JD. Laparoscopic gastric bypass after antireflux surgery for the treatment of gastroesophageal reflux in morbidly obese patients: initial experience. Obes Surg 2004;14(10):1373–1380.

Schauer PR, Gourash W, Hamad GG, Ikramuddin S. Operating room setup and patient positioning for laparoscopic gastric bypass and laparoscopic gastric banding. In: Whelan RL, Fleshman JW, Fowler DL, eds. The SAGES Manual: Perioperative Care in Minimally Access Surgery. New York: Springer-Verlag, 2006:76–84.

# Suggested Readings

Carlson MA, Frantzides CT. Complications and results of primary minimally invasive antireflux procedures: a review of 10,735 reported cases. J Am Coll Surg 2001;193(4):428–439.

D'Alessio MJ, Arnaoutakis D, Giarelli N, Villadolid DV, Rosemurgy AS. Obesity is not a contraindication to laparoscopic Nissen fundoplication. J Gastrointest Surg 2005;9(7):949–954.

Fraser J, Watson DI, O'Boyle CJ, Jamieson GG. Obesity and its effect on outcome of laparoscopic Nissen fundoplication. Dis Esophagus 2001;14(1):50–53.

Frezza EE, Ikramuddin S, Gourash W, et al. Symptomatic improvement in gastroesophageal reflux disease (GERD) following laparoscopic Roux-en-Y gastric bypass. Surg Endosc 2002;16(7):1027–1031.

Nguyen NT. Instrumentation, room setup, and adjuncts for laparoscopy in the morbidly obese. In: Scott-Conner CEH, ed. The SAGES Manual: Fundamentals of Laparoscopy, Thoracoscopy, and GI Endoscopy. New York: Springer-Verlag, 2006:288–292.

Ortega J, Escudero MD, Mora F, et al. Outcome of esophageal function and 24–hour esophageal pH monitoring after vertical banded gastroplasty and Roux-en-Y gastric bypass. Obes Surg 2004;14(8):1086–1094.

Perry Y, Courcoulas AP, Fernando HC, Buenaventura PO, McCaughan JS, Luketich JD. Laparoscopic Roux-en-Y gastric bypass for recalcitrant gastroesophageal reflux disease in morbidly obese patients. JSLS 2004;8:19–23.

Smith SC, Edwards CB, Goodman GN. Symptomatic and clinical improvement in morbidly obese patients with gastroesophageal reflux disease following Roux-en-Y gastric bypass. Obes Surg 1997;7:479–484.

# 14. Achalasia of the Esophagus

## A. Introduction

Achalasia is a motility disorder in which peristalsis is decreased in the body of the esophagus and the distal esophageal sphincter fails to relax properly during swallowing. The combination results in progressive inability to swallow. Early in the disease process, lower esophageal hypertrophy and failure to relax dominate the clinical picture, and hence the initial treatment is directed at this location. Various methods have been employed to disable or weaken the sphincter mechanism. Surgical therapy is employed when medical therapy or pneumatic dilatation are ineffective. This chapter explores alternatives in surgical therapy of uncomplicated achalasia. Chapter 15 discusses fundoplication as an adjunct to laparoscopic myotomy.

## B. Case

### *Carol E.H. Scott-Conner*

A 65-year-old woman developed progressive dysphagia over a period of about 2 years. She had lost an estimated 20 pounds over the past 6 months. The onset had been insidious and she had learned to drink carbonated soda with meals to assist swallowing. She reported an occasional sensation of food sticking in the substernal region, accompanied by an aching sensation. She could sometimes relieve this sticking sensation by standing up and hyperextending her chin. At times she regurgitated undigested food.

Her past medical history was otherwise unremarkable. Her family history was unobtainable, as she was adopted. She had not had any prior surgery. She was on no medications and had no known drug allergies.

The patient was a retired certified public accountant. She had a 10-pack-per-year history of smoking, but had stopped 30 years ago. She did not drink alcoholic beverages. The review of systems was unremarkable except as noted above.

On physical examination, the patient was a slender female, alert and oriented, in no acute distress. She had stigmata of recent weight loss.

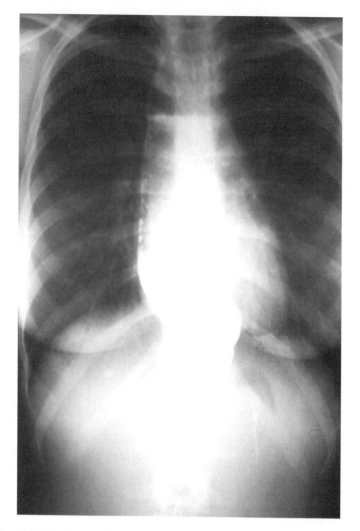

Fig. 14.1. Esophagram from upper gastrointestinal (GI) series shows birds beak deformity of distal esophagus. Proximal esophagus is dilated.

Vital signs included a temperature of 37.4 °C, pulse 65, blood pressure 145/90, height 169 cm, and weight 60 kg. Head and neck and cardiopulmonary examinations were negative.

The abdomen was soft and scaphoid without masses or tenderness. Bowel sounds were normal. There were no hernias. Rectal examination revealed no masses. Stool was guaiac negative. Laboratory results were normal. Chest x-ray was normal.

Upper gastrointestinal series showed a "bird's beak" deformity of the distal esophagus with some proximal dilatation consistent with achalasia (Fig. 14.1). Upper gastrointestinal endoscopy and esophageal manometry confirmed this finding.

**What surgical approach would you recommend?**

# C.  Laparoscopic Esophagomyotomy

*Jason M. Johnson*

In 1674 Sir Thomas Willis, faced with a starving patient unable to swallow, devised a mechanism by which a whalebone with a sponge attached to the end was repeatedly advanced through the mouth and down the esophagus to dilate a narrow distal esophagus. Thus was the first patient successfully treated for what is now call achalasia. Since the condition was originally described by Willis, we have a better understanding of achalasia and the resultant progressive inability of patients to nourish themselves due to a combination of a hypertensive lower esophageal sphincter (LES) and esophageal aperistalsis. Ultimately individuals who suffer severe achalasia have to resort to either surgical or nonsurgical therapeutic interventions that will enable them to eat and drink.

Nonsurgical management of achalasia has been debated over the years, and includes modalities such as endoscopic forceful dilation, pneumatic dilation, and botulinum toxin (Botox) injections. Although these modalities have proven somewhat effective in the short term, their efficacy over the long term does not compare to surgical intervention. It has also been well documented that individuals who have been exposed to numerous nonoperative modalities have an increased incidence of intra- and perioperative morbidity. However, nonsurgical management of achalasia is still vital in patients who are not good operative candidates, or it can be used as a bridge to definitive surgical therapy.

Due to the limited efficacy of medical and nonsurgical management, most patients with achalasia ultimately come to surgical intervention for treatment. Ernest Heller, in 1913, reported successful management of patients with achalasia by performing a cardiomyotomy. Heller's originally described procedure included both parallel anterior and posterior myotomies that extended for at least 8 cm along the distal esophagus and proximal gastric cardia. Only a few years later De Brune Groenveldt and Zaaijer recognized that only one anterior myotomy was necessary. The modified Heller myotomy and the basic concepts described in Heller's original procedure have remained for over 90 years the standard by which all other procedures and modalities are compared.

Traditionally a Heller myotomy was performed through a transthoracic approach. Proponents of this procedure argue that the esophagus traverses both chest and abdomen and that equal access can be obtained by using a thoracic approach. They have also argued that by keeping their intervention limited to the thoracic cavity there is minimal disruption of the inherent antireflux barrier and thus patients have a lower incidence of post-Heller myotomy gastroesophageal reflux disease (GERD). However, Abir et al. note that the incidence of GERD varies with a transthoracic approach (0% to 52%; mean 10%) and is not statistically different from a transabdominal approach (0% to 5%; mean 12.3%). The advent of minimally invasive techniques enabled thoracic surgeons to perform Heller myotomies via a thoracoscopic approach, and this is how the first minimal access procedures were performed.

Recent data, however, suggest that thoracoscopic Heller myotomy is associated with a higher rate of GERD and dysphagia, and so this approach is coming under question and has been abandoned by many in favor of the transabdominal laparoscopic approach.

As our experience with laparoscopy has increased, surgeons have become more adept at modifying the traditionally open technique so that it can be performed with minimal access techniques. This is the case with the Heller myotomy. The postoperative morbidity associated with a thoracotomy or a laparotomy is almost eliminated by performing a Heller myotomy via laparoscopy.

A transabdominal approach to a Heller offers several noticeable advantages to a transthoracic approach. First, by approaching the gastroesophageal (GE) junction from the abdomen, one can get a good feel that the myotomy has indeed crossed the LES adequately and well onto the stomach. Some would argue that proximal extension of the myotomy onto the esophagus is more difficult; however, with adequate esophageal mobilization one can ensure that the myotomy is complete. Most authors suggest taking the myotomy 5 to 6 cm onto the esophagus, across the LES, and then onto the stomach for 2 cm. By extending the myotomy well onto the stomach it ensures that all fibers of the LES are transected, and by doing so one decreases the incidence of postoperative dysphagia. When the procedure is performed thoracoscopically, it becomes difficult to ensure that the myotomy has been extended adequately onto the stomach, and as a result the thoracoscopic approach is associated with a higher rate of postoperative dysphagia.

The second advantage of performing Heller myotomies from the laparoscopic approach is the ease in which an antireflux procedure can be added to the procedure. Whether or not to add an antireflux procedure to a Heller myotomy has been continually debated over the past years, but more data suggest that the incidence of postoperative, asymptomatic acidic reflux remains high in individuals who do not undergo a concomitant antireflux procedure. In a randomized trial comparing Heller without Dor to Heller with Dor, Richards and his group from Vanderbilt University found that the incidence of pathologic gastroesophageal reflux (GER), defined as acid exposure greater than 4.2% per 24-hour period, decreased from 47.6% to 9.1% with the addition of a Dor, or anterior, fundoplication after the completion of a laparoscopic Heller myotomy. So many in the field advocate the addition of a fundoplication because of the potential adverse consequences of prolonged acid exposure to the distal esophagus.

The type of fundoplication to perform is also debated. Many authors argue that a Dor fundoplication is adequate for the treatment of post-Heller GER, while others contended a better result is obtained by adding a Toupet, or 270-degree, posterior fundoplication at the completion of the Heller myotomy. It appears that the majority of patients obtain relief from their dysphagia and have good postoperative control of their GER with the addition of a 270-degree posterior fundoplication. However, there are no head-to-head studies available to compare whether an anterior or posterior fundoplication is better after Heller myotomy (these issues are further explored in Chapter 15). Some authors contend that GER can be prevented with the addition of a complete Nissen type fundoplication to a laparoscopic Heller myotomy. Others, including myself, feel that the data do not support the use of a complete fundoplication due to the higher incidence of postoperative dysphasia.

Until the advent of minimally invasive surgery the standard of care for treatment of achalasia was thoracotomy. The postoperative morbidity caused by a thoracotomy has challenged minimal access surgeons to develop techniques that treat achalasia that are less invasive and associated with lower perioperative morbidity while providing long-term efficacy, and ultimately the ability to eat.

In my practice I perform a laparoscopic Heller myotomy with the concomitant use of endoscopy. Once I have created a myotomy and extended it 5 to 6 cm onto the esophagus and down onto the stomach 2 cm, I then introduce an endoscope to ensure the myotomy has completely traversed the LES. Endoscopic examination also provides the opportunity to ensure that there are no inadvertent mucosal perforations. Many times the patient who are referred to me have undergone either botulinum toxin injection, pneumatic dilatation, or a combination thereof, and so the correct planes are often difficult to identify and small mucosal injuries are not uncommon. By using the laparoscope in conjunction with the endoscope, it is possible to visualize the entire myotomy and repair what would be an otherwise missed full-thickness injury. At the completion of the Heller I add a Dor fundoplication, as the evidence is rather convincing that an antireflux procedure should be added after a laparoscopic Heller myotomy. Additionally, the anterior fundoplication using stomach can serve as a natural patch and buttress on top of the myotomy.

In summary, patients who suffer from achalasia are best served with a Heller myotomy, which by far provides the best long-term relief of symptoms. Over the past decade as the field of minimal access surgery has expanded, we have continually pushed the envelope with the diseases that are treated laparoscopically. It has been well established that in the right hands a laparoscopic Heller myotomy is a safe procedure and produces equivalent, and in some instances better, long-term results when compared to nonsurgical and other surgical modalities. For good surgical candidates a laparoscopic Heller myotomy should be offered as the first line of treatment. However, further studies are needed to delineate the appropriate type of fundoplication to perform along with the laparoscopic myotomy.

# D.  Thoracoscopic-Assisted Esophagomyotomy

## Zane T. Hammoud and Kenneth A. Kesler

As there is no effective therapy to correct the absence of motility in the esophageal body, efforts to palliate the symptoms of achalasia have focused on division of the hypertonic LES muscle. Ellis first described Heller myotomy performed through an open left thoracotomy approach with a limited myotomy carried onto the gastric cardia. The main advantage of the transthoracic approach, as compared to an open transabdominal approach used at the time, was avoiding the disruption of the phrenoesophageal ligament, therefore eliminating significant GERD or the need for an antireflux procedure. In 1993, Ellis reported his

22-year experience involving 185 patients with 93% improvement after primary procedures and a 4.8% incidence of significant GERD. Although Ellis also found a tendency for the development of recurrent symptoms after 10 years, these data arguably establish the open left thoracotomy approach as a gold standard against which short- and long-term results of other techniques should be compared.

With the relatively recent advent of video endoscopic technology, several minimally invasive surgical techniques have been described to eliminate the short-term morbidity of open thoracotomy. Unfortunately, attempts at a pure thoracoscopic approach not uncommonly lead to incomplete LES division, and this approach therefore has largely been abandoned. The technique of laparoscopic Heller myotomy was introduced in 1991, which resulted in more complete division of the LES as compared to the pure thoracoscopic approach. Not surprisingly, however, similar to the open laparotomy approach, a high incidence of significant GERD has prompted most surgeons to combine a laparoscopic myotomy with a partial fundoplication, the anterior (or "Dor") currently being the most popular.

Many variations of the laparoscopic approach have been described. In general, this technique involves placing the patient in the lithotomy position with four or five ports strategically placed through the upper abdominal wall. Dissection begins by dividing the gastrohepatic omentum and identifying the right diaphragmatic crus. The phrenoesophageal ligament is then incised, exposing the anterior wall of the esophagus and left diaphragmatic crus. Additional mediastinal dissection is carried out to expose an adequate length of distal esophagus. An anterior myotomy is performed using a hook cautery cephalad onto the esophagus for a length of 4 to 6 cm and caudad onto the stomach for 2 to 4 cm while carefully avoiding injury to the anterior vagus nerve. Usually an anterior fundoplication is accomplished in conjunction with tacking the right and left myotomized muscle edges to their respective crus, which is intended to minimize an early "scar over" phenomenon of the divided LES muscle. Most single-institution experiences utilizing a laparoscopic approach report 84% to 93% symptomatic improvement but have less than 2 years of follow-up. A few reports with longer follow-up have appeared in the literature, with good to excellent results maintained in 73% to 84% of patients. More recently, a robot-assisted laparoscopic approach has been described. Robotic systems have superior magnification and three-dimensional optics as compared to standard two-dimensional laparoscopic imaging. Moreover, robotic surgery allows "wrist-like" movements with motion scaling enabling more precise dissection. These features may reduce the incidence of mucosal perforation as well as allow better identification of any undivided LES fibers through a minimally invasive abdominal approach.

Since 1998, our institution has utilized a minimally invasive thoracoscopic-assisted technique, which allows a Heller myotomy to be performed under direct visualization without rib spreading or rib reapproximation. Thoracoscopic-assisted myotomy is performed under selective lung ventilation with the patient in the right lateral decubitus position. The operating table is "jack-knifed," which widens the lower left-sided intercostal spaces. A 10- to 12-cm incision is established over the rib superior to the estimated level of the diaphragm dome, which usually represents the sixth or seventh interspace depending on the patient's body habitus. Self-retaining retractors are used to separate the chest wall soft tissues only. The opening through the interspace can be further widened by judicious intercostal muscle retraction, with one arm of the self-retaining retractor applied to the superficial fascial layer of the intercostal muscle and the other arm of the retractor applied to the chest wall soft tissues inferiorly. Attention must be given to avoiding placement of the retractor teeth deep near the intercostal neurovascular bundle, which may result in intercostal neuralgia common after rib spreading and one of the main causes of postthoracotomy morbidity. Two 10-mm trocar ports are placed just cephalad to the diaphragm insertion on the costal margin. An endoscopic fan-type retractor is deployed through the one-trocar port to retract the diaphragm caudally, and a thoracoscope is placed through the other trocar port. Alternatively, a self-retaining laparoscopic liver retractor can be used for caudal diaphragmatic retraction. The thoracoscope is used to help illuminate the operative field for the primary surgeon and provides video-imaging for the assistants from a monitor placed above the patient's head. The primary surgeon additionally uses headlight illumination and optical loupe magnification.

The vast majority of the procedure is performed by the surgeon under direct visualization through the interspace without assistance. The inferior pulmonary ligament is divided with an extended electrocautery unit. A laparotomy sponge is packed against the deflated lung to keep it rotated cephalad and out of the operating field. With the primary surgeon standing on the left side of the operating table (assuming right hand dominance), the parietal pleura overlying the esophagus is secured with a forceps then divided with electrocautery from the inferior pulmonary vein to the crus of the diaphragm. The posterior esophageal margin is identified, and then secured with a Russian-type forceps 2 to 3 cm above the crus. Judicious division of the longitudinal and the circular muscle layers at this level is then accomplished with the electrocautery unit until the submucosal layer is identified. A submucosal plane is established with a long right-angle clamp in the cephalad direction. The primary surgeon continues to apply downward traction on the posterior margin of the esophagus with the forceps while elevating the muscular wall off the submucosa with the right-angle clamp. The primary surgeon then looks to the video screen and confirms satisfactory clamp positioning. The first assistant divides the elevated muscle using electrocautery under direct visualization. This dissection technique is continued superiorly to within 1 to 2 cm of the inferior pulmonary vein.

The primary surgeon then moves to the right side of the operating table. Although more cumbersome, we prefer to utilize upward and outward countertraction with forceps held by both the primary surgeon and first assistant who are working under direct visualization and video-assistance, respectively, as the plane between the muscular and submucosal layers typically becomes more difficult to dissect inferiorly onto the cardia. Of equal importance, the upward esophageal retraction along with simultaneous downward retraction on the diaphragm at this point in the procedure makes the gastric cardia easily identified as compared to the pure thoracoscopic approach. This sequence of right-angle clamp dissection by the primary surgeon and then muscular wall division by the first assistant is continued inferiorly 1 to 2 cm onto the gastric cardia. The primary surgeon returns to the left side of the operating table and again secures the posterior margin of the divided esophageal muscle wall at the cardia level with forceps. Using freehand dissection with gentle use of the electrocautery tip and application of electrocautery, any remaining circular muscle fibers are disrupted over the proximal cardia. A submucosal plane is then developed posteriorly using mainly blunt dissection with the tip of the electrocautery unit for the entire length of the myotomy. A 5- to 7-mm strip of dissected muscle wall is removed longitudinally, carefully avoiding the posterior vagus nerve to prevent an early "scar over" phenomenon. The pleura overlying the myotomized esophagus is closed with a running monofilament suture. As ribs have not been separated, no intercostal sutures are needed and only the chest wall soft tissues are closed after lung reinflation. A chest tube is placed and usually removed on the second or third postoperative day. A liquid diet is begun on the first postoperative day and advanced on an as-tolerated basis.

Our institutional series from 1998 to 2005 includes 46 patients ranging in age from 21 to 89 years (mean 47 years). Two patients early in our experience required conversion to open thoracotomy due to bleeding in one case and perforation in the other. After an average of 24 months, 87% of patients report good to excellent results. Only two patients have been medically treated for significant GERD. For the first half of our series, the average operating time was 97 minutes; however, our average operating time is now under 1 hour. We have documented that patients experienced significantly less pain and a shorter time interval before returning to work compared to an open thoracotomy approach. We believe that advantages to the thoracoscopic-assisted Heller myotomy include eliminating the need for fundoplication and a relatively lower risk of mucosal perforation as compared to the laparoscopic approach. Although long-term results are pending, we anticipate that they would not be dissimilar to the results of the open thoracotomy approach.

The thoracoscopic-assisted approach may be preferable in cases of previous laparotomy and vigorous achalasia where a relatively higher myotomy is necessary. Thoracoscopic-assisted myotomy may also be preferable in cases where severe submucosal scarring is anticipated due to multiple previous Botox injections. The laparoscopic approach does offer advantages over the thoracoscopic-assisted approach including easier exposure of the gastroesophageal junction and gastric cardia. Intraoperative management is less complex without the need for a double-lumen endotracheal tube. Potentially there might be decreased postoperative pain and length of hospital stay due to the presence of a chest tube used for the thoracoscopic-assisted approach.

Given the limitations of nonsurgical therapy and the refinement of minimally invasive technology and techniques, the treatment paradigm for achalasia is rapidly shifting toward initial surgical therapy for most patients. It appears that both laparoscopic and thoracoscopic-assisted Heller myotomy approaches have good to excellent short-term results. Unfortunately, current data are limited to retrospective single institution series using inconsistent quality of life instruments, which makes evidence-based decisions difficult. Moreover, long-term results of minimally invasive approaches are lacking. Although either a laparoscopic or a thoracoscopic-assisted approach may have advantages in specific cases, in general thoracic surgeons familiar with an open thoracotomy approach may prefer a thoracoscopic-assisted myotomy. Similarly, abdominal surgeons will have a quicker learning curve and initially feel more comfortable with a laparoscopic approach.

# E.  Conclusions

*Carol E.H. Scott-Conner*

Relatively early in the development of minimal access surgery, laparoscopic surgeons recognized that the magnification and precise dissection characteristic of laparoscopy might be advantageous during the performance of myotomy for achalasia. The first attempts were thoracoscopic, but it rapidly became evident that it was difficult to attain adequate exposure of the distal esophagus and proximal stomach. In part, this is an example of how a minimal access technique may be similar to, but not quite the same as, its open counterpart. During open transthoracic myotomy, the esophagus is encircled and elevated from the mediastinum. Significant traction can be applied to the esophagus and the proximal stomach is thus delivered into the surgical field. During thoracoscopic myotomy, it was difficult if not impossible to duplicate this exposure.

Simultaneously, techniques were developed for exposure of the distal esophagus for performance of laparoscopic Nissen fundoplication. It was obvious that the exposure attained in this manner was quite adequate for esophageal myotomy, and the thoracoscopic approach was largely superseded. Because of the extensive hiatal dissection, it became customary to add a partial fundoplication (see also Chapter 15).

When spasm is limited to the distal esophageal sphincter, as in the case presented, the laparoscopic approach is the preferred approach for most surgeons. The thoracoscopic-assisted approach provides a useful alternative in those cases where an extended thoracic myotomy is required, or where prior surgery in the left upper quadrant might render laparoscopy difficult.

# References

Abir F, Modlin I, Kidd M, et al. Surgical treatment of achalasia: current status and controversies. Dig Surg 2004;21:165–176.

De Brune Groenveldt JR. Over cardiospasmus. Ned Tijdschr Geneeskd 1918;54:1281–1282.

Ellis FH Jr. Oesophagomyotomy for achalasia: a 22-year experience. Br J Surg 1993;80:882–885.

Heller E. Extramucöse Cardioplastie beim chronischen Cardiospasmus mit Dilatation des Oesophagus. Mitt Grengeb Med Chir 1913;2:141–149.

Richards WO, Torquati A, Holzman MD, et al. Heller myotomy versus Heller myotomy with Dor fundoplication for achalasia. Ann Surg 2004;240:405–415.

Zaaijer JH, Cardiospasm in the aged. Ann Surg 1923;77:615–617.

# Suggested Readings

Anselmino M, Perdikis G, Hinder RA, et al. Heller myotomy is superior to dilation for the treatment of early achalasia. Arch Surg 1997;132:233–240.

Bansal R, Nostrant TT, Scheiman JM, et al. Intrasphincteric botulinum toxin versus pneumatic balloon dilation for treatment of primary achalasia. J Clin Gastroenterol 2003;36:209–214.

Bonatti H, Hinder RA, Klocker J, et al. Long-term results of laparoscopic Heller myotomy with partial fundoplication for the treatment of achalasia. Am J Surg 2005;190:874–878.

Csendes A, Braghetto I, Burdiles P, et al. Very later results of esophagomyotomy for patients with achalasia: clinical, endoscopic, histologic, manometric, and acid reflux studies in 67 patients for a mean follow-up of 190 months. Ann Surg 2006;243:196–203.

Ellis FH Jr, Olsen AM, Holman CB, et al. Surgical treatment of cardiospasm: consideration of aspects of esophagomyotomy. JAMA 1958;166:29.

Gockel I, Junginger T, Eckardt VF. Long-term results of conventional myotomy in patients with achalasia: a prospective 20-year analysis. J Gastrointest Surg 2006;10:1400–1408.

Horgan S, Galvani C, Gorodner MV, et al. Robotic-assisted Heller myotomy versus laparoscopic Heller myotomy for the treatment of esophageal achalasia: multicenter study. J Gastrointest Surg 2005;9:1020–1029.

Kesler KA, Tarvin SE, Brooks JA, et al. Thoracoscopic-assisted Heller myotomy for the treatment of achalasia: results of a minimally invasive technique. Ann Thorac Surg 2004;77:385–392.

Khajanchee YS, Kanneganti S, Leatherwood AE, Hansen PD, Swanstrom LL. Laparoscopic Heller myotomy with Toupet fundoplication: outcome predictors in 121 consecutive patients. Arch Surg 2005;140;9:827–833.

Leyden JE, Moss AC, MacMarhuna P. Endoscopic pneumatic dilation versus botulinum toxin injection in the management of primary achalasia. Cochrane Database of Systematic Reviews 2006;4:CD005046.

Park, W, Vaezi MF. Etiology and pathogenesis of achalasia: the current understanding. Am J Gastroenterol 2005;100(6):1404–1414.

Patti MG, Arcerito M, DePinto M, et al. Comparison of thoracoscopic and laparoscopic Heller myotomy for achalasia. J Gastrointest Surg 1998;2:561–566.

Pereira-Graterol F, Moreno-Portillo M. Distal esophageal perforation repair during laparoscopic exophagomyotomy: evaluation of outcomes and review of surgical technique. J Laparoendosc Adv Surg Tech A 2006;16:587–592.

Rakita SS, Villadolid D, Kalipesad C, Thometz D, Rosemurgy A. BMI affects presenting symptoms of achalasia and outcome after Heller myotomy. Surg Endosc 2007;21:258–264.

Ramacciato G, Mercantini P, Amodio PM, et al. The laparoscopic approach with antireflux surgery is superior to the thoracoscopic approach for the treatment of esophageal achalasia: experience of a single surgical unit. Surg Endosc 2002;16:1431–1437.

Ramacciato G, Mercantini P, Amodio PM, Stipa F, Corigliano N, Ziparo V. Minimally invasive surgical treatment of esophageal achalasia. JSLS 2003;7:219–225.

Rosetti G, Brusciano L, Amato G, et al. A total fundoplication is not an obstacle to esophageal emptying after Heller myotomy for achalasia. Ann Surg 2005;241:614–621.

Stewart KC, Finley RJ, Clifton JC, et al. Thoracoscopic versus laparoscopic modified Heller myotomy for achalasia efficacy and safety in 87 patients. J Am Coll Surg 1999;189:164–170.

Torquati A, Lutfi R, Khaitan L, et al. Heller myotomy vs Heller myotomy plus Dor fundoplication: cost-utility analysis of a randomized trial. Surg Endosc 2006;20:389–393.

Tsiaoussis J, Athanasakis E, Pechlivanides G, et al. Long-term functional results after laparoscopic surgery for esophageal achalasia. Am J Surg 2007;193:26–31.

# 15. Laparoscopic Management of Achalasia

## A. Introduction

The first minimal access procedures for achalasia were performed thoracoscopically, by analogy with the open Heller myotomy. As laparoscopic surgeons became facile at operating around the esophageal hiatus, it became evident that an adequate myotomy could be done laparoscopically in most cases. Today, the vast majority of laparoscopic surgeons add a partial fundoplication to their myotomy. The choice of a posterior partial fundoplication (Toupet) or an anterior partial fundoplication (Dor) remains a matter of surgeon preference and discussion.

## B. Case

### Samad Hashimi

A 45-year-old man with a long history of achalasia presented for surgical evaluation of his current problem. His symptoms began when he was in his early twenties and included dysphagia to solids more than liquids, chest pain (negative cardiac workup), and heart burn. These symptoms progressively worsened to the point that he regurgitated food, and required the head of his bed to be elevated in order to sleep. He reported a 20-lb unintentional weight loss over the past year. His wife stated that he had suffered from halitosis for as long as she can remember. He had tried calcium channel blockers and nitrates with no benefit. He had also undergone multiple pneumatic dilations by his local internist. His symptoms resolved temporarily but then recurred. He wanted to pursue a more permanent solution to his problem.

His past medical history was significant for hyperlipidemia, controlled by medication. He had a previous tonsillectomy and an appendectomy when he was a teenager. He has been married 15 years and has two children, ages 12 and 9, both healthy. He is a social drinker and never smoked cigarettes, but he enjoyed an occasional cigar on the weekends. He is an active business manager who frequently travels on business to Europe and Canada. He exercises regularly.

His physical examination was completely normal, with the exception of a well-healed right lower quadrant transverse appendectomy scar. Barium swallow demonstrated a dilated esophagus (7 cm) terminating in a beak-like narrowing.

Manometry following an overnight fast demonstrated lower esophageal sphincter (LES) pressure of 27 mm Hg, with absent relaxation in response to swallowing. Esophageal primary peristalsis was absent.

Endoscopy demonstrated a dilated esophagus with residual food particles. Esophageal mucosa appeared normal with some mild areas of irritation (biopsies revealed mild inflammatory changes). The LES was traversed easily with the endoscopy. Retroflexed views of gastric fundus demonstrated normal appearing mucosa without masses or grossly abnormal findings. No strictures were identified.

A 24-hour ambulatory pH monitoring was negative for gastroesophageal reflux.

**What intervention would you offer this patient?**

# C. Laparoscopic Myotomy with Toupet (Posterior) Fundoplication

*Jo Buyske*

This patient would benefit from a laparoscopic myotomy and fundoplication. He has already undergone pneumatic dilatation with recurrence of his symptoms. This failure is not surprising, since we know that younger patients (those under 65) and male patients are the least likely to have a good long-lasting result from pneumatic dilatation for achalasia.

The therapeutic approach to achalasia is primarily directed at the LES. Treatment options include endoscopic injection of botulinum toxin, balloon dilatation, and surgical myotomy of the LES. Treatment has two goals: to improve esophageal emptying, and to minimize the unpleasant symptoms of a dysfunctional foregut. These are not perfectly correlated. Some patients with very severe achalasia and an end-stage esophagus have surprisingly few symptoms, and may even be obese. Some patients with early achalasia and a relatively well-preserved esophagus are highly symptomatic, with chest pain, dysphagia, weight loss, and regurgitation.

Botulinum toxin injection into the LES is effective in paralyzing the muscles of the LES. This effect is temporary. Botulinum toxin can be a useful tool in atypical cases. Take, for example, the patient who has a motility disorder with symptoms of dysphagia and chest pain and has esophageal manometry that shows some peristalsis or a normal LES pressure. A trial of botulinum toxin may help predict if this patient will respond to myotomy. We extrapolate from a good response to one form of sphincter-directed therapy (in this case, botulinum toxin) to predicting a good response to a more definitive sphincter-directed therapy (myotomy or pneumatic dilatation). Botulinum toxin can also be useful as a temporizing measure. We have used it for a patient who wanted to attend a family wedding in 2 weeks, which seemed to be too tight a time frame in which to have surgery and recover safely. We have also used it when patients have had a crisis of achalasia, specifically the acute inability to manage even liquids. If a qualified surgeon is not immediately available, botulinum toxin may allow a more elective treatment plan.

Pneumatic dilatation of the LES is effective in a significant number of patients. The risk of rupture and the high long-term failure rate (at least 50% have failed by 10 years) have discouraged practitioners and patients from pursuing this route. Several studies have demonstrated that men are more likely to fail this approach than women, and young men are the most likely to fail. It is important that the patient have a true pneumatic dilatation. Many patients report being "dilated" and in fact have had a series of graduated size dilators passed. This is not a true trial of pneumatic dilatation for achalasia, and will have a lower rate of success than the real thing.

There are several features to this patient's history that favor surgical myotomy over an endoscopic approach. He is known to have achalasia and has had a good symptom response to previous sphincter-directed therapy in the form of pneumatic dilatation. Assuming that he is free of any complicating time constraints, there is no indication for botulinum toxin at this point. His gender, age, and previous history of recurrence after pneumatic dilatation predict a limited benefit from any future dilatations.

The LES can be approached through either the chest or the abdomen. The benefits of a minimally invasive approach have been well described, with shorter hospital stays and more rapid recovery. The thoracoscopic approach to esophagomyotomy has proved more cumbersome than the laparoscopic approach and has been largely abandoned. A laparoscopic approach to esophageal myotomy is in order for this man with no prior history of upper abdominal surgery.

To wrap or not to wrap? And if we wrap, which wrap? It is important to note that gastroesophageal reflux can be asymptomatic. Using patient-reported heartburn as a measure of the presence or absence of reflux has been shown to be unreliable. Although some authors have reported good results from myotomy without fundoplication, these reports rely primarily on reported symptoms, not objective measures of reflux. Those studies that have used 24-hour pH studies as a measure of postoperative reflux in patients who have had a myotomy show that the prevalence of reflux is much higher than is expected by patient report alone. This is true both in patients who have undergone a concomitant antireflux procedure and those who have not. Those patients who have had a wrap along with their myotomy are less likely to have reflux than those who have not, but nevertheless may have reflux with or without associated symptoms.

Patients with achalasia have an amotile or dysmotile esophageal body. They frequently empty their esophagus by gravity alone. In a normal esophagus an episode of reflux is met with a stripping peristaltic wave, which quickly flushes acid back out of the esophagus. Patients with achalasia may not have this response, so that any given episode of reflux will last longer than in a normal esophagus. If the reflux occurs at night when the patient is supine, the duration of a given episode of reflux might be very long indeed.

Given the high prevalence of reflux in patients who are studied after myotomy, in combination with the poor symptom correlation and poor esophageal clearance, we strongly recommend that an antireflux procedure be a routine addition to a surgical myotomy.

Both anterior and posterior fundoplication have been used in the setting of achalasia. A 360-degree fundoplication creates resistance to esophageal emptying that may be impossible for the dysmotile achalasic esophagus to overcome, and so is not recommended. The advocates of a Dor anterior fundoplication cite its ease of use as well as its limited resistance to esophageal emptying. They also propose an advantage to leaving the posterior attachments of the distal esophagus undisturbed. Proponents of a Toupet posterior wrap state that it is a more effective antireflux procedure. They also propose that suturing the hemifundoplication to the cut edges of the myotomy helps to keep the myotomy from closing. Neither approach has been definitively proven to be superior. We prefer a posterior wrap because it includes full mobilization of the esophagus, allowing for a long and easily seen myotomy within the abdomen. We reserve a Dor fundoplication for those cases in which an inadvertent esophagotomy was made, in which case the Dor serves as a buttress for the repair. In these circumstances we also leave a drain behind the esophagus.

# D.  Laparoscopic Myotomy with Dor Fundoplication

*Marco G. Patti and James W. Ostroff*

We would perform laparoscopic myotomy with anterior (Dor) fundoplication. Esophageal achalasia is a primary esophageal motility disorder of unknown origin characterized by lack of esophageal peristalsis and inability of the LES to relax properly in response to swallowing. The goal of treatment is to relieve the functional obstruction caused by the LES, therefore allowing emptying of food into the stomach by gravity. However, the elimination of the LES may be followed by reflux of gastric contents into the aperistaltic esophagus, with slow clearance of the refluxate and the risk of developing esophagitis, strictures, Barrett's esophagus, and even adenocarcinoma. For this reason a fundoplication should always be performed after a Heller myotomy.

In 1992 we described our initial experience with a thoracoscopic Heller myotomy. We performed a left thoracoscopic myotomy with the guidance of intraoperative endoscopy, which extended for only 5 mm onto the gastric wall. The long-term follow-up in the first 30 patients confirmed the excellent outcome of the initial report: almost 90% of patients had relief of dysphagia, the hospital stay was short, the postoperative discomfort was minimal, and the recovery was fast. Unfortunately, the operation was followed by a very high incidence of postoperative reflux (60%, by pH monitoring), which was asymptomatic in most patients. In addition, we were unable to help patients with dysphagia who had developed abnormal reflux secondary to pneumatic dilatation. These were probably the key reasons that made us switch to a laparoscopic myotomy and Dor fundoplication.

Today it is accepted that a fundoplication is necessary to prevent reflux after a laparoscopic Heller myotomy, by performing a Dor fundoplication, a Toupet fundoplication, or a Nissen fundoplication. This approach is based on some retrospective studies and two prospective randomized trials comparing laparoscopic myotomy alone versus myotomy and fundoplication. In 2003 Falkenback and colleagues reported the results of a prospective randomized trial comparing myotomy alone versus myotomy and Nissen fundoplication. Postoperative reflux was present in 25% of patients who had a myotomy and fundoplication but in 100% of patients who had a myotomy alone. Twenty-percent of the patients in the latter group developed Barrett's esophagus.

In 2004 Richards and colleagues reported the results of a prospective randomized trial comparing laparoscopic myotomy alone versus laparoscopic myotomy and Dor fundoplication. Postoperative ambulatory pH monitoring showed reflux in 48% of patients after myotomy alone but in only 9% of patients when a Dor fundoplication was added to the myotomy. The incidence and degree of postoperative dysphagia were similar in the two groups.

In esophageal achalasia the pump action of the esophageal body is completely absent, as there is no peristalsis. Therefore, a total fundoplication might create too much resistance at the level of the gastroesophageal junction, impeding the emptying of food from the esophagus into the stomach by gravity, and eventually causing persistent or recurrent dysphagia. Although some groups still claim good results from adding a total fundoplication after a myotomy, most have abandoned this approach and switched to a partial fundoplication. This decision was based on the results of long-term studies that demonstrated eventual esophageal decompensation and symptom recurrence in most patients.

There are no published prospective randomized trials comparing a partial posterior (Toupet) versus an anterior (Dor) fundoplication in association with a Heller myotomy in patients with achalasia. Some groups feel that a posterior fundoplication is better as it keeps the edges of the myotomy separated and it is a more effective antireflux operation. Others, however, feel that a Dor fundoplication is simpler to perform as it does not need posterior dissection, and it adds the advantage of covering the exposed mucosa.

Our philosophy at the University of California at San Francisco during the last 12 years has been to perform a laparoscopic Heller myotomy and Dor fundoplication. The myotomy is about 9 cm in length and extends for about 2 cm onto the gastric wall. We do not perform intraoperative endoscopy. After the short gastric vessels are divided, an anterior 180-degree fundoplication (Dor) is performed. There are two rows of sutures, one right and one left. The left row has three stitches. The first stitch incorporates the stomach, the esophagus, and the left pillar of the crus. The second and the third stitches incorporate only the stomach and the esophageal wall. Subsequently, the fundus is folded over the exposed mucosa, so that the greater curvature of the stomach is next to the right pillar of the crus. Similar to the left row, the right row has three stitches and only the uppermost stitch incorporates the fundus, the esophagus, and the right pillar of the crus. Finally, two additional stitches (apical stitches) are placed between the anterior rim of the esophageal hiatus and the superior aspect of the fundoplication. After laparoscopic Heller myotomy and Dor fundoplication, excellent or good results for dysphagia were obtained in 91% of patients, with a 15% incidence of postoperative reflux.

The application of minimally invasive surgery to the treatment of esophageal achalasia has determined an unexpected change in the treatment algorithm of this disease, whereby today a laparoscopic Heller myotomy is considered by most gastroenterologists and surgeons the primary treatment modality for esophageal achalasia, reserving pneumatic dilatation to the few failures of this operation

# E.  Conclusions

## *Samad Hashimi*

Achalasia is the most common primary motility disorder of the esophagus. It is characterized by the absence of esophageal peristalsis, incomplete relaxation of the LES, and elevated lower esophageal resting pressure. Etiology of this disorder is unknown. The underlying pathophysiology appears to be a loss of ganglion cells in the myenteric plexuses of the esophagus, resulting in absence of peristalsis of the lower esophageal body, failure of the LES to relax with swallowing, and normal or elevated resting LES pressures. Consequently, a functional obstruction at the level of the LES develops. Progressive dysphagia to liquids and solids is the primary symptom. If the patient does not undergo adequate treatment, regurgitation of food and weight loss can develop, as in the current case.

A number of treatment options, both surgical and medical, have been devised whose sole purpose is to balance relief of esophageal outflow obstruction and destruction of the normal mechanism that prevents reflux. One question that has plagued the surgical community for a while has been whether a limited myotomy without an antireflux procedure could provide long-term relief of symptoms without associated complications of reflux. Other questions that have been posed are if an antireflux procedure is needed and, what type of procedure (Dor vs. Belsey vs. Nissen) would accomplish the desired results.

Malthaner et al. followed 35 achalasia patients for a minimum of 10 years. Twenty-two patients underwent a myotomy and Belsey hemifundoplication. Excellent results were achieved in 95% of patients at 1 year, declining to 67% at 20 years. Two of the patients underwent early reoperation for dysphagia secondary to incomplete myotomy. Three patients underwent esophagectomy, one patient underwent antrectomy, and Roux-en-Y diversion for complications from reflux disease. The study concluded that although there was deterioration of excellent results, those deteriorations were secondary to reflux disease.

Bonavina et al. reported excellent results with transabdominal myotomy and Dor fundoplication. The patients were followed for an average of 5.4 years and 94% had excellent outcomes. Patti, Molena, et al.'s comparison of thoracoscopic Heller myotomy (no antireflux procedure) versus laparoscopic Heller myotomy plus Dor fundoplication demonstrated that a laparoscopic approach with an antireflux procedure significantly reduced postoperative reflux and even corrected reflux present preoperatively. In addition, the patients in the laparoscopic group were reportedly more comfortable and left the hospital earlier.

Unfortunately, most of the long-term studies (10 to 20 years' follow-up) were performed in an era where most procedures were open procedures. There have been numerous studies that have shown a lower incidence of gastroesophageal reflux (GER) by 24-hour pH study in patients undergoing Heller myotomy plus Dor fundoplication (Anselmino et al., Bonavina et al., Patti, Molena, et al.). There have been numerous studies discussing treatment options for achalasia, but the follow-up has been less than 10 years.

Richards et al. randomized 43 patients to receive either myotomy alone or myotomy plus Dor fundoplication for achalasia. Patients were then studied for 24 hours via a pH study and then a manometry at 6 months postoperatively. Pathologic reflux was noted in 47.6% of patients with the Heller myotomy vs. 9.1% in those who underwent Heller myotomy plus Dor fundoplication. The authors did not note any significant difference between the two techniques with respect to postoperative LES pressure or postoperative dysphagia scores. The study also noted sustained acid exposure times in the distal esophagus of patients who underwent myotomy alone. This could lead to severe acid erosion of the esophagus. Based on these data it should not be surprising to conclude that the addition of a Dor fundoplication after a myotomy could potentially prevent long-term complications associated with GER. Most surgeons, as previously noted, routinely add a partial fundoplication to myotomy for just these reasons.

Two questions remain to be answered:

- What is the optimal length of the myotomy on the gastric cardia and is intraoperative endoscopy necessary?
- Does the type of fundoplication (Dor versus Toupet) matter?

Until long-term studies are available to guide surgeons, the type of partial fundoplication will remain a matter of surgeon preference.

# References

Anselmino M, Zaninotto G, Costantini M, et al. One-year follow-up after laparoscopic Heller-Dor operation for esophageal achalasia. Surg Endosc 1997;11:3–7.

Bonavina L, Nosadinia A, Burdini R, Baessato M, Percchia A. A primary treatment of esophageal achalasia: long-term results of myotomy and Dor fundoplication. Arch Surg 1992;127:222–226.

Malthaner RA, Todd TR, Miller L. Perason FG. Long-term results in surgically managed esophageal achalasia. Ann Thorac Surg 1994;58:1343–1347.

Patti MG, Molena D, Fisichella PM, et al. Laparoscopic Heller myotomy and Dor fundoplication for achalasia: analysis of successes and failures. Arch Surg 2001;136:870–877.

Richards W, Torquati A, Holzman M et al. Heller myotomy versus Heller myotomy with Dor fundoplication for achalasia: a prospective randomized double-blind clinical trial. Ann Surg 2004;240(3):405–415.

# Suggested Readings

Falkenback D, Johansson J, Oberg S, et al. Heller's esophagomyotomy with or without a 360 degrees floppy Nissen fundoplication for achalasia. Long-term results from a prospective randomized study. Dis Esophagus 2003;16:284–290.

Farhoomand K, Connor J, Richter J. Predictors of outcome of pneumatic dilation in achalasia. Clin Gastroenterol Hepatol 2004;2(5):389–394.

Khajanchee Y, Kanneganti S, Leatherwood A, et al. Laparoscopic Heller myotomy with Toupet fundoplication: outcomes predictors in 121 consecutive patients. Arch Surg 2005;140(9):827–833.

Lyass S, Thoman D, Steiner J, Phillips E. Current status of an antireflux procedure in laparoscopic Heller myotomy. Surg Endosc 2003;17:554–558.

Oddsdottir M. Laparoscopic cardiomyotomy. In: Scott-Conner CEH, ed. The SAGES Manual: Fundamentals of Laparoscopy, Thoracoscopy, and GI Endoscopy. New York: Springer-Verlag, 2006:238–245.

Oelschlager B, Chang L, Pellegrini C. Improved outcome after extended gastric myotomy for achalasia. Arch Surg 2003;138(5):490–497.

Patti M, Pellegrini C, Horgan S. Minimally invasive surgery for achalasia: an 8-year experience with 168 patients. Ann Surg 1999;230:587–594.

Patti MG, Fisichella PM, Perretta S, et al. Impact of minimally invasive surgery on the treatment of esophageal achalasia. A decade of change. J Am Coll Surg 2003;196:698–703.

Pellegrini CA, Wetter LA, Patti MG, et al. Thoracoscopic esophagomyotomy. Initial experience with a new approach for the treatment of achalasia. Ann Surg 1992;216:291–296.

Peters J. An antireflux procedure is critical to the long-term outcome of esophageal myotomy for achalasia. J Gastrointest Surg 2001;5(1):17–20.

Rossetti G, Brusciano L, Amato G, et al. A total fundoplication is not an obstacle to esophageal emptying after Heller myotomy for achalasia: results of a long-term follow up. Ann Surg 2005;241:614–621.

Topart P, Deschamps C, Taillefer R, Duranceau A. Long-term effect of total fundoplication on the myotomized esophagus. Ann Thorac Surg 1992;54:1046–1051.

West R, Hirsch D, Barelsman J, et al. Long-term results of pneumatic dilation in achalasia followed for more than 5 years. Am J Gastroenterol 2002;97;1346–1351.

Zaninotto G, Costantini M, Molena D, et al. Treatment of esophageal achalasia with laparoscopic Heller myotomy and Dor partial fundoplication: prospective evaluation of 100 consecutive patients. J Gastrointest Surg 2000;4:282–289.

# 16. Preoperative Staging
# for Esophageal Carcinoma

## A. Introduction

Squamous carcinoma of the esophagus must be accurately staged before treatment. Although multimodality therapy is the current standard of care, the timing of surgery with respect to chemotherapy and radiation depends critically on the stage of disease. Staging modalities include laparoscopy, thoracoscopy, computed tomography (CT), magnetic resonance imaging (MRI), positron emission tomography (PET), and endoscopic ultrasound. In this chapter, several experts discuss their preferred staging algorithms.

## B. Case

### *Samuel M. Maurice*

A 77-year-old man presented with an 8-month history of progressive dysphagia, associated with a 30-pound weight loss. Over the past 2 months his dysphagia had progressed from an inability to swallow solid foods to difficulty swallowing thickened liquids. A barium swallow showed a nearly obstructing distal esophageal mass. Upper endoscopy revealed an approximately 7-cm mass in the distal esophagus. Biopsy showed poorly differentiated squamous cell carcinoma. He was referred for surgical evaluation.

His past medical history was significant for hypertension and chronic obstructive pulmonary disease. His past surgical history included bilateral cataract operations, and an open right inguinal hernia repair. His mother died at age 75 from breast cancer, and his father died at age 85 from heart disease. One sister was alive, with hypertension, at age 74.

He was a married, retired steelworker. Two children were alive and well. He smoked two packs per day for approximately 50 years. He was a recovered alcoholic who had stopped drinking 20 years earlier.

The patient was on metoprolol, Combivent metered dose inhaler (MDI), and aspirin. He was allergic to sulfa drugs. His review of systems was otherwise negative. On physical examination, his pulse was 77, and blood pressure was 142/80. He was cachectic but in no acute distress. He was not icteric. His head and neck examination was negative. There was no lymphadenopathy. His chest was clear to auscultation. His abdomen was soft, without masses or tenderness. Digital rectal exam was negative, and stool was Hemoccult negative.

His laboratory results, including liver function tests, were all normal. His chest x-ray was negative, and CT of the abdomen and pelvis confirmed a nearly obstructing distal esophageal mass measuring $10 \times 11$ cm. No lymphadenopathy or metastatic disease was noted.

**What additional studies should be done to stage his malignancy before treatment?**

# C. Our Preferred Staging Algorithm

*Beate Rau*

Surgery with complete resection and no residual tumor (R0—resection, according to the Union Internationale Contre le Cancer [UICC]) is still recommended as the best treatment option for esophageal carcinoma. This can be performed easily in early lesions but may be difficult in locally advanced cancers. The treatment of advanced esophageal cancer with disseminated disease must be directed toward palliation of symptoms. The primary goal of palliation is the restoration of swallowing and the relief of pain. In principle, this can be achieved by radio-(chemo)-therapy, and endoscopic treatment. Therefore, precise staging is necessary to choose the right treatment direction and includes the evaluation of resectability and curability.

For resectability of esophageal cancer, localization and infiltration depth is the most important factor. To achieve curability, distant metastases that mainly belong to extra-regional lymph nodes (e.g., hepatoduodenal ligament, paraaortic), liver and pulmonary metastases, and peritoneal carcinomatosis have to be excluded.

## Assessment of Resectability

Extension of esophageal cancer depends on location (upper, middle, lower third) and the infiltration of the surrounding structures and organs. Loco-regional staging of cancer are accurately identified by CT and endoscopic ultrasound (EUS). The accuracy of tumor, node, metastasis (TNM) staging is not influenced by the type of ultrasound used. Curved array or radial scanner in EUS demonstrated accuracy for the T category of 72% or 73% and for the N category of 70% or 77%, respectively. Positron emission tomography is able to detect esophageal cancer, but cannot precisely demonstrate the infiltration depth of the tumor.

Lerut et al. reported that locally advanced tumors (T3/T4) were accurately identified by CT in 15/16 (94%) and by endoscopic ultrasound (EUS) in 14/16 (88%). Laparoscopy was not able to detect tumors above the diaphragm, but in visible tumors the accuracy was 10/12 (83%). Endoscopic ultrasound was the best modality for assessing early tumors and locoregional nodal involvement with accuracies of 8/13 (62%) and 21/29 (72%), respectively.

Thoracoscopy, especially when combined with endoluminal ultrasound, might be useful to predict resectability in tumors localized in the middle third of the esophagus. With the attempt of thoracoscopic esophageal resection in four of 22 patients (18%) conversion to thoracotomy was necessary. Prediction of resectability is limited with tumors infiltrating surrounding structures. In these cases the risk of uncontrollable bleeding or damage of mediastinal structures is very high.

Prediction of resectability with laparoscopy, therefore, is limited to esophageal cancer of the distal third, especially when infiltrating the esophagogastric junction.

## Recommendation: Assessment of Resectability in Esophageal Cancer

- EUS is the best locoregional staging technique.
- CT scan can predict locally advanced cancer (T3/T4).
- The prediction of resectability of esophageal cancer by means of staging thoracoscopy or laparoscopy is limited and therefore not necessary.

## Assessment of Disseminated Disease

### Lymph Node Metastases

The prognostic value of lymph node metastases in esophageal cancer has been well described. Tumors of the upper esophagus metastasize primarily to cervical lymph nodes and the supraclavicular nodes. These may be accurately predicted with ultrasound in 88% of patients. Involvement of celiac nodes may occur in 10% of cancers located in the cervical and upper region and up to 44% of patients with middle third tumors. Tumors of the middle and distal third spread to mediastinal, celiac, and perigastric nodes. Mediastinal lymph nodes belong to the regional lymph nodes and are included in an en bloc resection.

All lymph nodes localized to the paraaortic region or in the hepatoduodenal ligament are classified as distant metastases according to the UICC. Consequently, staging must focus on these regions to avoid unnecessary exploratory laparotomies.

In a prospective trial in esophageal adenocarcinoma, Sihvo et al. staged patients with PET, spiral CT, and EUS, and the results were compared with histopathology. The accuracy in detecting locoregional lymph node metastasis did not differ significantly among EUS (72%), PET (60%), and CT (58%). Even when PET was added to standard staging, the accuracy of N staging was not improved. Regarding lymph node metastasis, PET had 32% sensitivity, 99% specificity, and 93% accuracy for individual lymph node group evaluation. However, the overall lymph node staging evaluation revealed 55% sensitivity, 90% specificity, and 72% accuracy. The accuracy in detecting locoregional lymph node metastasis did not differ significantly among EUS (72%), PET (60%), and CT (58%).

Staging laparoscopy accurately predicted intraabdominal lymph nodes in 65% compared with percutaneous ultrasound in 34% or CT in 45% in a study by Kato et al. Laparoscopy including laparoscopic ultrasound showed a higher sensitivity than US and CT in detecting macroscopic nodal metastases (78% vs. 11% vs. 55%). When staging laparoscopy was combined with thoracoscopy, Krasna, Jiao, et al. reported that the accuracy in detecting lymph node metastases rose to 94%. In their trial including 134 patients with esophageal cancer, systematic sampling of lymph nodes was performed in a minimally invasive fashion at different levels of lymph nodes (LNs). Three noninvasive imaging (CT, MRI, EUS) modalities each incorrectly identified LN staging as noted by missed-positive or false-negative LN or metastatic disease found at minimally invasive staging in 50%, 40%, and 30% of patients, respectively. In 80 patients with esophageal cancer who were ready to go for curative resection staging, laparoscopy combined with laparoscopic ultrasound revealed a high number of distant lymph node (nine patients) and liver metastases (nine patients). Especially for distal esophageal cancer, the inclusion of laparoscopic ultrasound appears to improve accuracy.

## Recommendation: Assessment of Lymph Node Metastases in Esophageal Cancer

- The prediction of lymph node metastasis of esophageal cancer by means of staging laparoscopy alone is limited and therefore not necessary. Only the combination with laparoscopic ultrasound is effective for lymph nodes in the coeliac axis and especially in distal esophageal cancer (grade B).
- Assessment of lymph node metastases with laparoscopic ultrasound is very effective detecting additional suspicious lymph nodes in over 15%. In locally advanced cancer (T3/T4) or adenocarcinoma in the distal esophagus, the detection rate is higher (grade B).
- PET, CT, EUS for untreated esophageal cancer are equally effective. Combination of PET with EUS or with CT improves the accuracy of staging of up to 90% (grade B).

## *Peritoneal Spread*

In disseminated disease the distribution between squamous carcinoma and adenocarcinoma might be interesting to consider, but there are no valuable data. Isolated peritoneal carcinomatosis in squamous cell carcinoma of the esophagus is rare. We reported an incidence of 10% to 20% peritoneal carcinomatosis found on staging laparoscopy but not detected by conventional imaging (CT, US). Bonavina, Incarbone, and Peracchia reported similar results. In contrast, O'Brien et al. did not find any peritoneal metastases in 30 patients with squamous cell cancer. Although PET is the best diagnostic tool to detect distant metastases compared with CT and EUS, the sensitivity for isolated peritoneal carcinomatosis is nearly 0%.

## Recommendation: Assessment of Peritoneal Spread in Esophageal Cancer

- The prediction of peritoneal spread of esophageal cancer by means of staging laparoscopy is very precise, while histology is easily possible (grade B).
- CT, EUS, and PET are not useful to detect peritoneal carcinomatosis, although isolated peritoneal carcinomatosis is very rare in squamous cell carcinoma of the esophagus (grade B).

## Liver

Liver metastases occur in squamous cell carcinoma of the esophagus. The frequency depends on the localization of the tumor. Bosch et al. reported that liver metastases were found at autopsy in 16% of patients with upper-third tumors, 29% with middle-third tumors, and 43% with distal-third tumors. O'Brien et al. performed a prospective comparison of laparoscopy and combined imaging (CT and ultrasound) in the preoperative staging of distal esophageal and gastric cancer in patients who were selected for surgery. Metastatic disease outside the potential field of resection was found in 27% of patients. Metastases were detected preoperatively by laparoscopy with a sensitivity of 77%. Combined imaging reached a sensitivity of only 38%. Liver metastases were found by laparoscopy with a sensitivity of 60% and by combined imaging with a sensitivity of 47%.

Staging laparoscopy in esophageal cancer revealed additional information in 21%. Disseminated disease was not found in early cancer. With increasing depth of tumor infiltration, the percentage of additional lesions rises. In two of 10 uT2-tumors (20%) and 10 of 39 uT3-tumors (26%), we found additional distant metastases, indicating the benefit of staging laparoscopy in locally advanced esophageal cancers.

The role of PET in detection of distant metastasis is well documented. Compared with CT and EUS, PET demonstrated a major impact in detection of distant metastasis.

### Recommendation: Assessment of Liver Metastases in Esophageal Cancer

- Assessment of disseminated disease by means of staging laparoscopy is rare, at 10% to 20% (grade B).
- Staging laparoscopy is recommended in locally advanced (T3/T4) esophageal cancer or adenocarcinoma in the distal esophagus (grade B).
- PET for detection of distant metastases is recommended (grade B).

## Restaging After Preoperative Radiochemotherapy in Esophageal Cancer

After preoperative treatment to reduce tumor size, the tumor must be restaged. Nearly 20% of patients achieve complete remission of the tumor, and some tumors are decreased to less than 10% of viable tumor cells. Therefore, even detection of esophageal cancer after pretreatment is difficult. Cerfolio et al. reported on a prospective trial on a consecutive series of patients for restaging integrated EUS combined with fine-needle aspiration (EUS-FNA), CT, and PET-CT. The accuracy for distinguishing pathologic T4 from T1 to T3 disease is 76%, 80%, and 80% for CT, EUS-FNA, and PET-CT, respectively. PET-CT is more accurate than EUS-FNA and CT for predicting nodal status and complete responders. Out of 15 patients with complete response (pCR) PET-CT accurately predicted pCR in 89%, EUS-FNA in 67%, and CT alone in 71%.

Accurate determination of response after neoadjuvant therapy is of major interest for many reasons. Comparison to pretherapeutic staging is important. This aspect was elucidated by Swisher et al. in a retrospective trial comparing the results by CT (reduction of wall thickness in millimeters), by EUS (reduction of mass size in centimeters), and by PET (reduction of SUV [standardized uptake value]). All three aspects significantly predicted response.

## Recommendation: Assessment of Response in Esophageal Cancer

- Response to preoperative treatment in esophageal cancer PET is recommended, with an accuracy ranging between 75% and 90% (grade B).
- Staging laparoscopy or thoracoscopy are not recommended to predict response (grade B).
- The accuracy of EUS and CT to predict response is less than PET, if done only after preoperative treatment. Reduction of wall thickness and mass size described by CT or EUS is also relevant staging information (grade B).

# D.  Nonsurgical Staging of Esophageal Cancer

*Prasad S. Adusumilli and Amit N. Patel*

Identification of early-stage esophageal cancer allows surgical curative therapy. Depth of tumor penetration and nodal involvement determine the eligibility for surgical resection and are the two most important prognostic indicators in the management of esophageal cancer. Following diagnosis by barium swallow or through upper endoscopy with biopsy, CT, PET, and EUS all have important roles in the staging of patients with esophageal cancer. Endoscopic ultrasound is the most accurate technique for the locoregional tumor size (T) and nodal involvement (N) staging. In addition, EUS-FNA allows tissue diagnosis of lymph nodes and liver metastases. Computed tomography is most valuable at detecting metastatic (M) distant disease, particularly in the liver, lungs, and periaortic lymph nodes. Optimal staging strategies for esophageal cancer combine EUS-FNA with CT scan. Whereas CT infers T staging by measuring esophageal wall thickness (normal esophageal thickness by CT scan is less than 5 mm), EUS can predict more accurately the level of submucosal and transmural involvement and the morphologic regional node characteristics worrisome for metastasis. Positron emission tomography facilitates noninvasive means of detecting primary, nodal, and distant metastatic disease by identifying areas of high glucose metabolism using 18F-deoxyglucose (FDG) as a tracer. The accuracy of PET scanning surpasses that of CT scanning in staging esophageal cancer with regard to nodal disease and metastatic involvement. Reed et al. performed a cost-effectiveness analysis and demonstrated that CT followed by EUS/FNA was the most inexpensive strategy and resulted in more quality-adjusted life years than other strategies with the exception of PET plus EUS/FNA, which was slightly more effective but also more expensive.

## T stage

In experienced hands, EUS provides a better evaluation of T stage when compared with other modalities (accuracy of 85% to 90%). Accuracy increases with deeper tumor penetration and with improved sensitivity as T stage increases. Furthermore, the accuracy of EUS was reported to be better in smaller tumors (<5 cm) compared with larger tumors (≥5 cm) and in staging esophageal tumors than in staging esophagogastric junction tumors. Overstaging by EUS may occur when inflammation surrounds the tumor. More recently, with smaller-caliber probes, such as the catheter miniature echo probe, evaluation of even high-grade obstructing lesions is facilitated by EUS. Normal esophageal wall thickness by CT is 3 mm, and any thickness greater than 5 mm is considered to be abnormal. The sensitivity of PET in detecting primary esophageal tumors ranges from 78% to 95%, with most false-negative tests occurring in patients with T1 or small T2 tumors. Both CT and PET do not provide definition of the esophageal wall and surrounding tissue and are therefore of no value for determination of the specific T stage. However, one recent study demonstrated increasing mean FDG uptake with increasing depth of invasion of esophageal cancer in PET scans.

## N Stage

Incidence of lymph node involvement is lower for high-grade dysplasia and intramucosal cancer (2% to 6%), which increases to 30% to 50% in adenocarcinoma penetrating into the submucosa. The accuracy of endoscopic ultrasound to determine nodal involvement (mediastinal, periesophageal, celiac, and perigastric lymph nodes) ranges from 65% to 86%. The depth of tumor invasion as assessed by EUS is a strong predictor of N1 disease. Malignant lymph nodes typically appear hypoechoic, with a round shape, discrete borders, and size greater than 1 cm. Lymph nodes that meet all four of these criteria have an 80% to 100% likelihood of malignancy; however, only approximately 35% of malignant nodes demonstrate all four criteria. Fine-needle aspiration by EUS improves the accuracy of staging. In addition, the size of lymph nodes at the celiac axis (>2 cm) determined by EUS has been strongly correlated with survival. Computed tomography readily visualizes lymph nodes in paraesophageal and retroperitoneal fat. Recent studies using high-resolution helical CT scanning have demonstrated sensitivities of 11% to 77% as well as specificities of 71% to 95%. Although an enlarged lymph node on CT scanning may suggest a metastasis, tissue confirmation is generally needed to justify a change in management. Furthermore, a review of the literature reveals 83% to 87% accuracy in the assessment of periesophageal abdominal nodes, but only 51% to 70% accuracy in assessing adenopathy in the chest associated with esophageal cancer by CT. The use of PET scan for detection of regional lymph nodes is hampered by the proximity of the primary tumor. Often the avidity of the uptake by the primary tumor overwhelms any uptake by locoregional lymph nodes. Thus, most studies have demonstrated very poor sensitivity of PET (28% to 39%) in detecting regional lymph node metastases. The sensitivity of PET for the detection of cervical, upper thoracic, and abdominal lymph node metastases appears to be better (78%, 82%, and 60% compared to 38% and 0% for middle and lower thoracic). On the other hand, the specificity of PET for detecting regional lymph node tumor deposits is very high, at 95% to 100%.

## M Stage

Patients with newly diagnosed esophageal carcinoma may present with metastases to the liver (35%), lung (20%), bone (9%), adrenal gland (2%), brain (2%), as well as rarely to pleura, pancreas, and spleen. Two potential sites where EUS could be useful are metastases to the left lateral segment of the liver and the retroperitoneum. Computed tomography scanning is most useful for the detection of distant metastases (non-nodal M1B status). The accuracy of detection of aortic, tracheobronchial, and pericardial invasion is greater than 90% with modern CT imaging. In most studies FDG-PET is superior to CT for detection of stage IV disease. FDG-PET detects radiographically occult distant metastases in 10% to 20% of patients; the combination of PET and CT is reported to avoid unnecessary surgery in 90% of patients with otherwise unsuspected metastatic disease. In addition, patients who were followed after induction chemoradiation and surgery and patients who had no evident disease after esophagectomy had a 2-year disease-free survival of 38% and an overall survival of 63% when SUV change was greater than 60%.

## Restaging

Endoscopic ultrasound generally performs poorly in the restaging of patients after induction chemoradiotherapy (CRT) in differentiating tumor from necrosis or inflammatory reaction (20% false-positive rate). Computed tomography also has poor accuracy for assessment of response to neoadjuvant therapy in patients with esophageal cancer. Fluorodeoxyglucose-PET seems to be a promising noninvasive tool for assessment of neoadjuvant therapy in patients with esophageal cancer and was able to predict both the responses to preoperative CRT and poor prognosis in a study by Westerp et al. One group correlated major PET response after induction CRT (80% reduction in tumor-to-liver ratio) to histopathology obtained during esophagectomy. In this series the sensitivity of serial PET for a major CRT response (1 month post-CRT) was 71% and its specificity was 82%. The median survival time of major PET responders after CRT was significantly increased at 16.3 months compared to 6.4 months for those who did not respond. For anastomotic recurrence, conventional workup was better than PET (accuracy of 96% vs. 74%) because endoscopy provided for direct visualization and biopsy of anastomotic lesions. On the other hand, PET was better than conventional workup at diagnosing regional and distant recurrence with accuracies of 87% versus 81%, respectively. Furthermore, FDG-PET is not only suitable for response evaluation after a full course of CRT, but can also be used for early response prediction. Wieder et al. have clearly shown that an FDG-PET that is performed as early as 14 days after initiation of the neoadjuvant radiochemotherapy protocol can reliably distinguish between responders and nonresponders.

In summary, rational use of imaging modalities can facilitate complete noninvasive evaluation and accurate preoperative staging in esophageal cancer. As the incidence of esophageal cancer increases, such noninvasive evaluation can not only facilitate rational use of available resources but also directs stage-dependent treatment algorithms.

# E. Conclusions

## Samuel M. Maurice

The incidence of esophageal cancer is increasing by about 10% per year in the United States. It was estimated that there would be 14,550 new cases of esophageal cancer and an estimated 13,770 deaths from esophageal cancer in 2006. Esophageal cancer is potentially curable in its earliest stages, but there are no curative options for patients with advanced disease. The proper selection of a treatment, whether palliative or curative in intent, and correct stratification of patients for clinical trials depend on accurate staging. Current basic staging for esophageal cancer combines EUS with CT. Despite advanced imaging techniques like CT and EUS, Romijn et al. found unresectable disease in up to 20% of patients at the time of laparotomy.

This approach is far from optimal, leading many clinicians to contemplate using the minimally invasive techniques of laparoscopy and video-assisted thoracoscopy to improve esophageal cancer staging and minimize the number of unnecessary laparotomies. Thoracoscopy allows evaluation of the entire thoracic esophagus and periesophageal lymph nodes when performed through the right hemithorax and evaluation of the aortopulmonary and periesophageal lymph nodes and lower esophagus when performed through the left hemithorax. Lymph nodes can be sampled, the pleura can be examined, and adjacent organ invasion can be confirmed. Laparoscopy allows visualization of peritoneal surfaces for carcinomatosis, inspection of the liver surface (and parenchyma if laparoscopic ultrasound is employed), examination of the stomach for tumor involvement, and sampling of lesser curve and celiac lymph nodes after entry into the lesser sac.

A number of studies have compared combined laparoscopic and thoracoscopic staging to conventional imaging techniques. Krasna, Reed, et al., in a preliminary report of a National Institutes of Health (NIH)-sponsored, prospective, multiinstitutional trial (CALGB 9380), reported that combined laparoscopic/thoracoscopic staging (LS/TS) was feasible in 73% of patients and doubled the number of metastatic lymph nodes identified by conventional noninvasive means. In comparison to conventional preoperative testing, thoracoscopy/laparoscopy identified involved lymph nodes or metastatic disease previously missed by CT in 50% of patients, by MRI in 40%, and by EUS in 30%. The LS/TS patients had a median hospital stay of 3 days, and they experienced no deaths or major complications.

Krasna, Jiao, et al. related their experience with TS/LS in 111 patients at the University of Maryland. They compared TS/LS with conventional imaging (CT, MRI, and EUS) in diagnosing T4 and N1 disease. When compared to final surgical pathologic staging, 100% specificity was achieved by TS/LS. TS/LS correctly downstaged 13 of 19 patients diagnosed as T4 by conventional imaging to T3 and correctly upstaged eight patients from T3 to T4. TS/LS was also significantly more accurate than CT, MRI, and EUS in diagnosing lymph node metastases in the chest (90.8% vs. 57.9%, $p < .001$) and in the abdomen (96.4% vs. 68.1%, $p < .001$).

A prospective study by Luketich et al. of 26 patients compared TS/LS to EUS. TS/LS proved to be superior in identifying lymph node metastasis and allowed evaluation of five of the 26 patients (19%) whose obstructing lesion prevented adequate EUS evaluation. In this study, TS/LS did not upstage any EUS-identified T3 disease. In regard to lymph node status, TS/LS found N1 disease in six of eight patients thought to be N0 by EUS. TS/LS identified N1 disease in 18 of 21 patients (86%), while EUS assigned N1 status to only 12 of 21 patients (57%). Furthermore, EUS did not detect any metastatic disease, while TS/LS identified small liver metastases in four of 26 patients. The authors found no mortality and only one major complication secondary to a small bowel obstruction caused by an incarcerated hernia at one of the 10-mm port sites.

These studies assert that TS/LS may offer advantages to conventional imaging in correctly identifying TNM status. The general application of these techniques, however, is debated. Wallace et al., using a decision analysis model, compared the cost-effectiveness of different staging strategies, including CT, EUS, PET, and TS/LS. They found the combination of PET and EUS with FNA to be the most cost-effective strategy followed by CT with EUS-FNA. Both of these staging strategies proved more effective and less costly than CT alone or combinations of CT with TS/LS.

Studies have also looked at laparoscopy alone in staging esophageal cancer. A number of prospective and retrospective studies have examined the sensitivity, specificity, and accuracy of laparoscopy and laparoscopic ultrasound in staging gastroesophageal cancers. Laparoscopy has been found to be 42% to 100% sensitive and 100% specific in detecting intraabdominal metastasis. In relation to conventional imaging techniques, many studies have found laparoscopy to be superior in detecting metastases and in preventing nontherapeutic laparotomies.

Bonavina, Incarbone, Lattuada, et al., in a prospective study of 50 patients with cancer of the esophagus or gastroesophageal junction, compared diagnostic laparoscopy with CT and ultrasound (US). Laparoscopy showed a higher sensitivity than US and CT in detecting peritoneal metastases (71% vs. 14% vs. 14%), macroscopic nodal metastases (78% vs. 11% vs. 55%), and liver metastases (86% vs. 86% vs. 71%), while adding no procedural mortality. A study by Watt et al. also showed laparoscopy to be superior to US and CT in detecting intraabdominal metastasis. In this prospective study of 90 patients with tumors of the esophagus or gastric cardia, the authors found that all modalities had a high specificity for detecting intraabdominal metastases ranging from 86 to 100%. However, laparoscopy was found to be significantly more sensitive and accurate in detecting hepatic metastases (88% and 96%) than ultrasound (48% and 83%) or CT (56% and 85%). Laparoscopy was also found to be more sensitive and accurate in detecting lymph node metastases (51% and 72%) than US (17% and 52%) or CT (31% and 57%). The difference between laparoscopy and CT in detecting lymph node metastases, however, just failed to reach statistical significance. While ultrasound and CT detected no peritoneal metastases, laparoscopy demonstrated a sensitivity of 89% and an accuracy of 98%.

In another prospective study of 145 patients with distal esophageal or gastric cancer, laparoscopy was found to be more sensitive than combined CT and US in detecting intraabdominal metastases (77% vs. 38%) and peritoneal metastases (96% vs. 21%). The difference in sensitivity between laparoscopy (64%) and combined CT and US (50%) in detecting hepatic metastases did not reach statistical significance in this study. Anderson et al., in a prospective study of 44 patients with gastroesophageal cancer, found laparoscopy with laparoscopic US significantly more accurate than CT and US in the assessment of the primary tumor (91% vs. 64%) and nodal status (91% vs. 62%).

As the above studies illustrate, laparoscopic staging may offer benefits over conventional imaging in staging esophageal cancer. Investigators have also looked at whether this greater accuracy of staging leads to changes in treatment. In both retrospective and prospective studies of patients with gastroesophageal tumors, laparoscopic staging has avoided unnecessary laparotomies in 5% to 24% of patients.

In designing studies, many investigators have included both patients with tumors of the esophagus and patients with tumors of the gastric cardia in their study populations. On subset analysis, the decrease in nontherapeutic laparotomies appears more pronounced in the patients with gastric cardia tumors than in those with more proximal esophageal tumors. In Clements et al.'s study of 255 patients with gastroesophageal cancer, laparotomy was avoided in 18% of patients: 35% with gastric cancer, 11.1% with cancer of the gastroesophageal junction, and 13.6% with cancer of the esophagus. Nieveen van Dijkum et al., in a prospective study, showed that laparoscopic staging avoided laparotomy in 20% of the patients with tumors of the gastroesophageal junction and in only 5% with cancer confined to the esophagus. These findings are similar to another prospective study of 56 patients in which laparotomy was avoided in 11% of patients with cancer of the gastric cardia but was avoided in only 3% of patients with cancer of the middle or lower esophagus. It appears that laparoscopy detects more metastases in cardiac tumors compared to more proximal esophageal tumors. This is consistent with Dagnini et al.'s observations that abdominal metastases are almost always absent in lesions of the upper third of the esophagus but progressively increase in frequency from the middle esophagus to the gastric cardia. In Dagnini et al.'s report of 369 cases, upper-third lesions were associated with intraabdominal metastases in 3.6% of the cases, middle-third lesions in 6.3%, lower-third lesions in 20.5%, and gastric cardia lesions in 55%. The yield of laparoscopy appears to increase from proximal to distal esophageal/cardiac tumors.

There is considerable debate about whether the addition of laparoscopic ultrasound to laparoscopic staging offers a clinically significant benefit. Finch et al. found that laparoscopic US significantly improved the accuracy of TNM staging (82%) versus laparoscopy alone (67%) and CT alone (47%). This improved staging has been shown to change therapy in some studies. In a prospective study of 93 patients by Smith et al. and in a retrospective study of 48 patients by Hulscher et al., laparoscopic US spared an additional 8% of patients in these studies from laparotomies over those deemed unresectable by laparoscopic staging alone. Laparoscopic ultrasound (LUS) may also provide additional prognostic information. In a prospective study of 44 patients with gastroesophageal cancer, LUS, in predicting the presence of metastatic lymph node disease, predicted poor prognosis and early recurrence during long-term follow-up of these patients. This may prove useful in selecting patients for neoadjuvant and adjuvant therapies. Other studies have not shown a benefit of LUS over laparoscopy alone.

Laparoscopic staging and laparoscopic ultrasound are rarely associated with complications. Many studies report no procedural morbidity or mortality. Complications have been reported. For example, Bemelman et al. reported a morbidity rate of 3.5%, all secondary to wound infections. Nieveen van Dijkum et al., in a study of laparoscopic staging for esophageal, gastric, pancreatic, and hepatobiliary cancers, reported a 1% major complication rate, 3% minor complication rate, and 0% mortality rate. Port-site metastases were observed in 2% of their patients, all of whom had extensive peritoneal metastases at the time of diagnosis. Port-site metastasis after laparoscopic staging of an esophageal cancer, albeit rare, is more than a theoretical risk, as it has been reported in the literature.

In many studies TS/LS has proven to be superior for accessing TNM status compared to conventional imaging alone. However, the exact role of laparoscopy and thoracoscopy in staging esophageal cancer is currently debated. Whether laparoscopy/thoracoscopy will become the general practice in evaluating locoregional disease as mediastinoscopy has done for lung cancer staging remains to be determined. The principal disadvantages of TS/LS are its high cost and its requirement of hospitalization. To better clarify its role, a prospective multiinstitutional study, CALGB 9380, is currently underway to access the efficacy, accuracy, and cost of minimally invasive surgical staging. It is hoped that the final results of this study will better clarify the role of TS/LS in esophageal cancer staging.

# References

Anderson DN, Campbell S, Park MGM. Accuracy of laparoscopic ultrasonography in the staging of upper gastrointestinal malignancy. Br J Surg 1996;83:1424–1428.

Bemelman WA, van Delden OM, van Lanschot JJB, et al. Laparoscopy and laparoscopic ultrasonography in staging of carcinoma of the esophagus and gastric cardia. J Am Coll Surg 1995;181:421–425.

Bonavina L, Incarbone R, Lattuada E, Segalin A, Cesana B, Peracchia A. Preoperative laparoscopy in management of patients with carcinoma of the esophagus and of the esophagogastric junction. J Surg Oncol 1997;65:171–174.

Bonavina L, Incarbone R, Peracchia A. Staging by immediate preoperative laparoscopy in adenocarcinoma of the distal esophagus and cardia. Ann Chir 1999;53(9):850–853.

Bosch A, Frias Z, Caldwell WL, Jaeschke WH. Autopsy findings in carcinoma of the oesophagus. Acta Radiol Oncol 1979;18:103–106.

Cerfolio RJ, Bryant AS, Ohja B, Bartolucci AA, Eloubeidi MA. The accuracy of endoscopic ultrasonography with fine-needle aspiration, integrated positron emission tomography with computed tomography, and computed tomography in restaging patients with esophageal cancer after neoadjuvant chemoradiotherapy. J Thorac Cardiovasc Surg 2005;129(6):1232–1241.

Clements DM, Bowrey DJ, Havard TJ. The role of staging investigations for oesophagogastric carcinoma. Eur J Surg Oncol 2004;30:309–312.

Dagnini G, Caldironi MW, Marin G, et al. Laparoscopy in abdominal staging of esophageal carcinoma. Gastrointest Endosc 1986;32:400–402.

Finch MD, John TG, Garden OJ, Allan PL, Paterson-Brown S. Laparoscopic ultrasonography for staging gastroesophageal cancer. Surgery 1997;121:10–17.

Hulscher JBF, Nieveen van Dijkum EJM, de Wit LT, et al. Laparoscopy and laparoscopic ultrasonography in staging carcinoma of the gastric cardia. Eur J Surg 2000;166:862–865.

Kato H, Miyazaki T, Nakajima M, et al. The incremental effect of positron emission tomography on diagnostic accuracy in the initial staging of esophageal carcinoma. Chirurg 2005;103(1):148–156.

Krasna MJ, Jiao X, Mao YS, et al. Thoracoscopy/laparoscopy in the staging of esophageal cancer: Maryland experience. Surg Laparosc Endosc Percutan Tech 2002;12(4):213–218.

Krasna MJ, Reed CE, Nedzwiecki D, et al. CALGB 9380: a prospective trial of the feasibility of thoracoscopy/laparoscopy in staging esophageal cancer. Ann Thorac Surg 2001;71:1073–1079.

Lerut T, Nafteux P, Moons J, et al. Three-field lymphadenectomy for carcinoma of the esophagus and gastroesophageal junction in 174 R0 resections: impact on staging, disease-free survival, and outcome: a plea for adaptation of TNM classification in upper-half esophageal carcinoma. Ann Surg 2004;240(6):962–972.

Luketich JD, Schauer P, Landreneau R, et al. Minimally invasive surgical staging is superior to endoscopic ultrasound in detecting lymph node metastases in esophageal cancer. J Thorac Cardiovasc Surg 1997;114:817–823.

Nieveen van Dijkum EJ, de Wit LT, Delden OMv, et al. Staging laparoscopy and laparoscopic ultrasonography in more than 400 patients with upper gastrointestinal carcinoma. J Am Coll Surg 1999;189: 459–465.

O'Brien MG, Fitzgerald EF, Lee G, Crowley M, Shanahan F, O'Sullivan GC. A prospective comparison of laparoscopy and imaging in the staging of esophagogastric cancer before surgery. Am J Gastroenterol 1995;90:2191–2194.

Romijn MG, Van Overhagen H, Spillenaar Bilgen EJ, et al. Laparoscopy and laparoscopic ultrasonography in staging of oesophageal and cardial carcinoma. Br J Surg 1998; 85(7):1010–1012.

Sihvo EI, Rasanen JV, Knuuti MJ, et al. Adenocarcinoma of the esophagus and the esophagogastric junction: positron emission tomography improves staging and prediction of survival in distant but not in locoregional disease. J Gastrointest Surg 2004;8(8):988–996.

Smith A, Finch MD, John TG, et al. Role of laparoscopic ultrasonography in the management of patients with oesophagogastric cancer. Br J Surg 1999;86:1083–1087.

Swisher SG, Maish M, Erasmus JJ, et al. Utility of PET, CT, and EUS to identify pathologic responders in esophageal cancer. Ann Thorac Surg 2004;78(4):1152–1160.

Wallace MB, Nietert PJ, Earle C, et al. An analysis of multiple staging management strategies for carcinoma of the esophagus: computed tomography, endoscopic ultrasound, positron emission tomography, and thoracoscopy/laparoscopy. Ann Thorac Surg 2002;74:1026–1032.

Watt I, Stewart I, Anderson D, et al. Laparoscopy, ultrasound and computed tomography in cancer of the oesophagus and gastric cardia: a prospective comparison for detecting intra-abdominal metastases. Br J Surg 1989;76:1036–1039.

Westerp M, van Westreenen HL, Reitsma JB, Hoekstra OS, Stoker J. Esophageal cancer: CT, endoscopic ultrasound, and FDG PET for assessment of response to neoadjuvant therapy—systemic review. Radiology 2005;236:841–851.

Wieder HA, Beer AJ, Lordick F, et al. Comparison of changes in tumor metabolic activity and tumor size during chemotherapy of adenocarcinomas of the esophagogastric junction. J Nucl Med 2005;46:2029–2034.

## Suggested Readings

Abdalla EK, Pisters PWT. Staging and preoperative evaluation of upper gastrointestinal malignancies. Semin Oncol 2004;31:513–529.

Espat NJ, Jacobsen G, Horgan S, Donahue P. Minimally invasive treatment of esophageal cancer: laparoscopic staging to robotic esophagectomy. Cancer J 2005;11:10–17.

Flett ME, Lim MN, Bruce D, et al. Prognostic value of laparoscopic ultrasound in patients with gastro-esophageal cancer. Dis Esophagus 2001;14:223–226.

Freeman RK, Wait MA. Port site metastasis after laparoscopic staging of esophageal carcinoma. Ann Thorac Surg 2001;71:1032–1034.

Hünerbein M, Rau B, Hohenberger P, Schlag PM. The role of laparoscopic ultrasound for staging of gastrointestinal tumors. Chirurg 2001;72:914–919.

Jemal A, Siegel R, Ward E, et al. Cancer statistics 2006. CA Cancer J Clin 2006; 56:106–130.

Larson SM, Schoder H, Yeung H. Positron emission tomography/computerized tomography functional imaging of esophageal and colorectal cancer. Cancer J 2004; 10:243–250.

Menon KV, Dehn TCB. Multiport staging laparoscopy in esophageal and cardiac carcinoma. Dis Esophagus 2003;16:295–300.

Natsugoe S, Yoshinaka H, Shimada M, et al. Assessment of cervical lymph node metastasis in esophageal carcinoma using ultrasonography. Ann Surg 1999;229:62–66.

Patel AN, Buenaventura PO. Current staging of esophageal cancer. Surg Clin North Am 2005;85:555–567.

Rau B, Hunerbein M. Diagnostic laparoscopy: indications and benefits. Langenbecks Arch Surg 2005;390:187–196.

Siemsen M, Svendsen LB, Knigge U, et al. A prospective randomized comparison of curved array and radial echoendoscopy in patients with esophageal cancer. Gastrointest Endosc 2003;58(5):671–676.

Stell DA, Carter CR, Stewart I, Anderson JR. Prospective comparison of laparoscopy, ultrasonography and computed tomography in the staging of gastric cancer. Br J Surg 1996;83:1260–1262.

Wakelin SJ, Deans C, Crofts TJ, Allan PL, Plevris JN, Paterson-Brown S. A comparison of computerised tomography, laparoscopic ultrasound and endoscopic ultrasound in the preoperative staging of oesophago-gastric carcinoma. Eur J Radiol 2002; 41(2):161–167.

Yau KK, Siu WT, Cheung HYS, et al. Immediate preoperative laparoscopic staging for squamous cell carcinoma of the esophagus. Surg Endosc 2006;20:307–310.

# 17. Esophageal Carcinoma

## A. Introduction

Before advanced minimal access techniques were developed, surgery for esophageal carcinoma required either a transthoracic approach or a transhiatal approach. Both had advantages and disadvantages. Currently, there are several minimal access approaches that can be used for surgical resection of esophageal malignancies. Robotic surgery, not included in this manual, is also being applied. This chapter explores several alternative approaches that may be used to resect esophageal carcinoma for potential cure.

## B. Case

### Paul B. Tessmann

A 61-year-old man presented with a 2-month history of dysphagia. This began as dysphagia for solid foods approximately 6 months ago, but over the past month this had rapidly progressed to the point where he could only eat soft foods such as mashed potatoes, noodles, and shakes. His wife noted that his energy was slightly diminished, and he had lost approximately 10 pounds over the past several months.

His past medical history was significant for gastroesophageal reflux disease for the past 20 years, controlled on a proton pump inhibitor. He also had type 2 diabetes mellitus, hypertension, and benign prostatic hypertrophy. His past surgical history was significant for an appendectomy at age 19. He did not have a family history of cancer.

His medications included aspirin, omeprazole, glimepiride, metformin, rosiglitazone, lisinopril, metoprolol, and terazosin. He had no known drug allergies.

He was a retired schoolteacher. He had a 60-pack-a-year smoking history, but had stopped smoking 12 years earlier, and there was no alcohol use in the past 35 years.

The review of systems was positive for dysphagia and weight loss as noted above. He did not have any symptoms of heartburn, nausea, vomiting, chest pain, cough, change in bowel habits, melena, or bright red blood per rectum.

On physical examination, he was a well-developed white male with stigmata of recent weight loss. His height was 182 cm and he weighed 73 kg. His vital signs, head and neck, and cardiopulmonary examinations were all normal. There was no supraclavicular or cervical lymphadenopathy.

On abdominal examination, there was a well-healed right lower quadrant scar, consistent with previous appendectomy. There were no hernias. The abdomen was soft, without masses or tenderness. Bowel sounds were normal.

Rectal examination revealed a smooth, slightly enlarged prostate, and no mucosal lesions. Stool was guaiac negative.

Laboratory studies were remarkable only for an hematocrit of 34%. Liver function tests were normal.

Barium swallow study showed a 5-cm irregular stricture in the distal esophagus. Esophagoscopy revealed a friable, partially obstructing, noncircumferential mass at approximately 30 cm from the incisors. Barrett's metaplasia was noted to 27 cm. Biopsy of the mass revealed a moderately differentiated adenocarcinoma.

Endoscopic ultrasound revealed a T3 tumor and one paraesophageal mediastinal lymph node measuring 6 × 3 mm, appearing oval and hypoechoic, with well-defined margins.

Chest x-ray was negative. Computed tomography scan showed irregular thickening of the distal esophagus, with no other involved lymph nodes or evidence of distant metastasis.

The impression was moderately differentiated 5-cm adenocarcinoma of the distal esophagus, clinically staged as T3 N1 M0, stage III.

The patient was entered into a clinical trial of neoadjuvant chemoradiation therapy. Follow-up studies showed a favorable response and he was referred for surgical resection. He was interested in a minimal access approach.

**How would you approach this tumor?**

# C. Minimally Invasive Esophagectomy

*Michael Kent and James Luketich*

Resection of esophageal cancer is most commonly performed through either an open transhiatal or transthoracic (Ivor Lewis) approach. Several alternatives, such as en-bloc esophagectomy or thoracoabdominal esophagectomy, have also been proposed in an effort to either improve survival or minimize postoperative morbidity. In many cases, the choice between these approaches is one of personal preference. A transthoracic approach may be preferred by surgeons with experience in other intrathoracic procedures, such as pulmonary resection. On the other hand, a transhiatal esophagectomy is often the procedure of choice of surgeons with expertise in open foregut surgery, such as gastrectomy. However, no study has conclusively shown a survival benefit of one form of esophagectomy over the other. Indeed Hulscher et al., in a randomized study comparing transhiatal with Ivor Lewis esophagectomy for patients with esophageal cancer, demonstrated equivalent survival at 5 years.

While survival may be equivalent, it is clear that the morbidity following esophagectomy is greatly influenced by the operative approach. For example, in the randomized study mentioned above, the incidence of pulmonary complications was 57% in the transthoracic group compared to 27% in the transhiatal group. This is certainly related to the impact that synchronous thoracotomy and laparotomy incisions have on pulmonary function in the perioperative period. The development of pneumonia is significant, as the risk of death in these patients is reported to be as high as 20%.

Conversely, anastomotic stricture and leak are more common in patients with a cervical anastomosis. In addition, injury to the recurrent laryngeal nerve is less common if dissection in the neck is avoided. This injury may significantly impact on a patient's quality of life, and has also been shown to be associated with a decreased 5-year survival following esophagectomy.

In an attempt to lower morbidity, we and other centers have explored minimally invasive approaches to esophageal resection. A potential benefit of these techniques is the improvement in pain control and pulmonary function by avoiding synchronous thoracotomy and laparotomy incisions. Although the operation is technically challenging, portions of the operation are quite familiar to surgeons with minimally invasive training in other areas. For example, creation of the gastric tube is not unlike what is required for Roux-en-Y gastric bypass. The mobilization of the abdominal esophagus is the same as that performed during laparoscopic fundoplication. Because of this, interest in minimally invasive esophagectomy will only increase, as greater numbers of surgeons complete their training with experience in other advanced laparoscopic cases.

There is another reason to persist in efforts to improve the technique of esophagectomy. Open esophagectomy is well known to be associated with the highest morbidity and mortality among any elective operation. This has led to increasing interest among medical oncologists in treating patients with definitive chemoradiation alone. Two recent studies on squamous cell cancer of the esophagus lend some support to this practice. The impact of these reports has been to recommend nonoperative therapy for marginal surgical candidates, such as the elderly or those with multiple comorbidities. Indeed, the National Comprehensive Cancer Network in its recent guidelines now considers definitive chemoradiation to be an acceptable alternative to esophagectomy. Unfortunately, some of these data have been extrapolated to healthy patients with high-grade dysplasia or early-stage esophageal cancer in whom very high 5-year survival rates can be anticipated after esophagectomy. Consequently, it is incumbent on surgeons to refine the technique of esophagectomy, lest the paradigm of treatment of esophageal cancer gradually move away from surgical resection.

## Technical Considerations

The technique of minimally invasive esophagectomy (MIE) has evolved as our experience with other minimally invasive foregut procedures, such as laparoscopic Heller myotomy, repair of giant paraesophageal hernias, and staging for esophageal cancer, has grown. Currently, we have performed over 500 MIEs at the University of Pittsburgh Medical Center.

The early efforts with minimally invasive esophageal resection were hybrid approaches, combining thoracoscopic mobilization of the esophagus, an open laparotomy for creation of the gastric tube, and a cervical anastomosis. No conclusive benefit was seen with this approach compared with standard esophagectomy, although the number of patients studied was small and the authors had likely not yet surpassed the learning curve with this procedure.

Since these early reports several modifications have been proposed, including laparoscopic transhiatal esophagectomy and robotic-assisted esophagectomy. An entirely laparoscopic esophagectomy, without the need for thoracoscopy, would seem to have significant benefits. The entire procedure may be performed with the patient in the supine position and with a standard single-lumen endotracheal tube. However, we have found that the disadvantages of this approach far outweigh these benefits. The working space through the hiatus is quite small, and allows only limited access to the middle and upper third of the esophagus. As a consequence any thoracic lymph node dissection is extremely difficult through this approach. Because of this we prefer to first mobilize the thoracic esophagus through a right video assisted thoracic surgery (VATS) followed by laparoscopy to prepare the gastric tube. Although early in our experience MIE was only offered to patients with Barrett's disease and early-stage tumors, we now offer MIE to patients with more advanced disease, including those who have undergone induction chemoradiation therapy. Patients found to have bulky nodal metastases by computed tomography (CT) or staging laparoscopy are not felt to be candidates for MIE, and consideration is given to either an open operation or definitive chemoradiation. A brief description of the operation follows.

## Thoracoscopy

The initial step in MIE is an on-table esophagogastroduodenoscopy (EGD) to confirm the tumor's location and the suitability of the stomach as a conduit for reconstruction. Significant extension onto the cardia of the stomach will often require a wider gastric resection margin and may prevent the construction of a gastric conduit that will reach the neck. For these cases, we prefer a high chest anastomosis, generally performed thoracoscopically (see below). Laparoscopic staging may also be of use in these patients to more accurately define the degree of cardia involvement before proceeding with resection.

After endoscopy patients are then turned to the left lateral decubitus position for thoracoscopy. The surgeon stands on the right side and the assistant on the left. Four thoracoscopic ports are used (Fig. 17.1). A 10-mm camera port is placed in the seventh or eighth intercostal space, just anterior to the midaxillary line. A 5-mm port is placed at the eighth or ninth intercostal space, posterior to the posterior axillary line, for the ultrasonic coagulating shears (U.S. Surgical, Norwalk, CT). A 10-mm port is placed in the anterior axillary line at the fourth intercostal space and is used to insert a fan-shaped retractor to retract the lung anteriorly and expose the esophagus. The last 5-mm port is placed just anterior to the tip of the scapula and is used for retraction by the surgeon. A key initial step in exposure is to place a retracting suture through the central tendon of the diaphragm, which is brought out through the anterior chest wall via a 1-mm incision. This suture retracts the diaphragm inferiorly and allows excellent visualization of the gastroesophageal junction (GEJ).

The inferior pulmonary ligament is then divided and the mediastinal pleura overlying the esophagus divided to the level of the azygos vein. The azygos vein is then ligated using an endoscopic stapler (U.S. Surgical). We are careful at this point to preserve the mediastinal pleura

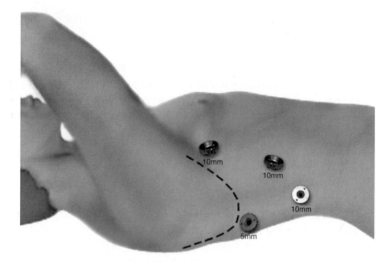

Fig. 17.1. Placement of ports for thoracoscopic phase of dissection.

above the junction of the azygos vein and the superior vena cava. We believe this maintains the gastric conduit in a mediastinal location and may seal the plane between the stomach and the thoracic inlet, minimizing any downward extension of a cervical anastomotic leak into the chest. We then proceed to circumferentially mobilize the esophagus up to 2 cm above the carina, sweeping all periesophageal nodes and fat into the specimen. We do not attempt to include the thoracic duct in the resected specimen. However, any lymphatic branches arising from the duct are carefully clipped and divided, to prevent chylothorax. A Penrose drain placed around the esophagus greatly aids in subsequent mobilization (Fig. 17.2). The entire thoracic esophagus is then mobilized from the thoracic inlet to the diaphragm. It is important not to carry the dissection too low into the peritoneal cavity, which would hinder the creation of pneumoperitoneum during laparoscopy. Also, we keep the dissection plane close to the esophagus at the superior extent of the dissection, to avoid injury to either the airway or the recurrent laryngeal nerves. We specifically divide the vagus trunks at the level of the azygous vein, to prevent any possible traction injury to the recurrent laryngeal nerves.

After the esophagus is completely mobilized, a single 28-French (F) chest tube is placed and the patient is turned to the supine position for laparoscopy. Prior to turning we reintubate the patient with a single-lumen endotracheal tube. We have found that dissection of the cervical

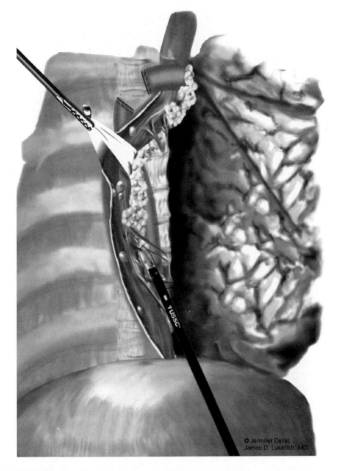

Fig. 17.2. Mobilization of thoracic esophagus.

esophagus is much more difficult with the larger, double-lumen tube in place. In addition, bronchoscopy can be performed through the single-lumen tube prior to extubation.

## Laparoscopy and Cervical Anastomosis

The five abdominal ports used for gastric mobilization are in the same configuration we use for benign esophageal cases, although they are placed somewhat lower so we can visualize the entire stomach (Fig. 17.3).

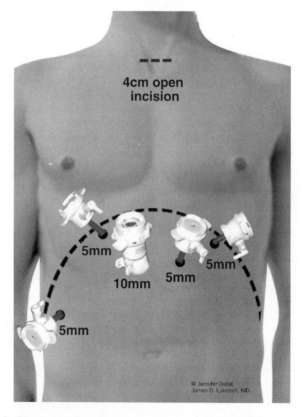

Fig. 17.3. Placement of ports for laparoscopic phase of dissection.

The gastrohepatic ligament is first divided and the right and left crura are dissected. Unlike other foregut operations, we do not divide the phrenoesophageal ligament until the conclusion of the laparoscopy. This allows us to maintain the pneumoperitoneum for the duration of the procedure. The stomach is then mobilized by dividing first the short gastric vessels and then the gastrocolic omentum, carefully preserving the right gastroepiploic vessels. The stomach is then retracted superiorly and the left gastric artery is divided using a vascular stapler.

The laparoscopic mobilization of the pyloroantral area must be meticulous. During this part of the procedure, we periodically grasp the antrum, near the pylorus and carefully lift it toward the diaphragmatic hiatus. When sufficiently mobilized, the pylorus should be easily elevated to the right crus in a tension-free manner. If this cannot be accomplished, or there is tension during this maneuver, further Kocherization is needed. After mobilization, a pyloroplasty is then created by opening the pylorus with the ultrasonic shears and closing the pylorus transversely using the Endostitch (US Surgical, Division of Tyco, Ltd, Princeton NJ) (Fig. 17.4). In our experience a laparoscopic pyloromyotomy is difficult to perform and often leads to insufficient gastric emptying.

The gastric tube is then created by dividing the stomach at the lesser curve using a 4.8-mm stapler, preserving the right gastric vessels (Fig. 17.5). This tube is created to be 5 to 6 cm in diameter. Early in our experience we created a tube of 3 to 4 cm and found a significant increase in gastric tip necrosis and anastomotic leaks. During this step, we have found it beneficial to have the first assistant grasp the tip of the fundus and gently stretch it toward the spleen, while a second grasper is placed on the antral area and a slight downward retraction is applied. This places the stomach on slight stretch, and facilitates a straight staple line application, which should be parallel to the gastroepiploic arcade. The most superior portion of the gastric tube is then attached to the resection specimen using two Endostitches. These stitches maintain correct orientation of the stomach as it is delivered into the mediastinum and neck.

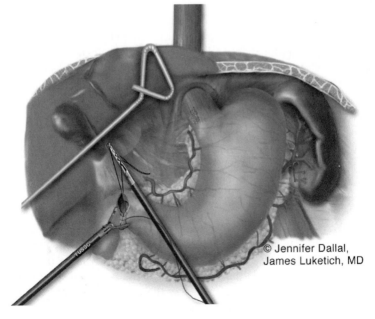

© Jennifer Dallal,
James Luketich, MD

Fig. 17.4. Closure of pyloroplasty.

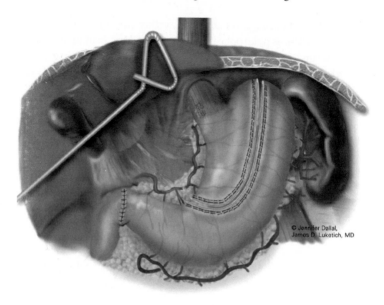

Fig. 17.5. Creation of gastric tube.

A feeding jejunostomy is then placed using a needle catheter kit (Compat Biosystems, Minneapolis, MN). A limb of jejunum is first tacked to the anterior abdominal wall using an Endostitch. An additional 10-mm port may be placed in the right lower quadrant to facilitate this step. The needle and guidewire are then passed into the jejunum under laparoscopic vision. Proper positioning of the catheter is confirmed by observing distention of the jejunum as air is insufflated into the needle catheter. The jejunum is then completely tacked to the abdominal wall using several additional Endostitches. Laparoscopy is concluded by division of the phrenoesophageal membrane. We also partially divide the right and left crura to allow easy passage of the stomach into the mediastinum.

Next a horizontal neck incision is made to expose the cervical esophagus. We typically leave the Penrose drain around the esophagus during VATS mobilization and push this drain into the neck at the conclusion of thoracoscopy. This allows quick identification of correct dissection plane. The specimen is then pulled out of the neck and the cervical esophagus is divided 1 to 2 cm below the cricopharyngeus. We then perform a side-to-end esophagogastrostomy using a 25-mm end-to-end anastomosis (EEA) stapler.

After the neck anastomosis is completed, we return to the laparoscopic view. Attention is directed to reducing any excess gastric conduit pulled into the thoracic cavity, which invariably occurs during the pull-up and anastomosis. This can be achieved by grasping the antral area firmly, but carefully and gently tugging downward toward the abdomen; often several centimeters will reduce before the anastomosis is observed to move slightly caudad. When this occurs, one can generally assume the redundant gastric tube in now within the abdomen. Failure to perform this step may lead to a slight sigmoid curve of the redundant gastric antrum within the chest that may lead to poor gastric emptying and the need for subsequent revision.

Finally, three tacking sutures are placed between the gastric tube and the diaphragm to prevent hiatal herniation. Usually one suture is placed between the left crus and the stomach just anterior to the greater curve arcade, the second on the right side of the gastric tube just above the right gastric vessels, and the third stitch anteriorly between the stomach and the diaphragm. Figure 17.6 illustrates the completed reconstruction.

We close the neck incision very loosely. Meticulous closure of the platysma will invariably allow a leak, should one occur, to track into the mediastinum rather than out the neck. To prevent this we usually leave the neck incision open except for a single staple to oppose the skin edges. The horizontal incision that we use is created in the lines of a skin fold and heals remarkably well, without the need for meticulous closure.

## Minimally Invasive Ivor Lewis Esophagectomy

As described above, our standard MIE is concluded with a cervical esophagogastric anastomosis. However, creation of an intrathoracic anastomosis does carry some benefits. Avoiding dissection in the neck significantly lowers the risk of injury to the recurrent laryngeal nerves. In addition, a small group of patients will develop significant problems with esophageal transit and aspiration, despite intact recurrent laryngeal nerves (Easterling et al., Martin et al.). Although these complications are rarely reported as fatal, they may have a profound impact on the risk of aspiration pneumonia, clearance of pulmonary secretions, and overall quality of life. In addition, creation of a lower anastomosis may be necessary in patients with significant gastric extension of GEJ tumors to involve the cardia. In these cases, more stomach must be resected to obtain an adequate margin, and the remaining gastric tube may not have sufficient length to reach the neck.

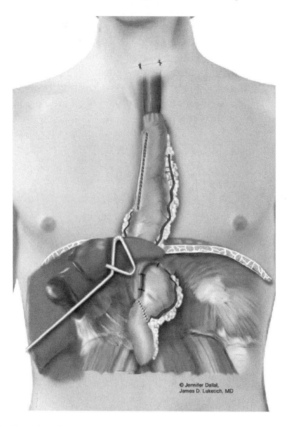

Fig. 17.6. Completed reconstruction.

The concern with an Ivor Lewis esophagectomy is the significant increase in pulmonary complications with this approach. It would seem that a minimally invasive Ivor Lewis esophagectomy would combine the advantages of avoiding dissection in the neck with the benefits of a reduction in pulmonary morbidity seen with minimally invasive surgery. A brief description or our operative approach is given below.

The conduct of the operation is similar to a standard MIE, although we begin this procedure with laparoscopy. Once the abdominal phase has been completed the patient is turned to the left lateral decubitus position. We use the same port sites for thoracoscopy that have been described. The only modification is to enlarge the posterior-inferior eighth intercostal port site to 3 to 4 cm to allow the introduction of the

EEA stapler (U.S. Surgical) and removal of the specimen. A laparo-scopic wound protector is used at this site to minimize the risk of port-site contamination. Once the esophagus has been mobilized to a level 4 to 5 cm above the azygos vein, the distal esophagus and stomach are brought through the hiatus into the chest, along with the gastric tube that has been sutured to the specimen. The esophagus is elevated and transected 2 to 3 cm above the level of the azygos vein. The specimen is removed using an endo-catch bag (U.S. Surgical) to prevent wound contamination. The anvil of a 25-mm EEA stapler is then placed into the proximal esophagus and secured using a purse-string Endostitch (U.S. Surgical). The stapler is then placed through the enlarged port, introduced into the tip of the newly created gastric conduit, and a circu-lar anastomosis (side of gastric conduit to end of esophagus) is created at the level of the azygos vein. The redundant portion of the gastric con-duit is trimmed using an articulating, linear stapler (Endo-GIA II, U.S. Surgical), and a 28F chest tube and a Jackson-Pratt drain are placed by the anastomosis. The potential space between the conduit and the right crus of the diaphragm is then closed with interrupted stitches to prevent delayed herniation.

We have recently reported our initial experience with this procedure. Early in the series, we had performed a hybrid operation combining laparoscopy with a right thoracotomy. As our experience increased, we began to construct the anastomosis thoracoscopically. Among a total of 50 patients, we noted a mortality of 6% and a leak rate of 6%. No patient developed injury to the recurrent laryngeal nerves, and the incidence of pneumonia was 8%. We have found these early results to be encourag-ing, although a larger series with longer follow-up will better define the benefits and any unique complications of this approach.

# D. Hybrid Video-Assisted Esophagectomy

*Satoshi Yamamoto, Katsunobu Kawahara, and Takayuki Shirakusa*

We utilize a hybrid approach in which the thoracic dissection is accomplished using VATS, and the abdominal dissection is performed with a minilaparotomy. We perform a cervical neck dissection and place the anastomosis in the neck. This technique has been described by Kawahara et al. and we will describe our procedure here.

We begin with the patient under single (left lung) ventilation in the left lateral decubitus position. We insert five to six thoracoscopic ports from the fourth to eighth intercostal spaces in the anterior, middle, and posterior axillary lines. A 30-degree visual thoracoscope is inserted through the port placed in the seventh intercostal space at the midaxillary line, and dissection of the esophagus and periesophageal tissues commences. When difficulties are experienced, for example, if the esophageal tumor is too large or severe adhesion to the bronchus or left atrium is observed, we perform a 6-cm thoracotomy in the auscultation triangle.

We dissect the thoracic esophagus and mediastinal nodes with a harmonic scalpel. The lymph nodes along the left recurrent laryngeal nerve are dissected with bipolar electric coagulator scissors to prevent heat injury to the nerve. After total dissection of thoracic esophagus, the esophagus is divided at the upper thoracic esophagus. A chest tube is inserted, and the patient turned to the supine position.

A collar incision is made in the neck and a bilateral neck lymph node dissection is performed. Some teams perform this dissection simultaneously with the abdominal phase of surgery.

An 8-cm upper-midline abdominal incision is then made. A perigastric lymph node dissection is then performed. The dissection of the lower thoracic and abdominal esophagus is performed via the transhiatal route. The esophagus is then pulled into the abdominal cavity. A thin gastric tube is made and pulled up through the retrosternal route and anastomosed end-to-end to the cervical esophagus using 4-0 monofilament absorbable suture.

In 101 (90.2%) of our 112 patients, a thin gastric tube was used for reconstruction. In 11 (9.8%) patients who had undergone a distal gastrectomy for a gastric cancer or peptic ulcer, the reconstruction was performed with use of the left colon in five (4.5%) patients and the ileocolon in six (5.4%).

Our results with this approach have been quite good. Lymph node metastasis was found in 65 (58.0%) patients. A thoracoscopic esophagectomy was performed on 65 (58.0%) patients, and a video-assisted esophagectomy was performed on 47 (42.0%) patients. All 112 patients were extubated in the operating room after surgery. Two (1.8%) patients with emphysema were reintubated for ventilator support in the intensive care unit (ICU). The average thoracoscopic time was 111 minutes (range 45 to 210 minutes), and average intrathoracic blood loss was 134 mL (range 20 to 490 mL). The average number of mediastinal dissecting nodes was 28 (range 5 to 79 nodes).

Intraoperative complications occurred in four (3.6%) patients. Azygos vein arch injury occurred in one (0.9%) patient. Hemostasis was achieved using an endoclip. The membranous portion of the trachea was injured in three (2.7%) patients. In two (1.8%) patients, the laceration was repaired with direct suture closure and wrapped with the right lobe of the thymus. In one (0.9%) patient with a large defect in the membranous portion of the trachea, we switched to an open thoracotomy and the tracheal defect was patched with a latissimus dorsi muscle flap.

Early postoperative complications occurred in 29 (25.9%) patients. Major anastomotic leakage occurred in four (3.6%) patients who required reanastomosis. Chylothorax improved by fasting and intravenous hyperalimentation for 2 to 3 weeks after surgery.

The overall 5-year survival rate was 52%. All patients with stage 0 disease were alive after 4 years. The 5-year survival rate was 87% in stage I disease, 70% in stage IIA disease, 68% in stage IIB disease, and 27% in stage III disease. There were no patients with stage IV disease who survived 4 years or longer. The 5-year survival rate of the patients with node-negative disease was 75%, and for these with node-positive disease it was 31%.

To sum up, several minimally invasive approaches have been tried for treatment of esophageal cancer. The majority of surgeons have shown that a thoracoscopic esophagectomy is feasible and can be performed safely for select patients; however, no clear advantages over a traditional open thoracotomy have been shown.

For thoracoscopic resection of the esophagus, the reported mean thoracoscopic procedure time have ranged from 104 to 198 minutes in several published series, the mean blood loss was 165 to 450 mL, and the mean number of thoracic lymph nodes was 7 to 12 (Gossot et al., Law et al., Peracchia et al.). The mean thoracoscopic procedure time and the blood loss amount in our series were similar to the finding in these reports, whereas the mean number of thoracic lymph nodes was greater in our series. Paratracheal node dissection may have contributed to the increased number of dissecting nodes.

Intraoperative complications, such as intercostal artery, azygous vein or aortic arch laceration, and bronchial injury, have been reported to be associated with this approach. In our series, injury to the azygous vein arch and the membranous portion of the trachea occurred. In one patient, the thoracoscopic approach was converted to open surgery, and the lacerated trachea was repaired. Dissection should be performed with care, and the prompt recognition of the necessity to convert to open surgery in difficult cases is important.

Postoperative mortality and morbidity rates are reported to range from 0% to 11% and 0% to 38.9% in published series, respectively. The incidence of postoperative respiratory complications is reported to range from 0% to 36%, recurrent laryngeal nerve palsy ranges from 0% to 29.4%, and anastomotic leakage ranges from 0% to 17.6%. In our series, the rate of major postoperative complications was similar to the rate noted in these reports.

There have been few reports of long-term survival of patients with a thoracoscopic esophagectomy for esophageal cancer. Smithers et al. reported an overall 5-year survival rate of patients who underwent thoracoscopic esophagectomy for esophageal cancer of 40%. In our series, the survival of patients with stage 0, I, II, and III disease compared satisfactorily with those reports.

In conclusion, both thoracoscopic and video-assisted esophagectomies are thus considered to be feasible and safe options for treatment of esophageal cancer, and the survival time of patients with stage I, II disease has been found to be satisfactory.

# E. Mediastinoscope-Assisted Transhiatal Esophagectomy

*Akira Tangoku, Junichi Seike, Junko Honda, Takahiro Yoshida, and Atsushi Umemoto*

Transhiatal esophagectomy (THE) avoids thoracotomy and shortens surgical time, but the risk of intraoperative morbidity such as massive bleeding stresses the surgeon, and lymph node sampling is not possible. Mediastinoscopy supplies a clear visualization of anatomic structures of the mediastinum. With the mediastinoscope, transhiatal esophagectomy can be performed safely under direct vision. Lymph node sampling is feasible due to clear visualization of the mediastinum. Patients with superficial esophageal cancer and preoperative medical risk factors are good candidates for this procedure. In our experience, bleeding is minimal and operative time short. Morbidity and mortality are decreased, compared with more extensive operative approaches. For properly selected patients, mediastinoscope-assisted transhiatal esophagectomy (MATHE) is a safe and minimally invasive technique that allows direct visualization of mediastinal structures.

As lymphatic spread and lymph nodes metastases are common even in the case of superficial cancer, transthoracic (abdominothoracic) en bloc esophagectomy (TTE) with radical lymphadenectomy has improved the survival of patients with esophageal cancer not only in squamous cell carcinoma but also in adenocarcinoma. Unfortunately, operative morbidity and mortality rates are high due to the radical mediastinal lymphadenectomy and single lung ventilation. Pulmonary complications after TTE are common, and these morbidities are life-threatening. Many patients with esophageal cancer are elderly and have compromised medical risks preoperatively.

Transhiatal esophagectomy (THE) avoids thoracotomy and shortens operation time. It has been adopted for palliative treatment of esophageal cancer. However, operative risks of bleeding and mediastinal injury due to blind manipulation stress the surgeon, and reported postoperative morbidity and mortality are not small (Wong). Lymph nodes status, which is the best indicator for prognosis and postoperative therapy, is not known. The mediastinoscope avoids these risks and allows lymph node sampling under direct vision.

## Indications and Contraindication

Endoscopic mucosal resection (EMR) is indicated for localized, superficial (lesions limited to the epithelial layer and the proper mucosal layer) cancer in which no lymphatic metastases are expected. Widespread or multiple mucosal lesions require wide EMR, which may result in postoperative stenosis or perforation of the esophagus. Mediastinoscope-assisted transhiatal esophagectomy is recommended in such widespread or multiple superficial cases. It is also preferred for patients with preoperative medical risk factors, such as heart disease, pulmonary dysfunction, cirrhosis, diabetes mellitus, malnutrition, age over 80, and synchronous malignancy at another site.

This procedure is contraindicated for advanced tumors such as T3 or T4 disease, bleeding tendency, and body deformity. The mediastinal space is very small, and such a large tumor occupies the space. Therefore, safe dissection under clear vision is difficult. We have safely performed MATHE for advanced disease in patients with severe comorbidities that precluded alternative approaches, such as profound thrombocytopenia, amyotrophic lateral sclerosis, and postpoliomyelitis syndrome.

## Technical Considerations

We use a 5-mm-diameter mirror scope attached to a retractor with a transparent flat tip (Subcu-dissector, Endopath Saphenous Vein Harvest Tray, Ethicon Endosurgery, Inc., Cincinnati, OH) (Fig. 17.7) as a

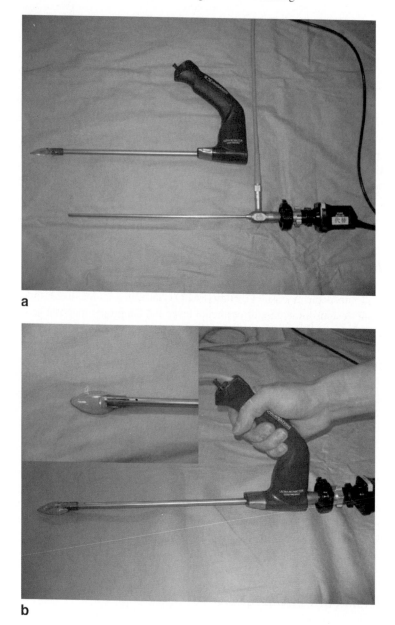

Fig. 17.7. (A) Mediastinoscope. (B) A transparent cap. A 5-mm-diameter mirror scope was used. A transparent cap is placed on the tip to prevent soiling with blood. The flat retractor is necessary to create a mediastinal operating space.

mediastinoscope. The mediastinal operating space is made by retracting the trachea and the esophagus with this mediastinoscope (Fig. 17.8).

The patient is placed in the supine position on the operating table with both arms tucked. An operator and an assistant (cervical team) perform MATHE with the mediastinoscope via the neck while the other surgeons (abdominal team) simultaneously prepared the interposition graft and dissected the terminal esophagus, and the abdominal and lower esophageal lymph nodes.

Mediastinoscope-assisted transhiatal esophagectomy is started via a left cervical approach. A collar incision is made in the left anterior neck. The anterior edge of the sternocleidomastoid muscle is divided and retracted, and the anterior cervical muscles divided transversely. The cervical esophagus is circumferentially exposed and elevated with a rubber tube. The mediastinoscope is inserted carefully from the left side of the esophagus and pushed gently into the mediastinum (Fig. 17.9). The surgical space is created by retracting the esophagus with the mediastinoscope. The thoracic duct is easily retrieved on the left posterior side of the esophagus (Fig. 17.10). Lymphatic and blood vessels are

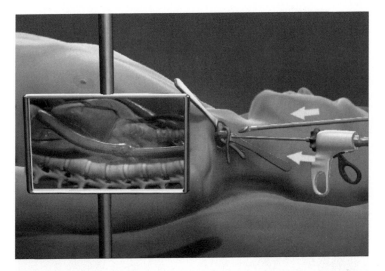

Fig. 17.8. Mediastinoscope-assisted transhiatal esophagectomy (MATHE) is started via a left cervical approach. The mediastinoscope is inserted into the mediastinum via the neck and sometimes from the hiatus. The surgical space is made by retracting the esophagus with the mediastinoscope. The esophagus is dissected under direct vision.

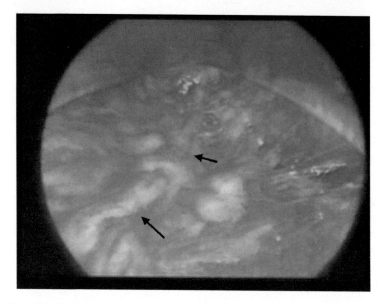

Fig. 17.9. Mediastinoscopic view of thoracic duct. The esophagus is retracted anterior with the mediastinoscope. The thoracic duct (arrows) is then easily retrieved on the left posterior side of the esophagus.

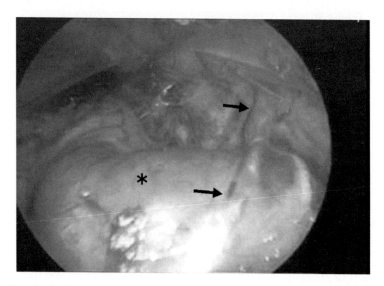

Fig. 17.10. Mediastinoscopic view of azygos arch and right bronchial artery. The esophagus is dissected carefully to avoid damaging the small vessels and lymph vessels. The azygos arch (*) and right bronchial artery (arrows) are exposed clearly on the right posterior side of the esophagus.

safely exposed and coagulated with Laparosonic Coagulating Shears (LCS) (Harmonic Scalpel, Ethicon) and a coagulator that simultaneously suctions and irrigates (Endopath Probe Plus II, Ethicon). On the right side, the esophagus is dissected gently with the LCS, and the azygos arch and bronchial artery exposed (Fig. 17.11). On the anterior side of the esophagus, the tracheoesophageal ligament is divided sharply, and the tracheal bifurcation and pulmonary hilar nodes become visible. The esophagus is dissected by coagulating small vessels with a hooked coagulator (Endopath), that simultaneously suctions and irrigates (Fig. 17.12). On the posterior side, the esophageal artery is coagulated with LCS while suctioning the mist. The upper thoracic paraesophageal and the lower paraesophageal lymph nodes are exposed and dissected together with the esophagus.

During this procedure, which is performed by the cervical team, the abdominal team prepares the interposition graft. The stomach was used as the graft in all but four of our patients who had previously undergone

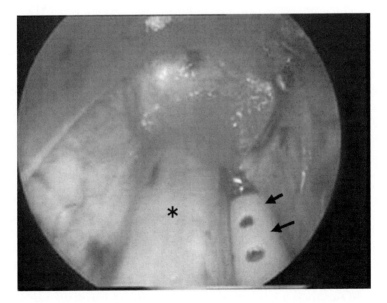

Fig. 17.11. Mediastinoscopic view of lower esophageal dissection. The tracheoesophageal ligament is divided, and the mediastinoscope is inserted more deeply, the esophagus (*) is then observed in a wide surgical field. Lymphatic and blood vessels are safely exposed and coagulated with a hooked coagulator (arrows) that can suction and irrigate simultaneously.

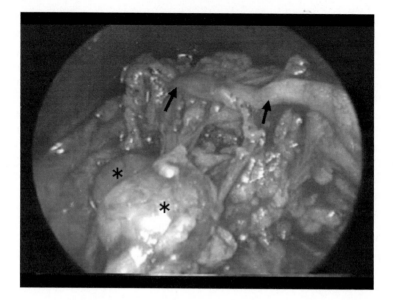

Fig. 17.12. Mediastinoscopic view of left recurrent laryngeal nerve. The left recurrent nerve (arrows) is visible under the left side of the trachea. The para-recurrent nerve nodes (*) are carefully dissected.

gastrectomy and three patients with synchronous gastric cancer. The gastric lymph nodes (right cardiac, left cardiac, lesser curve, left gastric artery) and the lower thoracic paraesophageal lymph nodes, diaphragmatic nodes, and posterior mediastinal nodes are dissected. The esophagus is divided in the neck with a linear cutter (Proximate Linear Cutter, Ethicon) and pulled through from the mediastinum toward the abdomen as the dissection is completed. The mediastinoscope is inserted again to confirm hemostasis and to dissect the remnant lymph nodes. The heart, azygos vein, and vagus nerve are easily seen. The left recurrent-laryngeal nerve is visible under the aortic arch and the left side of the trachea. The gastric tube is pulled up to the neck, and the anastomosis made with a detachable circular stapler (Endopath ILS, Ethicon). The suction drain is inserted in the neck and the abdomen, and then the incision is closed.

In summary, it has been reported that THE is most hazardous for tumors in the middle third of the esophagus; therefore, THE has been considered contraindicated for tumors in this location. Mediastinoscope-assisted transhiatal esophagectomy avoids many of these hazards by allowing dissection to proceed under direct visual control. It can be converted easily to a more radical surgery if lymph node metastases are found. To aid in this determination, we have developed a sentinel lymph node navigation method with multidetector CT scan using a nonionic water-soluble contrast medium, and examined it in the patients with superficial esophageal cancer (Hayashi et al.).

# F.  Conclusions

## *Paul B. Tessmann*

The Ivor Lewis procedure was the first widely practiced surgery for esophagectomy. It employs a combined laparotomy and right posterolateral thoracotomy through the fifth rib interspace. The anastomosis is performed in the chest. This procedure is not indicated for proximal carcinomas due to difficulty in obtaining adequate proximal margins, and it may be difficult to perform in patients with a previous right thoracotomy.

The Ivor Lewis procedure was subsequently criticized by some due to the complications and risks it posed, such as atelectasis, respiratory insufficiency, pneumonia, and devastating thoracic anastomotic leaks. The leaks occurred in 3.6% of cases, but carried an approximately 50% mortality. Orringer et al. then proposed a transhiatal approach, with an upper midline abdominal incision, a left oblique anterior neck incision, and esophagogastrostomy in the neck. Proposed benefits included decreased incidence of the above-listed complications, especially the problematic anastomotic leaks. Leaks could be easily treated by opening the neck incision and creating a spit fistula.

Both procedures, as well as variations on them, have been widely performed successfully, and have been studied. However, there are few good randomized controlled studies comparing the two. Large series of both have been reported, providing survival data, as well as rates of complications.

The Ivor Lewis carries a 12.3% incidence of pneumonia, a recurrent laryngeal nerve palsy rate of 0.9%, an anastomotic leak rate of 3.6% with approximately 50% mortality, anastomotic stricture in about one third of patients, a medial survival of 1.9 years, a 5-year survival of 25.2%, and a local recurrence rate of 5%.

The transhiatal approach carries a 5% incidence of pneumonia, an anastomotic leak rate of 10% to 15% in some series (less than 3% in Orringer et al.'s latest report) with nearly zero deaths, anastomotic stricture in about half the patients, less biliary reflux, a 3-year survival of 56%, and a local recurrence rate of 5.6%.

Recent advances in minimal access surgery have allowed comparable procedures to be performed without the morbidity associated with thoracotomy. The approaches presented in this chapter provide three different variations on this theme.

Location of tumor, extent of disease, and patient comorbidities are crucial factors to consider when choosing an operative approach. Neoadjuvant chemoradiation therapy may allow significant downstaging, facilitating surgery. Issues such as extent of necessary lymphadenectomy and impact on overall survival have yet to be resolved. Despite these uncertainties, minimal access procedures have virtually supplanted open surgery for treatment of esophageal carcinoma. Robotic surgery, not included in this chapter, is being applied in this disease as well.

# References

Gossot D, Cattan P, Fritsch S, Halimi B, Sarfati E, Celerier M. Can the morbidity of esophagectomy be reduced by the thoracoscopic approach? Surg Endosc 1995; 9:1113–1115.

Hayashi H, Tangoku A, Suga K, et al. CT lymphography-navigated sentinel lymph node biopsy in patients with superficial esophageal cancer. Surgery 2006;139:224–235.

Hulscher JB, van Sandick JW, de Boer AG, et al. Extended transthoracic resection compared with limited transhiatal resection for adenocarcinoma of the esophagus. N Engl J Med 2002;347:1662–1669.

Kawahara K, Maekawa T, Okabayashi K, et al. Video-assisted thoracoscopic esophagectomy for esophageal cancer. Surg Endosc 1999;13:218–223.

Law S, Fok M, Chu KM, Wong J. Thoracoscopic esophagectomy for esophageal cancer. Surgery 1997;122:8–14.

Orringer MB, Marshall B, Iannettoni MD. Transhiatal esophagectomy: clinical experience and refinements. Ann Surg 1999;230:392–403.

Peracchia A, Rosati R, Fumagalli U, Bona S, Chella B. Thoracoscopic esophagectomy: are there benefits? Semin Surg Oncol 1997;13:259–262.

Smithers BM, Gotley DC, McEwan D, Martin I, Bessell J, Doyle L. Thoracoscopic mobilization of the esophagus. A 6 year experience. Surg Endosc 2001;15:176–182.

Wong J. Esophageal resection for cancer: the rationale of current practice. Am J Surg 1987;153:18–24.

# Suggested Readings

Akaishi T, Kaneda I, Higuchi N, et al. Thoracoscopic en bloc total esophagectomy with radical mediastinal lymphadenectomy. J Thorac Cardiovasc Surg 1996;112: 1533–1541.

Altorki N. En-bloc esophagectomy—the three field dissection. Surg Clin North Am 2005;85:611–619.

Atkins B, Shah A, Hutcheson K, et al. Reducing hospital morbidity and mortality following esophagectomy. Ann Thorac Surg 2004;78:1170–1176.

Azagra JS, Ceuterik M, Goergen M, Jacobs D, Gilbart E. Thoracoscopy in oesophagectomy for oesophageal cancer. Br J Surg 1993;80:320–321.

Bodner J, Wykypiel H, Wetscher G, Schmid T. First experiences with the da Vinci operating robot in thoracic surgery. Eur J Cardiothorac Surg 2004;25:844–851.

Bumm R, Feussner H, Bartels H, et al. Radical transhiatal esophagectomy with two-field lymphadenectomy and endodissection for distal esophageal adenocarcinoma. World J Surg 1997;21:822–831.

Collard JM, Lengele B, Otte JB, Kestens PJ. En bloc and standard esophagectomies by thoracoscopy. Ann Thorac Surg 1993;56:675–679.

Easterling C, Bousamra M, Lang I, et al. Pharyngeal dysphagia in postesophagectomy patients: correlation with deglutitive biomechanics. Ann Thorac Surg 2000;69(4):989–992.

Espat NJ, Jacobsen G, Horgan S, Donahue P. Minimall invasive treatment of esophageal cancer: laparoscopic staging to robotic esophagectomy. Cancer J 2005;11:10–17.

Gockel I, Heckhoff S, Messow CM, Kneist W, Junginger T. Transhiatal and transthoracic resection in adenocarcinoma of the esophagus. Does the operative approach have an influence on the long-term prognosis? World J Surg Oncol 2005;24:40.

Kato H, Tachimori Y, Watanebe H, Yamaguchi H, Ishilkawa T, Itabashi M. Superficial esophageal carcinoma: surgical treatment and the results. Cancer 1990;66: 2319–2323.

Law S, Wong J. Use of minimally invasive oesophagectomy for cancer of the oesophagus. Lancet Oncol 2002;3:215–222.

Liao Z, Zhang Z, Jin J, et al. Esophagectomy after concurrent chemoradiotherapy improves locoregional control in clinical stage II or III esophageal cancer patients. Int J Radiat Oncol Biol Phys 2004;60:1484–1493.

Luketich JD, Alvelo-Rivera M, Buenaventura PO, et al. Minimally invasive esophagectomy: outcomes in 222 patients. Ann Surg 2003;238:486–496.

Martin R, Lestos P, Taves D, et al. Oropharyngeal dysphagia in esophageal cancer before and after transhiatal esophagectomy. Dysphagia. 2001;16(1):23–31.

McAnena O, Rogers J, Williams N. Right thoracoscopically assisted oesophagectomy for cancer. Br J Surg 1994;81:236–238.

National Comprehensive Cancer Network Guidelines. Version 1. 2003. www.nccn.org.

Rizk NP, Bach PB, Schrag D, et al. The impact of complications on outcomes after resection for esophageal and gastroesophageal junction carcinoma. J Am Coll Surg 2004;198:42–50.

Tangoku A, Hayashi H, Kanamura S, et al. Lymph node metastases identified with medi-astinoscopy in patient with superficial carcinoma of the esophagus. Surg Endosc 2000;14:595.

Tangoku A, Yoshino S, Abe T, et al. Mediastinoscope-assisted transhiatal esophagectomy for esophageal cancer. Surg Endosc 2004;18(3):383–389.

# 18. Gastric Adenocarcinoma

## A. Introduction

Gastric cancer is rare in the United States, but still common in other parts of the world. The diagnosis is often not suspected until the disease is fairly advanced. When gastric adenocarcinoma is diagnosed, accurate staging and careful multidisciplinary management improve the chances of success. This chapter addresses issues of preoperative staging and choice of surgical procedure.

## B. Case

### *José E. Torres*

A 62-year-old Chilean woman presented with a 6-month history of dyspepsia, bloating, nausea, and postprandial pain and vomiting. She had lost 15 pounds over the past 2 months. For the previous 3 years, she had been treated for presumed gastric ulcers with proton pump inhibitors. She did not have any history of bright red blood per rectum and denied changes in her bowel habits.

Her past medical history was significant for gastric ulcers as noted above, hypertension, migraine headaches, and arthritis. She had not had any prior surgery. Her family history was significant for a mother who died at age 78 from gastric carcinoma.

She was a married schoolteacher, who had never smoked or drank alcoholic beverages. Her medications included Imitrex, enteric coated aspirin, a proton pump inhibitor, and verapamil. She had no known drug allergies.

The review of systems was negative except as noted above. On physical examination, she was thin, alert and oriented, and in no acute distress. Her height was 160 cm and she weighed 50 kg. Head and neck examination was negative, as was cardiopulmonary examination. There was no supraclavicular adenopathy.

Abdominal examination revealed a soft, nondistended abdomen, without masses. Mild epigastric tenderness was noted. Bowel sounds were normal. Rectal examination revealed no masses and stool was trace guaiac positive. Laboratory examination was significant for a hematocrit of 30%. Liver function tests were normal.

Upper gastrointestinal series revealed an ulcerated mass in the distal stomach, suspicious for malignancy (Fig. 18.1). Upper gastrointestinal endoscopy confirmed the presence of a friable mass just proximal to the pylorus with a central ulcerated crater. Biopsies of the edge of the mass revealed adenocarcinoma.

Computed tomography (CT) scan showed thickening of the distal stomach but was negative for other masses, lymphadenopathy, or metastatic disease.

The impression was gastric carcinoma, limited to the stomach.

**Would you do laparoscopic staging before surgery? Would you consider laparoscopic gastric resection or opt for an open surgical procedure?**

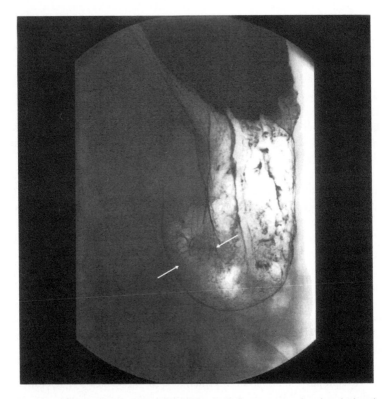

Fig. 18.1. Frame from upper gastrointestinal fluoroscopy showing lesion in distal stomach (arrows).

# C. Preoperative Staging Laparoscopy

## *Georgios C. Sotiropoulos and Christoph E. Broelsch*

A wide variety of multimodal treatment approaches are available for the treatment of advanced primary tumors and metastatic disease. Therefore, sensitive staging procedures are required to provide a rational basis for stage-adapted therapy of gastrointestinal tumors. One of the major goals of staging in surgical oncology is to identify patients with nonresectable or disseminated disease in whom curative surgery is not feasible, thus avoiding nontherapeutic laparotomy.

Imaging methods such as transcutaneous ultrasonography (US) and CT, as well as endoscopic methods such as esophagogastroscopy and endosonography, are used with a reported accuracy in the detection of intraabdominal metastases of gastric carcinoma up to 90%. However, the sensitivity of these methods for tumors <1 cm is poor, succeeding in detecting small intraabdominal metastases in only about the half of the cases. Staging laparoscopy is being used more commonly, particularly in combination with laparoscopic ultrasound, giving additional information in tumor staging and resulting in better evaluation of patients with abdominal cancer.

Although radical resection is supposed to be the only curative treatment of gastric cancer, it can be performed in less than 60% of all patients evaluated. Even newly diagnosed gastric cancer patients will be found at subsequent laparotomy to have been understaged in more than 25% of the cases, with several ethical, financial, and quality of life implications. Perioperative complications occur in 12% to 23% of unresectable patients undergoing exploratory laparotomy, with a reported mortality rate up to 21%. As many studies indicate that preoperative chemotherapy may increase the resectability rate and improve survival in patients with advanced gastric cancer, staging laparoscopy could guide the multimodal therapy planning and either lead to a reasonable surgery or avoid an unnecessary surgery. The high diagnostic efficacy of video-laparoscopy as regards the M factor (metastasis) has been reported by many investigators; preoperative laparoscopy, therefore, helps avoid unhelpful open surgical exploration in cases of peritoneal dissemination of tumor or liver metastases undetected by conventional staging.

In a consecutive series of 45 patients with locally advanced gastric tumor (T3–4, N1–2), who underwent staging laparoscopy in our department, peritoneal seeding was first found during staging laparoscopy in 22% of cases. Locoregional lymph node tumor involvement

Table 18.1. Clinical and laparoscopic rumor-staging according to the TNM System of the UICC. Disseminated disease was first detected during laparoscopy in 14 patients, leadings to changes in the therapy planning.

| n = 45 | | Laparoscopic staging | | | | | | | clinical staging total n |
|---|---|---|---|---|---|---|---|---|---|
| | | II | IIIA | | IIIB | IV | | | |
| UICC Stage | TNM classificatio | $T_3N_0M_0$ | $T_3N_1M_0$ | $T_4N_0M_0$ | $T_3N_2M_0$ | $T_4N_{1-3}M0$ | $T_{1-3}N_3M_0$ | $T_xN_xM_1$ | |
| Clinical Staging — II | $T_3N_0M_0$ | 4 | 1 | – | – | – | – | – | 5 |
| IIIA | $T_3N_1M_0$ | – | 14 | – | 4 | – | 1 | 2 | 21 |
| IIIA | $T_4N_0M_0$ | – | – | – | – | – | – | 2 | 21 |
| IIIB | $T_3N_2M_0$ | – | – | – | 3 | 1 | 2 | 3 | 9 |
| IV | $T_{1-3}N_3M_0$ | | | | | | | | |
| IV | $T_xN_xM_1$ | | | | | | | | |
| laparoscopic staging total n | | 4 | 15 | – | 7 | 2 | 3 | 14 | 45 |
| Accuracy of clinical staging | | 100% | 93.4% | | 42.9% | | | 5.3% | |

was additionally detected in two patients (5%). Liver metastasis and Krukenberg's tumor were each found in one patient. Sensitivity of clinical imaging was very poor for stage IIIB and IV gastric carcinoma (43% and 5%, respectively; Table 18.1). Staging laparoscopy improved staging in 14 patients (31%), leading to change of the multimodal therapy planning in all cases. Unnecessary laparotomy was avoided in these patients.

Cytologic examination confirmed the intraoperative diagnosis of peritoneal seeding in four of the 12 patients with peritoneal seeding, but gave no additional information in comparison to laparoscopy findings. The usefulness of cytologic workup during staging laparoscopy for gastrointestinal malignancies is controversial in the literature. Conversion to open surgery was not necessary in our series. No laparoscopy-related morbidity was observed. Mean hospital-stay was 3 days.

In conclusion, laparoscopy has a feasible value of improving preoperative staging in patients with gastric cancer. It is a safe method that permits the identification of patients who are suitable for curative surgery and can optimize the multimodal therapy planning, offering the best therapeutic approach: radical gastrectomy, neoadjuvant therapy, or nonsurgery and palliative treatment.

# D. Gastrectomy for Carcinoma

## *Carol E.H. Scott-Conner*

In the United States, gastric carcinoma is rare and the diagnosis is rarely made when the disease is still stage I or II. Surgical resection is rarely indicated as a palliative procedure, but is generally reserved for patients whose disease has not extended beyond the field of surgical resection. It is thus performed with potentially curative intent, despite the grim prognosis of the disease. The goal is an R0 resection, that is, no residual tumor left behind.

Preoperative laparoscopy enables laparotomy to be avoided in patients with unsuspected spread. It may be performed as a separate procedure or as the first phase of surgical therapy (same anesthesia), depending on surgeon scheduling preference. As noted in the previous chapters, when no such spread is found, the next step is to plan resection.

The standard operation for carcinoma of the distal stomach is radical subtotal gastrectomy. Five-centimeter margins above and below the tumor are recommended (National Comprehensive Cancer Network

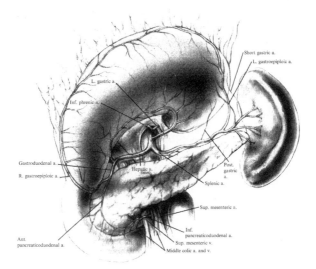

Fig.18.2. Regional anatomy. Lymph nodes cluster around named arteries. (From Scott-Conner CEH. Chassin's Operative Strategy in General Surgery, 3rd ed. New York: Springer-Verlag, 2002, with permission.)

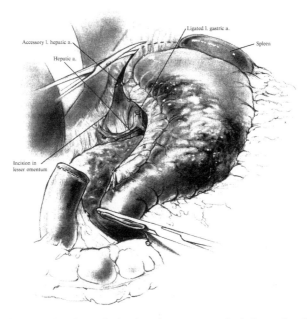

Fig. 18.3. Resection for radical subtotal gastrectomy includes regional lymph nodes and omentum. (From Scott-Conner CEH. Chassin's Operative Strategy in General Surgery, 3rd ed. New York: Springer-Verlag, 2002, with permission.)

[NCCN] guidelines). When this can be achieved by subtotal gastrectomy, complication rates are slightly less. Sometimes total gastrectomy is required for tumors of the distal stomach; it is commonly needed for more proximal lesions.

Regional nodes cluster around the named vessels in the area (Fig. 18.2). A radical subtotal gastrectomy is designed to remove these nodes (Fig. 18.3). The extent of nodal dissection is a major factor in staging, and accurate staging affects treatment and outcome. Brennan stressed, in a recent review, that at least 15 regional nodes should be sampled.

The Japanese Research Society for the Study of Gastric Cancer has developed standardized terminology for lymph node stations. Perigastric nodes along the greater and lesser curvature are termed N1. Those around the left gastric artery, common hepatic artery, celiac artery, and splenic artery are grouped together as N2, and more distant nodes (such as paraaortic) are considered distant metastases. The recommended D2 resection encompasses the nodes mentioned above.

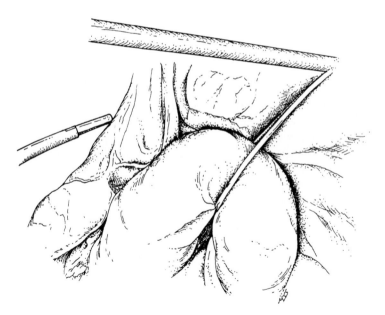

Fig. 18.4. Stomach being retracted with sling preparatory to division during laparoscopic gastrectomy. (From Scott-Conner CEH. The SAGES Manual: Fundamentals of Laparoscopy, Thoracoscopy, and GI Endoscopy. New York: Springer-Verlag, 2006.)

No benefit has been found to more extensive lymphadenectomy or resection of adjacent structures such as spleen or pancreas unless involved by direct extension. Such cases are generally apparent on preoperative imaging studies. Reconstruction is most commonly performed as a Billroth II. I prefer to make this an antecolic reconstruction, to keep the reconstruction away from the bed of the tumor.

In countries where gastric cancer is common and where screening programs detect early lesions, endoscopic mucosal resection of very early lesions may be performed. Laparoscopic gastrectomy has also been perfected. This operation is designed to mimic the open operation and equivalent resections, and node harvests have been documented. Because of the rarity of gastric cancer in the United States, most surgeons prefer traditional open techniques. Excellent descriptions of the endoluminal and laparoscopic techniques (Fig. 18.4) may be found in the SAGES manual.

# E. Conclusions

## José E. Torres

Worldwide, the incidence of gastric cancer has decreased significantly, but the prognosis still remains poor, with a 5-year survival rate ranging between 10% and 20%. In the United States, the median age of patients with gastric cancer is 65 years, and the majority of patients are male.

If gastric cancer is identified early, it may be cured by surgical resection. Optimal therapy of more advanced disease is typically multimodal, and requires accurate patient selection and careful tumor node, metastasis (TNM) staging. In a study of 32 T3 and T4 cases, Yano and colleagues found that 40.6% of the patients had inapparent peritoneal metastases detected at laparoscopy. The positive predictive value for staging laparoscopy was 100% and the negative predictive value was 89%.

The particular strength of laparoscopic staging lies in its ability to identify small masses not seen with other staging modalities. In two studies, D'Ugo and colleagues compared laparoscopy to ultrasound and CT scanning. Their 1996 study demonstrated that laparoscopy had an overall staging accuracy of 68.6% compared to 32.8% for ultrasound and CT, and that laparoscopy was the most sensitive method to detect peritoneal seeding. In 1997, they demonstrated that laparoscopy detected 21 cases of unsuspected metastatic disease in 100 patients to be considered M0. Laparoscopy altered clinical staging in 58% of their cases. A prospective study performed by Hunerbein et al. demonstrated that laparoscopy was much more accurate in the detection of distant metastasis than ultrasound and computed tomography and altered the treatment strategy in 45% of patients.

The therapy of choice for gastric cancer in the absence of disseminated disease is surgical resection with wide margins and en-bloc resection of lymph nodes and any adherent organs. The type of resection depends on the location, stage, and type of tumor. Many tumors are located proximally and curative resection of these tumors is very difficult. Tumors of the gastroesophageal junction are treated with either a gastric pull-up or esophagogastrectomy. Tumors within 2 cm of the squamocolumnar junction and of the subcardial region are usually treated with a total or proximal subtotal gastrectomy. Total gastrectomies are usually required for midbody tumors, whereas for distal tumors a distal subtotal gastrectomy is required. Resection incorporated regional lymphadenectomy.

Until recent advances in laparoscopic surgery, the treatment of gastric cancer has been limited to the open technique. This has been due to the belief that the principles of oncologic surgery are not maintained with laparoscopic gastric cancer surgery. These principles include minimal manipulation of the tumor specimen, attainment of adequate surgical margins, and adequate lymph node dissection. Azagra performed the first laparoscopic gastrectomy for malignancy in 1993. Since that time, laparoscopic surgery for gastric malignancy has been refined by European and Japanese surgeons. Early screening programs in Japan have made laparoscopic surgery a viable option for early gastric cancers, whereas European surgeons have utilized laparoscopic surgery for the treatment of moderately advanced cancer.

Laparoscopic gastrectomy for malignancy has been demonstrated to be a viable alternative to open gastrectomy. Several studies have demonstrated that the attainment of clear margins, adequate lymphadenectomy, short-term survival, wound seeding, and trocar site metastases are identical. Lopez et al. demonstrated that the results of laparoscopic gastric resections in patients with adenocarcinoma were similar to those obtained in open surgery with respect to the duration of the surgery, lymph nodes obtained, and complications. In a retrospective review of 44 patients, Huscher and colleagues reported that laparoscopic radical total or subtotal gastrectomy with extended lymphadenectomy for gastric cancer is an oncologically safe procedure with a conversion rate of 7% and operative morbidity and mortality rates of 7% and 12% respectively. Most recently Dulucq and his colleagues completed a prospective analysis of totally laparoscopic total and partial gastrectomies that included 31 patients. This study demonstrated that these procedures were safe and that the totally laparoscopic approach yielded adequate margins and followed oncologic principles.

# References

Brennan MF. Current status of surgery for gastric cancer: a review. Gastric Cancer 2005;8:64–70.

D'Ugo, Coppola R, Persiani R, Ronconi P, Caracciolo F, Picciocchi A. Immediately preoperative laparoscopic staging for gastric cancer. Surg Endosc 1996;10:996–999.

D'Ugo DM, Persiani R, Caracciolo F, Ronconi P, Coco C, Picciocchi A. Selection of locally advanced gastric carcinoma by preoperative staging laparoscopy. Surg Endosc 1997;11:1159–1162.

Dulucq JL, Wintringer P, Perissat J, Mahajna A. Completely laparoscopic total and partial gastrectomy for benign and malignant disease: a single institution's prospective analysis. J Am Coll Surg 2005;200:191–197.

Hunerbein M, Rau B, Hohenberger P, Schlag PM. The role of staging laparoscopy for multimodal therapy of gastrointestinal cancer. Surg Endosc 1998;12:921–925.

Lopez CB, Ruggiero R, Poves I, Betonnica C, Procaccini E. The contribution of laparoscopy to the treatment of gastric cancer. Surg Endosc 2002;16:616–619.

National Comprehensive Cancer Network. NCCN Clinical Practice Guidelines in Oncology. Gastric Cancer, vol. 1, 2007. www.nccn.org.

# Suggested Readings

Ajani JA, Mansfield PF, Ota DM. Potentially respectable gastric carcinoma: current approaches to staging and preoperative therapy. World J Surg 1995;19:216–220.

Brennan MF, Karpeh MS. Surgery for gastric cancer: the American view. Semin Oncol 1996;23:352–359.

Conlon KC, Karpeh MS Jr. Laparoscopy and laparoscopic ultrasound in the staging of gastric cancer. Semin Oncol 1996;23:347–351.

Cushieri A. Gastric resections. In: Scott-Conner CEH, ed. The SAGES Manual: Fundamentals of Laparoscopy, Thoracoscopy, and GI Endoscopy, 2nd ed. New York: Springer Verlag, 2006:267–281.

Etoh T, Shiraishi N, Kitano S. Laparoscopic gastrectomy for cancer. Dig Dis 2005;23:113–118.

Gallardo-Rincon D, Onate-Ocana LF, Calderillo-Ruiz G. Neoadjuvant chemotherapy with P-ELF (cisplatin, etoposide, leucovorin, 5-fluorouracil) followed by radical resection in patients with initially unresectable gastric adenocarcinoma: a phase II study. Ann Surg Oncol 2000;7:45–50.

Gouma DJ, de Wit LT, Nieveen van Dijkum E, et al. Laparoscopic ultrasonography for staging of gastrointestinal malignancy. Scand J Gastroenterol Suppl 1996;218:43–49.

Hayashi H, Ochiai T, Shimada H, Gunji Y. Prospective randomized study of open versus laparoscopy-assisted distal gastrectomy with extraperigastric lymph node dissection for early gastric cancer. Surg Endosc 2005;19:1172–1176.

Hayes N, Wayman J, Wadehra V, Scott DJ, Raimes SA, Griffin SM. Peritoneal cytology in the surgical evaluation of gastric carcinoma. Br J Cancer 1999;79:520–524.

Hunerbein M, Ulmer C, Handke T, Schlag PM. Endosonography of upper gastrointestinal tract cancer on demand using miniprobes or endoscopic ultrasound. Surg Endosc 2003;17:615–619.

Huscher CG, Mingoli A, Sgarzini G, et al. Videolaparoscopic total and subtotal gastrectomy with extended lymph node dissection for gastric cancer. Am J Surg 2004;188:728–735.

Huscher CG, Mingoli A, Sgarzini G, et al. Laparoscopic versus open subtotal gastrectomy for distal gastric cancer: five-year results of a randomized prospective trial. Ann Surg 2005;241:232–237.

Lowy AM, Mansfield PF, Leach SD, Ajani J. Laparoscopic staging for gastric cancer. Surgery 1996;119(6):611–614.

Otsuka K, Murakami M, Aoki T, Lefor A. Minimally invasive treatment of stomach cancer. Cancer J 2005;11:18–26.

Ozmen MM, Zulfikaroglu B, Ozalp N, Ziraman I, Hengirmen S, Sahin B. Staging laparoscopy for gastric cancer. Surg Laparosc Endosc Percutan Tech 2003;13:241–244.

Ribeiro U Jr, Gama-Rodrigues JJ, Bitelman B, et al. Value of peritoneal lavage cytology during laparoscopic staging of patients with gastric carcinoma. Surg Laparosc Endosc 1998;8:132–135.

Sendler A, Dittler HJ, Feussner H. Preoperative staging of gastric cancer as precondition for multimodal treatment. World J Surg 1995;19:501–508.

Sotiropoulos GC, Kaiser GM, Lang H, et al. Staging laparoscopy in gastric cancer. Eur J Med Res 2005;10:88–91.

Stell DA, Carter CR, Stewart I, Anderson JR. Prospective comparison of laparoscopy, ultrasonography and computed tomography in the staging of gastric cancer. Br J Surg 1996;83:1260–1262.

Suga S, Iwase H, Shimada M, et al. Neoadjuvant chemotherapy in scirrhous cancer of the stomach using uracil and tegafur and cisplatin. Intern Med 1996;35:930–936.

Usi S, Yoshida T, Ito K, Hiranumo S, Kudo SE, Iwai T. Laparoscopy-assisted total gastrectomy for early gastric cancer: comparison with conventional open total gastrectomy. Surg Laparosc Endosc Percutan Tech 2005;15:309–314.

van Dijkum EJ, Sturm PD, de Wit LT, Offerhaus J, Obertop H, Gouma DJ. Cytology of peritoneal lavage performed during staging laparoscopy for gastrointestinal malignancies: is it useful? Ann Surg 1998;228:728–733.

Wakelin SJ, Deans C, Crofts TJ, Allan PL, Plevris JN, Paterson-Brown S. A comparison of computerised tomography, laparoscopic ultrasound and endoscopic ultrasound in the preoperative staging of oesophago-gastric carcinoma. Eur J Radiol 2002;41:161–167.

Wanebo HJ, Kennedy BJ, Chmiel J, Steele GJ, Winchester D, Osteen R. Cancer of the stomach. A patient care study by the American College of Surgeons. Ann Surg 1993;218:583–592.

Weber KJ, Leyes CD, Coagner M, Divino CM. Comparison of laparoscopic and open gastrectomy for malignant disease. Surg Endosc 2003:17:968–71.

Yano M, Tsujinaka T, Shiozaki H, et al. Appraisal of treatment strategy by staging laparoscopy for locally advanced gastric cancer. World J Surg 2000;24:1130–1136.

Yonemura Y, Sawa T, Kinashita K, et al. Neoadjuvant chemotherapy for high-grade advanced gastric cancer. World J Surg 1993;17:256–262.

# 19. Feeding Tube Placement, Gastrostomy Versus Jejunostomy

## A. Introduction

When long-term enteral access is required in a mentally compromised adult, there are several options to consider. One of the most fundamental considerations is whether to place a gastrostomy or a jejunostomy. This chapter explores those issues. Chapter 20 explores the related issues of percutaneous endoscopic feeding tube access versus laparoscopic placement of a feeding tube.

## B. Case

*Kent Choi*

A 50-year-old woman initially presented to her neurologist 1 month ago after an acute stroke involving the right middle cerebral artery. Carotid arteriogram demonstrated evidence of a subacute spontaneous dissection of the midcervical portion of the right internal carotid artery consisting of a pseudoaneurysm with subintimal hematoma and intimal irregularity. She also developed new right anterior and posterior watershed infarcts as well as punctate focus in the left occipital lobe. Further investigation demonstrated a right internal carotid artery petrous portion dissection with pseudoaneurysm. With worsening neurological status, she underwent right internal carotid artery stent placement by neurointerventional radiology 10 days earlier.

After that procedure, she had a sudden mental status decline. A computed tomography (CT) scan of the brain revealed right parietotemporal occipital intercerebral hemorrhage. She was taken emergently to the operating room and underwent craniotomy with evacuation of the hematoma. Postoperatively, her mental status did not improve. She remained unresponsive, and was judged unlikely to be able to eat normally for a long period of time. The general surgery department was consulted for evaluation for surgical placement of a feeding tube.

Her past medical history was significant for childhood asthma, dermatitis, and keratosis. Her past surgical history included laser eye surgery in 1997, pelvic laparoscopy in 1985, cesarean section in 1981, extraction of wisdom teeth in 1972, and tonsillectomy in 1958. Her father died at 85 of congestive heart failure. Her mother was alive at 83 with a history of cervical cancer.

Her medications included phenytoin 200 mg NG t.i.d., chlorhexidine oral rinse t.i.d., Colace 100 mg NG b.i.d., senna 1 tab NG q.d., Prevacid 30 mg NG q.d., Tylenol PRN, and codeine PRN. She had no known allergies.

She was a nonsmoker. She had one beer per day prior to this recent illness. The review of systems was unobtainable.

On physical examination, she was lying comfortably in bed, supported on a ventilator, and receiving tube feedings through a nasogastric tube. Her temperature was 37.7 °C, heart rate 96, respiratory rate 18, and blood pressure 145/80. $O_2$ saturation was 100% on 35% $FIO_2$. She responded only by localizing to painful stimuli. Head and neck exam was unremarkable. Cardiovascular and pulmonary exam was benign.

Abdomen was soft, nontender, and nondistended. Bowel sounds were present. There was a well-healed low transverse incision and an infraumbilical incision. Extremities were without edema.

Laboratory examination included a white blood cell count of 17.3, hemoglobin 9.9, hematocrit 30, platelets 563, phenytoin 11, magnesium 1.9, sodium 136, chloride 102, $CO_2$ 23, BUN 16, creatinine 0.6, and glucose 143.

**You agree that she will need long-term, stable access for feeding. Would you recommend a gastrostomy or a jejunostomy?**

# C. Gastrostomy

*Gill McHattie*

This patient has had severe brain injury from which the degree of recovery/disability is still unknown. This is a challenging problem in critical care and requires a coordinated multidisciplinary team approach. It is known that nutritional support is an important part of care for any patient in critical care and that injury to the brain results in hypermetabolism. The duration of this hypermetabolic state is unknown beyond the first 2 weeks, but early introduction of nutritional support is recommended. Enteral nutrition provides a more physiologic method of nutrient delivery. It may be provided via the nasogastric route, the gastrostomy route, or directly into the jejunum via a nasojejunal tube or percutaneous jejunostomy.

It is known that this patient originally presented 1 month ago, but no mention is made of when nutritional support commenced within this period. We assume that enteral nutritional support via the nasogastric tube is being absorbed as both nutrients and medication are being provided via this route. Although artificial nutrition support can be delivered via the nasogastric route for an indeterminate period, it is widely recognized that a gastrostomy should be considered if the period of support is anticipated to be longer than 4 weeks.

Patients requiring artificial nutrition support should be fed via a tube into the stomach unless there is an upper gastrointestinal dysfunction, when postpyloric feeding should be considered. It is known that gastrointestinal function can be compromised in mechanically ventilated patients, the most common abnormality being delayed gastric emptying. Patients with severe brain injury also demonstrate delayed gastric emptying and dysfunction of the cardiac sphincter, which can predispose to aspiration of gastric contents. In reviewing the literature to compare gastric versus jejunal feeding, the Eastern Association for the Surgery of Trauma (2003) found no significant differences between these routes of feeding following severe injury.

Percutaneous endoscopic jejunostomy (PEJ) is considered an alternative where the patient has delayed gastric emptying. The evidence to support jejunal feeding is less robust than that for gastric feeding. No indication of gastric dysfunction is given for the patient presented. In addition, percutaneous endoscopic gastrostomies (PEGs) can be converted to jejunal tubes should the gastric route not be tolerated; however, these converted tubes are associated with a higher rate of tube dysfunction. There may be alteration in the efficacy of any medication administered via the jejunal route; therefore, it is imperative that the pharmacist be consulted if the route of administration changes because of a change in the patient's condition.

Percutaneous endoscopic gastrostomies were first described by Gauderer et al. in 1980. With experienced personnel this procedure is considered to be safe, simple, and effective. Enteral feeding provided via this route has been found to be highly efficient. Prior to the insertion of a PEG, it is important to take into account the clinical situation and whether this method of feeding is likely to improve or maintain the patient's quality of life. The most common indications for PEG are neurologic conditions. Studies in patients following cerebral vascular accidents have demonstrated improved nutrition and rehabilitation following PEG placement.

Protocols for the insertion and subsequent management of PEG tubes and enteral feeding are paramount to ensure good practice and optimal nutrient delivery. These protocols provide a communication tool for staff in all acute and rehabilitation settings, and help establish goals that are achievable and that take into account patients' changing caregivers and care requirements as they progress through their treatment pathways.

In conclusion, it is expected that this patient will require long-term artificial nutrition support; the choice of route is determined by her current clinical status and tolerance of enteral feeding via the nasogastric route. Although PEG placement is relatively common, there are risks and complications associated with the procedure that must be weighed against the benefits that such a procedure will bring the patient. The decision for a PEG insertion must be made by a multidisciplinary team through informed discussion that includes family members, taking into account treatment goals, which in this patient's case will initially be short-term based on the efficient delivery of nutritional support.

# D. Jejunostomy

## *Desmond Birkett*

This patient has had a severe brain injury that has rendered her unresponsive and requiring ventilatory support. Her prognosis is extremely poor, and she is unlikely to improve for some time, if at all. Continued nutrition is of paramount importance. Parenteral nutrition is excellent for short periods of time, but since it is unlikely that she will be able to eat by herself or be fed by mouth for some time, enteral nutrition is the preferred route of access.

Enteral nutrition can be provided via a variety of routes to the gastrointestinal tract. Nasogastric feeling tubes provide excellent access to the gastrointestinal tract via a natural orifice and can be placed and replaced with ease. However, for long-term feeding it is not the route of choice, because of the complications. The major and immediate complications are clogging of the small enteral tubes, and the constant dislodgment of the feeding tubes, particularly by the tongue movements of a restless patient. Reinsertion is possible but this becomes time-consuming, and may interfere with administering the desired amount of feeds required. The more often a nasogastric tube has to be reinserted the higher the chance that the tube will pass into the trachea rather than down the esophagus into the stomach, resulting in pulmonary complications.

This can happen even in patients who have a tracheostomy or endotracheal tube in place.

As well as these short-term complications, there is the long-term complication of a tracheoesophageal fistula, brought about by compression of the anterior wall of the esophagus and the posterior wall of the trachea between a tracheostomy tube or endotracheal tube that is pressing on the posterior wall of the trachea. The entrapment of the tracheal wall and wall of the esophagus between the tracheostomy or endotracheal tube and the feeding tube leads to pressure necrosis and a resultant tracheoesophageal fistula. This latter complication is extremely serious and difficult to repair and must be avoided at all costs. As a result, this method of feeding should be considered only for short-term enteral feeding.

For long-term enteral support, a feeding tube must be placed as an invasive procedure into the gastrointestinal tract, either as a feeding gastrostomy tube or as a feeding jejunostomy tube. The former is an excellent approach; it can be placed either at an open operation or by an endoscopic percutaneous approach. However, a feeding gastrostomy can have possible drawbacks.

Gastroesophageal reflux is common, and can be a major problem. This can be exacerbated by large volumes of tube feed in the stomach. In addition, a high fat content slows gastric emptying, and hence further increases the chances of reflux. This reflux can be more significant in a patient lying supine, because of the ease with which the refluxed contents can reach the back of the pharynx and be aspirated. Even in the presence of a tracheostomy tube or endotracheal tube, there is a chance of reflux into the trachea, resulting in recurrent aspiration pneumonia. The incidence and amount of reflux can be modified by reducing the rates of gastric infusion of feeds, but this may result in infusion rates that fail to meet the desired daily nutrition requirements.

Another issue is that of gastroparesis or poor gastric emptying, a problem that has its highest incidence in diabetic patients. The presence of these issues are not easy to elicit from the history of patients admitted as an emergency with a major cerebral catastrophe, rendering them unconscious. It is therefore important to try and elicit a good history from family members before deciding on the route to the gastrointestinal tract.

An endoscopic percutaneous gastrostomy can be converted into a feeding jejunostomy by passing a long feeding tube through the gastrostomy tube and endoscopically placing it past the duodenum into the upper jejunum. There are several problems with this technique. The long tubes clog easily and have to be replaced often, which means another endoscopic procedure for the patient, and the tubes tend to move and back-up into the stomach.

A better approach is to place a feeding jejunostomy tube directly into the jejunum. Fan et al. found that feeding tube patency was significantly longer in patients who had a direct percutaneous jejunostomy rather than a percutaneous gastrostomy with jejunal extension. Over a 6-month period, five patients in the former group and 19 in the latter group required intervention for tube dysfunction. Montecalvo et al. studied patients with feeding gastrostomy and jejunostomy tubes and found aspiration pneumonia to occur less often in patients with a jejunostomy tube. They also found that the patients with jejunostomy tubes received more consistent nutrition and that prealbumin levels were higher in the jejunostomy patients.

In this patient with a poor prognosis and an uncertain gastric history, a very good option would be a feeding jejunostomy over a feeding gastrostomy tube, and this I would favor.

There are several techniques for placement of a feeding jejunostomy: one open technique and two minimal access approaches. The open technique entails placing a jejunostomy tube under a general anesthesia through a small upper abdominal midline incision. The proximal jejunum is located just below the ligament of Treitz. The bowel is run to an area of the proximal jejunum that will reach easily to the abdominal wall. The loop of bowel is then delivered into the wound. Two purse-string sutures are placed on the antimesenteric side of the jejunum, and a stab wound is made in the center of the purse-string sutures. A 14-French red rubber catheter is advanced into the jejunum, fed distally, and then secured in place by tying the purse-string sutures. The tube is then buried into the jejunal wall in a Witzel manner for approximately 4 cm. The catheter is then brought out through a stab wound in the left side of the abdominal wall. The jejunal loop is then secured to the anterior abdominal with four nonabsorbable sutures. There are other operative techniques for the placement of an open jejunostomy tube; one is to place a T-tube through the purse-string suture, and then secure the bowel loop to the anterior abdominal wall with nonabsorbable sutures. Other variants of the technique can be found, but the basic principle is the same.

There are two minimal access techniques that can be used. A jejunostomy tube can be placed laparoscopically under general anesthesia. The technique consists of placing a trocar at the umbilicus and inducing pneumoperitoneum in the usual fashion. Two 5-mm trocars are placed, one on either side of the abdomen. The small bowel is run, and a site in the proximal jejunum is chosen to place the jejunostomy tube. A purse-string suture is placed in the antimesenteric border of the jejunum, a catheter is introduced into the jejunal lumen through a hole made in the center of the purse-string suture, and the suture is tied. The catheter is brought out through a stab wound on the left side of the abdomen, and the loop of bowel is sutured to the anterior abdominal wall with nonabsorbable sutures. There are laparoscopic jejunostomy kits that can be used, which contain T-tags that are passed through the abdominal wall and into the lumen of the bowel to hold the jejunal loop in close apposition with the abdominal wall. A needle is then passed in the center of the T-tags into the jejunal loop, a guidewire is passed through the needle, the needle is withdrawn, and a catheter is passed through over the needle into the jejunal loop and secured to the abdominal wall.

Probably the best and simplest method is to place a feeding jejunostomy tube directly into the jejunostomy percutaneously using an endoscopic technique in a manner similar to the placement of an endoscopic placement of a feeding gastrostomy tube. Under intravenous sedation a flexible endoscope is passed through the stomach and through the duodenum into the proximal small bowel, and the light in the bowel is located through the abdominal wall. A needle is then placed through the abdominal wall into the jejunal loop. A guidewire is then passed through the needle, grasped by a snare, and brought out through the mouth. A feeding tube is then fed over the guidewire and pulled through the abdominal wall and pulled into place so that the small bowel loop is snug against the abdominal wall. One of the major advantages of endoscopic placement of a feeding jejunostomy tube is that it is simple and can be placed in the intensive care unit without having to move the patient to the operating room.

Jejunostomy feeding tubes can be used immediately. A saline infusion is started at a low infusion rate. If this does not result in abdominal distention, then the feeds can be started at a low rate and advanced as tolerated. Diarrhea may occur from too rapid infusion of hypertonic solutions, but this can be controlled with manipulation of the feeds and their rate. One of the common complications of feeding jejunostomy tubes is tube blockage. This can be guarded against by flushing of the tube on a regular basis with saline. Should a mature tube need changing, this can be done by withdrawing the old tube and replacing it with a new tube. If there is any problem, it can be done under radiologic control, or the position of the tube can be confirmed by the injection of radiologic contrast through the tube under fluoroscopic control.

Although this patient had a cesarean section in 1981, the chances of adhesions are extremely low, and therefore are unlikely to preclude any of the options for the placement of a jejunostomy feeding tube. In those patients who have had a previous laparotomy, or an operation in the upper abdomen, adhesions may limit the placement of a feeding tube either endoscopically or laparoscopically, but might not preclude these approaches. They can be tried, and if adhesions are a significant issue, then the procedure can be converted to an open procedure for placement of the feeding jejunostomy tube.

# E. Conclusions

*Kent Choi*

Percutaneous endoscopic gastrostomy (PEG) provides a durable enteric feeding access for patients with an intact and functional gastrointestinal tract. It has some advantage over jejunostomy. It is commonly performed at the bedside with monitory care under sedation and local anesthetics. It can be used to administer bolus feeding, which is physiologically more natural than continuous tube feed. It is regarded as the gold standard for enteric feeding enterostomy. The absolute and relative contraindications for this procedure are well recognized and have been published by the American Society for Gastrointestinal Endoscopy. Frequent indications for PEG placement include impaired swallowing associated with neurological conditions, and neoplastic diseases of the oropharynx, larynx, and esophagus.

When PEG placement is difficult or dangerous, because, for example, of a large hiatal hernia, large Zenker's diverticula, morbid obesity, or overlying bowel or liver, open or laparoscopic gastrostomy tube placement should be considered.

Enteral access is often initiated via a nasojejunal route in critically ill patients. It is often associated with dislodgment, malpositioning, and physical discomfort with or without sinusitis. Percutaneous endoscopic placement of a jejunal feeding tube is indeed possible, but it is technically more challenging than PEG. Surgical jejunostomy tube placement using open or laparoscopic techniques is more invasive in nature and carries higher risk of potential complications, but it is the best options in patients with recurrent aspiration secondary to gastroesophageal reflux disease because distal tip placement can be reliably achieved.

The most common indications for jejunostomy tube placement are failure to tolerate gastric feeding, severe gastroesophageal reflux resulting in repeat tube feed-related aspiration, and gastric outlet obstruction or severe gastroparesis. There may also be a decreased incidence of aspiration. The disadvantages of jejunal feeding access as compared to gastrostomy tubes are the inability to administer bolus feed, increased frequency of diarrhea, a tendency for these small-caliber tubes to become clogged, the potential risk of bowel obstruction, and tube dislodgment.

The potential risk of aspiration is the factor of greatest concern in mentally impaired patients. Combined gastric decompression and jejunal feed tube, in theory, should provide a decreased risk of aspiration; however, published studies have numerous shortcomings, and further study is warranted. There is no consensus as to the best route for feeding mentally impaired adults, and the current literature is inconclusive. Lack of a standardized definition of aspiration and large variation in study methods compound the difficulty in obtaining a clear consensus. It is difficult to differentiate aspiration of gastric contents or tube feeding materials versus aspiration of pharyngeal secretion. There are also tremendous variations in feeding delivery methods, such as patient positioning, bolus versus continuous feeding, timing of feeding initiation after access placement, and use of prokinetic agents.

In summary, there is no convincing evidence to support the notion of using altered mental status as an independent indication for jejunostomy tube placement in patients who need long-term enteric feeding access. Given the difference in potential risk profile, PEG tube is still the preferred route for long-term enteric nutrition. Jejunostomy tube placement should be reserved for patients with clinically documented gastroesophageal reflux or the inability to tolerate gastric feeding for whatever reason.

# References

Fan AC, Baron TH, Rumalla A, Harewood GC. Comparison of direct percutaneous endoscopic jejunostomy and PEG with jejunal extension. Gastointest Endosc 2002;56:890–894.

Gauderer MW, Ponsky JL, Izant RJ. Gastrostomy without laparotomy: a percutaneous endoscopic technique J Pediatr Surg 1980;15:872–875.

Montecalvo MA, Steger KA, Farber HW, et al. Nutritional outcome and pneumonia in critical care patients randomized to gastric versus jejunal tube feedings. The Critical Care Research Team. Crit Care Med 1992;20:1377–1387.

# Suggested Readings

American Society for Gastrointestinal Endoscopy. Role of PEG/PEJ in enteral feeding. Gastrointest Endosc 1998;48:699–701.

Baron TH. Direct percutaneous endoscopic jejunostomy. Am J Gastroenterol 2006; 101:1407–1409.

Cech AC, Morris JB, Mullen JL, Crooks GW. Long-term enteral access is aspiration-prone patients. J Intensive Care Med 1995;10:179–186.

Faries MB, Roumbeau JL. Use of gastrostomy and combined gastrojejunostomy tubes for enteral feeding. World J Surg 1999;23:603–607.

Fox KA, Mularski RA, Sarfari MR, et al. Aspiration pneumonia following surgically placed feeding tubes. Am J Surg 1995;170:564–566.

Gauderer MWL. Percutaneous endoscopic gastrostomy and the evolution of contemporary long-term access. Clin Nutr 2002;21(2):103–110.

Georgeson KE. Laparoscopic versus open procedures for long-term enteral access. Nutr Clin Pract 1997;12:S7–8.

Jacobs DG, Jacobs DO, Kudsk KA, et al., for the East Practice Management Guidelines. Practice management guidelines for nutritional support of the trauma patient. 2003. www.east.org/tpg/nutrition.

Liebert MA, for the American Association of Neurological Surgeons, Joint Section on Neurotrauma and Critical Care. Nutritional support of brain injured patients. J Neurotrauma 1996;13(11):721–729.

Loser C, Aschl G, Hebuterne X, et al., for ESPEN. ESPEN guidelines on artificial enteral nutrition—percutaneous endoscopic gastrostomy (PEG). Consensus statement. Clin Nutr 2005;24:848–861.

McHattie G. Practice and problems with gastrostomies. Proc Nutr Soc 2005;64:335–337.

McMahon MM, Hurley DL, Kamath PS, Mueller PS. Medical and ethical aspects of long-term enteral tube feeding. Mayo Clin Proc 2005;80:1461–1476.

Mellinger JD, Ponsky JL. Percutaneous endoscopic gastrostomy: state of the art, 1998. Endoscopy 1998;30:126–132.

Murayama KM, Johnson TJ, Thompson JS. Laparoscopic gastrostomy and jejunostomy are safe and effective for obtaining enteral access. Am J Surg 1996;172:591–595.

National Institute for Clinical Excellence. Nutrition support in adults. Clinical Guideline 2006;32(977). London. www.nice.org.uk.

Pearce CB, Duncan HD. Enteral feeding. Nasogastric, nasojejunal, percutaneous endoscopic gastrostomy, or jejunostomy: its indications and limitations. Postgrad Med J 2002;78:198–204.

Ponsky JL, Aszodi A. Percutaneous endoscopic jejunostomy. Am J Gastroenterol 1984;79:113–116.

Sleigh G, Brocklehurst P. Gastrostomy feeding in cerebral palsy: a systematic review. Arch Dis Childhood 2004;89:534–539.

Stroud M, Duncan H, Nightingale J, for the British Society of gastroenterology. Guidelines for enteral feeding in adult hospital patients. Gut 2003;52(suppl VII).

Teasell R, Foley N, McRae M, Finestone H. Use of percutaneous gastrojejunostomy feeding tubes in the rehabilitation of stroke patients. Arch Phys Med Rehabil 2001;82:1412–1415.

# 20. Percutaneous Versus Laparoscopic Feeding Tube Placement

## A. Introduction

Multiple options exist when permanent feeding tubes are required. This chapter explores the alternatives—specifically, whether the percutaneous or laparoscopic route is preferable. Obviously, the first decision that must be made is whether feedings can be given into the stomach or whether jejunal access is necessary. This was explored in more detail in Chapter 19.

## B. Case

*Andrew Nowell*

An 80-year-old man with a history of coronary artery disease was admitted to the hospital after presenting for evaluation of abrupt onset of weakness and diaphoresis while sitting down. As part of his evaluation, transthoracic echocardiography was performed, which showed a left ventricular ejection fraction of 30% and apical hypokinesis. Cardiac catheterization was performed, which demonstrated occlusion of his three prior vein bypass grafts.

The cardiothoracic surgery department was consulted, which moved the patient to the operating room where a redo two-vessel coronary artery bypass graft (CABG) was performed. The patient was then taken to the intensive care unit (ICU) postoperatively for management, and he was extubated on the first postoperative evening. Soon thereafter, he was noted to be demonstrating left-sided neglect and hemiparesis as well as altered mental status. Neurology was consulted, and the subsequent workup revealed a right cerebral hemisphere infarction.

No neurologic recovery had occurred by postoperative day 14. The patient demonstrated extremely poor swallow function on formal evaluation, and had been receiving tube feeds via a Dobhoff tube. A consultation for placement of long-term tube feeding access was requested.

The patient's past medical history was significant for coronary artery disease, status post–three-vessel CABG and redo two-vessel CABG as reported in the history of the present illness, right hemisphere cerebrovascular accident status post–redo CABG, hypertension, hypercholesterolemia, prostatic adenocarcinoma status post–brachytherapy in 1990 (no recurrence per surveillance PSA testing), and chronic obstructive pulmonary disease.

The patient's past surgical history included a left total hip replacement in 1991 and an open cholecystectomy in 1979. His family history included a mother deceased secondary to metastatic renal cell carcinoma and a father decreased secondary to carcinoma of unknown primary, metastatic to the liver.

The patient was married, and before this hospitalization he lived at home with his wife. He is a nonsmoker and does not drink alcohol.

His current medications included lansoprazole 30 mg daily, aspirin 325 mg daily, felodipine 10 mg daily, lisinopril 15 mg twice daily, metoprolol 50 mg twice daily, prazosin 1 mg daily, simvastatin 10 mg daily, and Isordil 20 mg twice daily. He has no known drug allergies. The review of symptoms was not available due to the patient's neurologic status.

On physical examination, he was frail, with significant neurologic impairment, unable to respond to questions, and wearing a diaper.

Vital signs included a temperature of 36°C, pulse 74, blood pressure 139/58, and $SaO_2$ 99% on room air. His height was 175 cm, weight 70 kg, and body mass index (BMI) 22.9.

He was alert but not oriented, and his response to commands was variable. He had a dense hemiplegia.

His head and neck and cardiopulmonary examination were negative. He had a Dobhoff tube in place in his left nares. His sternotomy wound was healing nicely, without evidence of breakdown or infection.

His abdomen was flat, soft, and nontender. There was a well-healed right subcostal incision. No hernias were present. Bowel sounds were normal. Rectal examination revealed no mucosal lesions. Prostate was firm and nodular, and stool was guaiac negative.

Laboratory results were significant for a hematocrit of 30%, a white cell count of 10.7, blood urea nitrogen (BUN) of 18, and creatinine of 1.4.

The assessment was that this 80-year-old man had sequelae of a perioperative cerebrovascular event, including markedly impaired swallowing. He required long-term access for enteral feeds.

**Which route of access would you choose—percutaneous endoscopic or laparoscopic? Gastrostomy or jejunostomy?**

# C. Percutaneous Endoscopic Placement of Feeding Tubes

## Edward Lin and Louis O. Jeansonne IV

The need for enteral feeding access is a common clinical problem, and there are multiple alternatives available to the surgeon. While flexible nasogastric or nasoenteric tubes are effective short-term measures, gastrostomy or jejunostomy tubes are the most appropriate choice for long-term nutritional support. Indications for long-term enteral feeding include neurologic disability, facial trauma, malignancy, or any other condition that impairs the ability to swallow or otherwise tolerate oral feedings. Options for placement of feeding tubes include percutaneous (either endoscopic or radiographic) and surgical (open or laparoscopic) routes.

The emergence of the percutaneous endoscopic gastrostomy (PEG) tube created a minimally invasive option for gastrostomy placement. The avoidance of the risks of general anesthesia with this procedure represents a major advantage over open or laparoscopic techniques. Other advantages of the PEG tube include the lack of incision and the capability to be performed outside of the operating room, resulting in markedly decreased procedure cost. The PEG tubes have also been shown to have a lower incidence of major complications than either radiologically or surgically placed feeding tubes. Disadvantages of this technique include the risk of dislodgment or injury to adjacent viscera, and the requirement of a patent upper gastrointestinal (GI) tract.

While a PEG tube provides excellent feeding access with a low risk of complications for the majority of patients, there are some instances in which the patient's inability to tolerate gastric feeding results in the necessity for a postpyloric feeding tube. Our procedure of choice in this case is a percutaneous endoscopic gastrostomy/jejunostomy tube (PEG/J). This is an endoscopically placed feeding tube that enters the stomach and has a tip that rests in the proximal jejunum. This procedure, while somewhat technically challenging, has the benefit of providing postpyloric feeding in a minimally invasive fashion for the patient with gastroparesis or delayed gastric emptying.

For the patient described in this scenario, an elderly postsurgical cardiac patient with multiple comorbidities and complications, feeding access should be obtained in the most minimally invasive fashion possible. In this situation we would advocate a PEG or PEG/J.

The procedure can be performed either in the operating room or at the bedside in a monitored setting. At our institution, it is most commonly performed in the surgical ICU or endoscopy suite, using a standard "pull" technique, by a single surgeon and a nurse assistant. After obtaining informed consent, the patient is placed in the supine position and is given appropriate sedation and pain control. Blood pressure, heart rate, respiratory rate, and oxygen saturation are monitored. An esophagogastroscopy is performed, and the stomach is insufflated. If a PEG/J is planned, the duodenum is entered and inspected prior to tube insertion, in order to ensure a patent GI tract and to facilitate entry into the duodenum later in the procedure. The endoscope is pulled back into the stomach, and the optimal location for tube placement is visualized and confirmed both by transillumination and manual pressure on the external abdomen (Fig. 20.1A). A hollow sheathed needle is used to puncture the skin and enter the stomach (Fig. 20.1B). The needle is removed and the sheath is left in place. A guidewire is placed through the sheath, and an endoscopic snare is used to catch the guidewire. The endoscope is then removed through the mouth along with the guidewire. A 1-cm incision

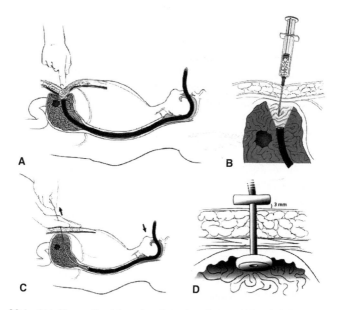

Fig. 20.1. (A) The optimal location for tube placement is visualized and confirmed both by transillumination and manual pressure on the external abdomen. (B) A hollow sheathed needle is used to puncture the skin and enter the stomach. (C) The gastrostomy is pulled into the stomach using the guidewire. (D) A T-bar is used to secure the tube in place. (From Ponsky JL. Percutaneous endoscopic gastrostomy. J Gastrointest Surg 2004;8(7):903–906, with permission.)

is made in the skin adjacent to the guidewire insertion point. The gastrostomy tube is attached to the guidewire, and using the wire it is pulled back into the stomach through the mouth (Fig. 20.1C). The tube is pulled through the skin until the disk is snug against the internal gastric wall. A T-bar is used to secure the tube in place (Fig. 20.1D).

Where indicated, a jejunal feeding tube can be introduced either through an existing gastrostomy tube or as a double-channel gastrojejunal tube. At our institution, a smaller jejunal tube is normally placed through the existing PEG tube and advanced into the jejunum endoscopically. The size of the jejunostomy tube is determined by the size of the PEG tube. For a 20-French (F) PEG tube, an 8F jejunostomy tube is used; for a 24F PEG tube, a 12F jejunostomy tube is used. Prior to insertion, the jejunal tube is prepared by attaching a looped silk suture to the distal tip. An endoscopic clip applier is advanced through the PEG tube from the inside, and is used to grasp the silk suture and pull the jejunal tube back through the PEG tube into the stomach (Fig. 20.2). While con-

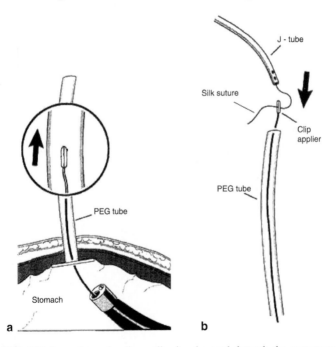

Fig. 20.2. (A) An endoscopic clip applier is advanced through the percutaneous endoscopic gastrostomy (PEG) tube from the stomach and (B) is used to grasp a silk suture attached to the J-tube. (Modified from Bumpers et al., A simple technique for insertion of PEJ via PEG, Surg Endosc, 1994;8:121–123, with permission.)

tinuing to grasp the suture with the clip applier, the endoscope is then advanced through the pylorus into the duodenum and proximal jejunum (Figs. 20.3 and 20.4). Once the tip is in the desired position, the endoscopic clip applier is used to secure the tip suture to the intestinal mucosa in order to prevent migration of the tip (Figs. 20.5 and 20.6). The tube is left to gravity drainage for 24 hours before feeding, but may be used for medications immediately.

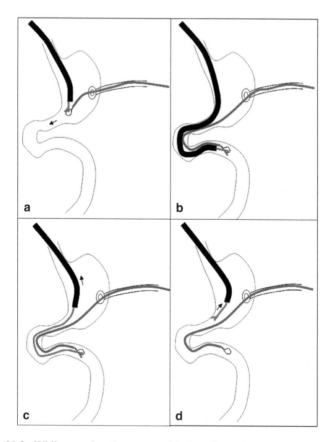

Fig. 20.3. While grasping the suture with the clip applier (A), the endoscope is advanced into the duodenum (B) or (C) proximal jejunum, and (D) the endoscopic clip applier is used to secure the tip suture to the intestinal mucosa.

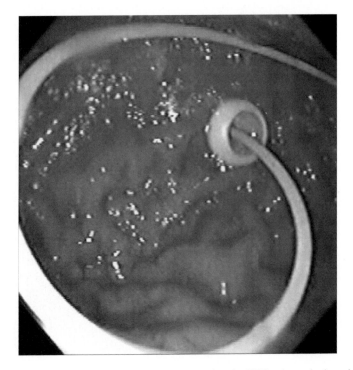

Fig. 20.4. The jejunostomy tube is shown entering the PEG tube and advancing distally into the duodenum.

In conclusion, the clinical scenarios that accompany the need for enteral feeding access often involve chronic, critical, terminal, or debilitating illness. In these patient populations, the need to minimize complications from invasive procedures is paramount. Therefore, we advocate percutaneous endoscopic placement of feeding access in a monitored setting whenever possible. The procedure can be performed by a single surgeon if adequate assistance is available. The presence of impaired gastric emptying does not preclude an endoscopic technique, since PEG/J placement is possible. The tip of a PEG/J can be endoscopically clipped to the intestinal mucosa to prevent migration, offering an advantage over radiographically placed tubes.

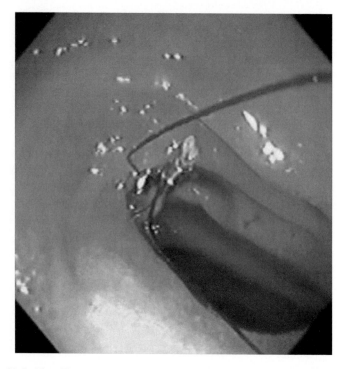

Fig. 20.5. The silk suture is seen clipped to the mucosa to prevent migration of the tip of the tube.

## D.  Laparoscopic Feeding Tube Placement

*Carol E.H. Scott-Conner*

Laparoscopic feeding tube placement should be considered as an alternative whenever the endoscopic technique described above is not feasible. In addition, there are specific areas in which the laparoscopic route may provide a more durable or better means of access.

The first of these is the situation in which a permanent, mucosa-lined gastrostomy is desired. This creates an extremely stable tract that can simply be cannulated whenever feeding is to be administered. Because the tract is mucosa-lined, premature dislodgment of the tube is not a concern. In the case described, where it is uncertain how much additional recovery might occur, a less durable route of access, more easily reversed, such as a Stamm gastrostomy, might be preferable. A Stamm gastrostomy can generally be "reversed" when it is no longer needed by simply pulling out

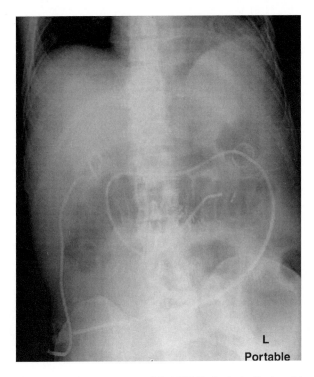

Fig. 20.6. Radiographic appearance of the PEG/J tube in its final position.

the tube. The same is true for a PEG, with the caveat that sufficient time must have elapsed for the stomach to be firmly adherent to the anterior abdominal wall.

The technique of laparoscopic Janeway gastrostomy mimics the equivalent open approach. Trocars are placed and an endoscopic linear stapler is used to create a tongue of gastric wall (Fig. 20.7). This tongue is then brought out through a strategically placed trocar site by simply grasping it and withdrawing the trocar, grasper, and tongue of stomach through the trocar site. It is then matured to the skin (Fig. 20.8). The main problem associated with Janeway gastrostomies has been leakage from the staple line. This may be particularly apt to occur at the "crotch" where the tongue of stomach takes a right-angle bend relative to the rest of the stomach, and may be related to traction on the staple line at this point. For this reason, it is customary to imbricate at least this part of the staple line. It is important to make the tongue wide enough to accommodate a tube.

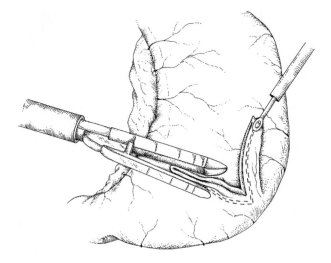

Fig. 20.7. Construction of the tongue of the stomach that will be passed out through the trocar site to provide a completely mucosal-lined (Janeway) gastrostomy for permanent enteral access. (From Scott-Conner CEH, ed. The SAGES Manual: Fundamentals of Laparoscopy, Thoracoscopy, and GI Endoscopy, 2nd ed. New York: Springer-Verlag, 2006, with permission.)

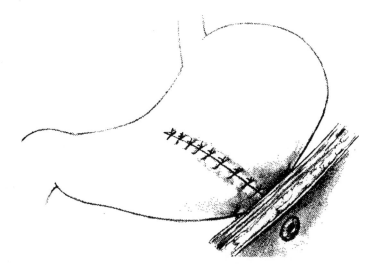

Fig. 20.8. Completed Janeway gastrostomy. (From Scott-Conner CEH, ed. Chassin's Operative Strategy in General Surgery, 3rd ed. New York: Springer-Verlag, 2002, with permission.)

When jejunostomy is chosen as the preferred route of access, a laparoscopic jejunostomy allows the surgeon to create a stable access portal that is securely sutured to the anterior abdominal wall. This technique requires facility with laparoscopic suturing; as with any jejunostomy, the possibility exists of volvulus, torsion, or internal hernia.

A relatively simple method, somewhat analogous to the needle-catheter jejunostomy technique used during open surgery, is shown in Figures 20.9 and 20.10 and described in detail in the SAGES manual.

# E. Conclusions

## *Andrew Nowell*

Enteral intake is the recognized preferred route of nutritional support in patients, with benefits including maintenance of gastrointestinal mucosal integrity and decreased infection rates. The patient's native

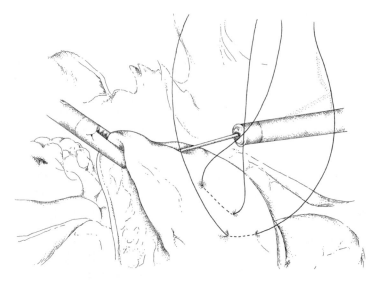

Fig. 20.9. Laparoscopic jejunostomy. Anchoring sutures have been placed and a needle is being advanced percutaneously into the lumen of the bowel. (From Scott-Conner CEH, ed. The SAGES Manual: Fundamentals of Laparoscopy, Thoracoscopy, and GI Endoscopy, 2nd ed. New York: Springer-Verlag, 2006, with permission.)

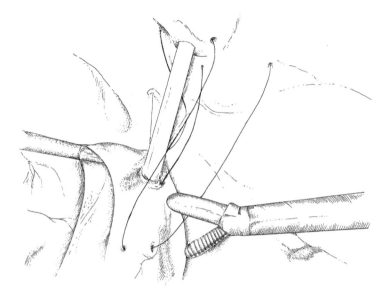

Fig. 20.10. A dilator is being passed through the abdominal wall into the lumen of the jejunum. Care is taken to pass the dilator just far enough to access the lumen, but not so far as to risk posterior perforation. (From Scott-Conner CEH, ed. The SAGES Manual: Fundamentals of Laparoscopy, Thoracoscopy, and GI Endoscopy, 2nd ed. New York: Springer-Verlag, 2006, with permission.)

ability to achieve adequate intake is often impaired, requiring use of an enteral access device to accomplish administration of nutrition, fluids, and medications. In the short term, a nasoenteric tube is commonly used due to relative ease of placement. However, these devices are prone to accidental dislodgment, frequently become occluded, can predispose to sinusitis, and can be perceived as uncomfortable. In patients who require enteral nutritional support for longer than 4 to 6 weeks, placement of some type of transcutaneous enteral access device is indicated.

For patients who require long-term enteral access, a variety of methods exist including gastrostomy and jejunostomy placed via open surgical technique or laparoscopically. Additionally, PEG, PEG-jejunostomy, or direct percutaneous endoscopic jejunostomy (DPEJ) can be utilized. Of these techniques, PEG has enjoyed success as a frequent method of enteral access due to the relatively noninvasive nature of the procedure and the ability to be placed successfully and without complication. Specific issues related to choice of gastrostomy versus jejunostomy were explored in Chapter 19, and will only be touched upon here. However, in some patients endoscopic access is impossible (for example, head and neck cancer patients), and alternate means of tube placement must be sought.

In such cases, a laparoscopic approach for placement of the gastrostomy or jejunostomy offers the potential advantages of smaller incisions, less postoperative pain, and better visualization of the peritoneal cavity. Both techniques can be accomplished safely, with a similar profile of complications.

Specific indications for PEG include patients with impaired swallow secondary to neurologic event, central nervous system or spinal cord deficits, cancer of the oropharynx/esophagus, and severe facial trauma. The PEG may also be used for long-term gastric decompression. Absolute contraindication to PEG includes inability to perform upper endoscopy, as in patients with severe facial trauma and head/neck malignancies, and inability to oppose the stomach to the anterior abdominal wall, as in planned use of the stomach in esophageal reconstruction. Relative contraindications include ascites, coagulopathy, morbid obesity, prior gastric/abdominal surgery, and neoplastic/inflammatory disease of the stomach. Additionally, in those patients with gastroparesis, severe gastroesophageal reflux, high risk of aspiration, and gastric outlet obstruction PEG is relatively contraindicated and jejunostomy preferred.

Intestinal obstruction is the absolute contraindication to jejunostomy, while relative contraindications include extensive abdominal adhesions, Crohn's disease, postradiation enteritis, ascites, and bowel edema.

Techniques for PEG placement are well established, and consist of two primary techniques: the pull type and the push type. Both require endoscopic visualization of the stomach, transillumination of the abdominal wall in the area of planned needle introduction so as to minimize the risk of interposed viscus, and endoscopic visualization of the needle placed percutaneously into the stomach to facilitate guidewire positioning. In the pull technique, after the guidewire is introduced into the stomach, it is secured to an endoscopic snare and passed back up through the esophagus and out the oropharynx. The PEG tube is then secured to the wire, and traction on the distal end of the guidewire protruding from the abdominal wall is used to carefully advance the PEG tube down through the upper digestive tract until the "mushroom" bolster of the tube is visualized to approximate gastric mucosa. The push technique uses an introducer tube that contains a central lumen designed to be placed over the guidewire. This tube is then pushed until it passes out through the abdominal wall, when it is then secured and used to advance the PEG to into final position under endoscopic guidance. A percutaneous technique can be used to access the jejunum via the gastrostomy tube, by advancing a specially designed tube into the small intestine.

Techniques for laparoscopic gastrostomy or jejunostomy are somewhat more varied. A standard Stamm gastrostomy can be performed laparoscopically. Alternatively, a more permanent gastrostomy can be created using the Janeway technique. No indwelling tube is required.

At least four different techniques for laparoscopic jejunostomy have been described in the literature. One method involves a laparoscopic-assisted jejunostomy, in which the jejunum is mobilized and the intended area of tube placement selected laparoscopically and then exteriorized at a small laparotomy incision or enlargement of a trocar site. The jejunostomy tube is then placed and secured under direct visualization as in a Witzel or Stamm technique.

Another technique involves the placement of transabdominal sutures placed laparoscopically to approximate a discrete area of the seromuscular layer of the jejunum to the anterior abdominal wall, similar to the final pexy of the gastric wall to the abdominal wall in a Stamm gastrostomy. Then, a feeding tube or needle catheter is placed through the center of the area demarcated by the sutures. The sutures have been described as either secured down at the fascial level, or alternatively tied over bolsters on the skin, and removed 2 weeks later, with the jejunum remaining adherent to the abdominal wall. A similar technique is described that utilizes T-fasteners in lieu of the transabdominal sutures. Originally designed for percutaneous gastrostomy, the T-fastener is inserted into the jejunal lumen via a slotted needle, and deployed by stylet. It is used to approximate the jejunal wall to the anterior abdominal wall, after which a feeding tube is placed into the jejunal lumen transabdominally using the Seldinger-type technique.

A completely intraabdominal laparoscopic technique has been described for placement of a jejunostomy tube. For this, intracorporeal knot tying is used to secure a purse-string suture around a feeding tube placed transabdominally into the jejunum under direct laparoscopic visualization. Additional sutures are placed laparoscopically to anchor the jejunum to the anterior abdominal wall.

Placement of the PEG can be accomplished in a majority of attempts, with a documented success rate ranging from 97% to 100% by experienced operators. Success rates are similar when resident physicians place these tubes under faculty supervision. Success rates for laparoscopic jejunostomy have similarly been reported to approach 100%.

Complications of PEG placement include those relating to the procedure itself as well as postplacement complications. Taken together, PEG-related morbidity has been reported to range from 0% to 17%. Mortality rates are described as approximately 1%. Procedure-related complications range from 1% to 4% of cases, and include acute hemorrhage (1%), laceration or through-and-through puncture of stomach or intestine (0.5% to 1.8%), and hematoma (<1%). Infection of the PEG site is the most common postplacement complication, ranging from 5% to 30%, but of these, less than 2% require intervention other than antibiotics.

One of the hallmark complications of PEG is premature displacement, particularly with delayed recognition. This is particularly apt to occur in neurologically impaired patients. The PEG tubes are accidentally dislodged at rates ranging from 1.6% to 4.4% of the time, with half of these displacements occurring prior to the 7 to 10 days required for maturation of the tract. Buried bumper syndrome, where the intragastric bolster migrates through a portion of the gastric or abdominal wall has been reported in up to 21.8% of cases, and is managed either through repositioning of the bolster back into the stomach or removal transabdominally. Other complications include leakage onto the skin (1% to 2%), and intraabdominal leakage (0.6%).

Complications of laparoscopic gastrostomy or jejunostomy are not as well documented, due to relatively fewer numbers of placements as compared to PEG. Individual case series have documented complication rates ranging from 1.7% to 50%. Han-Geurts et al. reviewed 21 studies describing experience with laparoscopic jejunostomy, in a total of 384 procedures using a variety of described techniques, and noted that the cumulative complication rate of all studies was approximately 21%. In this review, the most common complications were wound infection (5%) and dislodgement of the tube (4.2%). Reoperation and conversion to open procedure rates were approximately 1.8%. Other described complications included obstruction, perforation, and volvulus. Total mortality rate was 2.3%.

The PEG/J and laparoscopic gastrostomy/jejunostomy are complementary techniques that can be used to achieve enteral access in the patient requiring long-term nutritional support. The experience with PEG is the largest, and this device can reliably be placed by physicians with a variety of training backgrounds. Laparoscopic placement of gastrostomy or jejunostomy tubes is a relatively newer technique requiring the skills of a surgeon versed in laparoscopic technique. Complication rates seem to be similar, although the data are not as robust as those for PEG.

# References

Bumpers HL, Luchette FA, Doerr RJ, Hoover EL. A simple technique for insertion of PEJ via PEG. Surg Endosc 1994;8:121–123.

Han-Geurts IJM, Lim A, Stijnen T, Bonjer HJ. Laparoscopic feeding jejunostomy. Surg Endosc 2005;19:951–957.

# Suggested Readings

Allen JW, Ali A, Wo J, Bumpous JM, Cacchione RN. Totally laparoscopic feeding jejunostomy. Surg Endosc 2002;16:1802–1805.

American College of Surgeons. ACS surgery: principles and practice. 2006. http://www.acssurgery.com/.

Bosco JJ, Barkun AN, Isenberg GA, et al. Endoscopic enteral nutritional access devices. Gastrointest Endosc 2002;56(6):796–802.

DiSario JA, Baskin WN, Brown RD, et al. Endoscopic approaches to enteral nutritional support. Gastrointest Endosc 2002;55(7):901–908.

Gauderer MWL, Ponsky JL, Izant R. Gastrostomy without laparotomy: a percutaneous endoscopic technique. J Pediatr Surg 1980;15:872–875.

Goldman RK. Minimally invasive surgery: bedside tracheostomy and gastrostomy. Crit Care Clin 2000;16(1):113–128.

McClave SA, Chang WK. Complications of enteral access. Gastrointest Endosc 2003; 58(5):739–751.

Nagle AP, Murayama KM. Laparoscopic gastrostomy and jejunostomy. J Long-Term Effects Med Implants 2004;14(1):1–11.

Ponsky JL, Aszodi A. Percutaneous endoscopic jejunostomy. Am J Gastroenterol 1984; 79:113–116.

Ponsky JL, Gauderer MWL. Percutaneous endoscopic gastrostomy: a nonoperative technique for feeding gastrostomy. Gastrointest Endosc 1981;27:9–11.

Rustom IK, Jebreel A, Tayyab M, England RJ, Stafford ND. Percutaneous endoscopic, radiological and surgical gastrostomy tubes: a comparison study in head and neck cancer patients. J Laryngol Otol 2006;120(6):463–466.

Stiegmann GV, Goff JS, Silas D, Pearlman N, Sun J, Norton L. Endoscopic versus operative gastrostomy: final results of a prospective randomized trial. Gastrointest Endosc 1990;36(1):1–5.

# 21. Bariatric Surgery: Choice of Operative Procedure

## A. Introduction

Several options exist for minimal access bariatric surgery for morbid obesity. This chapter explores the specific choice between two procedures—the laparoscopic adjustable gastric band, and the laparoscopic Roux-en-Y gastric bypass. Details on both procedures and on laparoscopy in the morbidly obese are given in the SAGES manuals.

## B. Case

### *Joseph Y. Chung*

A 33-year-old woman with a body mass index (BMI) of 42 was referred for bariatric surgery. She had failed multiple supervised weight-loss programs over a span of 15 years. She had recently developed hypertension and diabetes, and also required bi-level positive airway pressure (BiPAP) at night for obstructive apnea. She had suffered from depression since grade school and had been on antidepressants for many years. She attributes her depression to her weight.

Her past medical history was also significant for chronic lower back pain and hyperlipidemia. She had no previous surgical procedures. She was on multiple medications including antihypertensives, antidepressants, lipid-lowering drugs, and an oral hypoglycemic agent.

She was married, with two children, and worked as an attorney. She had a 10-pack-a-year smoking history, but stopped smoking 6 years ago.

The review of symptoms was significant for dyspnea on exertion, which precluded exercise. She had chronic fatigue and joint pains. She had mild gastroesophageal reflux symptoms, which she controlled with Tums. She had some stress urinary incontinence.

Her physical examination revealed an obese (BMI of 42) female in no distress. Her abdomen was obese and without surgical scars. Her lower extremities had bilateral 1+ pitting edema. She strongly wishes to undergo surgery.

**Which procedure would you recommend?**

# C. Laparoscopic Adjustable Gastric Banding

*Jonathan A. Myers*

This patient is an ideal candidate for laparoscopic adjustable gastric banding (LAGB), which provides a safe, effective, adjustable, cost-efficient, and, if needed, reversible surgical option for weight loss.

The laparoscopic adjustable gastric band is a silicone band that is placed around the proximal portion of the stomach to create a small gastric pouch. After the patient ingests a small portion of food, the pouch becomes full, thus inducing a feeling of satiety. The band is connected via a catheter to a subcutaneous reservoir (port) secured to the anterior rectus sheath. A balloon situated in the lumen of the band can be gradually tightened with the addition of saline injected through the reservoir when the patient reports a cessation of weight loss and loss of satiety after meals. The LAGB is the most common bariatric procedure performed worldwide and is gaining popularity in the United States after receiving approval for use by the Food and Drug Administration in 2001.

Placement of the LAGB has consistently been shown to be one of the safest bariatric procedures available. The procedure is performed laparoscopically, without the need for bowel division, anastomosis, or rearrangement. Mortality from this procedure is reported to be one-tenth that of the laparoscopic Roux-en-Y gastric bypass (RYGBP). In the absence of suture lines, anastomotic leak is virtually nonexistent, and due to the minimal dissection required for this procedure, the incidence of inadvertent visceral injury is very low (0.80%). Other perioperative complications associated with LAGB include wound infection (0.28%) and injury to the spleen or liver (0.05%). Avoidance of electrocautery during the procedure reduces the risk of bowel injury. Confining the dissection to avascular planes minimizes the risk of bleeding. Long-term complications include pouch formation (3.97%), band slippage (1.62%), port flip (0.87%), catheter breakage (0.80%), and erosion of the band into the stomach (0.59%). The combination of improved surgical technique using the pars flaccida approach and diligent adjustment under fluoroscopic guidance has greatly reduced the incidence of these complications. Most pouch dilatations can be managed conservatively with band deflation while band slips can be managed laparoscopically with revision, or if needed band removal. Port and catheter complications have been minimized by design improvements, and, when they occur, are generally managed surgically under local anesthesia in an outpatient setting.

The purely restrictive nature of the LAGB eliminates the metabolic consequences of malabsorption associated with the gastric bypass. Maintaining continuity of the gastrointestinal tract allows for postoperative accessibility of the entire stomach by endoscopy, a benefit not available after RYGBP. Peptic ulcer disease, bleeding, or malignancy in the remnant stomach after gastric bypass may be difficult to diagnose or treat. Endoscopic access to the biliary tract via endoscopic retrograde cholangiopancreatography (ERCP) in patients with choledocholithiasis, cholangitis, or other disease processes is also hindered after RYGBP.

The LAGB provides an effective means of gradual weight loss over months to years. Several studies demonstrate that gastric bypass affords a rapid initial weight loss of greater than 70% of excess weight in the first year. This figure then tends to plateau, and many patients actually begin to gain some weight back after the 2- to 3-year mark. The pattern of weight loss exhibited by LAGB tends to be a steady rise with expectations of an average of 40% excess weight loss (EWL) after 1 year, and up to 50% to 70% EWL after 2 to 3 years. The general consensus is emerging that after 2 to 3 years the amount of weight loss with the LAGB or with gastric bypass is not statistically different and tends to be in the 50% to 60% EWL range. Thus it is important to emphasize that weight loss with the LAGB may not be as rapid as with the bypass, but is as effective over time. A further advantage of the band is that the more gradual pattern of weight loss has been shown to result in a lower incidence of symptomatic cholelithiasis, a common problem after gastric bypass that many feel necessitates simultaneous cholecystectomy or the use of choleretic agents in the postoperative period. As with other bariatric procedures, health and quality of life continue to improve after the weight loss achieved from LAGB. Marked improvement in diabetes, hypertension, dyslipidemia, reflux esophagitis, asthma, depression, and obstructive sleep apnea has been observed in postoperative patients.

The adjustability of the band is a major attribute of LAGB. Beginning several weeks after initial placement, patients return for sequential filling of the band to induce satiety and promote weight loss. We perform this under fluoroscopic guidance, although many institutions opt to perform adjustments using an office-based "palpation" technique with an algorithm for fill volume. We recommend fluoroscopy to access the subcutaneous port as well as to gauge the filling process by obtaining a limited esophagram during the fill. This protocol optimizes band tightness while minimizing complications such as erosion and band slippage from overtightening, and inadvertent injury to the reservoir or tubing from blind access with a needle. The entire process takes about 8 minutes and allows weight loss to be tailored to each individual patient. We strive to achieve a goal of 1 to 2 pounds of weight loss per week.

When patients note that they are able to ingest larger meals and fail to achieve adequate weight loss, they schedule an adjustment. In general, patients require an average of five or six adjustments in the first year, and two to four adjustments per year in subsequent years. Fluoroscopy allows us to determine if any pouch is present, and initial conservative management with temporary band deflation is employed. The adjustable nature of the band is also ideal for patients who are scheduled to undergo future endoscopy or surgery, as the band can be emptied prior to their procedure. Likewise, pregnant patients who are experiencing vomiting or insufficient weight gain during their pregnancy can have fluid removed to eliminate this problem, provided that appropriate shielding of the uterus is performed while accessing the reservoir. Patients who are ill, dehydrated, or merely wish to have less dietary restriction are also ideal candidates to take advantage of this benefit. The band can then be filled at a later date when appropriate to continue to achieve the patient's weight-loss goals.

Placement of the LAGB is the most cost-effective surgical bariatric option available today. The LAGB studies report an average operating room time of between 45 and 60 minutes and a mean hospital stay of 1.3 days. Many procedures are even being done in an outpatient setting. Laparoscopic RYGBP is a longer procedure, with reports approaching a minimum of 90 to 120 minutes of operating room time and an average length of stay of 2.5 days. It has been reported that normal activity can be resumed after nearly 18 days for the gastric bypass but after only 7 days for the LAGB. Thus patients undergoing LAGB will spend less time in the OR, less time in the hospital, and less time recovering from surgery. This enables them to resume normal daily activities and return to work sooner than patients undergoing gastric bypass, which translates into a substantial cost benefit.

A final advantage of LAGB over RYGBP is that, if needed, it is reversible. Although LAGB is intended to be permanent, certain circumstances, such as failed revision of a band slip or, rarely, patient intolerance warrant its removal. This is performed as a laparoscopic procedure and, after completion, the stomach usually returns to its original configuration. After removal, some patients may regain much of their original weight. Accordingly, they may consider another bariatric surgical option in the future.

In conclusion, LAGB offers a clear advantage over the laparoscopic RYGBP in the above patient. It provides the optimal balance of safety and efficacy without eliminating the possibility for subsequent procedures in the future should the need arise.

# D. Laparoscopic Roux-en-Y Gastric Bypass

*Mohammad Jamal*

We would offer this patient laparoscopic Roux-en-Y gastric bypass.

Obesity is a complex metabolic disorder influenced by the interaction of several genetic, endocrine, metabolic, and environmental factors. It has gained alarming epidemic proportions in the United States, with nearly 20% of the adult population affected, an estimated 40 million Americans overweight and nearly 11.5 million morbidly obese. With obesity comes an array of debilitating and life-threatening comorbidities including type 2 diabetes mellitus, hypertension, hypercholesterolemia, obesity hypoventilation and sleep apnea syndrome, venous stasis disease, cholelithiasis, cardiovascular disease, renal disease, and osteoarthritis. Necrotizing panniculitis, hypercoagulable states, psychosocial problems, and uterine, colon, and breast cancer are also found with an increasing frequency in the morbidly obese. Other obesity-related illnesses, including overflow incontinence, pseudotumor cerebri, sex hormone imbalance, and gastroesophageal reflux, may cause significant physical and emotional disability. Overall, obesity-related illnesses consume nearly 5% of the total health care costs in the United States—a staggering $100 billion.

The most accurate method of defining the relationship between body weight and frame size is the body mass index (BMI). Obesity is defined as a BMI of greater than 30. The 1991 National Institutes of Health (NIH) Consensus Panel on Gastric Surgery for Severe Obesity defined morbid obesity as a BMI of 35 or greater with severe obesity-related comorbidity, or 40 or greater without comorbidities. Superobese patients are defined as having a BMI of 50 or greater. Other definitions of morbid obesity include patients who weigh at least 200% of their ideal body weight (IBW). The patient in the above case scenario is an ideal candidate for bariatric surgery, and the following discussion further emphasizes the proven effectiveness of surgery as a cure for obesity related comorbidities.

Dietary and pharmacologic treatments for morbid obesity are known to have a high failure rate, whereas bariatric surgery seems to be the only available cure for morbid obesity, resulting in a significant sustained weight loss and resolution of obesity-related comorbidity. Most developed and affluent nations have seen a dramatic rise in the performance of bariatric surgical procedures with proven effectiveness at curing morbid obesity. The number of gastrointestinal surgeries performed annually for severe obesity in the United States alone has increased from about

16,000 in the early 1990s to about 103,000 in 2003. Laparoscopic bariatric surgical procedures are now among the most commonly performed operations worldwide. It must be borne in mind that an effective bariatric procedure is one that results in a sustained excess weight loss of greater than 50% as well as resolution of comorbid conditions. Any surgical procedure that does not achieve these goals cannot be classified as a successful weight loss operation.

Bariatric surgical procedures can be divided into two broad categories: restrictive and malabsorptive. The restrictive procedures (like the vertical banded gastroplasty and the adjustable gastric banding) have been known to have a high failure rate in the morbidly obese individuals, especially in those who regularly eat sweets. On the other hand, purely malabsorptive procedures (like the biliopancreatic diversion) as well as combination procedures (like the gastric bypass) have a long and proven history of successful weight loss and resolution of comorbidities. We now discuss the pros and cons of the two most common bariatric procedures performed in the United States—the Roux-en-Y gastric bypass (RYGBP) and the laparoscopic adjustable gastric banding (LAGB or Lap-Band).

First described by Mason and Ito nearly 30 years ago, the gastric bypass is considered the gold standard bariatric procedure. The National Institutes of Health Consensus Conference (NIHCC) in 1991 declared RYGBP and vertical band gastroplasty (VBG) to be the two most suitable weight loss procedures with excellent outcomes and low morbidity. This consensus led most bariatric surgeons to perform either VBG or RYGBP as the predominant weight loss procedures in the United States. The RYGBP is constructed using a small 15- to 20-mL gastric pouch and a Roux-en-Y gastrojejunostomy, a design that fundamentally creates malabsorption by bypassing the distal stomach, proximal duodenum, and a variable length of the jejunum depending on the length of the Roux limb, as well as restriction of food intake by creating a small gastric pouch. This operation is better classified as a hybrid procedure combining both restriction and malabsorption to differentiate it from truly malabsorptive procedures like the biliopancreatic diversion (BPD) with or without the duodenal switch (BPD-DS) procedure.

Several large randomized controlled trials report a significantly better and sustained weight loss as well as resolution of obesity-related comorbidities in subjects undergoing the RYGBP. Griffin et al. compared RYGBP and jejunoileal bypass (JIB), and clearly established the superior long-term weight loss benefits of RYGBP over JIB without the long-term complications of diarrhea and protein calorie malnutrition seen in the JIB group. In similar studies by Laws and Piantadosi and Pories et al., patients who underwent a gastric bypass were compared with those undergoing purely restrictive gastric partitioning procedures, such as vertical banded gastroplasty. The resulting data clearly suggest the superior weight loss benefits in RYGBP patients without the long-term sequelae of band erosion, reflux, and vomiting. Sugerman and colleagues similarly reported the results of their randomized prospective study comparing VBG and RYGBP. This study also documented the superior long-term weight loss benefits of RYGBP over VBG (EWL of 71% vs. 55%), though with a slightly higher complication rate in the RYGBP group. Most of the nutrient and vitamin deficiencies in the gastric bypass patients (iron deficiency anemia, and vitamin $B_{12}$ deficiency) were easily correctable with additional supplementation.

The development of laparoscopic surgical techniques has revolutionized the world of bariatric surgery. Several large studies documenting the safety and efficacy of laparoscopic Roux-en-Y gastric bypass (LRYGBP) are available in the surgical literature. These have paralleled the weight loss and resolution of comorbidities seen with the open approach. Data reported by Fernandez et al. suggest excellent weight loss results between laparoscopic and open gastric bypass over 12 months of follow-up. In terms of complications, the operative mortality for gastric bypass has been reported in the range of 0.5% to 1.0% in both open and laparoscopic gastric bypass series. Long-term nutritional issues include a similar risk of iron deficiency anemia as well as the need for vitamin $B_{12}$ supplementation. In contrast to purely malabsorptive procedures, protein calorie malnutrition is rare in gastric bypass patients. In terms of immediate postoperative complications, multivariate analysis of this series of 3000 open and laparoscopic gastric bypass patients suggest that older, heavier male patients with multiple comorbid conditions are at increased risk for anastomotic leak and higher mortality and therefore this procedure should be avoided by surgeons in the early part of their training.

Laparoscopic gastric bypass has also been compared to open gastric bypass in a prospective randomized trial by Nguyen et al. in which longer operative time for the laparoscopic group was found but with less overall blood loss and shorter hospitalization. Higher operating room expenses were offset by lower hospital costs in laparoscopic patients, and a significant reduction in wound complications including hernia and wound infections were recognized in the laparoscopic group. One-year follow-up data in this group showed a similar EWL between the two groups.

The outcomes data on the laparoscopic adjustable gastric banding (LAGB), however, are lacking long-term follow-up. Initial U.S. clinical trials sponsored by the Food and Drug Administration (FDA) with the Lap-Band system did not reproduce the results of studies performed elsewhere in the world. In both the FDA-monitored trials A and B, including several large academic U.S. centers, percentage excess weight loss (%EWL) was unimpressive and reported anywhere from 36% to 54% at the end of the 36-month follow-up period. Complication rates were high, and included band slippage, infection, leakage from the inflatable silicone ring causing inadequate weight loss, and esophageal dilatation. Several of these patients required removal of the devices as well as conversion to another bariatric procedure. Conversions were difficult and fraught with complications as reported by Doherty and DeMaria et al.

A comparative study of LAGB with RYGBP was reported by Biertho et al. In this analysis, 456 patients undergoing the LRYGBP at a U.S. center were compared to 805 LAGB performed in European institutions. Body mass index, complication rates, mortality, and excess weight loss after 3, 6, 12, and 18 months were obtained. The 805 patients selected for this study underwent the laparoscopic Swedish adjustable gastric banding (SAGB, Obtech) performed as the initial surgical treatment of their obesity. Patients with a BMI above 50 were usually considered for an open gastric bypass. Preoperative BMI was 49.4 in the RYGBP group and 42.2 in the LAGB group; perioperative major complication rates were 2.0% versus 1.3%, and the early postoperative major complication rates were 4.2% versus 1.7%, respectively. Mortality rate was 0.4% in the RYGBP group versus 0% in the LAGB group. The global EWL was 36.3% for RYGBP versus 14.7% for LAGB at 3 months, 51.6% versus 21.9% at 6 months, 67.0% versus 33.3% at 12 months, and 74.6% versus 40.4% at 18 months, respectively. Long-term follow-up for the LAGB group showed an EWL of 47% at 2 years, 56% at 3 years, and 58% at 4 years. The EWL at 3, 6, 12, and 18 months was statistically superior in the LGB group, for all BMI ranges studied. More recent experience with the LAGB suggests a slightly better excess weight loss with a lower complication profile. However, no long-term U.S. studies are currently available to advocate a large-scale use of the device for treatment of morbid obesity in the United States.

In all studies combined, comparing the open and laparoscopic approach, the gastric bypass produces comparable and sustained weight loss with an improvement in obesity related comorbidities. In most studies, the laparoscopic approach affords an improved short-term recovery from surgery, a shorter hospital stay, and a lower incidence of incisional hernias. The incidence of anastomotic strictures and increased hospital cost is reportedly higher in some clinical series. The current evidence suggests gastric bypass is the weight loss procedure of choice for morbidly obese patients with a good outcome and acceptable morbidity and mortality.

# E. Conclusions

## Joseph Y. Chung

Given the recent and explosive increase in demand for bariatric surgeries in the United States, the question arises as to which procedure to recommend to our patients. Unfortunately, there are currently no published randomized controlled trials directly comparing the two most common bariatric procedures presently being performed: laparoscopic gastric bypass and laparoscopic gastric banding. That being said, the contemporary literature, although far from conclusive, seems to strongly favor gastric bypass over gastric banding as the bariatric procedure of choice.

The 2005 clinical practice guidelines from the American College of Physicians (Snow et al.) notes that there is, as of yet, no conclusive evidence that one surgical procedure is superior to another for the management of morbid obesity. This is not surprising, given that case series dominate the surgical bariatric literature. Maggard et al. noted the significant limitations of the few randomized trials available. It is this lack of evidence, more than anything else, that seems to explain how the United States can have such a strong bias toward gastric bypass when, in contrast, Europe and Australia seem to clearly favor gastric banding. One should take note, however, that worldwide survey data from 2002–2003 seems to more closely mirror the American bias, with gastric bypass accounting for 65.1% of the bariatric surgeries performed, and laparoscopic adjustable banding accounting for only 24%.

To grasp how one bariatric surgery can be superior to another, it is helpful to begin by understanding that the surgical treatment of obesity achieves weight loss by two major mechanisms. The first is through restriction of oral intake, by limiting the volume of the proximal stomach. The second is through malabsorption, achieved by diverting the food stream to bypass segments of the small intestines. Procedures such as the adjustable gastric banding and the vertical banded gastroplasty work purely by restriction. On the other hand, procedures such as Roux-en-Y gastric bypass, biliopancreatic diversion, and duodenal switch work by a combination of both restriction and malabsorption.

Proponents of gastric banding, using devices such as the Lap-Band (which is the only one currently FDA approved for use in the U.S.), note that unlike gastric bypass, the procedure is simple and is relatively easy to learn and perform. The literature also seems to suggest that there is less mortality and morbidity associated with gastric banding, as compared to gastric bypass. And finally, proponents note that gastric banding is far more easily reversible and that recent data suggest that respectable weight loss can achieved in many patients.

Proponents of gastric bypass, on the other hand, note the complete absence of concerns regarding slippage, erosion, and the possible long-term complications of having a foreign body within the gastrointestinal track, which have been associated with the banding procedures. But most importantly, they note the seemingly superior short- and long-term weight loss results, which have a strong theoretical basis: gastric bypass has both a restrictive and malabsorptive component, making it more difficult to "cheat" by drinking large amounts of high-calorie liquids, which is a common reason cited for failures with the purely restrictive procedures.

Maggard et al. pooled data from 147 studies and performed a meta-analysis. First, they compared nonsurgical verses surgical treatment for weight loss and concluded that surgery was clearly more effective, especially for patients with a BMI of 40 or greater. However, they also attempted to compare the various surgical procedures available. Randomized controlled studies were rare, and only five such trials had sufficient data for pooling. Although none of these trials directly compared Roux-en-Y gastric bypass to the laparoscopic gastric banding, the authors of the meta-analysis concluded that gastric bypass procedures seemed to result in more, and lasting, weight loss than purely restrictive procedures, such as gastric banding. Moreover, they noted that there was no statistically significant difference in the mortality and morbidity among the various procedures.

In conclusion, the currently available evidence comparing gastric bypass to gastric banding is insufficient to say that one is clearly better than the other for the treatment of morbid obesity. However, the seemingly superior weight loss achievable with gastric bypass, and the lack of evidence that there is any greater morbidity or mortality, favors gastric bypass over gastric banding as the bariatric procedure of choice.

# References

Biertho L, Steffen R, Ricklin T, et al. Laparoscopic gastric bypass versus laparoscopic adjustable gastric banding: a comparative study of 1,200 cases. J Am Coll Surg 2003;197(4):536–544.

DeMaria EJ, Sugerman HJ, Meador JG, et al. High failure rate after laparoscopic adjustable silicone gastric banding for treatment of morbid obesity. Ann Surg 2001;233(6):809–818.

Doherty C, Maher JW, Heitshusen DS. Long-term data indicate a progressive loss in efficacy of adjustable silicone gastric banding for the surgical treatment of morbid obesity. Surgery 2002;132(4):724–727.

Fernandez AZ Jr, DeMaria EJ, Tichansky DS, et al. Experience with over 3,000 open and laparoscopic bariatric procedures: multivariate analysis of factors related to leak and resultant mortality. Surg Endosc 2004;18(2):193–197.

Griffin WO Jr, Young VL, Stevenson CC. A prospective comparison of gastric and jejunoileal bypass procedures for morbid obesity. Ann Surg 1977;186(4):500–509.

Laws HL, Piantadosi S. Superior gastric reduction procedure for morbid obesity: a prospective, randomized trial. Ann Surg 1981;193(3):334–340.

Maggard MA, Sugarman LR, Suttorp M, et al. Meta-analysis: surgical treatment of obesity. Ann Intern Med 2005;142:547–559.

Nguyen NT, Goldman C, Rosenquist CJ, et al. Laparoscopic versus open gastric bypass: a randomized study of outcomes, quality of life, and costs. Ann Surg 2001;234(3):279–289.

Pories WJ, Flickinger EG, Meelheim D, Van Rij AM, Thomas FT. The effectiveness of gastric bypass over gastric partition in morbid obesity: consequence of distal gastric and duodenal exclusion. Ann Surg 1982;196(4):389–399.

Snow V, Barry P, Fitterman N, et al. Pharmacologic and surgical management of obesity in primary care: a clinical practice guideline from the American College of Physicians. Ann Intern Med 2005;142:525–531.

Sugerman HJ, Londrey GL, Kellum JM, et al. Weight loss with vertical banded gastroplasty and Roux-en-Y gastric bypass for morbid obesity with selective versus random assignment. Am J Surg 1989;157(1):93–102.

# Suggested Readings

Chapman AE, Kiroff G, Game P, et al. Laparoscopic adjustable gastric banding in the treatment of obesity: a systematic literature review. Surgery 2004;135:326–351.

DeMaria EJ. Is gastric bypass superior for the surgical treatment of obesity compared with malabsorptive procedures? J Gastrointest Surg 2004;8(4):401–403.

Fisher BL. Comparison of recovery time after open and laparoscopic gastric bypass and laparoscopic adjustable banding. Obes Surg 2004;14:67–72.

Higa KD, Boone KB, Ho T, Davies OG. Laparoscopic Roux-en-Y gastric bypass for morbid obesity: technique and preliminary results of our first 400 patients. Arch Surg 2000;135(9):1029–1033.

Jones DB, Provost DA, DeMaria EJ, Smith CD, Morgenstern L, Shirmer B. Optimal management of the morbidly obese patient. Surg Endosc 2004;18:1029–1037.

NIH conference. Gastrointestinal surgery for severe obesity. Consensus Development Conference Panel. Ann Intern Med 1991;115(12):956–961.

O'Brien PE, Dixon JB. Lap-Band®: Outcomes and results. J Laparoendosc Adv Surg Tech 2003;13:265–270.

O'Brien PE, Dixon JB, Brown W. Obesity is a surgical disease: Overview of obesity and bariatric surgery. ANZ J Surg 2004;74:200–204.

Ren CJ, Horgan S, Ponce J. US experience with the LAP-BAND system. Am J Surg 2002;184(6B):46S–50S.

Rubenstein RB. Laparoscopic adjustable gastric banding at a U.S. center with up to 3-year follow-up. Obes Surg 2002;12(3):380–384.

Schauer PR, Ikramuddin S, Gourash W, Ramanathan R, Luketich J. Outcomes after laparoscopic Roux-en-Y gastric bypass for morbid obesity. Ann Surg 2000;232(4):515–529.

Shen R, Dugay G, Rajaram K, Cabrera I, Siegel N, Ren CJ. Impact of patient follow-up on weight loss after bariatric surgery. Obes Surg 2004;14:514–519.

Steinbrook R. Surgery for severe obesity. N Engl J Med 2004;350(11):1075–1079.

Weber M, Muller MK, Bucher T, et al. Laparoscopic gastric bypass is superior to laparoscopic gastric banding for treatment of morbid obesity. Ann Surg 2004;240:975–983.

Wittgrove AC, Clark GW. Laparoscopic gastric bypass, Roux en-Y-500 patients: technique and results, with 3–60 month follow-up. Obes Surg 2000;10:233–239.

Zinzindohoue FC, Chevallier JM, Douard R, et al. Laparoscopic gastric banding: a minimal invasive surgical treatment for morbid obesity. A prospective study of 500 consecutive patients. Ann Surg 2003;237:1–9.

# 22. Bariatric Surgery with Incidental Gallstones

## A. Introduction

Gallstones are common in the morbidly obese population. During the performance of open bariatric surgery, it was common practice to remove the gallbladder if gallstones were discovered during exploration. Some even advocated prophylactic cholecystectomy, reasoning that rapid weight loss was associated with lithogenic bile and the development of gallstones during the postoperative period.

Now most bariatric procedures are performed via a minimally invasive approach. This has resulted in a reexamination of the role of concomitant cholecystectomy. This chapter explores these issues.

## B. Case

### Robert Hanfland

A 26-year-old woman with morbid obesity presented for laparoscopic gastric bypass surgery. She had been obese for most of her life, with significant weight gain following her early teens and after the birth of a child 3 years earlier. She had tried numerous weight-loss programs, gaining all of her weight back after moderate losses. She suffered from a number of related illnesses, all of which have worsened as she gained weight.

She reported that she eats three meals per day, as well as two to three snacks per day (usually chips). She drinks two to three 12-ounce cans of diet soda per day.

Her past medical history was significant for obstructive sleep apnea, arthritis of the knee and hip joints, gastroesophageal reflux disease, polycystic ovary disease, depression, and morbid obesity. She had had one pregnancy, with a spontaneous vaginal delivery. She had not had any prior surgery.

With the exception of dyspnea on exertion, all systems were negative except as noted above. She was on no medications and had no allergies.

Her family history was significant for a father who had hypertension and a gastric bypass. Her mother had type 2 diabetes mellitus, breast cancer, and cervical stenosis. She had a sister who had had a cholecystectomy.

She was married, with one child (3 years old). She worked as a hair stylist. She did not smoke or drink alcoholic beverages.

On physical examination, she was a pleasant, cooperative, morbidly obese female. Her temperature was 35.9 °C, pulse 88, respiratory rate 18, blood pressure 136/86, height 161 cm, weight 134.1 kg, and body mass index (BMI) 50.6. Abdominal examination revealed an obese abdomen with significant pannus, no intertriginous dermatitis, no tenderness, no hepatosplenomegaly. The remainder of her physical examination was negative. Laboratory tests, including liver function tests, were normal.

The patient was referred for dietary counseling and was able to lose 18 pounds. She was reevaluated and determined to be a suitable candidate for bariatric surgery.

The alternatives, including adjustable laparoscopic gastric band and Roux-en-Y gastric bypass were discussed. Understanding the expected outcomes of each and the attendant risks, she chose to proceed with a laparoscopic gastric bypass.

During surgery, inspection revealed a lobulated gallbladder with multiple gallstones. There was no obvious inflammation or edema of the gallbladder wall.

**How should this be managed? Would you perform an incidental cholecystectomy or wait until she is symptomatic? What about pharmacologic management with bile salts?**

# C. Do Not Perform Incidental Cholecystectomy

*Satish N. Nadig and Benjamin E. Schneider*

The growing incidence of obesity in the United States brings with it a myriad of significant health risks, including diabetes mellitus, hypertension, hypercholesterolemia, osteoarthritis, cardiac disease, and atherosclerosis. Results with the medical management of obesity remain suboptimal, and surgical management has been recognized as the only effective method to treat severe obesity and its related comorbidities. Further, the use of laparoscopy in the surgical treatment of obesity has revolutionized postoperative management of patients by reducing pain, pulmonary impairment, wound infections and recovery time. Roux-en-Y gastric bypass (RYGBP) and laparoscopic banding procedures are now the most popular bariatric procedures performed.

Cholelithiasis is also a common problem in the Westernized world particularly in the obese patient population. The risk of gallstone formation is directly proportional to an increasing BMI. Further, rapid weight loss, as in the case of patients following gastric bypass, has been shown to increase bile lithogenicity and thus gallstone formation 32% to 42%. Treatment options for biliary stones following gastric bypass are limited by the fact that the excluded duodenum is extremely difficult to access endoscopically rendering endoscopic decompression (endoscopic retrograde cholangiopancreatography, ERCP) virtually impossible. It has therefore previously been suggested that routine cholecystectomy should be performed at the time of open gastric bypass.

The risk of gallstone formation in patients who undergo laparoscopic banding, however, is markedly less than in those patients status post-RYGBP. Further, the technical aspects of laparoscopic adjustable banding preclude convenient cholecystectomy at the time of operation. This chapter discusses the approach to gallbladder disease in patients facing bariatric surgery.

Many surgeons routinely screen patients undergoing laparoscopic RYGBP for gallstones either preoperatively or intraoperatively using intraoperative ultrasound (IOUS). Other groups have made it a practice to prophylactically perform cholecystectomy at the time of RYGBP. The use of IOUS has been shown to be not only feasible but also more sensitive than preoperative transabdominal ultrasound in the obese patient. In the first instance, the gallbladder is identified and examined by the surgeon using a 7.5-MHz transducer to determine the presence or absence of gallstones. If stones are present, a laparoscopic cholecystectomy is performed; if absent, the patient is advised about the risk of stone formation and placed on ursodiol (300 mg twice daily) therapy for 6 months with close postoperative follow-up and repeat transabdominal ultrasound if symptoms occur. The use of ursodiol therapy has been shown to reduce the risk of stone formation in a study of patients undergoing open RYGBP from 32% (placebo) to 13% (300 mg/day), 2% (600 mg/day), and 6% (1200 mg/day). These data suggest that medical therapy to reduce stone formation, as opposed to routine cholecystectomy, is a reasonable approach.

Simultaneous cholecystectomy is often performed at the time of open RYGBP. The midline incision of the open approach provides adequate exposure to the right upper quadrant and does not significantly increase hospital length of stay. This is not the case for the laparoscopic approach, however. Adequate exposure and visualization of the right upper quadrant is compromised in the laparoscopic RYGBP due to port placement and body habitus. Simultaneous cholecystectomy in the laparoscopic patient may lead to an increase in operative time, length of hospital stay, and unnecessary risk of biliary injury to the asymptomatic patient. Further, Villegas et al. found that only 7% of patients with gallstones after surgery become symptomatic requiring cholecystectomy. Therefore, IOUS with selective simultaneous cholecystectomy for gallstones and ursodiol therapy in conjunction with close follow-up (including repeat ultrasound) in stone-free patients is a rational approach to patients undergoing laparoscopic Roux-en-Y gastric bypass.

In contrast to the post-RYGBP patient, the incidence of gallstone formation after adjustable laparoscopic banding has been shown to be no different than the nonsurgical obese population. In a recent study of 1000 patients, wherein all preoperative patients were screened for symptoms of gallstones via ultrasonography, 191 patients underwent cholecystectomy prior to or at the time of gastric banding. The remaining 809 patients were followed closely postoperatively and 55 patients (6.8%) underwent uncomplicated elective cholecystectomy for symptomatic cholelithiasis. Three approaches to the management of gallstone disease appear in the literature. The first approach reported by Hamad et al. describes investigating all patients prior to bariatric surgery for gallstones and proceeding with empiric cholecystectomy if stones are found. As discussed previously, the second approach is the routine removal of the gallbladder, without any investigation, at the time of bypass or banding. Finally, O'Brien and Dixon describe an approach wherein only those patients expressing symptoms undergo screening for gallstones. Those patients with symptomatic cholelithiasis underwent laparoscopic cholecystectomy at the time of or before gastric banding. Laparoscopic cholecystectomy with banding adds approximately 30 minutes to the procedure and increases the technical difficulty of the cholecystectomy. The port sites used for the laparoscopic banding procedure are not ideal for cholecystectomy, and this increases the risk of injury to the patient. Our current approach is to perform laparoscopic cholecystectomy in symptomatic patients prior to the gastric banding procedure. This dual procedure approach allows for optimal exposure for both procedures and decreases the theoretical risk of band infection.

More than 50% of Americans are considered overweight, and the performance of bariatric procedures, especially laparoscopic Roux-en-Y gastric bypass and laparoscopic gastric banding, are on the rise. Patients who are status post–gastric bypass become calorically restricted, which thereby reduces bile acid secretion and results in supersaturated bile. The rapid weight loss in combination with a decrease in gallbladder contractility secondary to a decrease in cholecystokinin from duodenal bypass in this patient population predisposes them to an increased rate of gallstone formation. The increased rate of cholelithiasis is curbed by the use of ursodiol postoperatively. Ursodiol increases bile acid concentration and bolsters gallbladder contractility, thereby inhibiting stone formation by decreasing bile saturation and gallbladder stasis. With intraoperative ultrasound, any patients with stones may be surgically treated and the remainder of patients may be medically managed with ursodiol for 6 months and followed closely postsurgery. With this approach the incidence of symptomatic gallstones post–laparoscopic RYGBP is low. In the case of laparoscopic gastric banding we have found that preoperative screening for symptomatic cholelithiasis is best treated as two separate operations, with the laparoscopic cholecystectomy preceding gastric banding.

# D. Perform Concomitant Cholecystectomy Only for Symptomatic Stones

## Andras Sandor and John J. Kelly

One might initially argue that cholecystectomy should not be offered, lacking informed consent. If a surgeon is in the habit of examining the gallbladder intraoperatively with an algorithm that includes selective use of incidental cholecystectomy for a diseased or stone-laden gallbladder, then the surgeon should have prepared and informed the patient for this possibility before surgery. We will present evidence against incidental cholecystectomy at the time of planned laparoscopic bariatric surgery, when asymptomatic gallstones are found.

Four possible strategies exist: no concomitant cholecystectomy in any patient (nonselective), remove the gallbladder in all patients (nonselective), remove the gallbladder only if cholelithiasis is present (selective), and remove the gallbladder only if symptomatic cholelithiasis is present (selective). In the following discussion, we present our rationale for not performing cholecystectomy in the asymptomatic patient; neither preoperative nor intraoperative evaluation nor postoperative pharmacotherapy is recommended. We recommend postoperative management on a case-by-case basis if symptoms develop.

The incidence of preexisting cholelithiasis is substantial in the bariatric population (28% to 45% as opposed to 10% to 12% in the non-obese population). The vast majority of these patients with gallstones are asymptomatic. In addition, up to 40% of patients who experience rapid weight loss after gastric bypass will form gallstones, due to increased lithogenicity of bile. This propensity to develop stones led to prophylactic cholecystectomy as a widely accepted practice among surgeons performing open gastric malabsorption procedures. Miller et al. documented that intense use of ursodeoxycholic acid can reduce the incidence of postoperative stone formation from 22% to 3% at 12 months, and from 30% to 8% at 24 months.

Morbid obesity is no longer a contraindication for laparoscopic cholecystectomy. Although operative times were longer in several series, no statistically significant difference in conversion rates, complications, mortality, or length of stay were noted. Hamad et al. have documented the feasibility and safety of concomitant laparoscopy cholecystectomy and laparoscopic Roux-en-Y gastric bypass, but gave no information about the feasibility of intraoperative cholangiography in that setting.

The argument against performing cholecystectomy at the time of bypass is based on the additional time and surgeon fatigue due to the level of difficulty of exposure and dissection without altering port placement, which may potentially contribute to the theoretical risk of injury to major vascular or biliary structures. Placing an additional port in the right upper quadrant can substantially facilitate the procedure.

Analyzing the various management options, it is apparent that no rational argument can be made in favor of the two nonselective extremes cited above. What about selective cholecystectomy only for proven stones? Selection based on intraoperative findings such as in this case would be inaccurate. Stones in many patients would not be found by visual inspection or instrument palpation due to gallbladder distention. Even preoperative assessment can be faulty. Silidker et al. cited a 91% sensitivity and a 100% specificity for preoperative transabdominal ultrasonography (US) to predict cholelithiasis in the morbidly obese patient, but others have found this modality quite unreliable. Intraoperative laparoscopic US is the most accurate, but its widespread use is limited by availability and the lack of necessary expertise.

Although dissolution therapy is highly effective in present de novo stone formation, the duration of therapy is not clearly defined and patient compliance has generally been extremely poor.

We have previously reported the results of our study of the role of incidental cholecystectomy in which we followed 268 consecutive patients undergoing laparoscopic Roux-en-Y gastric bypass (LRYGBP) for morbid obesity. We excluded 71 patients with previous cholecystectomy. All patients had preoperative transabdominal US. In the first cohort of 123 patients, all patients with a positive US had concomitant cholecystectomy at the time of LRYGBP, if US showed gallstones. The second cohort of 74 patients did not have concomitant cholecystectomy, regardless of US results. After more than 2 years of follow-up, the rate of symptomatic gallstones (12.5% to 17.6%) was statistically similar in the two groups. The majority of patients who developed symptomatic gallstones had negative preoperative US studies. This observation supports the hypothesis that symptoms usually develop in patients with de novo, rather than preoperative, gallstone disease, and our selective approach did not significantly reduce the rate of symptomatic cholelithiasis.

An intact gallbladder with symptomatic gallstones certainly carries the risk of cholecystitis, choledocholithiasis, or pancreatitis. A second surgical procedure may have peri- and postoperative complications. However, the need to electively or urgently operate on such patients usually presents more than 6 months after the bariatric procedure. By that time, some comorbidities have undergone significant resolution, leading to a decrease in operative risk. Visceral fat shrinks, and the paucity of adhesions greatly facilitates exposure and dissection. The difficulty level of a laparoscopic cholecystectomy under these circumstances is the same as one in a nonobese individual. Access to the common bile duct can be accomplished, if needed, by laparoscopic common duct exploration or via ERCP.

In summary, in the asymptomatic patient, preoperative workup or intraoperative assessment for cholelithiasis is unnecessary and redundant. Selective cholecystectomy in this patient population would not significantly decrease the overall occurrence of symptomatic cholelithiasis after bariatric surgery. Incidental cholecystectomy should be reserved for patients whose stones were symptomatic before the bariatric procedure.

# E.  Conclusions

## Carol E.H. Scott-Conner and Robert Hanfland

The attitude of bariatric surgeons toward incidental cholecystectomy has evolved as surgery moved from an open to a minimally invasive approach. Whereas removing the gallbladder during open bariatric surgery simply requires repositioning some fixed retractors before proceeding with the additional dissection, incidental cholecystectomy during laparoscopic bariatric surgery requires placement of additional trocars and adds an additional procedure, with its own complications and difficulties, to an already long and rather difficult operation. It is worth recalling that laparoscopic cholecystectomy is significantly more difficult in the morbidly obese patient. Indeed, morbid obesity was at one time regarded as a relative contraindication to laparoscopic cholecystectomy.

There is no question that gallstones are common in the morbidly obese population. In addition, after effective bariatric surgery, bile stasis and a change in bile composition lead to sludge formation and, without intervention, the incidence of cholelithiasis approaches 50% in some series; however, the incidence of symptomatic gallstones requiring intervention is considerably lower.

Ursodeoxycholic acid treatment can be employed to decrease the incidence of cholelithiasis in this population, but is not well tolerated and compliance may be problematic. The risk is related to the rapidity of weight loss; accordingly, it is reportedly higher after Roux-en-Y gastric bypass than after gastric restrictive operations such as the adjustable laparoscopic band.

Additional considerations include the ease with which laparoscopic cholecystectomy can be performed after the patient has lost weight, if symptomatic cholelithiasis becomes problematic. Papavramidis reported his experience with patients who required cholecystectomy for complications of gallstones after successful bariatric surgery and confirmed that laparoscopic cholecystectomy was feasible in the majority.

Because ERCP may not be possible after Roux-en-Y gastric bypass (due to the length of the roux limb), careful assessment of the common duct with preparation for laparoscopic common duct exploration (either transcystic or via choledochotomy) at the time of cholecystectomy would seem prudent.

Techniques have even been developed to facilitate endoscopic management of choledocholithiasis after Roux-en-Y bypass. The simplest method involves accessing the distal stomach via gastrostomy. To facilitate such access, some surgeons tack the anterior wall of the defunctionalized stomach to the anterior abdominal wall, tagging it with a radiopaque circular marker. Pimentel et al. described laparoscopic gastrostomy formation, followed by endoscopic cannulation of the duodenum through the gastrostomy, as an alternative.

In conclusion, while there are no long-term prospective randomized series demonstrating clear superiority for one approach over another, many bariatric surgeons follow an algorithm similar to those discussed in the two previous sections of this chapter. Such an approach reserves cholecystectomy for patients with symptoms, and does not advocate it as a routine prophylactic measure. Patients are not screened preoperatively. The use of ursodeoxycholic acid during the period of rapid weight loss in patients without cholelithiasis is generally accepted as a potential preventive strategy. Intraoperative ultrasound may assist in identification of those patients likely to benefit from this therapy.

# References

Hamad GG, Ikramuddin S, Gourash WF, Schauer PR. Elective cholecystectomy during laparoscopic Roux-en-Y gastric bypass: Is it worth the wait? Obes Surg 2002;13:76–81.

O'Brien PE, Dixon JB. A rational approach to cholelithiasis in bariatric surgery. Its application to the laparoscopically placed adjustable gastric band. Arch Surg 2003;138:908–912.

Papavramidis S. Laparoscopic cholecystectomy after bariatric surgery. Surg Endosc 2003;17:1061–1064.

Silidker MS, Cronan JJ, Scola FH, et al. Ultrasound evaluation of cholelithiasis in the morbidly obese. Gastrointest Radiol 1988;13(4):345–346.

Villegas L, Schneider B, Provost D, et al. Is routine cholecystectomy required during laparoscopic gastric bypass? Obes Surg 2004;14:60–66.

# Suggested Readings

Amaral JF, Thompson WR. Gallbladder disease in the morbidly obese. Am J Surg 1985;149:551–557.

Broomfield PH, Chopra R, Sheinbaum RC, et al. Effects of urodeoxycholic acid and aspirin on the formation of lithogenic bile and gallstones during loss of weight. N Engl J Med 1988;319:1567–1572.

Erlinger S. Gallstones in obesity and weight loss. Eur J Gastroenterol Hepatol 2000;12:1347–1352.

Fobi M, Lee H, Igwe D, et al. Prophylactic cholecystectomy with gastric bypass operation: incidence of gallbladder disease. Obes Surg 2002;12:350–353.

Friedman GD, Kannel WB, Dawber TR. The epidemiology of gallbladder disease: observations in the Framingham study. J Chronic Dis 1966;19(3):273–292.

Kolecki R, Schirmer B. Intraoperative and laparoscopic ultrasound. Surg Clin North Am 1998;78:251–271.

Kral JG, Heymsfield S. Morbid obesity: definitions, epidemiology, and methodological problems. Gastroenterol Clin North Am 1987;16(2):197–205.

MacLure KM, Hayes KC, Colditz GA, Stampfer MJ, Speizer FE, Willett WC. Weight, diet, and the risk of symptomatic gallstones in middle aged women. N Engl J Med 1989;321:563–569.

Martin LF, Tan TL, Horn JR, et al. Comparison of the costs associated with medical and surgical treatment of obesity. Surgery 1995;118:599–607.

Mason EE, Renquist KE. Gallbladder management in obesity surgery. Obes Surg 2002;12(2):222–229.

Miller K, Hell E, Lang B, Lengauer E. Gallstone formation prophylaxis after gastric restrictive procedures for weight loss: a randomized double-blind placebo-controlled trial. Ann Surg 2003;238:697–702.

Nguyen NT, Goldman C, Rosenquist CJ, et al. Laparoscopic versus open gastric bypass: a randomized study of outcomes, quality of life, and costs. Ann Surg 2000;234:279–291.

Nguyen NT, Lee SL, Goldman C, et al. Comparison of pulmonary function and postoperative pain after laparoscopic versus open gastric bypass: a randomized trial. J Am Coll Surg 1999;188:491–497.

Pimentel RR, Mehran A, Szomstein S, Rosenthal R. Laparoscopy-assisted transgastrostomy ERCP after bariatric surgery: case report of a novel approach. Gastrointest Endosc 2004;59:325–328.

Schmidt JH, Hocking MP, Rout WR, et al. The case for prophylactic cholecystectomy concomitant with gastric restriction for morbid obesity. Am Surg 1988;54:269–272.

Shiffman M, Sugerman H, Kellum J, et al. Gallstone formation after rapid weight loss. A prospective study in patients undergoing gastric bypass surgery for treatment of morbid obesity. Am J Gastroenterol 1991;86:1000–1005.

Shiffman ML, Sugerman HJ, Kellum JM, et al. Gallstones in patients with morbid obesity. Relationship to body weight, weight loss and gallbladder bile cholesterol solubility. Int J Obes 1993;17:153–158.

Sugerman HJ, Brewer WH, Shiffman ML, et al. A multicenter, placebo-controlled, randomized, double-blind, prospective trial of prophylactic Ursodiol for the prevention of gallstone formation following gastric-bypass-induced rapid weight loss. Am J Surg 1995;169:91–97.

Wattchow DA, Hall JC, Whiting MJ, et al. Prevalence and treatment of gallstones after gastric bypass surgery for morbid obesity. Br Med J 1983;286:763.

Wudel LJ, Wright JK, Debelak JP, et al. Prevention of gallstone formation in morbidly obese patients undergoing rapid weight loss: results of a randomized controlled pilot study. J Surg Res 2001;102:50–56.

Yang H, Petersen GM, Roth MP, et al. Risk factors for gallstone formation during rapid loss of weight. Dig Dis Sci 1992;37(6):912–918.

# 23. Uncomplicated Adhesive Small Bowel Obstruction

## A. Introduction

The experience of performing an exploratory laparotomy for acute small bowel obstruction, and finding and snipping a single adhesive band, has caused some surgeons to wonder if laparoscopy would be a better way to explore and treat these patients. This chapter explores laparoscopy versus laparotomy for acute, uncomplicated, small bowel obstruction that is assumed to be due to adhesions.

## B. Case

### *José E. Torres*

A 78-year-old man presented to the emergency department with a 4-day history of severe, crampy, sharp, midabdominal pain. This began gradually and had increased in intensity. He was unable to define any precipitating or alleviating factors. He had not had a bowel movement for 3 days, and had not passed flatus in 2 days. He began vomiting the evening before.

His past medical history was significant for hypertension, peripheral vascular disease, transient ischemic attacks, arthritis, and chronic obstructive pulmonary disease. His past surgical history included coronary artery bypass surgery and an open appendectomy.

He was married, with three sons and a daughter. He still worked as a farmer. He had a 30-pack-a-year history of smoking, and occasionally used alcohol.

On physical examination, he was a slender male who lay supine, in no apparent distress. His abdomen was firm, distended, with voluntary guarding. Bowel sounds revealed occasional tinkles and rushes. No hernias were palpated. He had a well-healed McBurney incision. Pulses were full and equal bilaterally to dorsalis pedis and posterior tibialis. Digital rectal examination was normal.

Flat and upright x-rays of the abdomen revealed complete small bowel obstruction with multiple loops of dilated small bowel, and no gas in the colon. Upright chest x-ray did not show air under the diaphragm. Laboratory results, including electrolytes and complete blood count, were normal.

**What surgery would you recommend for this patient?**

# C.  Formal Laparotomy

*Vafa Shayani and Sharfi Sarker*

We would treat this patient by formal laparotomy and lysis of adhesions. Long before laparoscopic surgery gained acceptance by general surgeons, gynecologists utilized laparoscopy for lysis of pelvic adhesions in patients with chronic abdominal and pelvic pain. The laparoscopic approach to adhesiolysis may offer several advantages, such as decreased length of hospital stay, reduced need for narcotic analgesia postoperatively, and improved cosmesis. However, application of laparoscopy to management of intestinal adhesions in conjunction with acute small bowel obstruction (SBO) remains controversial. Several factors affect the safety and feasibility of this treatment modality. Advanced laparoscopic skills are necessary for what can be a technically challenging procedure. The high rates of conversion to laparotomy and variable rates of success attest to the complexity of the operation. Patient selection is a key component of successful and appropriate laparoscopic management of acute SBO.

Several factors inherent to the patient with acute SBO may render laparoscopy unfavorable. These include the limited intraabdominal working space secondary to distended loops of bowel and the fragility of dilated small bowel, predisposing it to injury, both during adhesiolysis and during manipulation of the intestine. In addition, visual cues available during laparoscopy may not be adequate for assessing the viability of ischemic bowel. Chosidow et al. compared 95 patients undergoing laparoscopy after resolution of SBO with 39 patients undergoing emergent laparoscopy for management of acute SBO, and reported higher rates of conversion (7% vs. 36%) and higher length of hospitalization (5.0 days vs. 6.6 days) when laparoscopy was performed emergently. Length of hospital stay was longest among those patients who were converted from laparoscopy to laparotomy.

Attempts at defining preoperative factors that lead to complications during laparoscopy for acute SBO have been generally unsuccessful. The conversion to laparotomy has been reported to be up to 46%. Intraoperative bowel injury during laparoscopy has been reported in up to 29% of the patients. Suter et al. reported increased length of operation ($p < .001$) and increased small bowel diameter $>4$ cm ($p = .02$) to be predictors of conversion to laparotomy. Furthermore, intraoperative enterotomy ($p = .008$) and need for conversion ($p = .009$) were independent factors predicting postoperative complications on multivariate analysis. However, no correlation has been shown between any preoperative laboratory values, number of scars, or number of previous operations and the need for conversion, which might facilitate selection of patients at high risk for perioperative complications. In our own reported series of patients undergoing laparoscopic lysis of intestinal adhesions, the only patients who suffered enterotomies were those who underwent urgent procedures in the face of acute SBO.

Although many patients with small bowel obstruction, requiring surgical intervention, may be successfully treated using the laparoscopic approach, considering the frequency and the serious nature of the complications associated with this procedure, early conversion to laparotomy may become necessary. Although no absolute contraindications to laparoscopy have been identified, severe abdominal distention and hemodynamic instability may be considered as relative contraindications to laparoscopic approach.

# D. Laparoscopic Exploration

*Brian T. Valerian and Steven C. Stain*

We would offer this patient laparoscopic exploration and lysis of adhesions. The indications for laparoscopic abdominal surgery are expanding, and the complexity of procedures able to be accomplished successfully has grown exponentially. Gastric bypass, colectomy, pancreatic, and ventral hernia surgery are all able to be performed via laparoscopy. As the number and variety of cases able to be performed laparoscopically have increased, skill sets, comfort level, and expertise have also increased. And as surgeons have become more technically adept, technology has also improved, allowing for better optics and safer, more effective laparoscopic instruments.

Twenty years ago this patient would require a laparotomy for exploration, likely lysis of adhesions, and release of the small bowel obstruction. Now it is reasonable to consider laparoscopic surgery for the management of this patient. Numerous reports and reviews in the recent literature support the use of laparoscopy in the treatment of acute small bowel obstruction. Ultimately, patient selection, surgeon expertise, and operative findings will contribute to the success of laparoscopy.

The evaluation of a patient with small bowel obstruction should include two position abdominal radiographs. Initial management should begin with nasogastric tube decompression, intravenous fluid resuscitation, placement of a Foley catheter to guide resuscitation, correction of electrolyte abnormalities, and consideration of computed tomographic imaging. Computed tomography has been shown to be a reliable tool (sensitivity >90%) in the evaluation of patients with suspected small bowel obstruction and may help localize the sight of obstruction. While the most likely cause for obstruction is adhesions from previous surgery, additional causes (especially in a 78-year-old) include neoplasm, bezoar, gallstone, inflammatory processes, and foreign bodies, to name a few. Preoperative imaging may help prepare for intraoperative findings and better guide therapy.

Once deemed to require surgical intervention, the decision for laparoscopic versus open surgery needs to be made. Previous abdominal surgery was a contraindication for laparoscopy in the past, but that dictum no longer holds true. Patient selection is an important variable for laparoscopic success. An absolute contraindication for laparoscopy is a hemodynamically unstable patient. Other factors may be relative contraindications, but in the hands of a skilled advanced laparoscopist few factors preclude an attempt at laparoscopy. Preparation of the patient is no different from that for open surgery, with the exception of patient positioning. Both arms should be tucked at the sides and the low lithotomy position should be considered to allow more versatility for the surgical team. In addition, the patient should be firmly strapped or belted to the operating table to allow for steep tilting and positioning intraoperatively.

Initial trocar insertion must be safe. In a patient with small bowel obstruction the open (Hasson) technique may be a safer option than the Veress needle technique. Port placement should be away from or opposite previous incisions if possible, minimizing the risk of injuring bowel during port placement and allowing for better visualization of the affected area. Additional ports can then be placed under direct vision. Lysis of adhesions, both to the abdominal wall and interloop adhesions, should proceed carefully using sharp scissor dissection. The use of energy, that is, electrical or ultrasonic, should be avoided during lysis of adhesions to prevent energy transfer or injury to adjacent tissues. Intraoperative injury to bowel or other intraabdominal structures is of utmost concern. Recognized enterotomies or seromyotomies can often be repaired laparoscopically, but unrecognized enterotomy remains a large stumbling block for laparoscopy in bowel obstruction.

Another challenge during laparoscopy for bowel obstruction is visualization. Improved optics, angled telescopes, and smaller telescopes with excellent clarity have helped overcome some of the early limitations of laparoscopy. Distended bowel can still obstruct full visualization of the abdominal contents. Improved laparoscopic instrumentation has made maneuvering distended bowel loops easier, but caution and finesse are still required.

Patients with a single adhesive band causing small bowel obstruction are the ideal candidates for laparoscopy, but unfortunately there is no accurate way to predict which patients these will be. Some factors can lend insight. Patients who have only undergone appendectomy may be a good example. Controversy exists regarding the need to examine the entire length of small bowel. Patients with multiple previous abdominal surgeries may have more extensive adhesions, making laparoscopy more difficult and evaluation of small bowel from the ligament of Treitz to the terminal ileum tedious. Some authors suggest that if one definitive band with proximally dilated and distally decompressed small bowel is encountered, full exploration may not be required. Unfortunately, it is often the patients with more extensive adhesions that require examination of all the small bowel. Preoperative imaging may also lend insight. Massively dilated loops of small bowel (>4 cm) and distal obstructions make laparoscopy more challenging, but not impossible.

The most common cause of small bowel obstruction in Western countries remains adhesions, but the surgeon must be prepared to handle all types of pathology. Minilaparotomies are often helpful in performing segmental small bowel resections or for handling other pathology. A low threshold for conversion needs to be maintained at all times. Dense adhesions, inability to visualize the site of obstruction, and accidental bowel injury remain the most common reasons for conversion to open laparotomy. Suter et al. report that conversion rates are quite variable in the literature, ranging from 6% to 54%.

As more surgeons become expert in the techniques of advanced laparoscopy, indications for laparoscopy are also expanding. The benefits of laparoscopy in the management of small bowel obstruction are similar to those for other diseases and include less pain, quicker return of bowel function, quicker return to activities and earlier discharge from the hospital. An additional benefit of laparoscopy in the treatment of small bowel obstruction may be less adhesion formation following laparoscopy than laparotomy, although there have not been any reports in the literature in support of this.

# E.  Conclusions

*José E. Torres*

Small bowel obstruction is a common surgical problem that accounts for approximately 2% of all surgical admissions for abdominal pain and approximately 3% of exploratory laparotomies in the United States. Approximately 60% of patients with adhesive-related small bowel obstruction require surgical lysis of adhesions, and approximately one third of these patients experience a recurrent small bowel obstruction. Laparoscopic surgery has been shown to result in decreased postoperative adhesions and quicker recovery of bowel function and appears to be well suited for the treatment of acute small bowel obstructions.

As advances in laparoscopic surgery have occurred, surgeons have broadened their use of laparoscopy in diagnosing and treating small bowel obstruction if conservative management fails or if complications such as perforation occur. Bailey et al. compared laparoscopic surgical management with open management of small bowel obstructions. They found that 45% of their patients were treated laparoscopically, and laparoscopy assisted in another 22% of patients. Additionally, patients treated laparoscopically were discharged earlier than patients treated with a laparotomy, but the risk of early, unplanned reoperation was increased.

Several other studies have been performed that demonstrate that laparoscopy is a viable option in the diagnosis and treatment of small bowel obstruction in carefully selected patients in whom a low threshold for opening if complications arise. In 65 patients the diagnostic accuracy was found to be 96%, and 52% were treated laparoscopically while 20% were treated in a laparoscopically assisted procedure, limiting laparotomy to 28% of their patients with a mechanical small bowel obstruction.

What must be noted from the above studies is that in order to be successful in treating acute small bowel obstruction, the practicing surgeon must be very selective when selecting patients. Intraoperative complications were encountered in patients who had significant intestinal distention and extensive adhesions that obscured the operative field. Wullstein and Gross found that laparoscopic management of small bowel obstruction is reasonable in patients who had fewer than two previous laparotomies.

Patients with a history of more than two laparotomies were found to have an unacceptably high risk of intraoperative bowel perforation (26.9% in the laparoscopic group versus 13.5% in the open group).

# References

Bailey IS, Rhodes M, O'Rourke N, Nathanson L, Fielding G. Laparoscopic management of acute small bowel obstruction. Br J Surg 1998;85:84–87.

Chosidow D, Johanet H, Montariol T, et al. Laparoscopy for acute small-bowel obstruction secondary to adhesions. J Lap Adv Surg Tech 2000;10(3):155–158.

Suter M, Zermatten P, Halkic N, Martinet O, Bettschart V. Laparoscopic management of mechanical small bowel obstruction. Are there predictors of success or failure? Surg Endosc 2000;14:478–483.

Wullstein C, Gross E. Laparoscopic compared with conventional treatment of acute adhesive small bowel obstruction. Br J Surg 2003;90:1147–1151.

# Suggested Readings

Borzellino G, Tasselli S, Zerman G, Pedrazzani C, Manzoni G. Laparoscopic approach to post-operative adhesive obstruction. Surg Endosc 2004;18:686–690.

Daneshmand S, Hedley C, Stain S. The utility and reliability of computed tomography scan in the diagnosis of small bowel obstruction. Am Surg 1999;65(10):922–926.

Kirshtein B, Roy-Shapira A, Lantsberg L, Avinoach E, Mizrahi S. Laparoscopic management of acute small bowel obstruction. Surg Endosc 2005;19:464–467.

Levard H, Boudet M, Msika S, et al. Laparoscopic treatment of acute small bowel obstruction: a multicenter retrospective study. Aust NZ J Surg 2001;71:641–646.

Liauw JJY, Cheah WK. Laparoscopic management of acute small bowel obstruction. Asian J Surg 2005;28:185–188.

Miller G, Boamn J, Shrier I, Gordon PH. Etiology of small bowel obstruction. Am J Surg 2000;180:33–36.

Nagle A, Ujiki M, Denham W, Murayama K. Laparoscopic adhesiolysis for small bowel obstruction. Am J Surg 2004;187:464–470.

Navez B, Arimont J-M, Guiot P. Laparoscopic approach in acute small bowel obstruction. A review of 68 patients. Hepatogastroenterology 1998;45:2146–2150.

Shayani V, Siegert C, Favia P. The role of laparoscopic adhesiolysis in the treatment of patients with chronic abdominal pain or recurrent bowel obstruction. J Soc Laparoendosc Surg 2002;6(2):111–114.

Strickland P, Lourie DJ, Suddleson A, Blitz JB, Stain SC. Is laparoscopy safe and effective for treatment of acute small-bowel obstruction? Surg Endosc 1999;13:695–698.

Yau KK, Siu WT, Law BKB, et al. Laparoscopic approach compared with conventional open approach for bezoar-induced small bowel obstruction. Arch Surg 2005;140:972–975.

# 24. Possible Appendicitis

## A. Introduction

Laparoscopic appendectomy was the second major laparoscopic operation adopted by many general surgeons. One obvious advantage was the exceptional ability to visualize the remainder of the abdomen, and thereby exclude other causes of right lower quadrant pain in patients with equivocal findings. Thus, laparoscopic appendectomy found early application to women of reproductive age with right lower quadrant pain.

Although some advocate leaving the normal appendix in situ when another cause for the pain was found, most surgeons remove it, reasoning that occult pathology is often found and that the patient benefits more from removal. It has thus been difficult to demonstrate that laparoscopic appendectomy has reduced the negative appendectomy rate.

As laparoscopic appendectomy found wider use, computed tomography (CT) scan improved in resolution and it became possible to use an appendiceal protocol scan to confirm or rule out acute appendicitis. The question then arises, should a patient with equivocal symptoms have a CT scan or be taken straight to laparoscopic exploration and appendectomy. That is the issue discussed here.

## B. Case

### Heidi H. Richardson

A 27-year-old woman presented to the emergency department complaining of abdominal pain. This pain awakened her from sleep at around 3 a.m. At that time, it was periumbilical. She went back to sleep, only to awaken later with worsening abdominal pain, which had migrated to the right lower quadrant. She described the pain as constant, dull, and escalating. She had lost appetite, become nauseated, and vomited once.

Her past medical history was significant for a right ovarian cyst causing intermittent abdominal pain. She characterized this pain as different from her current episode. She had not had any previous surgery.

She was single and not currently sexually active. She underwent menarche at age 13, and was G1P1 (gravida/para). Her last menstrual

period was 2 weeks prior to this episode. She smoked two or three cigarettes per day, and drank occasionally. She was otherwise healthy and
the review of systems was otherwise negative.

On physical examination, she was well developed and moderately
obese. She was in moderate distress. Her temperature was 35.9 °C, respiratory rate 16, pulse 66 beats per minute, and blood pressure 131/86.

Her abdomen was soft with tenderness to palpation in the right lower
quadrant. There was mild direct rebound tenderness, also localization to
the right lower quadrant. She did not have any costo vertebral angle (CVA)
tenderness. Her pelvic examination was negative. Digital rectal examination was negative. The remainder of her exam was unremarkable.

Laboratory results included a hematocrit of 44%, hemoglobin of
14 g/dL, and white blood count (WBC) of 11,100/mm$^3$. Urinalysis was
negative and urine chorionic gonadotropin was negative. Abdominal
x-rays showed a normal gas pattern.

The impression was possible appendicitis.

**How would you proceed? Would you obtain a CT scan with
appendiceal protocol or perform laparoscopy?**

# C. Computed Tomography

## Aytekin Oto and Randy D. Ernst

We would recommend performing a CT scan, as CT is the primary
imaging modality for evaluation of acute right lower quadrant pain.
Confirmation of the diagnosis of acute appendicitis by a CT has proven
to decrease the negative appendectomy rate. Computed tomography
provides a thorough cross-sectional examination of the entire abdomen and pelvis, allowing for the detection of alternative diagnosis for
acute abdominal pain and possible complications of acute appendicitis.
Acute diverticulitis, hollow organ perforation, Crohn's disease, typhlitis,
ureteral stones, pyelonephritis, intraabdominal abscesses, epiploic
appendicitis, colitis, colon carcinoma, and abdominal aortic aneurysm
leakage/rupture can mimic the clinical presentation of acute appendicitis
and can be effectively distinguished from acute appendicitis by CT.

In women of childbearing age, symptoms of acute gynecologic conditions, such as ovarian torsion, ovarian dermoid, ovarian cyst rupture,
ectopic pregnancy, and pelvic inflammatory disease, may manifest
similarly to appendicitis. Rao, Feltmate, et al. have found that CT can

confirm or exclude appendicitis or acute gynecologic conditions in 98% of female patients. In females, difficulty in clinical diagnosis has led to false-negative appendectomy rates as high as 47% in patients aged 10 to 39 years. Nakhgevany and Clarke reported that an acute gynecologic condition is diagnosed eventually in 56% of such patients.

Depending on the amount of intraabdominal fat tissue, multidetector CT (MDCT) displays the normal appendix in approximately 97% of patients. To identify the normal appendix, follow the hepatic flexure caudally until the cecum is located. The two tubular structures joining the cecum are the terminal ileum and the appendix. The normal appendix is usually less than 7 mm in diameter, has a thin wall of 2 to 3 mm, and contains air or oral contrast (Fig. 24.1). The criteria for CT diagnosis of acute appendicitis include dilated appendix (>7 mm) with thick (>3 mm), enhancing walls and periappendiceal inflammation (Fig. 24.2). An appendicolith may also be present. Periappendiceal inflammation presents as increased density of the fat surrounding the appendix, indistinctness of the appendiceal borders, or free or loculated fluid around the appendix. Size by itself is not a dependable criterion especially in the absence of the listed findings. Normal appendices measuring up to 16 mm have been reported. Since the etiology of appendicitis is obstruction, distention of the entire appendix by oral contrast or air can help to exclude the diagnosis of acute appendicitis. In subtle cases of appendicitis,

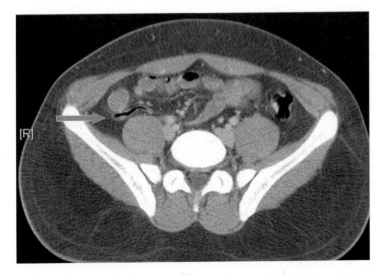

Fig. 24.1. Computed tomography scan showing normal appendix (arrow).

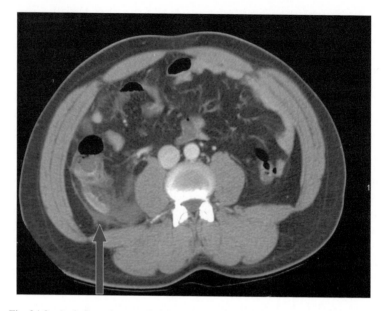

Fig. 24.2. An inflamed appendix is noted lateral to the psoas muscle (arrow). Peri-appendiceal inflammation and fluid are also seen in this 24-year-old woman.

focal thickening of the cecum at the base of the appendiceal orifice (cecal bar sign) may be the only sign of early appendicitis. It is important to examine the entire appendix, as the inflammation can be limited to only the tip of the appendix.

Careful attention to technique is essential. After the advent of spiral CT and now with the MDCT scanners available, the results of CT in the diagnosis of acute appendicitis have been excellent, with reported sensitivity, specificity, and positive and negative predictive values of over 95% and close to 100%. There is controversy in the literature about the use of oral and intravenous (IV) contrast for CT examinations. Use of rectal contrast is seldom indicated. Although acute appendicitis can often be diagnosed without oral and IV contrast, the use of contrast facilitates the diagnosis particularly in patients with limited peritoneal and retroperitoneal fat. In our institution, we use only IV contrast and have eliminated the routine use of oral contrast in emergency department abdominal CT examinations for the sake of improving patient through-put. Our experience has shown that CT with IV contrast alone is sensitive and specific for the confirmation or exclusion of acute appendicitis.

By eliminating the time required to administer oral contrast, the diagnosis might be made more rapidly.

Computed tomography is a very fast examination technique. With the current MDCT scanners, it takes only 10 to 30 seconds to scan the entire abdomen. Oral contrast administration requires approximately 1 to 2 hours before the study. However, for IV-contrast-only protocols, our experience indicates that the examination can be performed immediately, and the images are ready for review within minutes.

Radiation exposure and increased cost are the two disadvantages of the CT examination. In pregnant patients, magnetic resonance imaging (MRI) of the abdomen is a very promising technique that does not cause any radiation exposure to the fetus and still can detect acute appendicitis. Iodinated IV contrast needs to be cautiously used in allergic patients and in patients who are at high risk to develop contrast-induced nephropathy.

In conclusion, CT is the most reliable and the most commonly used imaging method in the evaluation of female patients with suspected acute appendicitis or acute gynecologic conditions. It provides fast and accurate diagnosis or exclusion of acute appendicitis and its complications.

# D. Laparoscopy

## *Michele McElroy and David Easter*

We would perform diagnostic laparoscopy with appendectomy. Acute appendicitis is a common disease in the United States, with a lifetime incidence of 7% to 8%. Accurate preoperative diagnosis can be particularly challenging in women of childbearing ages, as there are frequent atypical presentations and many potential diagnoses. Gynecologic processes can closely mimic the signs and symptoms of acute appendicitis and confuse the careful diagnostician. The negative appendectomy rate in women of childbearing age is approximately 2.5 times that of males from the same age group.

Computed tomography imaging has been used liberally in an attempt to improve the diagnostic accuracy in such women. For all types of patients, the positive predictive value of CT scan in the diagnosis of acute appendicitis can be as high as 95%. But not all patients need CT scans to augment a strong clinical suspicion. Flum et al. reported that population-based data from the last two decades have shown that, despite the increased use of CT to rule out appendicitis, the rate of negative appendectomy has not changed. Indeed, they reported that the false-positive rate of CT scans for the diagnosis of acute appendicitis in some settings is as high as 20%. If the overall rate of false-positive scans approaches 10%, and knowing that more CT scans are being ordered to rule out appendicitis, it follows that the liberal use of CT scans in this setting only increases the numbers of negative appendectomies in this difficult group. This management strategy can be improved upon.

We advocate the very selective—if not restrictive—use of CT scans in patients with suspected appendicitis (Fig. 24.3). Patients with obvious findings on CT scan also usually have obvious clinical signs and symptoms that easily warrant surgical exploration. When CT scans are negative or equivocal, there remains a very real possibility that early

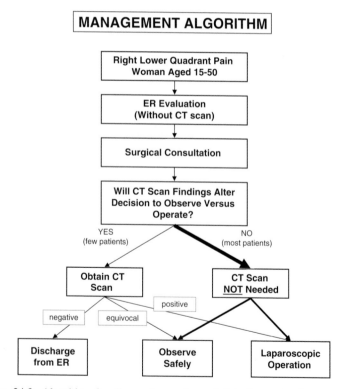

Fig. 24.3. Algorithm for diagnostic workup of right lower quadrant pain in women of childbearing age.

appendicitis or other serious surgical conditions are present. Therefore, many positive scans, some negative scans, and all equivocal scans are unhelpful to the clinician.

Prior to expensive imaging tests, we propose that a full consultation is completed by an experienced general surgeon. The consultant surgeon, after a careful history, physical exam, and simple lab tests, asks this critical question: Will a CT scan, if positive or negative, change the clinical recommendation? Equivocal CT results should not provoke a trip to the operating room!

Patients with significant clinical findings of acute appendicitis are those whose CT findings should be ignored. A trip to the operating room is warranted. In these circumstances, even if the appendix looks normal, it should be removed, because (1) future diagnostic confusion is avoided, and (2) a normal-appearing serosal surface may obscure significant mucosal ischemia.

Patients with a low clinical risk of acute appendicitis can be safely observed. Using CT scans very selectively can thereby clarify one's management strategy while avoiding unnecessary operations. Significant costs can be avoided by timely, competent surgical consultations.

In our experience, CT scans may be used in patients with suspected appendicitis specifically to speed emergency department transit times or to decide early on the need for surgical consultation. While this strategy may improve the efficiency of the emergency department, it most certainly shifts costs to radiology and surgical departments. In contrast, Gaitan et al. have shown diagnostic laparoscopy to be efficient and cost-effective when applied in women of reproductive age with acute abdominal pain, such as the patient described.

Nearly all general surgeons are currently very comfortable and proficient with laparoscopic operations, including diagnostic laparoscopy with appendectomy. Diagnostic laparoscopy is a useful tool in the evaluation of patients with acute abdominal pain, with a high degree of diagnostic accuracy. Even when the appendix is found to be normal, Golash and Wilson have reported that early laparoscopic evaluation for acute abdominal pain led to a significant and beneficial change of diagnosis/treatment in up to 30% of patients.

Diagnostic laparoscopy is also a safe option. When compared to open operations for similar indications, long-term follow-up of patients who had emergency laparoscopic operations revealed comparable rates of morbidity, mortality, readmission, and quality of life.

Technical considerations for laparoscopy in this group of patients include the following:

1.  Tuck both arms of the patient so as to preserve all options.
2.  Use urinary and gastric decompression in all patients to minimize organ injuries and facilitate visual access.
3.  Low stirrups (hips unflexed) and a full perineal/vaginal prep can be utilized in selected patients.
4.  Plan for many changes in table positions; expect to keep the anesthesiologists busy!
5.  Prepare to explore the entire abdominal cavity—pelvis, lesser sac, run the bowel—everything.
6.  Expect to use at least three ports, starting with a 5-mm port and scope in the left upper quadrant. This allows for sufficient distance between the entry site and the organs of suspicion. Two additional ports are placed after initial inspection.

Consensus statements advocate the use of diagnostic laparoscopy in patients with suspected appendicitis, particularly in women with severe nonspecific abdominal pain (Sauerland et al.). More liberal use of CT scans has failed to improve negative appendectomy rates. Our favored laparoscopic approach offers the opportunity for immediate treatment of both general surgical and gynecologic diseases and thus offers distinct clinical advantages.

# E.  Conclusions

## Heidi H. Richardson

Acute appendicitis may be a difficult clinical diagnosis, especially in women of reproductive age. Addiss et al. cite a lifetime risk of appendicitis is 8.6% for men and 6.7% for women, yet a lifetime incidence of appendectomy of 12% for men and 23.1% for women. The differential diagnosis of abdominal pain in women is broad, contributing to the difficulty in diagnosing acute appendicitis and necessitating further evaluation. Due to the concern for increased morbidity associated with a delayed diagnosis of appendicitis and appendiceal rupture, historically liberal appendectomies have been tolerated with a negative appendectomy rate of 20% to 40%. Improved diagnostic accuracy is needed to diagnose the true pathology and to decrease the number of unnecessary appendectomies, with associated anesthetic risk, iatrogenic injury, and prolonged recovery. Computed tomography and diagnostic laparoscopy have both been advocated as diagnostic tools in the diagnosis of acute abdominal pain in women of reproductive age.

Studies advocating the use of CT scan in the diagnosis of appendicitis have demonstrated sensitivities of 77% to 100%, specificities of 83% to 98%, and accuracies of 88% to 93%. Rao, Rhea, et al. published the results of their study of CT scans in 100 patients admitted for observation or operation for presumed appendicitis. Final outcomes were measured by pathology or follow-up 2 months after appendiceal CT scan. The radiologists' interpretation was 98% specific, 98% sensitive, with a 98% accuracy rate. Appendectomy was prevented in 13 patients, which demonstrated a cost savings. They concluded that routine appendiceal CT scan improves patient care and the use of hospital resources.

Several studies advocated the use of selective CT scan for diagnosing appendicitis. Antevil et al. retrospectively reviewed patients who underwent either appendectomy or CT scan for presumed appendicitis. There was a decrease in the negative appendectomy (NA) rate in those patients who received CT scan prior to appendectomy—15% versus 26%. Overall, women had a significantly higher NA rate when compared to men, 28% (72/253) versus 17% (66/380), and the use of CT was associated with a significantly lower NA rate in women, 42% (58/137) versus 12% (14/116), with no effect on the rates in men. The authors concluded that CT scan demonstrated the greatest benefit in women with reduction of the NA rate. Hershko et al. performed a prospective study of 308 patients with the presumed diagnosis of appendicitis. Those patients associated with a high index of suspicion for appendicitis (198 patients) underwent appendectomy without CT scan and had an NA rate of 17%. Women in this group had an NA rate of 24%, compared to 7% for men. Those associated with uncertain diagnosis or with low index of suspicion underwent CT scan, were admitted for observation, or were discharged. Computed tomography had a sensitivity of 91%, specificity of 92%, and accuracy of 91%, and it diagnosed other pathology in 23 patients and altered surgical management in 54 patients. The authors concluded that CT scan should be used in all women with a possible to definite clinical index of suspicion for acute appendicitis, and that it should be used selectively in men.

Many studies have demonstrated the value of diagnostic laparoscopy in the diagnosis of acute appendicitis, especially in fertile women. Van der Broek et al. performed a prospective study of 1050 patients with abdominal pain. Diagnostic laparoscopy reduced the overall NA rate from 25% to 14%. The NA rate for women with a preoperative questionable diagnosis of appendicitis who underwent diagnostic laparoscopy was reduced from 49% to 14% and for men from 22% to 11%. An alternate diagnosis was found in 54 patients, 72% of which were gynecological in nature. The authors concluded that women benefit most from diagnostic laparoscopy. Several other studies have confirmed that diagnostic laparoscopy is safe, decreases the negative appendectomy rates, and increases the accuracy of alternate diagnoses, especially in women. Others have emphasized the reliability of laparoscopic assessment of the appendix and the safety of leaving normal appendices behind.

Both CT scan and diagnostic laparoscopy have been found to be safe and effective methods for the diagnosis of acute appendicitis in women of reproductive age, yet both are associated with their own subset of advantages and disadvantages. Diagnostic laparoscopy may be used in patients with indeterminate CT findings, and ideally every operation should begin with a diagnostic laparoscopy and continue with appendectomy if deemed necessary. Studies have shown that leaving normal-appearing appendices can be safe and the laparoscopic assessment reliable, but most laparoscopists routinely remove the appendix, citing the possibility of a fecalith or other pathology. More studies are needed comparing the two diagnostic modalities in this subset of patients.

# References

Addiss DG, Shaffer N, Fowler B, Tauxe R. The epidemiology of appendicitis and appendectomy in the United States. Am J Epidemiol 1990;132(6):910–925.

Antevil J, Rivera L, Langenberg B, Brown C, The influence of age and gender on the utility of computed tomography to diagnose acute appendicitis. Am Surg 2004;70:850–853.

Flum D, McClure TD, Morris A, Koepsell T. Misdiagnosis of appendicitis and the use of diagnostic imaging. J Am Coll Surg 2005;201(6):933–939.

Gaitan H, Eslava-Schmalbach J, Gomez P. Cost effectiveness of diagnostic laparoscopy in reproductive aged females suffering from non-specific acute low abdominal pain. Rev Salud Publica 2005;7(2):166–179.

Golash V, Wilson PD. Early laparoscopy as a routine procedure in the management of acute abdominal pain. Surg Endosc 2005;19:882–885.

Hershko DD, Sroka G, Bahouth H, Ghersin E, Mahajna A, Krausz MM. The role of selective computed tomography in the diagnosis and management of suspected acute appendicitis. Am Surg 2002;68(11):1003–1007.

Nakhgevany KB, Clarke LE. Acute appendicitis in women of childbearing age. Arch Surg 1986;121:1053–1055.

Rao PM, Rhea JT, Novelline RA, Mostafavi AA, McCabe CJ. Effect of computed tomography of the appendix on the treatment of patients and use of hospital resources. N Engl J Med 1998;338(3):141–146.

Rao PM, Feltmate CM, Rhea JT, Schulick AH, Novelline RA. Helical computed tomography in differentiating appendicitis and acute gynecologic conditions. Obstet Gynecol 1999;93:417–421.

Sauerland S, Agresta F, Bergamaschi R, et al. Laparoscopy for abdominal emergencies: evidence-based guidelines of the European Association for Endoscopic Surgery. Surg Endosc 2006;20:14–29.

Van den Broek WT, Bijnen AB, VanEerten PV, DeRuiter P, Gouma DJ. Selective use of diagnostic laparoscopy in patients with suspected appendicitis. Surg Endosc 2000;14:938–941.

## Suggested Readings

Balthazar E, Rofsky N, Zucker R. Appendicitis: the impact of computed tomography imaging on the negative appendectomy and perforation rates. Am J Gastroenterol 1998;93:768–771.

Chung RS, Diaz JJ, Chari V. Efficacy of routine laparoscopy for the acute abdomen. Surg Endosc 1998;12:219–222.

Decadt B, Sussman L, Lewis MPN, et al. Randomized clinical trial of early laparoscopy in the management of acute non-specific abdominal pain. Br J Surg 1999;86:1383–1386.

Horton M, Counter S, Florence MG, Hart MJ. A prospective trial of computed tomography and ultrasonography for diagnosing appendicitis in the atypical patient. Am J Surg 2000;179:379–381.

Jan YT, Yang FS, Huang JK. Visualization rate and pattern of normal appendix on multi-detector computed tomography by using multiplanar reformation display. J Comput Assist Tomogr 2005;29:446–451.

Jones PF. Suspected acute appendicitis: trends in management over 30 years. Br J Surg 2001;88:1570–1577.

Kraemer M, Ohmann C, Leppert R, Yang Q. Macroscopic assessment of the appendix at diagnostic laparoscopy is reliable. Surg Endosc 2000;14:625–633.

Larsson PG, Henriksson G, Olsson M, et al. Laparoscopy reduces unnecessary appendicectomies and improves diagnosis in fertile women. Surg Endosc 2001;15:200–202.

Majewski WD. Long-term outcome, adhesions, and quality of life after laparoscopic and open surgical therapies for acute abdomen: follow-up of a prospective trial. Surg Endosc 2005;19:81–90.

Moberg AC, Ahlberg G, Leijonmarck CE, et al. Diagnostic laparoscopy in 1043 patients with suspected acute appendicitis. Eur J Surg 1998;164:833–840.

Moberg AC, Montgomery A. Introducing diagnostic laparoscopy in patients with suspected acute appendicitis. Surg Endosc 2000;14:942–947.

Mun S, Ernst RD, Chen K, Oto A, et al. Rapid CT diagnosis of acute appendicitis with IV contrast material. Emerg Radiol 2006;12:99–102.

Navez B, d'Udekem Y, Cambier E, Richir C, de Pierpont B, Guiot P. Laparoscopy for management of nontraumatic acute abdomen. World J Surg 1995;19:382–387.

Neumayer L, Kennedy A. Imaging in appendicitis: a review with special emphasis on treatment of women. Obstet Gynecol 2003;102(6):1404–1409.

Oto A, Ernst RD, et al. Right-lower-quadrant pain and suspected appendicitis in pregnant women: evaluation with MR imaging—initial experience. Radiology 2005;234:445–451.

Pieper R, Kager L, Nasman P. Acute appendicitis: a clinical study of 1018 cases of emergency appendectomy. Acta Chir Scand 1982;148:51–62.

Rennie ATM, Ctytherlerigh M, Theodoroupolou K, Farouk R. A prospective audit of 300 consecutive young women with an acute presentation of right iliac fossa pain. Ann R Coll Surg Engl 2006;88:140–413.

Thorell A, Grondal S, Schedvins K, Wallin G. Value of diagnostic laparoscopy in fertile women with suspected appendicitis. Eur J Surg 1999;165:751–754.

Van Dalen R, Bagshaw PF, Dobbs BR, Robertson GM, Lynch AC, Frizelle FA. The utility of laparoscopy in the diagnosis of acute appendicitis in women of reproductive age. Surg Endosc 2003;17:1311–1313.

Warren O, Kinross J, Paraskeva P, Darzi A. Emergency laparoscopy—current best practice. World J Emerg Surg 2006;1:24.

# 25. Acute (Retrocecal) Appendicitis

## A. Introduction

Laparoscopic appendectomy has evolved considerably from its origins as an incidental procedure, performed during gynecologic laparoscopy. Many surgeons now use it preferentially to treat acute appendicitis. When the appendix is known, by preoperative studies, to occupy a retrocecal position, it complicates both open and laparoscopic appendectomy. This chapter deals with the choice of approach in this situation.

## B. Case

### Hui Sen Chong

A 24-year-old man presented to the emergency department complaining of constant periumbilical pain of 5 hours' duration. The pain had gradually increased in intensity. He also felt nauseated and had vomited twice. He was anorexic. His last bowel movement was 2 days earlier. He had not passed flatus since the night before.

His past medical history was essentially negative. His only past surgery was removal of a lipoma from his forearm. He worked as an engineer. He smoked approximately half a pack of cigarettes per week. He did not use alcohol.

On physical examination, his temperature was 38.2 °C, pulse 90 beats per minute. His height was 6 feet and he weighed 103 kg. His abdomen was soft and nondistended. He had voluntary guarding and tenderness to light palpation in the right lower quadrant and periumbilical region. No masses or hernias were noted. Digital rectal examination was negative.

Laboratory studies were significant for a white cell count of 13.5. Computed tomography (CT) of the abdomen (Fig. 25.1) revealed an inflamed retrocecal appendix.

**What surgical procedure would you recommend for this patient?**

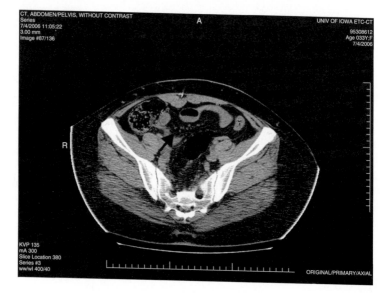

Fig. 25.1. Computed tomography scan showing inflamed retrocecal appendix (arrow).

## C.  Open Appendectomy

*Namir Katkhouda and Eric Pham*

We would perform open appendectomy. Since Fitz first described acute appendicitis in 1886, surgeons have become well aware of the presentation of appendicitis and the surgical options. Patients classically present with a history of periumbilical pain migrating to the right lower quadrant followed by vomiting or nausea. On physical exam, they may have a fever of >38 °C, tenderness at McBurney's point, or guarding in the right lower quadrant. Laboratory tests may show a mildly elevated leukocytosis above 10,000 cells/mL. However, due to the variable anatomy of the appendix, the patient with retrocecal appendicitis may not present with the classic symptoms.

The appendix's anatomy is well described. The average appendix is 9 to 10 cm in length with a diameter of 0.5 to 1.0 cm. The blood supply comes from the appendiceal artery, a branch of the ileocolic artery. It is usually located in the right lower quadrant and has been described as being medial, lateral, anterior, or posterior to the cecum. When the appendix is posterior, retrocecal appendicitis may not present with the classic symptoms due to overlying bowel. Instead of localized tenderness, patients with retrocecal appendicitis may have a dull aching tenderness because of the appendix's nonapposition to the anterior parietal peritoneum. One may be able to illicit abdominal pain on hip extension, the so-called psoas sign, with cases of retrocecal appendicitis. Consequently, patients with a variable anatomic position of the appendix may present late in the disease and are at higher risk for complicated appendicitis.

To prevent the morbidity from complicated appendicitis, surgeons aggressively perform appendectomies for suspected appendicitis. With over 250,000 cases of appendicitis a year in the United States, appendectomies are the second most common general surgery operation after laparoscopic cholecystectomies (Addiss et al.). Due to improved anesthesia, postoperative care, and advanced surgical techniques, the mortality of appendicitis has become less than 1% (Wagner et al.). However, the morbidity and mortality from cases of complicated appendicitis are higher. Postoperative complications and hospital stay in patients with complicated appendicitis are three times as long as those patients with less severe appendicitis (Guidry and Poole). Some studies suggest the main reason for complicated appendicitis is the delayed presentation of the patient to the hospital for care (Pittman-Walker et al.). One reason for delay includes the atypical nature of symptoms seen in patients with retrocecal appendicitis. The inflammation from retrocecal appendicitis may not come in contact with the anterior peritoneum, so patients may have pain and tenderness at a site other than the right lower quadrant.

Today, computed axial tomography (CAT) scans and ultrasounds aid with the diagnosis of retrocecal appendicitis. On CAT scan, the inflamed appendix may have a thickened wall (>2 mm). There could also be an appendicolith, target structure (concentric thickening of the appendiceal wall), free fluid, or mesenteric fat stranding. Findings on ultrasound suggesting appendicitis include a noncompressible tubular structure at the cecal base with a thickened wall (>2 mm), luminal distention with an increased diameter (>6 mm), and possibly free fluid in the pelvis.

When encountered with a complicated retrocecal appendicitis, the general surgeon has to decide not only when to operate but by which operation. Studies have shown the feasibility of initial conservative management with late-presenting complicated perforated appendicitis with an intraabdominal abscess (Nitecki et al.). These patients are placed on antibiotics, fluid resuscitated, have their abscess percutaneously drained, and are discharged with eventual follow-up for an interval appendectomy.

Candidates for such conservative management include patients who present more than 5 days after their initial symptoms, are not septic or have peritonitis, and respond to initial conservative management with fluids and antibiotics. If the patient does not improve after a 24-hour trial of conservative management or the abscess cannot be percutaneously drained, then the patient crosses over to the surgery arm.

Once the patient needs surgery, then two surgical options exist: laparoscopic versus open appendectomy. Absolute contraindications to the laparoscopic approach include patients with a large ventral hernia, a history of laparotomies for small bowel obstructions, and ascites with abdominal distention. Relative contraindications include those patients with a history of cirrhosis, coagulation defects, generalized peritonitis, shock on admission, and those who due to cardiac or pulmonary disease may not tolerate a pneumoperitoneum. A recent randomized prospective double-blinded study showed that compared to open appendectomies, laparoscopic appendectomies take on average 20 minutes longer with no difference in the overall complication rates (Katkhouda et al.). The choice of the operation should be based on surgeon or patient preference.

For open appendectomies, the classic incision is a 3- to 4-cm curvilinear incision overlying the point of maximal tenderness, usually McBurney's point. First, the external oblique aponeurosis is transected in the line of its fibers. Then the abdominal muscles are bluntly split open for sharp entry into the peritoneum. For more exposure, the incision can be extended into the rectus sheath. The cecum is gently mobilized to deliver the appendix onto the wound. The appendix is transected after the appendiceal base and mesoappendix are clamped and ligated. The stump may be coagulated or imbricated into the cecum using a purse-string stitch. After warm irrigation of the peritoneum and pelvis, the peritoneum and muscle aponeurosis are closed with absorbable sutures, leaving the skin to be closed with staples or sutures. For cases with perforated appendicitis, some surgeons prefer the skin to be left open for delayed primary or secondary closure. After surgery, patients are discharged when they tolerate a regular diet, have a normal white blood cell count, and are afebrile for 24 hours. In cases of complicated perforated appendicitis, antibiotics covering anaerobes and gram-negative enteric organisms are given for 7 to 10 days.

Several maneuvers may help find and mobilize the retrocecal appendix. First, the operating bed can be repositioned to bring the appendix closer to the incision. Second, a sweeping finger motion lateral to medial in the right paracolic gutter may help break up cecal adhesions or peritoneal attachments. Third, a laparotomy pad placed medially into the abdomen or sponge stick pushed medially may aid in retracting the small intestine out of the way to further isolate the appendix. To also help find the appendix, the anterior tenia coli may be followed to the cecal base.

In cases of complicated appendicitis with a difficult necrotic or inflamed appendiceal stump, a GIA (gastrointestinal anastomosis) stapler is helpful in performing a partial cecectomy. For a difficult retrocecal appendicitis, the appendiceal base may have to be transected first. The surgeon then works in a retrograde fashion ligating the mesoappendix. To lower wound infections, moist gauze sponges are used to wall off the peritoneal cavity and wound edges. Finally, the omentum should be brought over the site of the operation.

Some of the pitfalls in performing an open appendectomy include making an inappropriate incision. The incision should not be standardized. The surgeon needs to surmise the location of the appendix by the patient's point of maximal tenderness and adapt the incision for the best exposure. If one makes a too inferior incision and encounters an appendix higher than normal, it may be very difficult to mobilize the appendix out onto the wound.

# D. Laparoscopic Appendectomy

*Kamran Mohiuddin, Saira Nizami, Francis D'Souza, Iftikhar M. Khan, and Mohammed AshAaf Memon*

Our preference would be to do a diagnostic laparoscopy first, followed by a trial dissection to mobilize the cecum and right colon if we fail to see the appendix following various simple maneuvers such as positioning the patient and lifting the cecum with bowel graspers (see Operative Technique for Laparoscopic Appendectomy p. 313).

Appendicitis is one of the most common surgical emergencies every surgeon encounters during their career. The lifetime risk of developing appendicitis in an individual is 6%. The conventional method of doing an appendectomy is by the open method (open appendectomy, OA), which is a relatively quick and simple operation associated with short recovery time. It was first described in the 19th century and has remained unchanged since. Laparoscopic appendectomy (LA) was first introduced into clinical practice by Kurt Semm in the 1980s. However, the general surgical community has been slow to accept its benefits. Nonetheless, with an incidence of negative appendectomy approaching as high as

34% in women of reproductive age who frequently present with other conditions such as pelvic inflammatory disease, complicated ovarian cysts, endometriosis and ectopic pregnancy, diagnostic laparoscopy (prior to an appendectomy) allows for a more thorough examination of the abdomen and pelvis and it has been shown beyond doubt that it is an efficient tool in confirming the diagnosis and significantly reducing the number of histologically normal appendices as compared to a conventional open operation.

Many randomized controlled trials have now been published comparing LA to OA. Moberg et al. conducted a randomized blinded study comparing the two procedures. There was no significant difference between operating time, complication rate, median hospital stay, or time to full recovery, although a trend toward better performance of physical activity was noted after LA. Similar results were noted by Ignacio et al. in their randomized trial as well. However, the authors noted a significant difference in the cost of two procedures, which was significantly higher in the case of LA. Contrary to the above studies, many other trials do report a benefit for LA. Towfigh and colleagues analyzed the data from a prospective clinical pathway and reported a shorter length of stay especially for those undergoing LA for ruptured appendicitis using multiple regression analysis. Yet another recent report from a large administrative database showed a significant shorter hospital stay, lower rate of infections and overall complications, and a higher rate of routine discharge in patients undergoing LA versus OA. Katkhouda et al., in their randomized controlled trial, similarly revealed statistically better physical health and general scores on the quality of life assessment forms even though there were no other statistically important differences noted.

In terms of the location of the appendix, we were unable to find any evidence-based literature analyzing the success or failure of LA in the case of retrocecal appendix. However, it is the opinion of the surgical fraternity (anecdotal observation) that retrocecal appendix either when diagnosed by CT or during laparoscopy (when an appendix simply cannot be visualized) is an indication for the open procedure. In a recent randomized trial comparing LA versus OA, Moberg et al. excluded the patients from analysis whose appendix was not visible on diagnostic laparoscopy due to inflammation or being retrocecal. In one of the earliest studies published on LA by Browne, one patient was converted owing to difficulty in mobilizing a retrocecal appendix. A retrospective study performed to identify the CT predictors of failed laparoscopic appendectomy and subsequent conversion to OA did not find the retrocecal position of the appendix as a risk factor for conversion. However, the higher CT grade of inflammation was the main reason associated with higher rates of conversion to OA.

We propose the following simple and inexpensive method of LA, which requires only a monopolar diathermy scissors, part of the existing laparoscopic cholecystectomy set, and endoloops to accomplish this procedure safely and quickly without resorting to any costly and high-tech equipment such as Harmonic scalpel or endoscopic staplers.

## Operative Technique for Laparoscopic Appendectomy

### Patient and Surgeon's Position and Equipment Setup

The patient is placed in a steep Trendelenburg position and the operating table is tilted to the left. This position allows the small bowel to migrate in the left upper quadrant, thereby exposing the cecum and pelvis adequately for a thorough examination. The patient's arms are either tucked on the sides or placed flexed over the chest. The position of the surgeon, assistant, anesthetist, scrub nurse, instrument table, and video monitor is shown in Figure 25.2.

### Port Position

Following the creation of pneumoperitoneum (closed or open method), the first 10-mm port is placed infraumbilically. A 0- or 30-degree scope, whichever the surgeon prefers, is then introduced and the abdominal cavity is examined thoroughly. A second 5-mm port is introduced under direct vision just below the right costal margin just lateral to the midclavicular line, and the appendix is located using Johann atraumatic graspers. In case of nonvisualization of the appendix, we simply introduce a third 10- to 12-mm port in the left lower quadrant and use a bowel grasper to retract the cecum medially while using a monopolar diathermy scissor introduced via a second port to divide the lateral peritoneal fold, thereby mobilizing the cecum and right colon. This step does not require extensive mobilization of the right colon, as in the majority of cases once the cecum and right lower colon is fully mobilized, one is able to visualize even a true retrocecal appendix without much difficulty. In our experience this step is rarely required though.

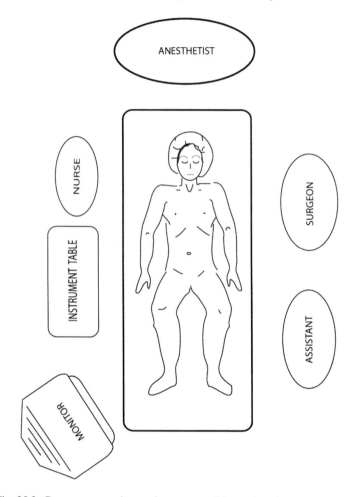

Fig. 25.2. Room setup, patient and surgeon position and equipment setup.

## Technique of Performing Laparoscopic Appendectomy

Once the appendix is discovered, it is grasped from the base and lifted up using the right upper quadrant port. A small window is created in the base of the mesoappendix close to the cecum using monopolar scissors introduced via the left lower quadrant port (Fig. 25.3). We then skeletonize the appendix by generously cauterizing in small increments right next to the wall of the appendix (Fig. 25.4). The entire meso-appendix can safely be divided this way without encountering any bleeding. On completion of this process, we routinely reinforce the divided mesoappendix with an endoloop (Fig. 25.5). The next step is to place two further endoloops on the appendix itself, one near the base and the second higher up, following which the appendix is divided (appendectomy) (Fig. 25.6). We then retract the appendix in the left lower quadrant port and remove the port along with the appendix. This prevents any skin contamination and subsequent port-site infection.

In conclusion, LA is a safe and effective procedure for removal of the appendix irrespective of its position such as retrocecal. Furthermore, it seems to be beneficial in terms of lesser wound infection rate, shorter hospital stay, and a better quality of life postoperatively. Moreover, the regular use of diagnostic laparoscopy as a first step in the management of

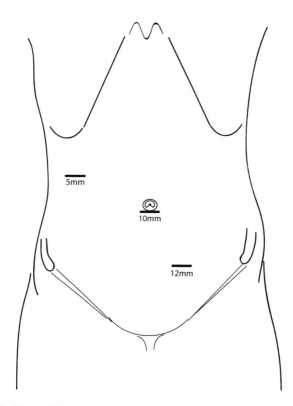

5mm

10mm

12mm

Fig. 25.3. Port positions.

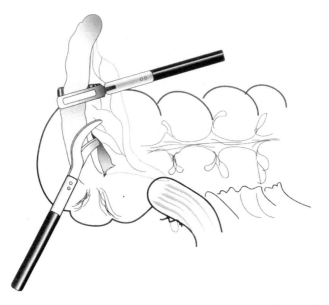

Fig. 25.4. Creation of small mesenteric window near the base of appendix with a laparoscopic scissors.

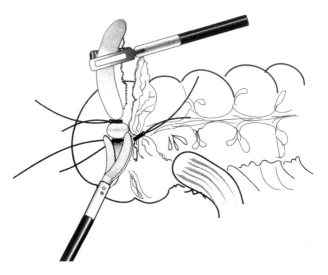

Fig. 25.5. Skeletonizing of appendix and application of endoloops on the mesoappendix and appendix.

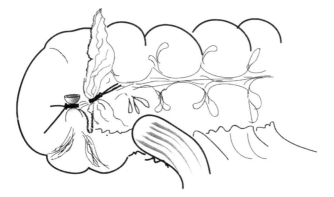

Fig. 25.6. Completion of laparoscopic appendectomy.

patients with suspected appendicitis, particularly in women of reproductive age, in obese patients, and in patients with diagnostic difficulties, prevents unnecessary OAs. This results in added savings by decreasing the number of hospital stays and morbidities associated with unnecessary surgery. In addition, we believe that the technique of LA as described above is simple, safe, inexpensive, and easily reproducible and can be introduced without the need for any additional expensive equipment. The strength of this technique is that it can be introduced in countries where financial and technological resources are limited.

# E. Conclusions

*Sen Chong*

In the years since laparoscopic appendectomy was first introduced by Semm, it has become an increasingly popular treatment modality for patients diagnosed with acute appendicitis. Nguyen et al. found that the utilization of LA increased more than twofold.

For laparoscopic appendectomy to be favored over open appendectomy, it should (1) decrease hospital stay, (2) lessen narcotic requirement, (3) speed return to normal activity, (4) be cost-effective, and (5) have fewer complications. Because open appendectomy is performed through a low incision with a relatively short stay in the hospital, it has been more difficult to demonstrate an advantage for this procedure than it was for laparoscopic cholecystectomy. The Kocher incision formerly used for open cholecystectomy was painful, and return to work was slow.

All meta-analysis of prospective randomized trials have concluded that laparoscopic appendectomy is at least as good as open appendectomy and sometimes a bit better, in terms of postoperative analgesia requirements, postoperative wound infections, length of hospital stay, return to work intervals, overall recovery, and patient satisfaction. Laparoscopic appendectomy is associated with a lower postoperative wound infection rate since the inflamed appendix is removed via a trocar or an endobag, thus preventing the inflamed appendix from coming in contact with the wound. Some studies have shown an increased rate of intraabdominal abscess formation after laparoscopic appendectomy compared with open appendectomy.

As for cost-effectiveness, laparoscopic appendectomy is associated with similar if not longer operative time and a higher operative cost especially if disposable equipment is used intraoperatively. However, the economic analysis done by Long et al. showed that when indirect costs are taken into account, the laparoscopic approach is relatively less expensive when compared to its counterpart.

Historically, laparoscopic appendectomy is associated with a 0% to 16% conversion rate to an open surgery. The most common reasons for LA to be converted to open are (1) dense adhesions from inflammation, (2) localized perforation, (3) peritonitis, and, in some cases, (4) a retrocecal appendix associated with difficult dissection or visualization. A relatively retrocecal appendix is found in 60% to 70% of the normal population, with a surgeon's skills and experience playing an important role in affecting the conversion rate. Difficulties arise when the appendix is densely retrocecal or bound to the cecum by peritoneal bands. Conversion of laparoscopic appendectomy to the open technique not only abolishes the advantages that LA has over the open technique but also incurs the added cost of equipment and operative time. When compared to patients who had had primary laparoscopic or open appendectomy, Hellberg et al. and Carbonell et al. found that converted cases had a significantly worse outcome in terms of time to full recovery, analgesic control, hospital stay, sick leave, and postoperative complications.

To conclude, patients with acute appendicitis diagnosed on CT scan, especially the female population and those with obesity, are excellent candidates for laparoscopic appendectomy. However, if there is an indication of complicated appendicitis, such as perforation or diffuse peritoneal signs, or if the surgeon lacks experience with laparoscopic appendectomy, open appendectomy should be performed since it has well-established excellent results and is associated with minimal morbidity. A densely retrocecal appendix will require some cecal mobilization, and should be attempted only by experienced laparoscopists. Conversion to open surgery may be required.

# References

Addiss DG, Shaffer N, Fowler BS, Tauxe RV. The epidemiology of appendicitis and appendectomy in the United States. Am J Epidemiol 1990;132:910.

Browne DS. Laparoscopic-guided appendicectomy. A study of 100 consecutive cases. Aust N Z J Obstet Gynaecol 1990;30:231–233.

Carbonell AM, Burns JM, Lincourt AE, Harold KL. Outcomes of laparoscopic versus open appendectomy. Am Surg 2004;70:759–765.

Guidry S, Poole G. The anatomy of appendicitis. Am Surg 1994;60:68.

Hellberg A, Rudberg C, Enochsson L, et al. Conversion from laparoscopic to open appendicectomy: a possible drawback of the laparoscopic technique? Eur J Surg 2001;167:209–213.

Ignacio RC, Burke R, Spencer D, Bissell C, Dorsainvil C, Lucha PA. Laparoscopic vs open appendectomy. What is the real difference? Results of a prospective randomized double-blinded trial. Surg Endosc 2004;18:334–337.

Katkhouda N, Mason RJ, Towfigh S, Gevorgyan A, Essani R. Laparoscopic versus open appendectomy. A prospective randomized double blind study. Ann Surg 2005;242:439–450.

Long KH, Bannon MP, Zietlow SP, et al. A prospective randomized comparison of laparoscopic appendectomy with open appendectomy: clinical and economic analyses. Surgery 2001;129:390–400.

Moberg AC, Berndsen F, Palmquist I, Petersson U, Resch T, Montgomery A. Randomized clinical trial of laparoscopic versus open appendicectomy for confirmed appendicitis. Br J Surg 2005;92:298–304.

Nguyen NT, Zainabadi K, Mavandadi S, et al. Trends in utilization and outcomes of laparoscopic versus open appendectomy. Am J Surg 2004;188:813–820.

Nitecki S, Assalia A, Schein M. Contemporary management of the appendiceal mass. Br J Surg 1993;80:18.

Pittman-Walker VA, Myers JG, Stewart RM, et al. Appendicitis: why so complicated? Analysis of 5755 consecutive appendectomies. Am Surg 2000;66:548.

Towfigh S, Chen F, Mason R, Katkhouda N, Chan L, Berne T. Laparoscopic appendectomy significantly reduces length of stay for perforated appendicitis. Surg Endosc 2006;20:495–499.

Wagner JM, McKinney WP, Carpenter JL. Does the patient have appendicitis? JAMA 1996;276:1589.

# Suggested Readings

Chung RS, Rowland DY, Li P, Diaz J. A meta-analysis of randomized controlled trials of laparoscopic versus conventional appendectomy. Am J Surg 1999;177:250–256.

Garbutt JM, Soper NJ, Shannon WD, et al. Meta-analysis of randomized trials comparing laparoscopic and open appendectomy. Surg Laparosc Endosc 1999;9:17–26.

Golub R, Siddiqui F, Pohl D. Laparoscopic versus open appendectomy: a meta-analysis. J Am Coll Surg 1998;186:545–553.

Guller U, Hervey S, Purves H, et al. Laparoscopic versus open appendectomy. Outcomes comparison based on a large administrative database. Ann Surg 2004;239:43–52.

Liu SI, Siewert B, Raptopoulos V, Hodin RA. Factors associated with conversion to laparotomy in patients undergoing laparoscopic appendectomy. J Am Coll Surg 2002;194:298–305.

Memon MA. Laparoscopic appendicectomy: current status. Ann R Coll Surg Engl 1997;79:393–402.

Pedersen AG, Petersen OB, Wara P, et al. Randomized clinical trial of laparoscopic versus open appendicectomy. Br J Surg 2001;88:200–205.

Sauerland S, Lefering R, Neugebauer EA. Laparoscopic versus open surgery for suspected appendicitis. Cochrane Database Syst Rev 2004;4:CD001546.

Siewert B, Raptopoulos V, Liu SI, Hodin RA, Davis RB, Rosen MP. CT predictors of failed laparoscopic appendectomy. Radiology 2003;229:415–420.

van Dalen R, Bagshaw PF, Dobbs BR, Robertson GM, Lynch AC, Frizelle FA. The utility of laparoscopy in the diagnosis of acute appendicitis in women of reproductive age. Surg Endosc 2003;17:1311–1313.

# 26. Perforated Appendicitis

## A. Introduction

Management of appendicitis has changed with the advent of laparoscopic appendectomy. Additional complexity is introduced into the algorithm when the history or imaging studies suggest that perforation and abscess formation have occurred. This chapter explores decision choices associated with that situation.

## B. Case

### *Evgeny V. Arshava*

A 22-year-old man was evaluated in the emergency department for abdominal pain and fever. He noted the onset of right lower abdominal pain 5 days earlier. He thought that he had fever at that time, but he did not measure his temperature. He experienced nausea without vomiting, had one episode of diarrhea, and experienced an ongoing sense of anorexia. He had never had symptoms like this before, and attributed his symptoms to "stomach flu." He treated himself with Tylenol and did not immediately seek medical attention. Over this period of time, his pain progressively worsened, to the point that he remained in bed for the past 2 days. The pain was aggravated by movement. His last bowel movement was 2 days prior to evaluation; it was small, soft, and without blood or mucous. The night before evaluation, he had chills and a temperature of 38.9 °C.

His past medical history was negative. Other than a tonsillectomy at age 6, his past surgical history was likewise negative. He was on no medications, and had no known allergies.

He lived with his parents and worked at his parents' farm. He smoked half a pack of cigarettes a day since age 19, drank alcohol socially, and denied recreational drug use.

The review of systems was negative with the exception of thirst.

On physical examination, he was a slender male, lying in bed, uncomfortable, with legs flexed on abdomen. His temperature was 39.0 °C, pulse 98, respiratory rate 22, blood pressure 128/80, and saturated 100% on room air. His mucous membranes were dry.

Abdominal examination was significant for a soft, nondistended abdomen, without bowel sounds. There was tenderness and guarding in the lower abdomen with mass palpated in the right lower quadrant. Rebound tenderness was noted in the right lower quadrant.

Digital rectal exam revealed normal tone, no masses, and right rectal wall tenderness. Guaiac test was negative.

His laboratory results included a hemoglobin of 15.4 g/dL, hematocrit of 46%, white blood count (WBC) of 22,000/mm$^3$, and 82% neutrophils with left shift. Microscopic examination of the urine revealed 5 to 10 WBC per high-power field (hpf), 4 to 6 RBC/hpf, and no bacteria.

A computed tomography (CT) scan of the abdomen and pelvis with IV and PO contrast showed 7×8 cm walled-off fluid collection in the right lower quadrant (RLQ) adjacent to the cecum. No extraluminal contrast was noticed. The base of the appendix was not visualized.

The impression was perforated appendicitis with appendiceal abscess.

**Which would you advise? Appendectomy (open or laparoscopic) versus percutaneous drainage followed by interval appendectomy?**

# C.  Laparoscopic Appendectomy or Nonoperative Management

## Michael A. Edwards and Bruce MacFadyen, Jr.

Acute appendicitis remains the most common intraabdominal surgical emergency and the second most common general surgical procedure performed in the United States. The first open appendectomy (OA) was performed by McBurney in 1889, and for over a century it has remained the gold standard for the surgical management of acute appendicitis. Kurt Semm, a German gynecologist, performed the first laparoscopic appendectomy in 1983. The introduction and logarithmic acceptance of minimal access surgery has challenged open appendectomy as the gold standard operation for acute appendicitis. Whether laparoscopic appendectomy (LA) is superior remains unknown and a topic of intense debate.

Multiple retrospective and prospective studies have highlighted the advantages and disadvantages of both open and laparoscopic appendectomy, often with conflicting results. Meta-analysis and systematic reviews of the published literature have failed to provide a consolidated consensus in favor of open or laparoscopic appendectomy because of the heterogeneity of outcome measures and other methodologic flaws of reported series. Reported design flaws include inadequate sample size, lack of power, lack of standardization in randomization and preoperative and postoperative care, inadequate reporting of surgeons' experience, and the exploratory nature of most studies. As a result, two decades following the introduction of LA, a consensus about its relative advantages remains controversial.

The safety and efficacy of laparoscopic appendectomy for acute appendicitis have been established by multiple prospective randomized trials. Advocates for open appendectomy argue that the incidence of intraabdominal abscess is lower, the operative time is shorter, and the direct costs are less. Advocates for laparoscopic appendectomy argue that there are fewer wound infections, less postoperative pain, reduced hospital length of stay, and improved quality of life. In addition, the ability to perform a complete exploratory laparoscopy is another advantage of the laparoscopic technique. In spite of these reported benefits for both techniques, neither option has evolved as superior to the other.

Whether laparoscopic appendectomy is superior to open appendectomy for complicated appendicitis (gangrenous or perforated with peritonitis) is also a point of controversy. Arguments against laparoscopic appendectomy included higher rates of intraabdominal abscess (IAA) and less cost-effectiveness. Multiple series have shown higher, lower, and similar rates of IAA following laparoscopic versus open appendectomy for perforated appendicitis. In a retrospective review, Kouwenhoven et al. reported no significant differences in IAA following laparoscopic versus open appendectomy for acute appendicitis (3.6% vs. 3.5%) and perforated appendicitis (7.7% vs. 9.5%). The variability in this outcome measure likely reflects study design flaws resulting in differences in patient selection, antibiotic regimen, extent of lavage, and surgical technique. Like all minimal-access operations, laparoscopic appendectomy is associated with a learning curve, and complication rates decrease as one ascends the learning curve. Katkhouda et al. reported a reduction in IAA rates from 2.4% to 0.4% by introducing a specialized laparoscopic team for laparoscopic appendectomy.

The second criticism is the poorer cost-effectiveness of laparoscopic appendectomy. The Cochrane Review of prospective randomized trials indicated that LA is less cost-effective, but it is difficult to draw definitive conclusions about cost-effectiveness because the studies reviewed were not without design flaws, including failure to consider the surgeons' learning curve. In a 5-year retrospective review of laparoscopic versus open appendectomy, Carbonell et al. reported no significant differences in the total hospital charges ($8801 vs. $9147) comparing LA to OA. Similarly, in a review of a large national administrative database of academic medical centers and teaching hospitals, Nguyen, Zainabadi, et al. reported no difference in mean cost per case of LA versus OA ($6242 vs. $6260). Whether the IAA rate and cost-effectiveness are legitimate arguments against LA remains unclear.

We routinely perform laparoscopic appendectomy for all patients with suspected acute appendicitis and appendicitis complicated by gangrene or perforation. Several advantages of LA have guided our practice. Most published series, including meta-analyses of randomized clinical trials, have shown that LA is associated with fewer overall complications, as well as less wound infection, postoperative pain, and a shorter hospital length of stay. Our experiences with LA have echoed the published literature.

There are other practical advantages to LA that should also be considered. First, it allows the surgeon to perform a complete exploratory laparoscopy. This is particularly helpful when the preoperative diagnosis is equivocal. As a diagnostic tool, laparoscopy is excellent for identifying other pathologies to explain the clinical presentation that may exist in conjunction with appendicitis. The literature suggests that this may be of particular benefit to female patients. We think that the laparoscopic technique would be of benefit to any patient with an equivocal diagnosis. It is also advantageous in patients with an appendix that is not located in its usual anatomic position. Second, the visualization afforded by laparoscopic exploration allows the surgeon to completely lavage the peritoneal cavity, and potentially minimizes the risk of postoperative infectious complications. Third, at an academic teaching center responsible for the training of the next generation of surgeons in the minimal-access surgical era, laparoscopic appendectomy can be safely performed by residents under the supervision of expert laparoscopic surgeons, as residents ascend their laparoscopic learning curve.

What about patients with appendiceal phlegmons and abscesses? We have had very good success with initial nonoperative management (antibiotics with/without percutaneous drainage) followed by an interval appendectomy for this patient population. At the time of interval appendectomy, a laparoscopic technique is utilized. For those patients who fail nonoperative management and require an operation, a laparoscopic appendectomy is attempted.

Laparoscopic appendectomy is safe and effective. Criticisms of the technique, including higher intraabdominal abscess rates and poorer cost-effectiveness, have not been conclusively borne out in the literature.

There are clear advantages to LA, including fewer overall complications and wound complications, less pain, shorter hospital stay, and the ability to perform a thorough exploration of the abdomen, resulting in identification of missed pathology and reducing the negative appendectomy rate. We have found laparoscopic appendectomy for acute and complicated appendicitis feasible and safe in our academic teaching setting and have made it a routine practice.

# D. Percutaneous Drainage and Interval Appendectomy

*Jared L. Antevil and Carlos V.R. Brown*

We would treat this patient initially with antibiotics, percutaneous drainage, and consider interval appendectomy (IA) 6 to 8 weeks after resolution of his symptoms. Immediate operative intervention in the setting of perforated appendicitis with an established abscess would be associated with greater morbidity and longer hospital stay.

Computed tomography (CT) imaging should be obtained in all patients with clinically suspected appendicitis and a palpable abdominal mass. It also should be strongly considered for those without a mass but with duration of pain greater than 48 to 72 hours. Various techniques of CT using combinations of oral, intravenous (IV), and rectal contrast have all demonstrated a high rate of diagnostic accuracy for acute appendicitis. However, we routinely employ both oral and IV contrast in the setting of suspected abscess to optimize the differentiation between intra- and extraluminal fluid collections (Figs. 26.1 and 26.2).

After the diagnosis of perforated appendicitis with intraabdominal abscess has been established, the patient should be admitted for IV fluids, analgesia, bowel rest, and IV antibiotics. The antibiotic regimen should be broad spectrum, with adequate coverage for gram-negative enteric and anaerobic organisms. We prefer to use the combination of a fluoroquinolone and metronidazole, as these agents have a favorable side-effect profile and facilitate transition to oral therapy with excellent bioavailability. Although some authors recommend subsequently tailoring antibiotic coverage based on drainage culture results, we modify antibiotics only for organisms resistant to initial empiric coverage. Abscesses are polymicrobial in the majority of cases, and should be treated as such.

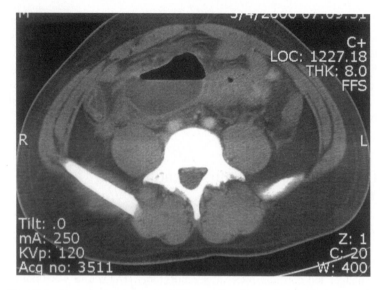

Fig. 26.1. Computed tomography (CT) scan showing well-defined abscess with air-fluid level.

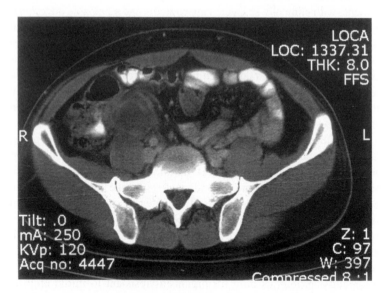

Fig. 26.2. CT scan image showing appendix with abscess formation and induration.

In our experience, patients presenting with a large abscess (>5 cm) accompanied by a systemic inflammatory response are unlikely to improve without drainage. Therefore, in the current case we would opt for primary CT-guided drainage. Sonographic guidance is an equally viable option for percutaneous treatment, albeit without the anatomic detail provided by CT. Percutaneous drains are removed after demonstrable clinical improvement and radiographic evidence of abscess resolution. However, in spite of the surgical dictum that all pus needs drainage, there is increasing evidence that many patients with appendiceal abscess may be adequately treated with antibiotic therapy alone. Rather than pursuing percutaneous aspiration and drainage in all patients in this setting, we reserve this intervention for those patients with large abscesses or who do not demonstrate prompt clinical improvement after the institutional of medical therapy. Patients who do not manifest a marked decrease in fever, leukocytosis, and tenderness within 48 hours of admission are referred for CT-guided drainage.

Nonoperative treatment of appendiceal abscess has a very high success rate, and morbidity is significantly lower than with early surgical intervention. Immediate operation in this setting is associated with higher rates of wound complications, recurrent abscess, and a greater incidence of overall complications. Furthermore, acute surgical intervention in the setting of perforated appendicitis with abscess formation may lead to a higher likelihood of cecectomy.

Once a patient is asymptomatic, the decision must be made whether to perform subsequent appendectomy. While IA was long considered a standard adjunct to prevent recurrence, recent evidence suggests recurrent appendicitis is not common. In the largest reported series of patients treated nonoperatively for appendicitis, Kaminski et al. examined 864 patients over a 13-year period, citing a 5% rate of recurrent appendicitis over a mean follow-up of 4 years. The authors did not note a higher rate of recurrence for patients who initially presented with perforation or abscess. Routine appendectomy in this setting, therefore, has no therapeutic benefit for the majority of patients.

Although recurrent appendicitis is uncommon, histopathologic studies show that in most cases the appendiceal lumen regains patency after clinical resolution of appendicitis. Because this dictates that most patients remain theoretically at risk for recurrence, and because IA may be performed with minimal morbidity and hospital stay, IA remains a reasonable treatment option. Operative exploration and treatment also avoids the risk of missing significant alternative pathology, such as appendiceal carcinoid or adenocarcinoma.

We make the decision whether to perform IA after successful nonoperative therapy on an individual basis, taking into account patient preference and comorbidities. In the present case, given the patient's young age and excellent health, we would offer laparoscopic IA 6 to 8 weeks after clinical resolution.

In conclusion, nonoperative therapy has clearly emerged as the preferred treatment modality for patients presenting with appendiceal abscess in the absence of generalized peritonitis. Percutaneous CT-guided drainage is an integral part of the nonoperative treatment algorithm, but may not be indicated in all cases. Current evidence is insufficient to support the routine practice of IA after successful nonoperative treatment, although we continue to feel that it is a reasonable treatment option in selected patients.

# E.  Conclusions

*Evgeny V. Arshava*

Untreated acute appendicitis may progress to gangrene and subsequent perforation of the appendix, leading to either diffuse peritonitis or a contained perforation. Omentum or adjacent bowel may form a phlegmon, which then progresses to a localized abscess in majority of patients. Two to six percent of patients with appendicitis present, usually 4 to 5 days after onset of disease, with a right lower quadrant mass, either phlegmon or abscess. These complications are more likely to occur in patients in whom a delayed diagnosis is more frequent—women, the elderly, and children.

The management of a ruptured appendix with a well-defined abscess has been controversial. Is it better to perform an immediate appendectomy with drainage of an abscess or to cool down the inflammation with antibiotics and perform later interval appendectomy? Others have argued that interval appendectomy may not even be necessary. Dialogue was complicated, in the pre-CT era, by the lack of accurate preoperative diagnosis and delineation of anatomy, as well as inability to safely drain an abscess percutaneously.

Because of substantial operative morbidity associated with surgery on complicated appendicitis, nonoperative management was introduced in the 1920s. These early studies lacked accurate imaging studies and percutaneous drainage. Bradley and Isaacs described 61 patients who underwent surgical drainage of the abscess, with a 28% complication rate and two deaths. Complications included wound infection, fecal fistula, small bowel obstruction, recurrent abscess, and sepsis. Paull and Bloom reviewed 60 patients with appendiceal abscess: 32 were treated by incision and drainage without appendectomy with 16% morbidity, and 17 patients had incision and drainage with appendectomy with 24% morbidity. Others were spared operation. Hoffman described 44 patients who had conservative treatment of an appendix mass without interval appendectomy and were followed for between 6 months and 22 years. Recurrent appendicitis developed in 20% of patients. Skoubo-Kristensen and Hvid followed 193 patients with an appendiceal masses that were treated conservatively for 10 years; 12% of patients underwent delayed surgical intervention for complications, with one death. Elective appendectomy was performed after 3 months, with a complication rate of 3.4%.

Preoperative imaging studies have been increasingly used during the last decade. Raptopoulos et al. noted that with liberal use of CT scan, patients have a significantly lower surgical-pathologic severity of appendiceal disease and hospital stay. Simultaneously, image-guided percutaneous drainage became established as a safe and effective therapeutic modality. Jamieson et al. reviewed 46 children with appendiceal abscesses. In 91%, image-guided drainage successfully treated an abscess. One patient developed a colonic fistula that resolved spontaneously. The application to complicated appendicitis was first established in the pediatric population. Gervais et al. described successful treatment of abdominal and pelvic abscess with percutaneous imaging-guided drainage in children in 85% to 90% of cases. Alexander et al. found that transrectal ultrasound (US)-guided drainage of deep pelvic abscesses is a safe and well-tolerated option if percutaneous transabdominal or transvaginal routes are not possible.

Bagi et al. presented 40 patients with appendiceal masses; 17 patients had an ultrasonically guided percutaneous drainage of an abscess and 16 had resolution of symptoms without further treatment or complications; 14 patients were treated conservatively without drainage, with resolution of symptoms without interference in 12. All nine patients with a phlegmon recovered without operative treatment. Oliak et al., in retrospective review of 155 consecutive patients with periappendicular abscess, found initial nonoperative management failed only in 5.8% and found an appendicitis recurrence rate of 8%. The complication rate was significantly higher in the operative group of patients (36% vs. 17%). Brown et al. compared immediate appendectomy versus expectant management including percutaneous drainage with or without interval appendectomy in 104 patients with periappendicular abscesses. The immediate appendectomy group had a higher rate of complications than the expectant management group at initial hospitalization (58% vs. 15%), for all hospitalizations (67% vs. 24%) with a significantly longer initial and overall hospital stay.

Yamini et al. reviewed treatment of 66 patients with 54 abscesses and 10 phlegmons, who were treated initially with intravenous antibiotics, and CT-guided drainage was used only if the patient failed to improve after 48 to 72 hours. Patients still not improving underwent appendectomy; 42% of patients did not require percutaneous drainage, and 51 patients improved without surgery. Interval appendectomy was carried out with 10% morbidity and a mean length of stay in the hospital of 1.4 days. A similar standardized approach was described by Helmer et al., who performed a retrospective study on 232 patients, both children and adults, with complicated appendicitis and showed a decrease in infectious complications (13% vs. 33%) using a standardized approach, which included US- or CT-guided percutaneous drainage of an abscess, appropriate antibacterial therapy, and interval appendectomy. Nitecki et al. also showed that with contemporary imaging and interventional radiologic techniques, 80% of patients presenting with an appendiceal mass can be safely spared an open operation. Tingstedt et al., in a retrospective review of 93 patients with appendiceal abscess, confirmed a high risk of more extensive surgical procedure and postoperative complications in patients who were operated on presentation.

One of the studies in the pediatric surgery literature suggested a superiority of immediate intervention. In prospective nonrandomized study of 82 pediatric patients with appendicular masses, Samuel et al. recommended early surgical intervention over nonoperative management, based on the failure of conservative management in 11% of patients and their higher morbidity. Persistent periappendicular abscess was present on interval appendectomies in 79% of patients treated conservatively. In this study the percutaneous drainage was not used. Larger studies, however, showed the superiority of a conservative approach in children with appendiceal masses. Gillick et al. reviewed records of 427 children with an appendix mass. Sixteen children had an immediate appendicectomy; 346 (84.2%) of the remaining children responded to initial conservative management and underwent elective appendicectomy 4 to 6 weeks later, with a complication rate of 2.3%.

It is essential to note, however, that in certain patients, usually elderly, radiologic imaging during the acute phase of the inflammatory process may not be accurate and can lead to diagnostic mistakes. Surgeons should consider other possible etiologies of right lower quadrant mass, including malignancy and Crohn's disease.

Thus, based on the available literature, it is generally accepted by most surgeons now that an appendiceal phlegmon can be managed with IV fluids and IV antibiotics, and a localized appendiceal abscess can be managed with CT- or US-guided percutaneous drainage. In most cases an appropriate clinical response can be achieved with resolution of abdominal pain and fever, and patients can be discharged. It is still controversial whether a delayed appendectomy is necessary.

Most patients after a conservatively treated appendiceal mass remain asymptomatic for the time of follow-up, although some develop a recurrence of appendicitis, requiring surgical intervention. Most studies report recurrence rates after resolution of an appendiceal mass as less than 20%, even with long-term follow-up. Most authors do not recommend routine appendectomy in all patients. Many surgeons advise against interval appendectomy in patients in whom operative risk is more significant than the 10% to 20% incidence of recurrent appendicitis.

Willemsen et al. performed a retrospective study involving 233 patients with appendiceal mass. At interval appendectomy, histologic examination showed a normal appendix without signs of previous inflammation in 30% of cases. Complications of interval appendectomy were observed in 18% of patients, including sepsis, bowel perforation, small bowel ileus, and various wound abscesses.

Obviously, in younger patients the lifetime risk of recurrent appendicitis is higher and the operative risk is lower. Therefore, most authors advocate interval appendectomy as a critical component of the conservative management of appendiceal mass in children.

The standard delay before interval appendectomy to allow the inflammatory changes to resolve is 6 to 10 weeks. In one study 15% of the patients in the delayed group had a recurrent acute episode during the waiting period. Despite the higher infection rate (17% versus 8%), the authors concluded that proceeding with appendectomy earlier may be safe and cost-effective.

Several studies addressed the effectiveness of a laparoscopic approach to interval appendectomy. Although laparoscopy provides visual inspection of the entire abdominal cavity, manipulation of tissues in the setting of postinflammatory changes can be technically challenging. Nguyen, Silen, et al. reviewed 56 patients treated conservatively for the periappendicular mass with interval appendectomy. There were no intraabdominal or wound infections after either open or laparoscopic appendectomy. There was no difference in operating time, but the hospital stay was much shorter in the laparoscopic group, with 59% of operations performed on an outpatient basis. Gibeily et al. reported that the laparoscopic approach was successful in 32 patients, with only 12% requiring elective conversion to an open procedure due to dense retrocecal fibrosis.

In conclusion, patients with periappendiceal masses generally improve with broad-spectrum antibiotics with or without percutaneous drainage. Available data on interval appendectomy may suggest that patients with lower operative risk, especially pediatric patients, should be considered for an interval procedure. The laparoscopic approach has been shown to be a safe alternative for interval appendectomy. If the risk of surgery is greater than the risk of recurrent appendicitis, and interval appendectomy is not chosen, then routine follow-up is necessary to rule out underlying malignancy.

# References

Alexander AA, Eschelman DJ, Nazarian LN, Bonn J. Transrectal sonographically guided drainage of deep pelvis abscesses. Am J. Roentgenol. 1994 May;162(5):1227–32.

Bagi P, Dueholm S. Nonoperative management of the ultrasonically evaluated appendiceal mass. Surgery 1987;101(5):602–605.

Bradley EL 3rd, Isaacs J. Appendiceal abscess revisited. Arch Surg 113:130–132, 1978.

Brown CV, Abrishami M, Muller M, Velmahos GC. Appendiceal abscess: immediate operation or percutaneous drainage? Am Surg. Oct; 69(10):829–32.

Carbonell AM, Burns JM, Lincourt AE, et al. Outcomes of laparoscopic versus open appendectomy. Am Surg 2004;70:759–765.

Ein SH, Shandling B. Is interval appendectomy necessary after rupture of an appendiceal mass? J Pediatr Surg. 1996 Jun;31(6):849–50.

Eriksson S, Granstrom L: Randomized controlled trial of appendicectomy versus antibiotic therapy for acute appendicitis. Br J Surg 1995;82:166–169.

Gahukamble DB, Gahukamble LD.: Surgical and pathological basis for interval appendicectomy after resolution of appendicular mass in children. J Pediatr Surg. 2000 Mar;35(3):424–7.

Gervais DA, Brown SD, Connolly SA, Brec SL, Harisinghani MG, Mueller PR. Percutaneous imaging-guided abdominal and pelvic abscess drainage in children. Radiographics 2004;24(3):737–754. Review.

Gibeily GJ, Ross MN, Manning DB, Wherry DC, Kao TC. Late-presenting appendicitis: a laparoscopic approach to a complicated problem. Surg Endosc 2003;17(5):725–729.

Gillick J, Velayudham M, Puri P. Conservative management of appendix mass in children. Br J Surg 2001;88:1539–1542.

Helmer KS, Robinson EK, Lally KP, et al. Standardized patient care guidelines reduce infectious morbidity in appendectomy patients. Am J Surg 183:2002;608–613.

Hoffman J, Lindhard A. Appendix mass: conservative management without interval appendectomy. Am J Surg 1984;148:379–382.

Jaffe TA, Nelson RC, Delong DM, Paulson EK. Practice patterns in percutaneous image-guided intraabdominal abscess drainage: survey of academic and private practice centers. Radiology. 2003 Feb;226(2):521–6.

Jamieson DH, Chait PG, Filler R. Interventional drainage of appendiceal abscesses in children. AJR Am J Roentgenol 1997;169(6):1619–1622.

Kaminksi A, Liu IA, Applebaum H, et al. Routine interval appendectomy is not justified after initial nonoperative treatment of acute appendicitis. Arch Surg 2005;140:897–901.

Katkhouda N, Friedlander MH, Grant SW, et al. Intraabdominal abscess rate after laparoscopic appendectomy. Am J Surg 2000;180:456–459.

Kouwenhoven EA, Repelear van Driel OJ, van Erp WFM. Fear for the intraabdominal abscess after laparoscopic appendectomy: not realistic. Surg Endosc 2005;19:923–926.

Nguyen DB, Silen W, Hodin RA. Interval appendectomy in the laparoscopic era. J Gastrointest Surg 1999 Mar–Apr;3(2):189–93.

Nguyen NT, Zainabadi K, Mavandadi S, et al. Trends in utilization and outcomes of laparoscopic versus open appendectomy. Am J Surg 2004;188(6):813–820.

Nitecki S, Assalia A, Schein M. Contemporary management of the appendiceal mass. Br J Surg 1993;80:18–20.

Marya SK, Garg P, Singh M, et al: Is long delay necessary before appendectomy after appendiceal formation? Can J Surg 1993;36:268–270.

Oliak D, Yamini D, Udani VM, Lewis JR, Arnell T, Vargas H, Stamos MJ. Initial nonoperative management for periappendical abscess. Dis Colon Rectum. 2001 Jul; 44(7):936–41.

Paull DL, Bloom GP. Appendiceal abscess. Arch Surg. 1982 Aug (8);117:1017–19.

Price MR, Haase GM, Sartorelli KH, Meagher DP Jr. Recurrent appendicitis after initial conservative management of appendiceal abscess.

Raptopoulos V, Katsou G, Rosen MP, Siewert B, Goldberg SN, Kruskal JB. Acute appendicitis: effect of increased use of CT on selecting patients earlier. Radiology 2003; 226(2):521–526.

Samuel M, Hosie G, Holmes K. Prospective evaluation of nonsurgical versus surgical management of appendiceal mass. J Pediatr Surg. 2002 Jun (6);37:882–6.

Skoubo-Kristensen E, Hvid I. The appendiceal mass. Ann surg 1982;196:584–587.

Thompson JE Jr, Bennion RS, Schmit PJ, Hiyama DT. Cecectomy for complicated appendicitis. J Am Coll Surg. 1994 Aug;179(2)135–8.

Riseman JA, Wichterman K. Evaluation of right hemicolectomy for unexpected cecal mass. Arch Surg. 1989 Sep;124(9):1043–4.

Tingstedt B, Bexe-Lindskog E, Ekelund M, Andersson R. Management of appendiceal masses. Eur J Surg 2002;168(11):579–582.

Willemsen PJ, Hoorntje LE, Eddes EH, Ploeg RJ. The need for interval appendectomy after resolution of an appendiceal mass questioned. Dig Surg 2002;19(3): 216–221.

Yamini D, Vargus H, Bongard F, Klein S, Stamos MJ. Perforated appencicitis: is it truly a surgical urgency? "Am Surg" 1998;64:970–975.

## Suggested Readings

Janik JS, Ein SH, Shandling B, Simpson JS, Stephens CA. Nonsurgical management of appendiceal mass in late presenting children. J Pediatr Surg 15:1980;574–576.

Jordan JS, Kovalcik PJ, Schwab CW: Appendicitis with a palpable mass. Ann Surg 1981. Feb;193(2):227–9.

Kapischke M, Caliebe A, Tepel J, et al. Open versus laparoscopic appendectomy: a critical review. Surg Endosc 2006;20:1060–1068.

Katkhouda N, Mason JR, Towfigh S, et al. Laparoscopic versus open appendectomy: a prospective randomized double-blinded study. Ann Surg 2005;242(3):439–450.

Lewin J, Fenyo G, Engstrom L. Treatment of appendiceal abscess. Acta Chir Scand 1988;154:123–125.

Mazziotti MV, Marley EF, Winthrop AL, et al. Histopathologic analysis of interval appendectomy specimens: support for the role of interval appendectomy. J Pediatr Surg 1997;32:806–809.

Sauerland S, Lefering R, Neugebauer EA. Laparoscopic versus open surgery for suspected appendicitis. Cochrane Database Systematic Review 2002;1:CD001546.

Sunil K, Sundeep J. Treatment of appendiceal mass: Prospective, randomized clinical trial. Indian J Gastroenterol 2004;23:165–167.

# 27. Large Bowel Obstruction Due to Carcinoma of the Rectum

## A. Introduction

Neoadjuvant radiation and chemotherapy are frequently employed for locally advanced rectal cancer. When the tumor is obstructing or near-obstructing, some sort of decompressive strategy is needed. Open colostomy was, for many years, the standard approach. Two minimal-access techniques of endoluminal stenting and laparoscopic colostomy have emerged and are explored in this chapter.

## B. Case

### Dionne Skeete

A 67-year-old man presented with a 1-month history of bright red blood per rectum, slightly formed liquid stools, and rectal pain. He had lost 30 pounds in 2 months despite a normal appetite. He also complained of increased passage of mucus per rectum over the past 2 months. He denied abdominal pain, bloating, nausea, emesis, dysuria, and hematuria.

He had a history of chest pain in 1972 with normal cardiac catheterization. His past medical history was otherwise negative. He had no previous surgery. His only medications were ibuprofen as needed for musculoskeletal pains. He had no allergies.

He was a retired iron worker, married, with three adult children. He had a 50-pack-a-year tobacco history, having stopped smoking 5 years ago. He consumed one six-pack of beer per week.

His mother died in her 70s from colon cancer. His father died at age 57 from a myocardial infarction, and one sister had coronary artery bypass surgery. The review of systems was otherwise negative.

Physical examination revealed a somewhat cachectic male. His height was 163 cm, and he weighed 58 kg. His pulse was 89 and his blood pressure was 134/69. Abdominal examination was negative for masses or tenderness. Rectal examination revealed a palpable rectal mass with gross blood. The remainder of the physical examination was normal.

Laboratories were significant for a hemoglobin of 11.5 g/dL and a hematocrit of 38%. Coagulation studies were normal. Carcinoembryonic antigen (CEA) was 1.5 ng/mL.

Rigid sigmoidoscopy showed an ulcerated friable fungating mass at 10 cm from the anal verge. The mass appeared to obstruct the lumen. Biopsy of the mass revealed moderately differentiated adeno-carcinoma.

A computed tomography (CT) scan of the abdomen and pelvis showed a 7.8 × 10 cm heterogeneous mass in the rectum with multiple small adjacent lymph nodes and presacral fat stranding, but no evidence of metastatic disease (Figs. 27.1 and 27.2). Chest x-ray was negative for metastatic disease.

**Which would you recommend for this patient with nearly obstructing rectal cancer: endoluminal stenting or laparoscopic colostomy?**

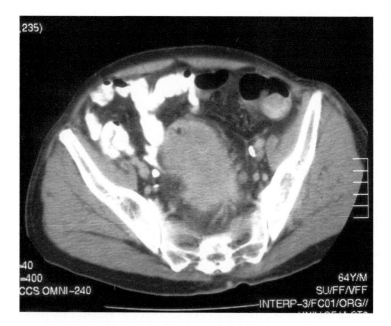

Fig. 27.1. Computed tomography (CT) scan showing rectal tumor with impinge-ment of colonic lumen.

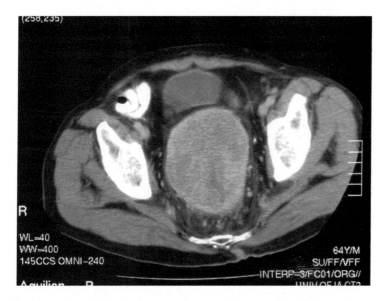

Fig. 27.2. CT scan showing large rectal mass with adjacent lymphadenopathy.

# C. Endoscopic Endoluminal Stenting

## *Maged Rizk and Henning Gerke*

We would place an endoluminal stent. Most malignant large bowel obstructions are due to masses on the left side of the colon, because the fecal material is more solid in the left side than the right. Acute colonic obstruction is an emergency that requires prompt attention because it can lead to electrolyte abnormalities, sepsis, and perforation. The surgical approach to colonic obstruction is to create a temporal diverting colostomy until a more definitive procedure can be performed at a later date. Because these patients are typically older and have medical comorbidities, there is an increased risk of complications, whether this is done by the traditional open or the newer laparoscopic technique.

Different nonsurgical modalities have been employed in the decompression of large bowel malignant obstructions. Among these are dilation, neodymium:yttrium-aluminum-garnet (Nd:YAG) laser ablation, electrocoagulation, cryotherapy, and photodynamic therapy. These methods may be effective in alleviating a malignant obstruction, but require repeated treatments, which are costly and time-consuming.

Restoration of luminal patency can also be achieved with self-expanding metal stents (SEMS). The current indications for colorectal stents are palliation of malignant colonic obstruction in patients who are not operative candidates, and preoperative decompression and adequate bowel preparation for a subsequent one-stage surgical procedure.

The SEMS are composed of a variety of metal alloys with varying shapes and sizes depending on the manufacturer. After deployment, the stent incorporates deep into the wall of the colon, causing a localized reaction that anchors the stent and helps to prevent subsequent dislocation. Rectal stents can be either coated or uncoated. Uncoated stents are usually preferred because of the lower risk of stent migration. Colonic SEMS can be placed using fluoroscopic guidance alone, endoscopic guidance alone, or a combination of endoscopic and fluoroscopic guidance. Stents with small-diameter introducer systems allow placement through the working channel of the endoscope. Other stents must be positioned over a guidewire that is placed endoscopically or under fluoroscopic guidance. The endoscope can be reinserted next to the guidewire to aid in positioning of the stent by direct endoscopic visualization.

Complications of stent placement include the following:

1.  Perforation (5–30%) from mucosal irritation, tumor friability, or pressure necrosis of the stent into the colonic mucosa
2.  Stent migration (10–50%), in which the stent may pass spontaneously, or require endoscopic removal
3.  Bleeding due to local wall irritation (12.5–50%)
4.  Pain (6.3–25%), typically from mucosal irritation and irritation of nerve endings at the squamocolumnar junction, which is usually mild, lasting for 3 to 5 days
5.  Occlusion (7–10%) from impaction of stool, or tumor ingrowth or overgrowth within a median time of 24 weeks in a pooled analysis

A barium enema may be helpful in defining the exact anatomy of the stricture prior to stent placement. However, there are other techniques including periprocedural injection of water-soluble contrast and direct measurement of the stricture length using a balloon catheter during the procedure.

In the case presented here, the patient is a relatively healthy man without substantial comorbidities. He has no evidence of metastases, thus the goal of surgical intervention should be for cure, which preoperative stenting may facilitate by allowing a single-stage surgical approach. Mainar et al. performed a multicenter retrospective review of preoperative stenting in 71 patients with malignant obstruction. Technical success in placing the stent was achieved in 90% of patients, with clinical improvement and resolution of the obstruction in 93% of patients within 96 hours. Sixty-five of these patients underwent elective single-stage surgery with a primary anastomosis a mean of 8.6 days later. There were no major complications. In another multicenter prospective randomized study comparing three different stent types, 26 patients underwent 31 stent placements with a technical success rate of 97%, and achieved clinical success as defined by successful palliation or ability to proceed with a single-stage procedure in 80%. In the preoperative group, 11 stents were placed in 10 patients. Bowel preparation was successful in all patients, and surgery was performed between 2 and 9 days after stent insertion.

Another study compared the outcome of patients undergoing placement of SEMS for relief of acute left-sided bowel obstruction followed by elective resection with the outcome of patients undergoing surgical intervention alone. In this study, 41 of 43 patients who were treated with colonic SEMS had alleviation of their symptoms, with 17 of these patients found to have unresectable disease after pre- or intraoperative staging; 22 of the 26 remaining patients were able to undergo primary anastomosis (85% vs. 41% in the surgical group). There was a decrease in total hospital days, days spent in the intensive care unit, and number of surgical procedures. Although the study was prospective, it was not randomized, with SEMS done in patients who presented with symptoms during radiology working hours, and surgical intervention alone done in patients who presented during the weekend, resulting in a greater number of patients in the SEMS group. Tumor stage using the Dukes criteria, tumor location, patient demographics, and comorbidities were similar in both groups.

The patient under discussion here has a rectal adenocarcinoma 10 cm from the anal verge. An abdominal CT and chest radiograph show no evidence of metastases. Placement of a rectal stent to alleviate the near-complete rectal obstruction is feasible and should be considered in this patient (Fig. 27.3). The above studies suggest that preoperative stent placement obviates the need for a second surgical procedure and decreases hospital stay and cost. However, stent placement followed by one-stage surgery has not been shown to reduce mortality compared to staged surgical resection. As for rectal stent placement with concomitant neoadjuvant chemoradiation, there is a paucity of literature on the topic. Aside from one case study in which no complications were reported (Adler et al.), no studies are currently available evaluating efficacy and complication rates. However, we believe that this is a viable option and may

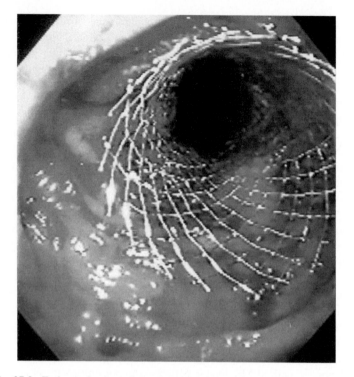

Fig. 27.3. Endoscopic view of rectal metal stent placed for a tumor stricture.

be considered in patients with a local tumor stage greater than T2 or perirectal lymph node involvement (N1) as in the presented patient.

# D. Laparoscopic Colostomy

*Manjula Jeyapalan*

This patient presented with moderately differentiated adenocarcinoma of the rectum. Workup has revealed an ulcerated rectal mass obstructing the lumen with multiple adjacent lymph nodes but no evidence of other metastases. He is under consideration for neoadjuvant therapy, but decompression is needed before therapy can begin to avoid complete obstruction during therapy. I would perform a laparoscopic colostomy. This patient is, I believe, an ideal candidate for this approach. He does not have prior abdominal surgery and his overall health is good, thus the risk of anesthesia and surgery should be minimal. The CT scan and chest x-ray do not show evidence of metastatic disease, but the laparoscopic approach may visualize tiny nodules on the peritoneal surface or liver, allowing more accurate staging. Any suspicious masses can be biopsied. If liver biopsy is required in a patient with known metastatic disease, biopsy can be done at the time of the procedure. Hemostasis is easily and securely obtained with electrocautery.

Olivieri et al. reported that laparoscopic colostomy is feasible in patients who have had prior abdominal surgery, but that operative times may be longer than in patients with virgin abdomens. The colon is easily mobilized laparoscopically; splenic flexure mobilization can be performed if necessary, and the condition of the proximal bowel easily assessed. Extensive intraabdominal metastatic disease, not present in this patient, may render this more difficult.

Laparoscopic colostomy formation involves less manipulation of tissues than the corresponding open procedure, and hence subsequent surgery is facilitated. The small incision facilitates recovery and speeds the time to the next phase of treatment, which, in the case presented, would be neoadjuvant chemotherapy.

I prefer to mobilize the colon as needed laparoscopically. I then identify the limb of bowel to mature and place a Babcock clamp on it, bringing it through the port site where I plan to mature the stoma. This technique is described in the SAGES manual (Mancino). It is easy to ensure that the limb reaches without excessive tension, and that it is not twisted. The abdomen is then desufflated and the stoma matured in the usual fashion.

# E. Conclusions

## *Dionne Skeete*

The traditional management of obstructing rectal cancers involved fecal diversion due to concerns of inadequate bowel preparation and technical issues given low pelvic anastomosis with thin dilated proximal large bowel. After recovery from the initial surgery, patients would undergo definitive resection or a course of neoadjuvant chemotherapy and radiation therapy followed by definitive surgical resection if initial staging revealed significant wall invasion or local lymphadenopathy.

With the development of minimally invasive techniques, laparoscopic stoma creation and colonic stenting have become reasonable alternatives to the traditional open operation.

Laparoscopy offers several advantages to an open approach. Laparoscopy can be used as a staging procedure as careful inspection of the peritoneal, serosal, and hepatic surfaces can be performed. Biopsies can be performed to rule out metastatic disease of suspicious lesions and lymph nodes seen on preoperative imaging. In addition, laparoscopy can allow for careful selection of the stoma site with mobilization of the colon as needed. There is limited handling of the intestines, which could potentially lead to earlier return of bowel function and decreased postoperative recovery. Limitations to laparoscopy include previous abdominal surgeries, obesity, and ascites, while complications include trocar injuries, stoma retraction, and incorrect maturation of the distal limb, parastomal abscess, and bleeding. Lui et al., in a review 80 patients undergoing laparoscopic stoma creation for fecal diversion at a single institution, reported a conversion rate of 1.3% with no procedure related mortality. There was an overall morbidity rate of 11.4% with six patients requiring reoperation for small bowel obstruction (two patients), parastomal abscess (one), port-site hernia (one), stoma retraction (one), and hemorrhage (one).

Colonic stenting was first described by Dohmoto and appears to gaining popularity as a treatment option in patients with obstructing lesions. Emergent surgery can be avoided, especially in the patient who is medically fragile and at high risk in surgery. Therefore, elective resection and primary anastomosis can be performed after resolution of bowel obstruction, completely avoiding the need for stoma creation. In addition, the stent can provide adequate palliation for patients with metastatic disease. Unfortunately, colonic stenting requires the availability of physicians with specialized training, and though the stent may be able to be deployed, clinical success is not always assured. Watson et al. performed a retrospective review of a single institution's experience with colonic stents, showing a 93% (100/107) technically successful stent deployment rate, with 97% of the patients having clinical relief from obstruction. There was a 9% complication rate including four stent migrations, three occlusions, and two perforations.

The management of obstructing rectal cancer depends on patient condition and status of disease, and institutional experience with less invasive techniques versus traditional approaches. The question remains what method of diversion is safest for the patient with the lowest morbidity and mortality, and what method is the most cost-effective. Targownik et al.

performed a decision analysis on a hypothetical patient with colonic malignancy–related obstruction. They concluded that stenting followed by definitive surgery was more cost-effective, required fewer operative procedures per patient, and had a lower procedure mortality than emergent surgery with a Hartmann's procedure or complete resection and anastomosis. To definitively answer this question, a prospective randomized controlled trial needs to be performed comparing the less invasive techniques of laparoscopic stoma creation and colonic stenting.

# References

Adler DG, Young-Fadok TM, Smyrk T, Garces YI, Baron TH. Preoperative chemoradiation therapy after placement of a self-expanding metal stent in a patient with an obstructing rectal cancer: clinical and pathologic findings. Gastrointest Endosc 2002;55:435–437.

Dohmoto M, Hünerbein M, Schlag PM. Palliative endoscopic therapy of rectal carcinoma. Eur J Cancer 1996;32A(1):25–29.

Lui J, Bruch HP, Farke S, Nolde J, Scwander O. Stoma formation for fecal diversion: a plea for the laparoscopic approach. Tech Coloproctol 2005;9(1):9–14.

Mainar A, Ariza MADG, Tejero E, et al. Acute colorectal obstruction treatment with self-expandable metallic stents before scheduled surgery and in palliation. Radiology 2000;216:492–497.

Mancino AT. Laparoscopic colostomy. In: Scott-Conner CEH, ed. The SAGES Manual: Fundamentals of Laparoscopy, Thoracoscopy, and GI Endoscopy, 2nd ed. New York: Springer-Verlag, 2006:357–361.

Targownik, L, Spegiel M, Sack J, et al. Colonic stent vs. emergency surgery for management of acute left sided malignant colonic obstruction: a decision analysis. Gastrointest Endosc 2004;60(4):865–873.

Watson A, Shanmugan V, Mackay I, et al. Outcomes after placement of colorectal stents. Colorectal Dis 2005;7:70–73.

# Suggested Readings

Fielding LP, Wells BW. Survival after primary and after staged resection for large bowel obstruction caused by cancer. Br J Surg 1974;61;16.

Fuhrman GM, Ota DM. Laparoscopic intestinal stomas. Dis Colon Rectum 1994;37(5):444–449.

Hallfeldt K, Schmidbauer S, Trupka A. Laparoscopic loop colostomy for advanced ovarian cancer, rectal cancer and recovaginal fistulas. Gynecol Oncol 2000;76:380–382.

Kang SG, Jung GS, Cho SG, Kim JG, Oh JH, Song HY, Kim ES. The efficacy of metallic stent placement in the treatment of colorectal obstruction. Korean J Radiol 2002;3(2):79–86.

Ludwig, KA, Milsom,JW, Garcia-Ruiz A, Fazio VW. Laparoscopic techniques for fecal diversion. Dis Colon Rectum 1996;39(3):285–288.

Martinez-Santos C, Lobato RF, Fradejas JM, Pinto I, Ortega-Deballon P, Moreno-Azcoita M. Self-expandable stent before elective surgery vs. emergency surgery for the treatment of malignant colorectal obstructions: comparison of primary anastomosis and morbidity rates. Dis Colon Rectum 2002;45(3):401–406.

Oliveira L, Reissman P, Nogueras J, Wexner S, Laparoscopic creation of stomas. Surg Endosc 1997;11:19–23.

Price AL, Rubio PA. Laparoscopic colorectal surgery: a challenge for ET nurses. J Wound Ostomy Continence Nurs 1994;21(5):179–182.

Roe AM, Barlow AP, Durdey P, Eltringham WK, Espiner HJ. Indications for laparoscopic formation of intestinal stomas. Surg Laparosc Endosc 1994;4(5):345–347.

Schwandner O, Schiedeck THK, Bruch HP. Stoma creation for fecal diversion: is the laparoscopic technique appropriate? Int J Colorect Dis 1998;13:251–255.

Sebastian S, Johnston S, Geoghegan T, et al. Pooled analysis of the efficacy and safety of self-expanding metal stenting in malignant colorectal obstruction. Am J Gastroenterol 2004;99:2051.

Seymour K, Johnson R, Marsh R, et al. Palliative stenting of malignant large bowel obstruction. Colorectal Dis 2002;4:240–245.

Spinelli P, Mancini A. Use of self-expanding metal stents for palliation of rectosigmoid cancer. Gastrointest Endosc 2001;53(2):203–206.

# 28. Carcinoma of the Cecum

## A. Introduction

For surgeons accustomed to performing right hemicolectomy through a small right transverse incision, the benefits of a laparoscopic approach to the right colon are not obvious. Such an approach requires an incision to deliver the specimen and to perform the anastomosis. This chapter explores the pros and cons of the minimal-access approach to this diagnosis, and gives tips for success with either technique.

## B. Case

*José E. Torres*

A 50-year-old woman began experiencing left-sided, cramping abdominal pain with a bout of diarrhea 2 months before seeking medical attention. Her initial episode resolved after 1 week, but the problem recurred, becoming nearly constant over the past several weeks. Colonoscopy revealed a nearly obstructing fungating mass at the cecum. Biopsies demonstrated moderately differentiated adenocarcinoma. The patient was referred for surgical evaluation.

Her past medical history was significant for fibromyalgia, depression, melanoma, and chronic neck pain. Her past surgical history included resection of a Clark's level I melanoma from the right leg in 1994, cervical fusion of C3 and C4 in 1995, and a laparoscopic left ovarian cyst removal in 1999. Her mother died at age 60 from throat cancer, and her father died from a myocardial infarction at age 84. One brother with ulcerative colitis underwent total proctocolectomy at age 30 and died at age 44.

The patient was on no medications and had no allergies. She was single, with two children. She was a recovering alcoholic and had stopped smoking in 1973. The review of systems was otherwise negative.

Physical examination revealed a slender pale woman, alert and oriented, in no acute distress. Pulse was 110, temperature 36.8 °C, respiratory rate 22, and blood pressure 126/69. She was 5 feet 4 inches in height and weighed 63 kilograms.

Her abdomen was soft and slightly distended, with active bowel sounds and diffuse tenderness greatest in the right lower quadrant; there were no masses. She had well-healed laparoscopy scars and no hernias. Rectal examination revealed no masses; brown stool was guaiac positive.

Chest x-ray was normal. A computed tomography (CT) scan of abdomen and pelvis demonstrated cecal carcinoma with lymphadenopathy, without evidence of liver metastases.

The impression was a 50-year-old woman with carcinoma of the cecum. Right colon resection was recommended.

**The patient asks if this can be done laparoscopically. What would you recommend?**

# C.  Laparoscopic-Assisted Right Colectomy

*James N. Lau and Sherry M. Wren*

We would recommend laparoscopic-assisted right hemicolectomy for this patient. Laparoscopic-assisted colectomy (LAC) has finally stepped from the shadows into the spotlight for the resection of non-metastatic colon cancer. Since the first use of minimally invasive surgical techniques for colectomy in 1991, there has been a fierce debate concerning the safety, utility, and ethics of laparoscopy for the treatment of malignant disease. Following years of retrospective analysis and single-institution experiences, there are now data from large multiinstitutional prospective randomized controlled trials (RCTs) that justify and even recommend LAC as the preferred method of addressing malignant colon lesions. This is the result of a coordinated effort by the American Society of Colon and Rectal Surgeons to organize prospective data collection of LAC for colon cancer after the initial disturbing reports of increased port-site recurrences. What has been important in the validation of LAC has been reproducible data showing that LAC is as safe and efficacious as open surgery (OS), and with equal or better long-term oncologic results. The apparent superior short-term results of the minimally invasive technique are why it should be the preferred method for colon resection of nonmetastatic disease. The Clinical Outcomes of Surgery Therapy Study Group of the Laparoscopic Colectomy (COST) trial is the groundbreaking multicenter prospective RCT that has legitimized laparoscopic colectomy over open surgery for colon cancer treatment.

In the early experience with LAC, more than 35 cases of port-site metastases were reported within a 2-year span. The true incidence was unknown, and despite the poor quality of the data at the time, it seemed that laparoscopic management of colon cancer compromised oncologic control. Since that time, there have been good single-center randomized trials and a multicenter prospective RCT that have definitively shown that there is not an increased wound implant rate following LAC over OS. Lacy, Delgado, et al., in a single center randomized trial, reported one port site recurrence in 106 LACs versus none from 102 open colectomies. The COST analysis, in which 872 patients were randomized to LAC or OS for cancer, reported only two patients with port recurrences (0.5%) in the laparoscopic arm while there was only one for the open arm (0.2% after a median follow-up of 4.4 years).

Safety can also be measured by the complications associated with a procedure. Reza et al., in a meta-analysis of RCTs from the years 2000 to 2005, report that seven of the analyzed RCTs examined complication rates and found no significant differences with respect to preoperative or postoperative morbidity. Lacy, Garcia, et al. reported 12/111 complications in patients treated with LAC compared with 31/108 in those who had OS, with wound infection and ileus more frequent with OS. The COST study verified what other studies have shown. The 30-day mortality of 428 undergoing LAC was four patients (1%), with one patient dying (of 435, <1%) in the OS group. The overall complication rate was 85/428 (20%) in the LAC arm with 92 (of 435, 21%) in the open arm.

The initial concern regarding port-site/wound recurrences has been proven to be unjustified in well-organized subsequent analyses. The perioperative mortality and morbidity are no different with LAC and OS. Therefore, minimally invasive colon resection is as safe to perform in patients with colon cancer as with open surgery.

In addition, demonstration that LAC and OS possess no difference in quality of oncologic resection refutes the unjustified technical concerns of adequacy of resection with LAC. The goals of an adequate oncologic resection involve appropriate vessel ligation, adequate resection with a minimum of 5 cm proximal and distal resection margins, and radical mesenteric lymphadenectomy (≥12 lymph nodes). Lacy, Garcia, et al.'s single institution experience yielded an average of 11 lymph nodes in the resected specimens in each arm of their study. In the COST study, the median number of recovered lymph nodes were 12 in both arms and the incidence of longitudinal resection margins <5 cm were 5% and 6% between the LAC and OS arms, respectively. Thus there appears to be no appreciable difference in oncologic outcomes between laparoscopic and open surgeries for cancer.

Until recently, there were no definitive data on intermediate or long-term outcomes of laparoscopic colon resections. These outcomes are best defined by tumor recurrence, disease-free survival, and overall survival. Most of the comparative studies published in the past showed the promise of no difference in long-term outcomes, and case series have found recurrence and survival data similar between LAC an OS. However, Lacy, Garcia, et al. published one of the first landmark RCTs at a single institution. Their median length of follow-up was 43 months. Their findings, when analyzed with the intention to treat, showed no significant difference in overall mortality, but the rates of cancer-related mortality favored the laparoscopic approach (9% for laparoscopic vs. 21% for open surgery). When analyzed by procedure actually performed and by cancer stage, the authors demonstrated that the probability of being free of recurrence, the overall survival, and the cancer-related survival in stage III tumors were superior in the laparoscopic colectomies (freedom from recurrence, $p = .04$; overall survival, $p = .02$; cancer-related survival, $p = .006$). Despite this report, LAC has only recently become an acceptable alternative to open colectomy following the report by the COST study. This analysis contained a larger sample, with multiple institutions, and with a median follow-up of 4.4 years. Of their 872 patients, 160 had a recurrence of their tumor (84 in the OS group and 76 in the LAC group), and 77 patients died before the tumor recurred (34 in OS and 43 in LAC). This indicates no advantage of open resection to laparoscopic colon surgery with respect to tumor recurrence. The estimated difference in the 3-year recurrence-free survival was 2.4 percentage points in favor of the laparoscopic surgery group. The overall survival and the disease-free survival were similar in the two groups. The absence of a difference in the time to recurrence, disease-free survival, and overall survival persisted in their multivariate analyses. This more comprehensive study refuted any advantages to LAC in stage III tumors previously seen in the study by Lacy, Garcia, et al. More than any other trial, the COST trial has indicated that there is no long-term difference in cancer outcomes between laparoscopic and open surgeries.

With safety, efficacy, and intermediate and long-term outcomes deemed equal with laparoscopic colon resection versus open resections, it is the short-term outcomes and the hint of improved quality of life with LAC that make it the overall preferred method of resection. Like other minimally invasive surgical procedures, LAC offers the benefits to the patient of a shorter length of stay in the hospital, less postoperative pain (in and out of the hospital), and quicker recovery of bowel function. Laparoscopic-assisted colectomy also offers the potential of a better short-term quality of life (QOL). Numerous studies have shown that while LAC had longer operative times, it was associated with less blood loss. The COST trial also possessed a QOL component published by Weeks et al. Their clinical outcomes validated previous studies by showing a shorter stay in the hospital with LAC (5.1 days vs. 6.4 days in the open arm) and less oral analgesic and parenteral narcotic/analgesic use (1.7 and 2.8 days, respectively, in LAC vs. 2.2 and 4.0 days, respectively, in the open group). However, those in the laparoscopic group who were converted to open (25.7%) had a longer hospital stay (6.5 days) and more oral analgesic and parenteral narcotic use (2.3 and 4.4 days, respectively) than both the true LAC and OS groups. Lacy, Garcia, et al. used a strict postoperative protocol and demonstrated a faster initiation of peristalsis and oral intake with those undergoing laparoscopic colectomy. Although Weeks et al. were able to show a significant difference in the number of days of oral and parenteral analgesia requirements, they did not find any significant differences in the QOL indices at 2 days, 2 weeks, and 2 months postoperatively, except for the global rating scale at 2 weeks in favor of the laparoscopic group.

Two issues warrant additional discussion. First, the conversion rate to open resection is 20% to 26%; second, the procedure should be performed in a stepwise, proctored fashion. The COST analysis reported the conversion rate of those intended for LAC and OS to be 26%; 7% of all patients intended for LAC required conversion due to tumor-related concerns (advanced disease). There were no differences in conversion rates between surgeons in their analysis as well as between those in the beginning of the trial and those at the end. All surgeons performing LAC in the COST trial were subject to quality control. Each surgeon had performed at least 20 LACs and submitted a videotape to be reviewed for oncologic technique, including vessel ligation, tumor handling, and thoroughness of exploration. The point of this discussion is that all the results arguing for an advantage to LAC are generated by qualified surgeons.

How do we ensure ourselves that we are qualified to perform LAC for colon cancer? There are some who believe that the initial high rates of wound implants from LAC were due to a lack of experience. Young-Fadok states, in her defense of the position that performance of LAC be in clinical trails only, that the lowering of these initially high rates of port recurrences came with the insistence of the surgical societies that LAC be performed only in trials. In this way, LAC was performed by those with experience or by those proctored by those with experience.

Since the compelling data of trials like the COST study, those without prior experience of LAC should gain this experience from courses at major societies, performing 30 procedures on benign disease, and by being proctored for these initial cases.

The goal in performing a right colectomy laparoscopically should always be to provide an adequate oncologic resection. Prior tissue diagnosis when possible is requisite, and if the area has been previously marked, then one may forgo colonoscopy and India ink identification of the tumor at the same venue. If intraoperative colonoscopy if performed, intestinal insufflation must be kept to a minimum lest the subsequent resection become more challenging. The patient must be strapped and padded in order to prepare for changing the position of the operating table. Both arms should be tucked and the monitor placed on the patient's right to provide the best working space and best view for the operating surgeon.

The abdomen is insufflated and the trocars (with or without a hand-assist device) placed in a fashion as to facilitate hepatic flexure takedown and ileocolic ligation. Inspection of the abdomen for carcinomatosis or distant metastasis should precede resection. Exposure of the mesenteric root is the key to an acceptable oncologic resection. The ileocolic and right colic vessels (if present) should be exposed in a window fashion prior to ligation and transection. Vessel ligation should be done prior to manipulation of the colon to comply with proper oncologic technique. The duodenum should be identified and protected during mesenteric mobilization and transection with the ligature device or other device.

After vascular division the colon can be mobilized. Exposure is enhanced by placing the table in the Trendelenburg right-side-up position. As mobilization of the ascending colon proceeds toward the hepatic flexure, the table should be gradually shifted to the reverse Trendelenburg position. The gastrocolic ligament is then taken down from the lateral to medial direction.

The devascularized and fully mobilized colonic segment can be exteriorized easily through a small incision (transverse right upper quadrant, periumbilical, or upper midline) after final mobilization of the colon off the retroperitoneum. The distal ileum and colon can be pulled through the incision with wound protection, and an extracorporeal anastomosis can be performed using the standard open technique. The bowel is then returned into the abdomen, the operative site inspected (some authors recommend irrigation with dilute Betadine saline solution to help prevent possible implantation), and then the fascia is closed. The mesenteric defect is closed at the surgeon's discretion.

Resection of the colon for nonmetastatic colon cancer should now be performed laparoscopically. The short-term outcomes of lower intraoperative blood loss, shorter hospital stays with a quicker return of bowel function, and significantly less need for oral and parenteral analgesics are convincing arguments in favor of LAC. The absence of any difference in safety, oncologic resectability, or short- and long-term outcomes between LAC and OS make LAC the preferred method in addressing colon cancer.

# D.  Open Right Colon Resection

## *Tzu-Chi Hsu*

I would offer this patient mini-incision open right hemicolectomy. Laparoscopy has been used as a treatment modality in various intraabdominal diseases following the success of laparoscopic cholecystectomy. Laparoscopic colectomy, without proven advantages and with unproven disadvantages, and partly commercially driven, has also been advocated as a treatment of choice for various colon and rectal diseases. However, there are still debates as to whether laparoscopic surgery is suitable for every type of colorectal disease and whether it is potentially harmful to some patients.

One advantage frequently mentioned by proponents of laparoscopy is the smaller incision size with a better cosmetic result. Surgeons using laparoscope only measure the largest incision, which is the incision used to remove the specimen. It is at least about 4 to 5 cm in length, sometimes even larger if the tumor or the specimen is bigger. In practice, an additional three to five incisions for trocars, with an average size of 1 cm each, are needed for a successful laparoscopic colectomy. This means that the overall length of incision would be the sum of the above and up to at least 7 to 10 cm. I have reported a series of 316 patients and have demonstrated that most colectomies, even radical resections, can be accomplished with an incision less than 7 cm without increased morbidity and mortality with good oncological resection, supported by an average number of more than 16 lymph nodes in the specimen. While it might be argued that only thin patients are suitable for mini-incision colectomies, we had reported mini-incision colectomies in obese patients with a body mass index (BMI) up to 38.

One additional reason to make this incision up to 6 to 7 cm is to allow adequate palpation of the intraabdominal organ with the hands, without losing tactile sensation. One is thus less likely to miss any synchronous intraabdominal pathology, which has frequently been found by me and reported in the literature. To accomplish a colectomy through a small incision, one should focus on and expose one area and ignore other areas while doing surgery. An analogy would be to concentrate on an individual word, phrase, or paragraph during reading.

Some proponents for laparoscope surgery claimed that laparoscopic surgery is less painful. I believe that the degree of pain is related to the length of the incision; smaller incisions are less painful. Patients who underwent laparoscopic surgery report that the pain is not entirely from the incision removing the specimen; the incision created for trocars, especially one for the trocar through the rectus muscle, is also painful. These realities are contrary to the general belief that laparoscopic surgery is painless. Since the mini-incision is actually not any longer than the laparoscopic colectomy, certainly it will be less painful than a regular 15-cm open colectomy incision and comparable to a laparoscopic surgical incision.

Proponents for laparoscopic colectomy also claimed that patients could be fed earlier following laparoscopic than open colectomy. A literature review suggests that this is not necessarily so. I also found 75% of patients who had an open colectomy could well tolerate feeding beginning from the second postoperative day. So, with mini-incision colectomy, it is simply a matter of when the surgeon wishes to feed the patient.

There is also an argument that the patients could be discharged earlier following laparoscopic than open colectomy. The timing of discharge is influenced by many factors. Many reports showed that there was no difference between laparoscopic and open colectomy groups.

Although it is still controversial, opponents of laparoscopic colectomy claim that cancer spread caused by pneumoperitoneum is possible. An open colectomy, especially mini-incision colectomy, will avoid this potential danger caused by pneumoperitoneum.

Once the procedure is perfected, mini-incision colectomy is less expensive, quicker, and less cumbersome. It does not require additional equipment such as laparoscope, ultrasonic shears, or Ligashear device.

My study suggests that the majority of colectomies can be accomplished by an incision less than 7 cm, no larger than the incision used in laparoscopic colectomy when multiple incisions made for trocars are added to the main incision length. The advantages of this mini-incision approach include lower cost, faster completion of procedure, reduced bulkiness of equipment, and the possibility of manually exploring the entire peritoneal cavity, thus taking advantage of tactile sensation. Table 28.1 compares the laparoscopic and mini-incision colectomies.

Table 28.1. Comparison of laparoscopic and mini-incision colectomy.

|  | Laparoscopy | Mini-incision |
|---|---|---|
| Feasibility | Feasible | Feasible |
| Cost | Expensive | Cheaper |
| Time spent | Longer | Shorter |
| Cumbersome | More | Less |
| Tactile sensation | Lost | Remain |
| Missing lesions | Likely | Less likely |
| Hazards of pneumoperitoneum | Yes | No |
| Spreading cancer by pneumoperitoneum | Likely | Less likely |
| Oncology result | Adequate(?) | Adequate |
| Local recurrence | Trocar site | Incision site |
| Size of incision | Smaller (?) | Similar |
| Pain | Less (?) | Similar |
| Feeding | Earlier (?) | No delay |
| Discharge | Earlier (?) | No delay |
| Limited by obesity | Possible | No limitation |
| Limited by tumor size | Possible | No limitation |
| Limited by tumor stage | Possible | No limitation |

# E. Conclusions

## José E. Torres

Colorectal carcinomas are one of the few malignancies that can be effectively cured if the surgical technique and approach are meticulous and the surgical oncologic principles are maintained. These principles include (1) attainment of adequate surgical margins and the removal of adjacent tissue and draining regional lymph nodes, (2) avoidance of tumor spillage, and (3) minimal surgical manipulation of the tumor. The use of laparoscopy in the treatment of colorectal tumors has been an issue of controversy. A moratorium on laparoscopic colon resections (LCRs) was agreed upon in 1994 when surgeons agreed that LCRs should be carried out only by surgeons participating in clinical trials. Critics raised questions: Was the adequacy of oncologic resection similar between open and laparoscopic colon resection? Were patterns of tumor dissemination altered by LCR techniques? Are the long-term survival rates similar between both types of surgery?

The indications for laparoscopically assisted colectomy are identical to those for open colon resection (OCR). Contraindications include metastatic disease and previous abdominal surgeries. The surgical procedure includes the placement of the laparoscopic ports for the dissecting instruments and the placement of the laparoscope. The surgeon explores the entire abdomen prior to beginning the dissection. Mesenteric resection and colon mobilization are performed with electrocautery or ultrasonic shears. The tumor and adjacent tissue are then removed in an endobag via a mini-laparotomy incision, which usually measures less than 7 cm. The anastomosis is then performed extracorporeally.

The complications of LCR are identical to those that occur during OCR, with the most serious being anastomotic leaks, bleeding, and wound infections.

Several studies have confirmed the advantages of LCR over OCR. Among these advantages are increased colonic motility, which leads to earlier initiation of oral feeds, decreased postoperative pain, decreased surgical site infections, and decreased blood transfusion requirements. The major disadvantages of LCR when compared to OCR are that LCR is significantly more expensive and requires increased operative times, but the financial disadvantages appear to be counterbalanced by the quicker recovery rates and earlier return to work, and the operative times decrease as surgeon experience with the procedures increase.

Several randomized control trials have been undertaken to answer these questions. With respect to adequacy of oncologic resection, Leung et al. published the results of a prospective randomized trial that demonstrated that the distal margins obtained and adequacy of lymph node resection were no different between the OCR and LCR groups. The Clinical Outcomes of Surgical Therapy Study Group, a multiinstitutional study and a randomized control trial by Lacy, Garcia, et al., demonstrated that the rates of recurrence, intraoperative complications, postoperative complications, and overall morbidity were nearly identical between patients undergoing LCR and OCR.

# References

Lacy AM, Delgado S, Garcia-Valdecasas JC, et al. Port site metastases and recurrence after laparoscopic colectomy: a randomized trial. Surg Endosc 1998;12:1039–1042.

Lacy AM, Garcia VJ, Pique JM, et al. Short-term outcome analysis of a randomized study comparing laparoscopic vs open colectomy for colon cancer. Surg Endosc 1995;9:1101–1105.

Leung KL, Kwok SPY, Lam SCW, et al. Laparoscopic resection of rectosigmoid carcinoma: prospective randomized trial. Lancet 2004;363:1187–1192.

Reza MM, Blasco JA, Andradas E, et al. Systematic review of laparoscopic versus open surgery for colorectal cancer. Br J Surg 2006;93:921–928.

Weeks JC, Nelson H, Gelber S, et al. Short-term quality-of-life outcomes following laparoscopic-assisted colectomy vs. open colectomy for colon cancer. JAMA 2002;287(3):321–328.

Young-Fadok TM. Colon cancer: trials, results, techniques (LAP and HALS), future. J Surg Oncol 2007;96(8):651–659.

# Suggested Readings

Bokey EL, Moore JW, Chapius PH, Newland RC. Morbidity and morality following laparoscopic-assisted right hemicolectomy for cancer. Dis Colon Rectum 1998;41:832–838.

Brown SR, Eu KW, Seow-Choen F. Consecutive series of laparoscopic-assisted vs. minilaparotomy restorative proctocolectomies. Dis Colon Rectum 2001;44:397–404.

Chapman AE, Levitt MD, Hewett P, Woods R, Sheiner H, Madden GJ. Laparoscopic-assisted resection of colorectal malignancies. Ann Surg 2001;234:591–606.

Chen WS, Lin WC, Kou YR, Kuo HS, Hsu H, Yang WK. Possible effect of pneumoperitoneum on the spreading of colon cancer tumor cells. Dis Colon Rectum 1997;40:791–797.

Clinical Outcomes of Surgical Therapy Group. A comparison of laparoscopically assisted and open colectomy for colon cancer. N Engl J Med 2004;350:2050–2059.

Goh YC, Eu KW, Seowchoen F. Early postoperative results of a prospective series of laparoscopic vs open anterior resections for rectosigmoid cancers. Dis Colon Rectum 1997;40:776–780.

Guller U, Jain N, Hervey, S, Purves H, Pietrobon R. Laparoscopic vs open colectomy. Outcomes comparison based on large nationwide Databases. Arch Surg 2003;138:1179–1186.

Hartley JE, Mehigan BJ, MacDonald AW, et al. Patterns of recurrence and survival after laparoscopic and conventional resections for colorectal carcinoma. Ann Surg 2000;232:181–186.

Hsu TC, Leu SC, Su CF, Huang PC, Tsai LF, Tsai SL. Assessment of intragastric pH value changes after early nasogastric feeding. Nutrition 2000;9:751–754.

Hsu TC. Feasibility of colectomy with mini-incision. Am J Surg 2005;190:48–50.

Hubens G, Pawels M, Hubens A, et al. The influence of pneumoperitoneum on the peritoneal implantation of free intraperitoneal colon cancer cells. Surg Endosc 1996;10:809–812.

Jacobi AC, Sabat R, Bohm B, et al. Pneumoperitoneum with carbon dioxide stimulates growth of malignant colonic cells. Surgery 1997;121:72–78.

Kasparek MS, Muller MH, Glatzle J, et al. Postoperative colonic motility in patients following laparoscopic assisted and open sigmoid colectomy. J Gastrointestinal Surg 2003;7(8):1073–1081.

Kim SH, Milson JW, Gramlich TL, et al. Does laparoscopic vs. conventional surgery increase exfoliated cancer cells in the peritoneal cavity during resection of colorectal cancer? Dis Colon Rectum 998;41:971–977.

Leung KL, Kwok SY, Lau WY, et al. Laparoscopic-assisted resection of rectosigmoid carcinoma: immediate and medium-term results. Arch Surg 1997;132:761–764.

Martel G, Boushey RP. Laparoscopic colon surgery: past, present and future. Surg Clin North Am 2006;86:867–897.

Nelson H, Sargent DJ, Wieand HS, et al. A comparison of laparoscopically assisted and open colectomy for colon cancer. N Engl J Med 2004;350(20):2049–2059.

Philipson BM, Bokey EL, Moore JE, et al. Cost of open versus laparoscopically assisted right hemicolectomy for cancer. World J Surg 1997;21:214–217.

SAGES Publication. Guidelines for laparoscopic resection of curable colon and rectal cancer. http://www.sages.org/sagespublication.php?doc=32.

Schlachta CM, Mamazza J, Gregoire R, Burpee SE, Poulin EC. Could laparoscopic colon and rectal surgery become the standard of care? A review and experience with 750 procedures. Can J Surg 2003;46(6):432–440.

Scott-Conner CEH. Right and left colon resections. In: Scott-Conner CEH, Dawson DL, eds. Operative Anatomy, 2nd ed. Philadelphia: Lippincott, 2003;470–483.

Stage JG, Schulze S, Moller P, et al. Prospective randomized study of laparoscopic versus open colonic resection for adenocarcinoma. Br J Surg 1997;84:391–396.

Tate JT, Kwok S, Dawson JW, et al. Prospective comparison of laparoscopic and conventional anterior resection. Br J Surg 1993;80:1396–1398.

Tomita H, Marcelo PW, Milson JW. Laparoscopic surgery of the colon and rectum [review]. World J Surg 1999;23:397–405.

Wexner SD, Cohen SM. Port site metastases after laparoscopic colorectal surgery for cure of malignancy. Br J Surg 1995;82:295–298.

Whelan RL, Young-Fadok TM. Should carcinoma of the colon be treated laparoscopically? Surg Endosc 2004;18:857–862.

# 29. Carcinoma of the Sigmoid Colon

## A. Introduction

Carcinoma of the colon is a common surgical problem. Laparoscopic techniques have been adapted to treatment of cancer of the sigmoid colon, and oncologic equivalence has been established if careful dissection principles are observed. This chapter explores some of the decisions that need to be made during this surgery. A related topic, management of carcinoma of the rectum, is discussed in Chapter 30.

## B. Case

### Carol E.H. Scott-Conner

A 58-year-old man consulted his family physician for progressive constipation over the past month and the occasional appearance of blood in his stool. He had not had any other abdominal symptoms, and his weight had remained stable.

His past medical history was significant for hyperlipidemia, hypertension, and chronic obstructive pulmonary disease. He had undergone coronary artery stenting 3 years previously and had a recent normal stress test. His past surgical history was significant for bilateral inguinal hernia repairs, done approximately 20 years earlier. His father died from prostate cancer, and his mother had uterine cancer. There is no other family history of cancer.

His medications included Zocor, atenolol, Plavix, and an angiotensin-converting enzyme (ACE) inhibitor. He had no known drug allergies.

He was a former smoker, having stopped smoking 5 years earlier after a 40-pack-a-year history. He worked as a used-car salesman, and walked 3 miles per day in good weather.

On examination, he was a well-developed, well-nourished, moderately obese white male. His height was 178 cm, he weighted 109 kg, and his body mass index (BMI) was 34. His vital signs were normal. Head and neck examination was negative, as was cardiopulmonary examination.

On abdominal examination, bilateral well-healed inguinal hernia repair incisions were noted. The abdomen was soft without masses or tenderness. Bowel sounds were normal. No hernias were detected. Rectal examination revealed a smooth prostate and no masses. Brown stool was strongly guaiac positive.

Laboratory results were significant for hematocrit of 35%. Liver function tests, electrolytes, blood urea nitrogen (BUN), and creatinine were all normal.

Colonoscopy revealed an ulcerated fungating lesion at 30 cm. A pediatric scope traversed the lesion with difficulty and the remainder of the colon was normal. Biopsies indicated moderately differentiated adenocarcinoma.

A computed tomography (CT) scan confirmed a mass in the mid-sigmoid colon with no other lesions and no suggestion of adenopathy. Sigmoid colon resection was recommended. The patient desired a minimal-access procedure.

**How would you proceed? Would you use a hand-assisted approach?**

# C. Laparoscopically Assisted Sigmoid Colon Resection

*David A. Vivas and Steven D. Wexner*

In this case we would advocate the minimally invasive, laparoscopically assisted approach. The cumulative experience at our institution and its acceptance as a safe and advantageous technique has made this approach our first choice.

Although at the beginning of the laparoscopic era medical comorbidities and obesity were considered either relative or absolute contraindications for the minimally invasive approach, this is no longer the case and currently patients with higher American Society of Anesthesiologists (ASA) classification and greater BMI are recruited for laparoscopic resections. Previous abdominal surgery does not preclude the laparoscopic approach, and at the present, in only a few instances would this technique be contraindicated. Repeated abdominal surgeries with severe intraabdominal adhesions and advanced malignant disease would be the most important contraindications. We do not perform hand-assisted laparoscopic surgery (HALS); our preferred technique is the laparoscopic assisted resection.

The patient is positioned in the supine modified lithotomy position using Allen® (Allen Medical Systems, Acton, MA) stirrups, with both arms tucked and well padded to avoid any injury. Bilateral ureteral stents may be placed if deemed beneficial. The surgeon and the camera assistant stand on the patient's right side while the first assistant stands on the left. If necessary, during the splenic flexure take down, the surgeon can stand in between the patient's legs. Two monitors are set in the room—one to the left and the other to the right side. We prefer to place a 10- to 12-mm supraumbilical port using the Hasson technique and two 10- to 12-mm working ports in the right upper and lower quadrant, lateral to the rectus muscle, using transillumination to identify and avoid the epigastric vessels. These ports should be placed at least one handbreadth apart to allow ample space for maneuvering the instruments. In some cases, it is necessary to place a fourth port in the left upper quadrant, left lower quadrant, or suprapubic midline position to help with retraction.

A 30-degree laparoscope is introduced through the supraumbilical port, and careful inspection of the intraabdominal cavity is carried out, looking for signs of advanced disease. Before the beginning of the dissection, the patient is placed in the steep Trendelenburg/right-side-down position, using gravity to mobilize the small bowel and left colon toward the right side and out of the pelvis.

We always use the lateral-to-medial approach. Two endoscopic Babcock clamps are placed through the two right-sided ports and the sigmoid colon is carefully grasped and medially retracted to expose the left gutter and define the white line of Toldt. At this point, we interchange the endo-Babcock placed in the right lower quadrant (RLQ) port (surgeon's right hand) for the ultrasonic scalpel and proceed to open the white line of Toldt in an avascular plane to the level of the splenic flexure, keeping gentle medial retraction with the right upper quadrant (RUQ) port endo-Babcock (Fig. 29.1). Dissection continues medially to identify and expose the left ureter and keep it out of harm's way. Having fully mobilized the left and sigmoid colon up to the sacral promontory, the surgeon can either stay on the patient's right side or move in between the patient's legs to commence splenic flexure mobilization. The patient is placed in the reverse Trendelenburg position, and again, using the endo-Babcock, the splenic flexure is caudally and medially retracted. Attachments between the spleen and the left colonic angle and the gastrocolic ligament are scored using the EnSeal™ (SurgRx, Inc., Palo Alto, CA) or the Ligasure (Tyco Inc., Norwalk, CT). The omentum can be either dissected free from the transverse colon or divided distal to the gastroepiploic vessels. The extent of the proximal

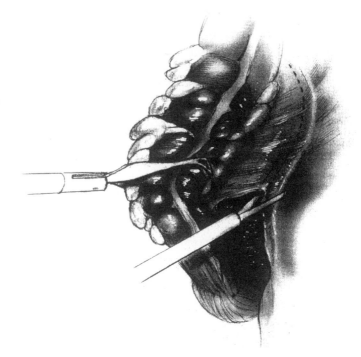

Fig. 29.1. Mobilization of the left colon begins with medial reflection and incision along the white line of Toldt. (From Wexner SD. Laparoscopic left hemicolectomy. In: Scott-Conner CEH, ed. Chassin's Operative Strategy in Colon and Rectal Surgery. New York: Springer-Verlag, 2006, with permission.)

dissection should be determined by the ability to subsequently create a tension-free anastomosis.

The mobilization is generally to the right of the middle colic vessels. After satisfactory mobilization of the colon is achieved, the medial aspect of the colonic mesentery is scored and the sigmoid vessels are identified. Windows at both sides are created and blood vessels are isolated (Fig. 29.2). At this point, the left ureter is once again identified through these windows, and the inferior mesenteric artery and vein are separately divided using an endoscopic stapler with a vascular cartridge, introduced through the RLQ port. It is important to visualize the tip of the stapler to avoid the inclusion of undesired structures in the staple line. Similarly, control of the proximal portion of the vessels should be maintained with the endo-Babcock prior to division to facilitate any further hemostasis,

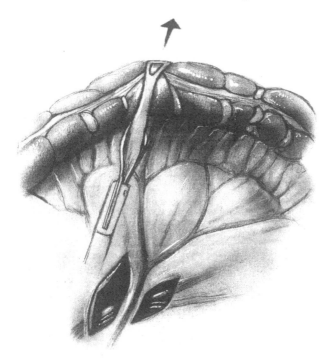

Fig. 29.2. A window is made in the mesentery preparatory to vascular division. Note that the ureter is visualized through the window and protected from harm. (From Wexner SD. Laparoscopic left hemicolectomy. In: Scott-Conner CEH, ed. Chassin's Operative Strategy in Colon and Rectal Surgery. New York: Springer-Verlag, 2006, with permission.)

as necessary. In case of persistent bleeding or oozing, additional measures can be implemented including the use of the ultrasonic scalpel and endoscopic clips or endoloops.

The level of the distal resection has to be determined, and in this particular case, given the mid-sigmoid location of the lesion, we would advocate division at the sigmoid-rectal junction. As anatomic landmarks for its identification, we use the confluence of the taenia coli, the level of the sacral promontory, and the obliteration of the appendices epiploicae; flexible or rigid sigmoidoscopic evaluation can also be helpful to verify the position of intended transection. Through the RLQ port, an endoscopic 45-mm articulating linear stapler is introduced and applied to the bowel, ensuring that the colonic wall is clear of fat and that no other structures are included; the stapler is then fired (Fig. 29.3) After stapling

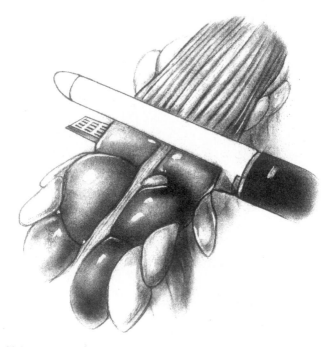

Fig. 29.3. The linear endoscopic stapler is used to transect the bowel at the rectosigmoid junction. Care is taken not to include any extra tissue in this staple line. (From Wexner SD. Laparoscopic left hemicolectomy. In: Scott-Conner CEH, ed. Chassin's Operative Strategy in Colon and Rectal Surgery. New York: Springer-Verlag, 2006, with permission.)

and transecting the rectosigmoid junction, the pelvis is filled with saline, and a proctoscopy is performed to verify staple line integrity.

The site of the proximal margin is determined at the junction between the descending and sigmoid colon and marked with endoscopic clips, ensuring that the resulting anastomosis between the descending colon and the rectum will be tension-free. The base of the colonic mesentery can be divided as necessary up to the middle colic vessels to ensure a tension-free anastomosis.

At this point, the incision site for specimen extraction is made depending on previous abdominal scars and body habitus. Usually, we prefer to place a suprapubic 10- to 12-mm port at the Pfannenstiel's incision site due to its satisfactory cosmetic results. However, if during the course of the dissection it was necessary to place any additional ports, we use that site for specimen retrieval. An endo-Babcock is introduced through the chosen site, and the distal colonic margin is gently grasped. A 5-cm incision is made using this port as a guide, and a wound protector is placed around it. The endo-Babcock is carefully withdrawn through the wound, along with the port and the gently held colon up to the level of proximal transection, which can be recognized by the previously placed endoscopic clips. The colon is then extracorporeally transected, placing a noncrushing clamp proximal at the site of transection to control spillage of intestinal contents. The specimen is withdrawn from the field and the cutting edges are cleared of appendices epiploicae, and a purse-string suture is performed using 0 polypropylene suture. A 33-mm circular stapler anvil is inserted in the proximal end of the bowel and the purse-string is secured (Fig. 29.4). The use of a 33-mm stapler helps ensure adequate luminal size and absence of significant descending colon muscular hypertrophy. The colon is then returned into the abdomen, the incision is closed, and pneumoperitoneum reestablished.

At this point, the surgeon carefully introduces the circular stapler through the anus to the level of the distal staple line. Under laparoscopic

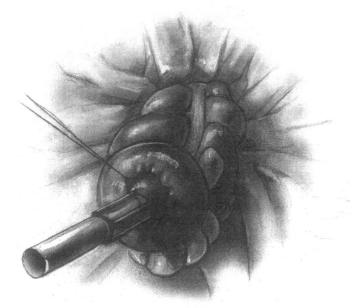

Fig. 29.4. The anvil and purse-string suture are placed under direct vision in the proximal end of the exteriorized bowel. (From Wexner SD. Laparoscopic left hemicolectomy. In: Scott-Conner CEH, ed. Chassin's Operative Strategy in Colon and Rectal Surgery. New York: Springer-Verlag, 2006, with permission.)

visualization, the stapler anvil is deployed through or near the distal staple line. The anvil shaft is gently grasped using the anvil grasper placed through the RUQ port and is attached to the circular stapler trocar. The camera can be moved to the RLQ port for a better view of stapler closure to ensure exclusion of extraneous structures and that the proximal bowel and mesentery are straight; the circular stapler is slowly closed and fired (Fig. 29.5). The stapler is withdrawn from the anus and both donuts are inspected and sent to the laboratory for pathologic evaluation. An atraumatic, noncrushing clamp is placed proximal to the anastomosis, and the pelvis is again filled with saline. Air is insufflated during repeat flexible sigmoidoscopy to ensure anastomotic integrity. After verification of hemostasis, the ports are closed. We do not routinely divert or use drains.

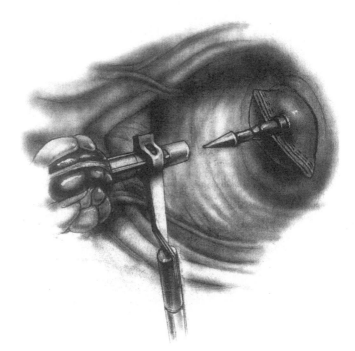

Fig. 29.5. The bowel is returned to the abdomen and pneumoperitoneum reestablished. Stapler and anvil are mated under direct vision. (From Wexner SD. Laparoscopic left hemicolectomy. In: Scott-Conner CEH, ed. Chassin's Operative Strategy in Colon and Rectal Surgery. New York: Springer-Verlag, 2006, with permission.)

# D. Laparoscopic Sigmoid Colon Resection

*George M. Eid and Carol McCloskey*

Since the minimally invasive approach to colorectal surgery was described in the early 1990s, the number of laparoscopic colorectal procedures has continued to increase. Laparoscopic colorectal surgery offers many advantages in comparison to open procedures, including decreased length of stay, improved cosmesis, and a more expedient recovery without compromising oncologic outcome. As the laparoscopic approach to colorectal surgery evolved, the hand-assisted laparoscopic technique was developed to overcome the technical limitations and the steep learning curve of laparoscopy. This hybrid approach bridged the gap between open and laparoscopic surgery for advanced procedures. Today, a totally laparoscopic approach is technically feasible. However, there is still debate over which method is superior, as it remains a matter of surgeon preference. We prefer the totally laparoscopic approach because we feel that the hand-assisted approach has many disadvantages, as described below.

Hand-assisted laparoscopic surgery requires placement of a hand port device into a minilaparotomy incision, allowing the surgeon to insert a hand into the peritoneal cavity while maintaining a pneumoperitoneum. This preserves tactile sensation, and allows use of the hand for atraumatic exposure, blunt dissection, and manual hemostasis, giving the surgeon a sense of control. Advocates of this approach feel that it is easier to learn and perform. Despite these advantages, the hand-assisted approach does have major shortcomings for both the surgeon and patient. For the surgeon, a hand in the laparoscopic operating field can limit the view, especially when operating in narrow spaces, such as the lesser pelvis. This difficulty cannot be totally solved by adjusting the angle of laparoscope. Also, the unnatural position of the surgeon's hand may cause significant hand fatigue and pain, which can decrease precision or create the need for frequent breaks, possibly prolonging the operation. Furthermore, this approach in obese patients can be exceptionally challenging. Externalization of bowel can be difficult due to the limited length of mesentery and increased travel distance imposed by a thick abdominal wall. Additional tension may lead to mesenteric vascular injury. Therefore, further colon mobilization is often required, adding to increased operative time.

There are also several important disadvantages for the patient. A much larger incision is required for hand port placement compared to the incision size required in a totally laparoscopic approach. A larger incision can potentially lead to a higher incidence of wound infection, incisional hernias, and postoperative pain, and a longer recovery time. The more frequent handling of the bowel during a hand-assisted approach may prolong the postoperative ileus. More importantly, it compromises the oncological principle of the "no-touch" technique. In addition, Whelan et al. demonstrated that the tissue trauma related to open colon resection is associated with a significant suppression of the cell-mediated immune response in comparison to the laparoscopic approach. Such a compromise in immune function can theoretically enhance intraperitoneal tumor cell growth and increase the risk of metastasis, although further human studies are needed to verify these findings and establish their clinical significance.

On the other hand, wound-related complications are limited, and tumor "no-touch" principles are achieved in totally laparoscopic colon surgery. The laparoscope can reach narrow spaces and magnify the local vision, providing views that are unsurpassed by any open or hand-assisted laparoscopic techniques. In the pelvic cavity for example, it helps surgeons identify accurately the interspace of loose connective tissue between visceral and parietal pelvic fascia, making it is easier to identify and protect the pelvic autonomic nerves. Good laparoscopic visualization while performing an anastomosis has the potential to decrease the incidence of leaks related to technical factors. Hemostasis is better achieved in minimally invasive sharp dissection with minimal blood loss under excellent magnification. The major deficit with laparoscopic surgery is the loss of tactile feedback. During the procedure, the surgeon is unable to utilize a hand directly to assess organs, to localize vessels, retract, and dissect. Also, there is a steep learning curve for advanced procedures. However, the provision of many modern laparoscopic tools has enabled the surgeon to successfully perform more advanced colorectal procedures. Many disadvantages, such as longer operative time, have been overcome by increasing experience, due to growing volumes of cases and appropriate training. In addition, the advent of computer enhanced images (robotic surgery) will soon allow the techniques of open surgery to be completely duplicated by making a totally laparoscopic hand-sewn anastomosis more easily performed due to added dexterity and three-dimensional views.

In conclusion, we recommend a totally laparoscopic approach to sigmoid colon resection because it offers many advantages to both the surgeon and patient in comparison to hand-assisted laparoscopy. We feel that the continually increasing number of cases as well as evolving technology will allow many surgeons to overcome the learning curve and begin to adopt it as a routine approach.

# E. Conclusions

*Carol E.H. Scott-Conner*

There are several critical decision points when surgery is elected for carcinoma of the sigmoid colon. In a situation such as that described here, adequate resection is crucial to preserve the hope of a cure.

The first decision is: open procedure or laparoscopic? SAGES has published guidelines for laparoscopic resection of curable colon and rectal cancer, and set forth several tenets. In addition to proper patient selection and preparation, SAGES stressed that laparoscopic surgery should follow standard oncologic principles, including proximal ligation of primary arterial supply, adequate proximal and distal margins, and appropriate lymphadenectomy (a minimum of 12 lymph nodes harvested). Both the Clinical Outcomes of Surgery Therapy Study Group of the Laparoscopic Colectomy (COST) trial and Lacy et al. in a similarly randomized trial have demonstrated that well-trained laparoscopists can achieve equivalent proximal and distal margins, number of lymph nodes, and length of vascular pedicle obtained when open and laparoscopic procedures were compared. Adequate training and experience are crucial, as these are considered to be among the complex laparoscopic cases. Many surgical centers build their initial experience with colon resection for benign disease before moving on to colon resection for cancer (with associated oncologic issues).

The second decision is: hand-assisted or traditional laparoscopic? Advocates of the hand-assisted approach argue that in a procedure such as colon resection, where an incision will need to be made at some point in the procedure, why not make that incision at the beginning? Placement of a hand-assist device allows the surgeon to retain tactile feedback and retract the bowel with the gentlest of instruments—the human hand. Yet, both of the expert surgeons here argue in favor of a non-HALS approach in this situation. Table 29.1 summarizes the general pros and cons of HALS versus the traditional approach, and it appears that a small Pfannenstiel incision for specimen removal (rather than a larger incision for HALS) remains the procedure of choice.

The final decision is: lateral to medial (traditional approach) or the newer medial to lateral approach advocated by some? The traditional approach uses a dissection strategy exactly comparable to that commonly done during open surgery. The colon is mobilized by incising the white line of Toldt and then rotating it away from the retroperitoneum. This inevitably places it in the way of the laparoscope, and it would seem intuitive that dissection that could begin medially and progress laterally might be easier. Such an approach was initially described by several groups and has been tested in at least one randomized clinical trial. This approach is best suited for use in slender patients, and so the patient presented here, with a BMI over 32, would not be considered ideal. In the medial-to-lateral approach the vascular pedicles are divided first and the colon is then mobilized. This approach is reminiscent of the "no-touch" technique that some surgeons have advocated during traditional open colon surgery. The approach is nicely described in a paper by Liang et al.

One basic consideration bears mentioning. Particularly when colon resection is performed for early lesions, accurate identification of the involved segment is crucial. Colonoscopic distances can be misleading, when translated to a location within the conventional surgical fields. Endoscopic bowel tattooing facilitates this and should be used whenever the tumor is small and the location ambiguous.

Table 29.1. Advantages and disadvantages of hand-assisted laparoscopic surgery.

| Advantages | Disadvantages |
|---|---|
| Allows for tactile sensation | Hand encroaches upon intraabdominal working space |
| Specimen retrieval and anastomosis may be performed through hand port site | May reduce benefit of laparoscopic surgery secondary to larger hand port |
| Rapid control of bleeding by direct pressure | Device-dependent air leak |
| Improved depth perception and shortened learning curve | Ergonomically unfavorable, leading to shoulder and forearm fatigue and strain |
| Reduced operative time | May increase cost |

*Source:* Modified from Schneider BE. Hand-assisted laparoscopic surgery. In: Scott-Conner CEH, ed. The SAGES Manual: Fundamentals of Laparoscopy, Thoracoscopy, and GI Endoscopy, 2nd ed. New York: Springer-Verlag, 2006.

In summary, properly selected patients can benefit from laparoscopic left colon resection. Oncologic principles must be followed, and the surgical team must be experienced in the use of this modality.

# References

Lacy AM, Garcia-Valdecasas JC, Delgado S, et al. Laparoscopy-assisted colectomy versus open colectomy for treatment of non-metastatic colon cancer: a randomized trial. Lancet 2002;359:2224–2229.

Liang JT, Lai HS, Huang KC, et al. Comparison of medial-to-lateral versus traditional lateral-to-medial laparoscopic dissection sequences for resection of rectosigmoid cancers: randomized controlled clinical trial. World J Surg 2003;27:190–196.

Whelan RL, Franklin M, Holubar SD, et al. Postoperative cell mediated immune response is better preserved after laparoscopic vs open colorectal resection in humans. Surg Endosc 2003;17(6):972–978.

# Suggested Readings

Ballantyne GH, Leahy PF. Hand-assisted laparoscopic colectomy: evolution to a clinically useful technique. Dis Colon Rectum 2004;47:753–765.

Cera SM, Wexner SD. Minimally invasive treatment of colon cancer. Cancer J 2005;11(1):26–35.

Clinical Outcomes of Surgical Therapy Study Group. A comparison of laparoscopically assisted and open colectomy for colon cancer. N Engl J Med 2004;350(20):2050–2059.

Franklin ME Jr, Rosenthal D, Abrego-Medina D, et al. Prospective comparison of open vs. laparoscopic colon surgery for carcinoma. Five-year results. Dis Colon Rectum 1996;39(10 suppl):S35–S46.

Guidelines for Laparoscopic Resection of Curable Colon and Rectal Cancer. http://www.wages.org/sagespublication.php?doc=32

Jacobs M, Verdeja JC, Goldstein HS. Minimally invasive colon resection (laparoscopic colectomy). Surg Laparosc Endosc 1991;1:144–150.

Loungnarath R, Fleishman JW. Hand-assisted laparoscopic colectomy techniques. Semin Laparosc Surg 2003;10:219–230.

Plocek M, Geisler D, Glennon E, Kondylis P, Reilly J. Laparoscopic colorectal surgery in the complicated patient. Am J Surg 2005;190(6):882–885.

Reissman P, Cohen S, Weiss EG, Wexner SD. Laparoscopic colorectal surgery: ascending the learning curve. World J Surg 1996;20:277–281.

Sigel A, Zerz A, Molle B, et al. Medial mobilization of the left hemicolon. Chirurg 2004;75:605–608.

Weiss E, Wexner S. Laparoscopic segmental colectomies, anterior resection, and abdomi-
    noperineal resection. In: Scott-Conner CEH, ed. The SAGES Manual: Fundamentals
    of Laparoscopy and GI Endoscopy. New York: Springer, 1999:290–295.
Wolf JS Jr. Devices for hand-assisted laparoscopic surgery. Expert Rev Med Devices
    2005;2:725–730.

# 30. Low Anterior Resection for Carcinoma Below the Peritoneal Reflection

## A. Introduction

Low anterior resection presents several attractions for the laparoscopic surgeon. First, the unparalleled visualization and exposure that are attained when laparoscopic surgery goes well would seem to facilitate careful dissection in the deep recesses of the pelvis (where visualization during open surgery can be problematic). Second, the anastomosis can be performed by transanal insertion of a circular stapling device, minimizing the length of incision required to complete the procedure.

However, the procedure is fraught with potential complications, including the long-term risk of local recurrence. This chapter explores the issues related to choice of laparoscopic versus open approach for carcinoma below the peritoneal reflection.

## B. Case

### Nora A. Royer

An 82-year-old woman presented with a 5-month history of bright bleeding per rectum and weight loss of 20 pounds. She had been feeling progressively weaker and sought medical attention after she became light-headed during a church service.

Her past medical history was notable for diabetes mellitus, hypertension, and coronary artery disease, which had been medically managed after myocardial infarction. Her past surgical history was significant for an appendectomy at the age of 10. Her father developed colon cancer at the age of 75.

Her medications included glipizide, metoprolol, aspirin, simvastatin, and lisinopril. She reported no allergies.

She never smoked and did not use alcohol. She walked half a mile to church on a near daily basis and lived independently.

On physical examination, she appeared her stated age, and was conversant and appropriate. Her heart rate was 64, blood pressure 110/64, and body mass index (BMI) 21. Head, ears, eyes, nose, and throat (HEENT) were normal cephalic and atraumatic (NCAT), the oropharynx was pink and moist without lesions, and the mucosa were pale. The neck was supple, with a normal range of motion.

Cardiovascular exam revealed regular rate and rhythm with no murmurs. Lungs were clear to auscultation bilaterally.

Her abdomen was soft, nondistended, and nontender with no palpable masses. Rectal examination revealed no masses. Stool was strongly guaiac positive. Flexible sigmoidoscopy revealed a fungating mass at 18 cm from the dentate line. Pathology showed moderately differentiated adenocarcinoma.

Evaluation included a computed tomography (CT) scan, which demonstrated thickening in the wall of the rectosigmoid colon. No enlarged lymph nodes were noted, and no lung or liver densities were present.

Endoscopic ultrasound showed a mass without extension outside the wall of the rectum. Her labs were significant for a creatinine of 1.4 and hemoglobin of 10.

In summary, this patient has a rectal cancer below the peritoneal reflection with comorbidities including coronary artery disease and diabetes. She was stable on medication and with good functional status. Low anterior resection was recommended.

**What would be your preferred approach: laparoscopic or open?**

# C. Laparoscopically Assisted Low Anterior Resection for Cancer

## *Bashar Safar and Steven D. Wexner*

Based on the evaluation this patient has undergone, this represents a case of early rectal cancer involving the upper rectum. We are strong advocates of the minimally invasive approach. There have been many trials in the last century showing the equivalence of the minimally invasive approach to conventional surgery for colon cancer from the oncologic standpoint and its superiority when short-term outcomes are measured, including less pain, faster return of bowel function, and faster recovery. The technical feasibility of laparoscopic rectal cancer surgery has been clearly demonstrated in recent reports; however, long-term outcomes from randomized controlled trials are still awaited.

A recent publication by Leung et al. addressed laparoscopic resections for cancer at the rectosigmoid junction; 403 patients were randomized to undergo laparoscopically assisted ($n = 203$) or conventional open ($n = 200$) resection of the tumor. After curative resection, the probabilities of survival at 5 years of the laparoscopic and open resection groups were 76.1% (standard error [SE] 3.7%) and 72.9% (4.0%), respectively. The probabilities of being disease free at 5 years were 75.3% (3.7%) and 78.3% (3.7%), respectively. The operative time of the laparoscopic group was significantly longer, whereas postoperative recovery was significantly better than for the open resection group, but these benefits were at the expense of higher direct cost. The distal margin, the number of lymph nodes found in the resected specimen, overall morbidity, and operative mortality did not differ between groups.

## Surgical Procedure

The patient is placed in the modified lithotomy position using Allen® (Allen Medical Systems, Acton, MA) stirrups with both arms tucked and well padded to avoid any injury especially at the bony prominence. The patient is secured to the operating table with particular attention to the shoulders to prevent the patient from slipping with extreme position changes that may be needed to perform the procedure. We routinely place ureteral stents for laparoscopic pelvic dissection; this aids in the identification of the ureters and prevents inadvertent injury. Rectal irrigation is performed using Betadine, and the abdomen is prepped and draped in the usual manner.

The team consists of the operating surgeon, first assistant, camera assistant, and a scrub technician. The surgeon stands to the patient's right with the camera assistant to his/her left. The first assistant stands on the left of the patient and the scrub technician stands with the Mayo table next to the right leg. Two monitors are used, one over the left leg for the surgeon and camera assistant, and the other over the right shoulder for the first assistant. The abdominal cavity is entered using the open Hasson technique above or below the umbilicus depending on the distance from the pubis. Pneumoperitoneum up to 15 mm Hg is created, and using a 30-degree scope a careful exploration of the entire abdominal cavity is undertaken, including the liver and all peritoneal surfaces to rule out tumor dissemination. Two 10- to 12-mm ports are then inserted as the main working ports for the surgeon, one in the right lower quadrant, which is used as the dissecting port, and the other in the right upper quadrant, which is used by the left hand for retraction. Both ports should be placed lateral enough to avoid injury to the hypogastric vessels and far enough apart (one handbreadth) to allow for easy maneuverability. A third port may need to be placed in the left lower quadrant or in the suprapubic region to aid in retraction during the rectal dissection. This extra port, if needed, will be later employed as the extraction site.

The patient is then placed in the steep Trendelenburg position with the left side up as much as possible, allowing gravity to keep the small bowel and the omentum out of the operating field. The sigmoid and descending colon is mobilized utilizing the lateral to medial approach. The sigmoid colon is grasped with an atraumatic grasper and retracted medially with the left hand, making sure not to handle the tumor itself and not to use the locking function of the grasper in order to avoid injury to the bowel. The white line of Toldt is identified, and dissection is carried out with the right hand using the ultrasound harmonic scalpel (Ultracision, Ethicon Endosurgery, Cincinnati, OH) in the avascular plane between the mesocolon and posterior peritoneum. The dissection is then continued medially until the ureter is identified and caudally until the mesocolon is separated from splenic attachments and Gerota's fascia.

The splenic flexure is next mobilized, either with the surgeon standing between the patient's legs or remaining on the patient's right side. The patient is placed in the reverse Trendelenburg position. Starting to the right of the middle colic vessels, the omentum is dissected off the colon, and the lesser sac is entered. The dissection is then extended toward the spleen using the harmonic scalpel, making sure to free all the attachments of the spleen to the colon. Once the splenic flexure is fully mobilized the colon is retracted laterally to expose the medial aspect of the mesocolon, an extra port in the left lower quadrant or suprapubically may be needed at this point as described above. A window is created in the base of the mesocolon at the level of the sacral promontory. The avascular plane is once again identified along with the left ureter. The mesocolon is dissected off the aorta until the inferior mesenteric artery (IMA) is identified. A window is created in the mesentery and the artery is divided close to the aorta (high ligation) using the ETS Flex45 Endoscopic Linear Cutter (Ethicon Endo-Surgery; Cincinnati, OH) with vascular stapler (2.5-mm staple height). It is crucial to be able to see the ureter while closing the stapler and avoid trapping it in the jaws of the stapler. After divided the IMA, the fourth portion of the duodenum is now identified at the ligament of Treitz with the inferior mesenteric vein (IMV) running to the left of it. The vein is then divided using a reload of the vascular stapler. Careful inspection of the anastomosis line is undertaken to ensure adequate hemostasis. Extra measures such as a laparoscopic endo-loop or clips may be required.

Next, the distal extent of the dissection has to be determined. This level can be identified either through preoperative marking or intraoperative sigmoidoscopy. Dissection is undertaken in the avascular areolar plane surrounding the mesorectum between the parietal and visceral facial planes of the pelvis and continued for a distance 5 cm beyond the distal margin of the tumor. We start the dissection posteriorly in a plane anterior to the hypogastric and autonomic nerves and then move on to the lateral stalks, leaving the anterior dissection last. The uterus may need to be retracted anteriorly to facilitate exposure; this can be done by securing it to the anterior abdominal wall or using a laparoscopic retractor to push it out of the way. The level of intended transaction can be confirmed by gently clamping the rectum and repeating the sigmoidoscopy. Once the level of transaction is determined, the scalpel can be used to divide the mesorectum; care must be taken to avoid conning during this part of the procedure, and the mesorectum must be divided at the same level as the rectal transaction. The endoscopic articulating linear stapler is reloaded with a gastrointestinal (GI) load, introduced through the right lower quadrant (RLQ) port, and the rectum is transected at the predetermined level; more than one firing of the stapler may be needed to get across the rectum. The suture line is inspected and sigmoidoscopy is repeated at this stage with the pelvis filled with saline to verify the competency of the staple line. The descending/sigmoid colon, which should be completely free, is brought down to the pelvis, and the proximal margin of transaction is determined and marked with two endoscopic clips for future identification.

The extraction site is chosen next. An extra 10- to 12-mm port is inserted two finger-breadths above the pubis, unless a port was inserted in the left lower quadrant (LLQ) for retraction, which can be used as the extraction site. The suprapubic position is preferred for cosmetic reasons. An endoscopic Babcock is inserted through the port, and the transected end of the bowel is grasped across the staple line and the ratchet is locked fully to avoid dislodgment. This is the only part of the procedure where the locking function of the instrument is used. The skin incision around the port is enlarged to accommodate the width of the specimen. Using the port as a guide, the incision is extended into the abdominal cavity either side of the port and then a wound protector is inserted around the port. The port along with the grasper and the bowel is extracted through the wound. The bowel is pulled out until the endoscopic clips placed earlier in the procedure to mark the location of transaction are identified. A proximal bowel clamp is applied, the bowel along with the mesentery is divided, and purse-string suture is performed using 0 polypropylene. A 33-mm circular anvil is inserted, the purse-string suture is secured around it, and the bowel is prepared for the anastomosis by clearing the mesentery and the appendices epiploicae off the anvil. The bowel is dropped back into the abdominal cavity, the incision is closed with a running PDS suture, and pneumoperitoneum is reestablished.

The anastomosis is then performed under direct vision. The circular stapler shaft is introduced through the anus after gentle dilatation and guided into the desired location with the endoscopic Babcock. We prefer to deploy the stapler at or near the staple line. The anvil shaft is guided with the endoscopic anvil grasper introduced through the RLQ into the stapler. Care must be taken to ensure that the bowel mesentery is not twisted and no extra tissues have been caught in the stapler while closing. The mesenteric edge is traced from the origin of the middle colic artery to the free edge of the bowel. Once the stapler is deployed, it should be very gently withdrawn and the two "donuts" inspected. The pelvis is filled with saline once again; the proximal bowel clamped with an atraumatic grasper and the anastomotic integrity is verified by direct vision through sigmoidoscopy and by an air-leak test. A drain can be placed through the lower quadrant port.

The trocars are removed and the fascia of the paraumbilical incision closed using PDS suture. We do not routinely close the fascia of lateral incisions. The subcutaneous tissue is irrigated and the incision closed with subcuticular absorbable suture.

The patient is allowed a liquid diet on the day of operation and is encouraged to mobilize.

# D.  Open Low Anterior Resection for Cancer

*Amanda Ayers and Jeffrey L. Cohen*

For carcinoma below the peritoneal reflection, we would do open (as opposed to laparoscopic) resection.

Laparoscopy for colorectal disease is now a common, widely accepted standard in many parts of the country. Recent trials have demonstrated equivalent safety and efficacy from an oncologic perspective of laparoscopic resection versus open colectomy for colon cancer. In addition, the previously described advantages of laparoscopy persist, specifically improved cosmesis, shorter length of stay, reduced pain, and earlier return of bowel function. More recently, several centers have started to publish data on the outcomes of the laparoscopic approach to rectal cancer.

However, rectal carcinoma below the peritoneal reflection remains a challenging entity to treat. Prior to the description of total mesorectal excision (TME) in 1982, recurrence rates were high. Since its inception, numerous studies have demonstrated TME to be superior in terms of local recurrence and overall survival, reducing recurrence rates from as high as 47% to between 4% and 11%. Total mesorectal excision is now the gold standard of surgical therapy for rectal cancer. The consequences of local recurrence extend beyond the issue of curability, to include managing the significant symptoms that may develop. Recurrences may result in difficult-to-control chronic pelvic pain. In addition, patients can develop large bowel obstructions, as well as possible ureteral obstructions, requiring decompressive procedures. Finally, the close proximity of the iliac vessels can result in venous obstruction and resultant leg edema.

The tenets of TME, namely direct visualization and sharp dissection, are required in order for complete excision of the tumor and the lymph node basin. This remains a technically difficult procedure even in experienced hands, given the complex anatomy and difficulty in avoiding the hypogastric nerves.

The advantages of laparoscopy for colorectal disease have led many surgeons to pursue newer and broader applications. Most recently that has included laparoscopic approaches for low pelvic disease. However, considerable caution must be used in the application of this newer technology to rectal cancer for general surgeons in practice.

The learning curve for laparoscopic colon resections has been estimated at between 55 and 80 cases. Complication rates have also been demonstrated to be higher for surgeons who perform these procedures less frequently, suggesting that laparoscopic colectomy represents a technically difficult procedure. For the general surgeon in practice who may perform 15 resections per year, the learning curve is not achieved for at least 4 years. Furthermore, the advancement to pelvic procedures represents another subset of skills in addition to those for colectomy and the necessity for further experience. With the knowledge that "open" TME represent a technically demanding and complex procedure, the laparoscopic total mesorectal excision is even more demanding.

The confines of the bony structure of the pelvis create an additional level of difficulty for laparoscopic surgery. First, due to the anatomic proximity to many of the pelvic organs, rectal cancer has the capability of contiguous spread. While TME necessitates direct visualization, the tactile sensation of the planes between structures in addition to visualization may assist in dissection. This problem is further complicated by patients with large, bulky tumors, which limit room for both manipulation and visualization. These situations may necessitate palpation of the planes and tumor morphology, which is lost in laparoscopy.

Second, the bony pelvis restricts distal resection capabilities. Unlike in open procedures in which the stapler can be passed into the pelvis from above, the stapler must be passed from a lower quadrant incision in laparoscopic resections. The pelvic brim may impede the manipulation of the stapler to a level below the tumor to a point in which an adequate resection margin is attainable. This problem is further accentuated in men who typically have narrower pelvises and increased amounts of intraabdominal fat. The inability to adequately place the stapler and achieve an adequate resection margin should preclude laparoscopic resection.

For rectal tumors below the peritoneal reflection, several facts are clear. First, total mesorectal excision represents the gold standard method of dissection and resection for improved oncologic outcomes. This represents a complex and difficult open procedure even in experienced hands, and when transitioned into laparoscopic resection, an even more demanding one. Second, the loss of tactile sensation can be a significant limitation in the pelvis. Third, current technology may limit our ability to perform TME with adequate resection margins. As laparoscopic technology and experience advance, so will its applications. However, until then, the principles of technically adequate oncologic resections cannot be sacrificed.

# E. Conclusions

## Nora A. Royer

Rectal cancer, part of the spectrum of diseases under the umbrella of colorectal cancer, represents a potentially treatable condition using surgical resection techniques. The cure rates using surgical therapy alone for noninfiltrative disease are often cited as being 45% to 50%. There will be approximately 40,000 new cases of rectal cancer diagnosed this year and approximately 56,000 deaths from colorectal cancer this year alone. Colorectal cancer is the third most common cancer and leading cause of cancer death in both men and women. The known risk factors for colon cancer include a family history of colon cancer in a first-degree relative, hereditary nonpolyposis colon cancer, familial adenomatous polyposis, prior colorectal cancer or dysplastic polyps in another region of colon, inflammatory bowel disease, and possibly exposure to radiation therapy in the pelvis.

The most important prognostic factors for rectal cancer are the nodal status and the level of penetration through the wall of the rectum. Because a significant cure rate and benefit can be achieved by surgical resection with or without neoadjuvant chemotherapy and radiation, most patients with local disease are candidates for resection of their tumor. The procedure used for resection of rectal cancer often depends heavily on surgeon preference and the tumor's distance from the anus, with the goal of the procedure generally being total mesorectal excision. Much of the variation in treatment has to do with the lack of a consensus definition on even a basic point such as what the rectum entails. The rectum is often defined by an anatomic landmark, usually the peritoneal reflection, or by a defined distance, which varies depending on the surgeon, from the anal verge or dentate line. The amount of variability in the procedure is now further increased with the growth in the number of laparoscopic cases being attempted for cancer.

Laparoscopic surgery for resection of colorectal cancer is a relatively new field. The laparoscopic approach to many surgeries is often favored because it uses smaller incisions, which many people feel leads to less pain and infection. Studies have variably shown that laparoscopic approaches may lead to decreased postoperative ileus, decreased chance of incisional hernia due to smaller fascial defects, and a lesser chance of adhesions and subsequent bowel obstruction. Recent interest in laparoscopic approaches for elderly patients has increased after studies showed that there were less pulmonary and cardiac effects from laparoscopic approaches, which is important in elderly patients who often have significant comorbidities that could affect perioperative and postoperative events. For rectal cancer specifically, the laparoscope can often offer a magnified and illuminated view of the deep pelvis, which can be difficult to achieve during any open procedure.

There are certain contraindications to a laparoscopic approach. For rectal cancer specifically, direct invasion or a tumor size greater than 8 to 10 cm can prevent a laparoscopic approach due to the difficulty of dissection and difficulty removing the specimen via a laparoscopic port site. Obesity is a relative contraindication as instrument placement and visualization are much more difficult with thicker subcutaneous tissues and with more visceral fat.

Studies specifically comparing the open versus laparoscopic approach for rectal cancer resection are small thus far but have shown consistent findings that favor the laparoscopic approach, especially for high-risk patients such as the elderly or those with multiple other comorbidities. Wu et al., in a nonrandomized trial of 38 patients with low rectal cancer, demonstrated that the laparoscopic cases had a longer operative time but decreased blood loss and fewer postoperative complications, such as ileus, urinary problems, and wound infection. This study also demonstrated one fifth of the postoperative morbidity in the laparoscopic group when compared with the open group. Zhou et al. conducted a randomized prospective trial of 171 patients with rectal cancer below the peritoneal reflection and obtained similar findings of less blood loss, earlier recovery of bowel function, and shorter hospitalization times for the patients treated with a laparoscopic approach. Both studies demonstrated a conversion rate to an open procedure after an initial laparoscopic attempt of around 15%.

The laparoscopic approach for colorectal cancer or any cancer resection requires special techniques to ensure good oncologic technique and full resection with margins. Early case experience had rates as high as 40% for port-site metastases when tumor contaminated specimens were removed via port sites. The use of sealable specimen bags and chemotherapeutic peritoneal washes as well as advances in surgical technique that allow for hand-assisted laparoscopic approaches with the maintenance of pneumoperitoneum have allowed for complete resection with a very low risk of port-site metastasis. The general consensus in the literature is that only surgeons with significant laparoscopic experience in nononcology colon and rectal resection cases consider undertaking oncologic procedures using the laparoscopic approach, as these cases require precision, clean margins, and careful dissection.

In conclusion, the laparoscopic approach for the total mesorectal excision of noninfiltrative rectal cancer below the peritoneal reflection is a valid approach in that it attains adequate surgical margins, has a lower complication rate, decreased blood loss, and a lower risk of pulmonary complications than the traditional open approach. It is best only attempted by highly experienced surgeons in the area of laparoscopic colorectal surgery. It also requires specialized equipment and a longer operative time. The longer operating times mean a longer period of exposure to general anesthesia and its inherent risks for patients with significant medical comorbidities. The risks and benefits of resection in general and in the type of complication that may most greatly impact the patient's long-term functional status should be carefully balanced prior to a laparoscopic low anterior resection for rectal cancer.

Although studies have demonstrated oncologic equivalence in trained hands, the learning curve for laparoscopic colon surgery is extensive. Unless the surgeon is well trained, oncologic principles may be sacrificed when low anterior resection is performed as a laparoscopic-assisted procedure. For the majority of surgeons, open low anterior resection with TME remains the safest option.

# References

Leung KL, Kwok SP, Lam SC, et al. Laparoscopic resection of rectosigmoid carcinoma: prospective randomized trial. Lancet 2004;363:1187–1192.

Wu WX, Sun YM, Hua YB, Shen LZ. Laparoscopic versus conventional open resection of rectal carcinoma: a clinical comparative study. World J Gastroenterol 2004;10(8):1167–1170.

Zhou ZG, Hu M, Li Y, et al. Laparoscopic vs open total mesorectal excision with anal sphincter preservation for low rectal cancer. Surg Endosc 2004;18:1211–1215.

# Suggested Readings

Barlehner E, Benhidjeb T, Andres S, Schicke B. Laparoscopic resection for rectal cancer: Outcomes in 194 patients and review of the literature. Surg Endosc 2005;19: 757–766.

Bretagnol F, Lelong B, Laurent C, et al. The oncological safety of laparoscopic total mesorectal excision with sphincter preservation for rectal carcinoma. Surg Endosc 2005;19:892–896.

Breukink SO, Grond AJK, Pierie JPEN, Hoff C, Merijerink WJHS. Laparoscopic vs open total mesorectal excision for rectal cancer: an evaluation of the mesorectum's macroscopic quality. Surg Endosc 2005;19:307–310.

Breukink SO, Pierie JPEN, Grond AJK, Hoff C, Wiggers T, Merijerink WJHS. Laparoscopic versus open total mesorectal excision: a case-control study. Int J Colorectal Dis 2005;20:428–433.

Clinical Outcomes of Surgical Therapy Study Group. A comparison of laparoscopically assisted and open colectomy for colon cancer. N Engl J Med 2004;350:2050–2059.

Dahlberg M, Glimelius B, Pahlman L. Changing strategy for rectal cancer is associated with improved outcome. Br J Surg 1999;86:379–384.

Davies MM, Larson DW. Laparoscopic surgery for colorectal cancer: the state of the art. Surg Oncol 2004;13:111–118.

Dincler S, Koller MT, Steurer J, Bachmann LM, Christen D, Buchmann P. Multidimensional analysis of learning curves in laparoscopic sigmoid resection eight-year results. Dis Colon Rectum 2003;46:1371–1379.

Dulucq JL, Wintriger P, Stabilin C, Mahajna A. Laparoscopic rectal resection with anal sphincter preservation for rectal cancer. Surg Endosc 2005;19:1468–1474.

Heald RJ, Karnajia ND. Results of radical surgery for rectal surgery. World J Surg 1992;16:848–857.

Kapiteijn E, van De Velde CJ. European trials with total mesorectal excision. Semin Surg Oncol 2000;19:350–357.

Lai PBS, Lau WY. Laparoscopic resection of rectosigmoid carcinoma: prospective randomized trial. Lancet 2004;363:1187–1192.

Leung KL, Kwok SPY, Lam SCW, et al. Laparoscopic total mesorectal excision for rectal cancer surgery. Dig Dis 205;23:135–141.

McMullen, TP, Easson AM, Cohen Z, Swallow CJ. The investigation of primary rectal cancer: current pattern of practice. Can J Surg 2005;48(1):19–26.

Morino M, Allaix ME, Giraudo G, Corno F, Garrone C. Laparoscopic versus open surgery for extraperitoneal rectal cancer: a prospective comparative study. Surg Endosc 2005;19:1460–1467.

Pikarsky AJ, Rosenthal R, Weiss EG, Wexner SD. Laparoscopic total mesorectal excision. Surg Endosc 2002;16:558–562.

Reza MM, Blasco JA, Andradas E, Cantero R, Mayol J. Systemic review of laparoscopic versus open surgery for colorectal cancer. Br J Surg 2006;93:921–928.

Scheidbach H, Rose J, Huegel O, Yildirim C, Kockerling F. Results of laparoscopic treatment of rectal cancer: analysis of 520 patients. Tech Coloproctol 2004;8(Suppl 1): s22–s24.

Tekkis PP, Senagore AJ, Delaney CP, Fazio V. Evaluation of the learning curve in laparoscopic colorectal surgery: comparison of right-sided and left-sided resections. Ann Surg 2005;42:83–91.

# 31. Splenectomy for Massive Splenomegaly

## A. Introduction

Laparoscopic splenectomy has become the procedure of choice for elective removal of the spleen. Technical difficulty arises when the spleen is massively enlarged. This chapter explores options for management in that situation, including preoperative embolization, technical tips to facilitate laparoscopic splenectomy, and minilaparotomy (open) splenectomy.

## B. Case

### *Dionne Skeete*

A 60-year-old man was referred for elective splenectomy. Over the past year he had developed progressive pancytopenia, and experienced a 30-pound weight loss, night sweats, and fatigue. Ten months earlier, a computed tomography (CT) scan performed for workup of nephrolithiasis had demonstrated splenomegaly. Bone marrow biopsy was suspicious for non-Hodgkin's lymphoma, but not diagnostic. Splenectomy was requested for diagnosis and treatment.

His past medical history was significant for right lower extremity deep venous thrombosis with bilateral pulmonary emboli 2 years earlier. He was recently diagnosed with type 2 diabetes mellitus. He had nephrolithiasis and had required cystoscopy for stone removal. His past surgical history included an open reduction and internal fixation on the left ankle, and amputations of several digits due to an accident with a grain augur (he worked as a farmer). His father died at age 72 from brain cancer. His mother died age 76 from metastatic pancreatic cancer. One brother died at age 10 from leukemia, and three brothers had type 2 diabetes mellitus.

Medications included Glucophage 1000 mg PO b.i.d. He had no known medication allergies.

He was married with six adult children. He had a 28-pack-a-year smoking history; he stopped smoking 15 years ago but still chewed tobacco. He occasionally had a glass of beer or wine.

The review of systems was remarkable only for mild abdominal pain, early satiety, and frequent nausea with occasional emesis, and myalgias. He denied easy bruising or lymphadenopathy.

Physical examination revealed a well-developed, well-nourished male, alert and oriented, in no acute distress. He appeared somewhat pale and showed signs of recent weight loss. His pulse was 81, temperature 35.1 °C, blood pressure 124/77, weight 105.6 kg, and height 184 cm. Cardiopulmonary examination was negative. No lymphadenopathy was appreciated.

Abdominal examination revealed a palpable, firm, tender left upper quadrant mass that extended down into the left lower quadrant. Rectal examination was negative and stool was guaiac negative.

Laboratory examination was significant for a white cell count of 3700/mm³, hemoglobin 11.2 g/dL, hematocrit 34%, and platelets 127,000/mm³. Blood urea nitrogen (BUN), creatinine, electrolytes, and coagulation studies were normal.

Abdominal and pelvis computed tomography (CT) scan (Figs. 31.1 and 31.2) showed an enlarged spleen measuring 26 cm in the craniocaudal dimension, without focal lesions. The liver was enlarged, measuring 24 cm. A 2.1-cm lymph node was identified in the porta hepatis and a 2.0-cm node in the portocaval regions.

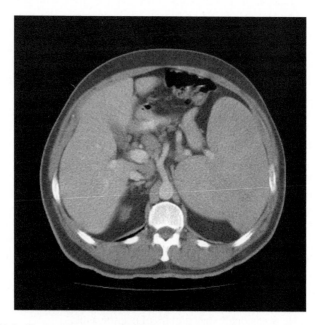

Fig. 31.1.  Computed tomography (CT) scan showing splenomegaly.

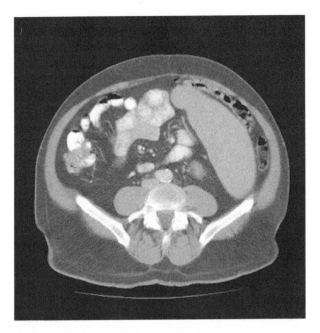

Fig. 31.2. CT scan showing extensive of spleen into pelvis.

The impression was pancytopenia and splenomegaly with bone marrow biopsy suspicious for lymphoma. Splenectomy to determine diagnosis and to decrease pancytopenia by eliminating splenic destruction was indicated.

**Would you perform the splenectomy laparoscopically or by an open approach? What about preoperative splenic artery embolization to facilitate the surgery and decrease blood loss?**

## C. Laparoscopic Splenectomy

*Lee Swanström*

Laparoscopy has become the established approach for most cases of splenectomy. The reason for this is the documented benefit that removing the spleen laparoscopically provides to patients: decreased pain, lessened hospital stay, lower wound complication rates, rapid return to preoperative activities, and minimal scarring. Because this is an extirpative procedure similar to laparoscopic cholecystectomy, the instrumentation needed and skills required are fairly basic and the learning curve fairly short. In the early experiences with laparoscopic splenectomy, splenic enlargement was generally regarded as a contraindication to the laparoscopic approach. In common with the usual evolution of laparoscopic procedures, this "contraindication" rapidly fell to the increasing experience and skill of practitioners who desired to bring the advantages of the laparoscopic procedure to as many patients as possible. Today, I would propose that splenomegaly should not be an indication for the laparoscopic approach, although it does make the procedure somewhat more difficult and requires some modification of technique as compared to the approach to the normal-sized spleen.

*Splenomegaly* is a relative term, and for the purposes of surgical approach I tend to describe two categories of splenic enlargement that require slightly different approaches. The first is *simple splenomegaly*, which I define as a spleen more than 50% enlarged from the average (<18 cm, <200 g) adult organ. A second category would be that of *massive splenomegaly*, defined as an adult spleen more than 25 cm in length or 900 g in weight. Simple splenomegaly requires minimal modification to the standard lateral or supine approaches that have been described. Several reports document that the success rates of laparoscopic removal is the same as that for average-sized spleens. Massive splenomegaly, such as that presented in the case described, requires more careful preoperative planning, more alterations in the approach, and consideration of alternatives such as hand-assisted laparoscopic surgery (HALS) approaches. Nonetheless, removing the spleen laparoscopically provides tremendous advantages for the patient, and perhaps even more for the big spleen, which would require a larger open incision, and thus is worth the added effort. This is supported by the literature where multiple reports describe successful laparoscopic or hand-assisted laparoscopic resection of spleens as large as 4800 g. These reports stress that the laparoscopic approach takes longer than open and that the complication rate for giant spleens can be increased as might be expected from the comparable open experience.

## Preoperative Evaluation

Where a standard laparoscopic splenectomy requires little in the way of preoperative imaging, such evaluation is important for splenomegaly. My preference is for a CT scan with a three-dimensional (3D) reconstruction, which shows the relationship of the spleen and its vessels to other intraabdominal organs and external landmarks (costal margin and iliac crest). In addition, I like to have a laparoscopic ultrasound available in the operating room as well. After positioning and prepping the patient, the ultrasound is used to map spleen position and determine the placement of the access ports. For massive splenomegaly we also type and crossmatch the patient for blood, as the splenic vessels can be large and the spleen itself carries significant blood volume.

## Operative Approach

For standard splenomegaly no alteration in patient position is needed, and for the most part the right lateral decubitus, or "hanging spleen," position is used. The critical procedural difference is that the position of the ports must be tailored to the splenic position, rather than placed in the typical subcostal location. Ultrasound is used to mark the location of the lower pole and hilum of the spleen on the skin. Ports must be placed below and medial to the spleen; this often pushes them away from the costal margin. An additional subcostal port may need to be placed later in the procedure to mobilize the upper pole if it is out of reach.

Dissection and mobilization is done in the standard fashion with ultrasonic coagulation and vascular staplers. One must be careful not to totally detach the large spleen from the diaphragm too early, as the heavy organ may fall into the pelvis or right upper quadrant and be hard to manipulate. We also try to keep a pedicle of tissue either at the hilum or peritoneal attachments to provide a "handle" to manipulate the organ after it is freed. Standard 15-cm impermeable tissue sacks are used to remove the enlarged spleen. If thinner, plastic bags are used, we would prefer to double-bag the spleen to avoid spillage during morcellation. Typically we would morcellize and remove the spleen through the 10-mm camera port, although with large spleens this can be a slow and tedious task.

For massive splenomegaly, additional alterations in the approach and technique are needed. The full lateral decubitus position is not possible, as the ports are often positioned at the midline or even on the patient's right. Likewise, a supine approach is not optimal as it can be difficult to lift the massive spleen out of the deep retroperitoneum. We favor a semilateral position with the patient approximately 45 degrees upright. Once again, ultrasound helps with the port placement. It is often impossible to position the lateral port below the lower pole of the spleen, which may be deep in the pelvis, and it is best placed as low as possible. One fortunate aspect of the massively enlarged spleen is that the hilar vessels are elongated and separated from the spleen, stomach, and retroperitoneum, which makes them easier to isolate and divide early in the case. Laparoscopic liver retractors, either 5 or 10 mm, are useful to manipulate the spleen, especially to divide the retroperitoneal attachments.

Once completely mobilized, the periumbilical camera port either is enlarged to 20 mm or converted to a hand port, and the specimen retrieval sack is introduced. No commercially available laparoscopic sack is available for the truly giant spleen, and I use a plastic bowel bag that is used during open procedures to contain the eviscerated small bowel during procedures such as aortic aneurysmectomy. Maneuvering the spleen into the bag tends to be the most difficult part of the procedure and requires some patience and coordinated effort with the assistant. It is made somewhat easier if a hand port is used, although there is not a lot of room for a giant spleen and a hand in these cases.

Complications are the same for standard laparoscopic splenectomy, although parenchymal injury is a bigger issue because of the forces needed to move the heavy organ. Bleeding is also always a concern as enlarged spleens tend to have larger blood vessels as well. Surgeons should be prepared to add a hand-port device or convert to open, although in our experience it is rare to need either.

## Conclusion

Splenomegaly, even massive splenomegaly, is not a contraindication to a laparoscopic approach. With a few modifications of the standard laparoscopic splenectomy, enlarged spleens can be safely removed and patients can benefit from the advantages of a minimally invasive approach.

# D.  Minimal-Access Open Splenectomy

## Marco Casaccia

Laparoscopic splenectomy (LS) is the procedure of choice in case of normal-sized spleens or in moderate splenomegaly. In massive splenomegaly, minimal-access splenectomy (MAS) may offer the same benefits of minimally invasive surgery while allowing safe manipulation and splenic dissection.

Extremely large spleens present special technical problems that test the current limits of laparoscopic surgery. However, as laparoscopic techniques, surgical skills, and instrumentation have improved, so have the safety and efficacy of this procedure even in the presence of splenomegaly. Open splenectomy (OS) in patients with hematologic disorders had a high morbidity and mortality but still represents the standard of care for malignant disease. We consider all patients with massive splenomegaly to be potential candidates for laparoscopic splenectomy. Since September 2002 we attempted a new approach in cases of severe splenomegaly not eligible for laparoscopy. The technique of splenectomy through a minimal access is here reported in detail.

The patient is placed in the supine decubitus position with a sandbag under the left flank. A left 14-cm incision under the costal margin is made. The operation is conducted under direct vision. Field exposure is achieved by conventional abdominal wall retractors. The Ultrasonic dissector is the only laparoscopic instrument necessary for the operation. Optional laparoscopic tools consist of a clip applier and a vascular stapler.

First, the stomach is retracted medially to expose the spleen. A thorough search is then made for accessory spleens. The first step is the identification of the gastrosplenic ligament and the opening of the lesser sac in its lateral portion. Next, the short gastric vessels lying over the splenic hilum are divided by using the Ultrasonic dissection or eventually over clips (Fig. 31.3). The uppermost vessels of the gastrosplenic ligament will be isolated and divided only after the isolation of the splenic artery and vein.

Then the dissection reaches the hilum, and the vessels are isolated from the pancreas and the surrounding tissues by combining a careful digital dissection with the use of the Ultrasonic dissector.

If a distributed anatomy is present, the splenic branches are usually dissected and divided between silk ligatures or clipped. In cases of magistral anatomy (early branching of splenic bilar vessels), after ensuring that the tail of the pancreas is identified and dissected away, we perform separate silk ligation of the splenic vessels with a delayed ligature of the vein to allow the spleen to empty out.

At this point, the volumetric reduction of the spleen enables the surgeon to complete the division of all the attachments. The short gastric vessels are very short and enlarged in splenomegaly, and they are located in the immediate vicinity of the diaphragm. Access to these vessels

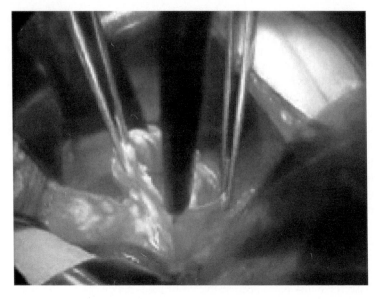

Fig. 31.3. Division of the short gastric vessels by using the Ultrasonic dissection.

requires combined dislocation of the stomach to the right, and gentle retraction of the upper splenic pole to the left.

The dissection continues with an incision carried slightly into the left side of the gastrocolic ligament; then the splenic flexure is partially mobilized by incising the splenocolic ligament, the lower part of the phrenicocolic ligament, and the sustentaculum lienis.

Finally, the phrenicocolic ligament is incised all the way to the left crus of the diaphragm by the Ultrasonic dissector. A sterile organ-retrieval bag is used for the extraction of the spleen. This bag is introduced into the abdominal cavity and the spleen is manually slipped inside to prevent splenosis during the subsequent manipulations. Grasping forceps are used to hold the edges of the bag and to effect partial closure. At the end of the procedure, a nasogastric tube and an abdominal drain in the left hypochondrium are left in place.

## Pearls

The use of the nondominant hand is of major importance in every step of the procedure:

- It retracts the spleen medially to free the splenodiaphragmatic ligament.
- It pulls the spleen downward to dissect the upper pole and to divide the uppermost short gastric vessels.
- It pulls the spleen upward to dissect the lower pole and the splenocolic ligament.
- During all the above-mentioned maneuvers, the hand carries out a sort of gentle "squeezing" of the spleen, thus obtaining an enlargement of the abdominal "working space."

Ligature of the splenic artery (magistral type) or arteries (distributed type) causes darkening of the entire spleen and warrants achieving ischemia of the whole organ. To have a further volumetric reduction of the spleen, it is necessary to isolate the splenic vein and to perform a distal ligature and a proximal venting of it. This maneuver has two advantages:

- A quicker emptying of the spleen
- Immediate intraoperative blood recuperation ready, after being processed, to be reinfused in the patient

## Pitfalls

If you are not sure about complete ischemia of the spleen after arterial obstruction, do not perform venting of the splenic vein but keep a loop on it to control possible bleeding during dissection.

## Discussion

Massive splenectomy virtually always relates to hematologic malignancies. In these patients, the local discomfort from massive splenomegaly and the risks of refractable thrombocytopenia and anemia are conventional indications for splenectomy. Open splenectomy has been associated with substantial morbidity and mortality, and the rates may be higher in patients with splenomegaly, patients with myeloproliferative disorders, and the elderly. Laparoscopic resection has become the standard means for removal of normal-sized spleens in many medical centers. The application of minimally invasive techniques in the setting of splenomegaly is less well defined and was previously considered a contraindication to the laparoscopic approach. As OS still represents the standard of care for malignant disease with massive splenomegaly, the MAS technique is intended to be a possible option to either OS and fully LS.

Many parameters play a role in the decision whether to use a laparoscopic or a minimal-access approach. We consider body habitus of the patient (body mass index [BMI] and body surface area [BSA]) and the three splenic diameters as measured by ultrasound (US) or computed tomography (CT) to be of practical relevance. Although spleen CT volumetric study (Fig. 31.4) with 3D vascular reconstruction may provide valuable information for planning the surgical strategy, it is still difficult to obtain and seems not to be cost-effective. The spleen length diameter (SLD) measurement, taken by a simple preoperative ultrasonography, represents the easiest parameter available.

The last analysis before going to a minimal-access or a laparoscopic approach is the preoperative clinical examination to assess the dimensions of the abdominal "working space" in case of a laparoscopic access. In particular, this parameter may play a critical role, being strongly

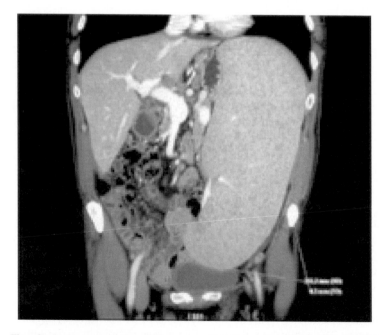

Fig. 31.4. A preoperative CT scan with spleen length diameter (SLD) measurement.

related to both body habitus and abdominal wall relaxation. Spleen size might be associated with abdominal dimensions in order to give some idea of the room available to move our laparoscopic instruments.

It is obvious that a spleen extending into the midline, as in the majority of our MAS patients, does not even allow placing the trocars in the correct left subcostal position without the risk of damaging the spleen.

Furthermore, two considerations have to be made when approaching a splenomegaly for malignancy. First, in the laparoscopic approach, a service minilaparotomy is always performed when pathologic examination of the surgical specimen is required to document the hematologic disease. Second, laparoscopic-assisted removal of the entire spleen via an accessory minilaparotomy does not affect the duration of surgery, rate of complications, or length of hospital stay.

We consider all patients with massive splenomegaly to be potential candidates for laparoscopic splenectomy, and the laparoscopic approach has been used since June 1997. Since September 2002, in 24 cases of massive splenomegaly not eligible for laparoscopy, we have adopted the MAS technique.

In our experience the operative time ranged from 60 to 225 minutes (mean, 105 minutes). The average weight of the spleen was 2467 g (range, 860 to 4800 g). The average SLD was 28 cm (range, 21 to 45 cm). Postoperative complications occurred in six cases, and none required reintervention. One perioperative death occurred 15 days after the operation in a patient affected by idiopathic myelofibrosis as a consequence of secondary blast crisis.

Comparing these data with a series of LS performed at our center for the same pathologies, we noted that the patients in the MAS group and in the LS group were comparable in age, American Society of Anesthesiologists (ASA) class, BMI, and BSA. Mean splenic weight exceeded 2 kg in both groups, but greater splenic dimensions were registered in the MAS group with a statistical significance as regards the transverse diameter measured at the splenic hilum.

Estimated intraoperative blood loss was similar in both groups, while operative time was shorter in the MAS group, but the difference was not statistically significant. The morbidity rate was similar in both groups. The mean length of hospital stay for MAS and LS was respectively 8 and 6 days. This difference was partly due to the 14-cm laparotomy that was used in the MAS approach versus the 7- to 8-cm accessory incision that was commonly used in the fully laparoscopic approach to retrieve the spleen.

Concerning the technical aspects of the operation, a 14-cm minilaparotomy was used in all cases. This measure corresponded to the

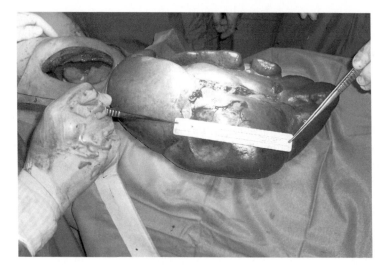

Fig. 31.5. A 4-kg (SLD = 35 cm) spleen after retrieval.

splenic transverse diameter in the first two cases of MAS. Later, this measure was adopted successfully in all the other cases regardless of this parameter (Fig. 31.5).

Many authors advocate the use of hand-assisted laparoscopic splenectomy in case of massive splenomegaly with results that are comparable
to or even better than those with conventional LS. Hand assistance, by
regaining tactile feedback, also increases the safety of the procedure,
since it enables the surgeon to rapidly identify vascular structures and,
in the case of accidental bleeding, allows immediate hemostatic control by digital compression. Furthermore, manual manipulation of the
spleen, particularly when it is a large one, is probably safer and easier
than manipulation with laparoscopic instruments.

Similarly, our MAS approach makes extensive use of the surgeon's
nondominant hand. Analogies with the fully laparoscopic approach are
represented by the use of laparoscopic instruments like the ultrasonic
dissector, the clip applier, and the vascular stapler.

This MAS technique stays on the border among OS, HALS and LS,
retaining all the advantages of a minimally invasive approach. We believe
that experience with laparoscopic splenectomy is necessary to perform
MAS since the laparoscopic skills of the surgeon greatly facilitate dissection with this approach.

Minimal-access splenectomy in patients with severe splenomegaly
represents an additional tool in surgeon's armamentarium. It couples the

advantages of the hand assistance, such as shorter operative times and increased safety of the procedure, with the classic benefits of minimal invasive surgery.

# E. Preoperative Splenic Artery Embolization

## *Melhem Sharafuddin*

Transcatheter arterial embolization is increasingly being performed to treat traumatic splenic injuries and aneurysms, providing a viable alternative to open surgery while allowing splenic salvage. The role of arterial embolization in the primary management of splenomegaly and hypersplenism remains the subject of debate. Proponents of this approach insist that, when used for hypersplenism, splenic embolization can improve the hematologic parameters in patients who otherwise would be unable to undergo high-dose chemotherapy or immunosuppressive therapy. Some have also advocated the use of splenic embolization to reduce splenic blood flow, thus lowering portal pressure and preventing sequelae in patients with portal hypertension. This approach has also been used to treat splenic artery steal syndrome and improve liver perfusion in liver transplant recipients. Avoidance of surgery is preferred in certain patient populations such as those with cirrhosis with severe portal hypertension and in pediatric patients where splenic function preservation is desired.

When surgery is elected, preoperative embolization may be considered. This approach attempts to decrease the risks associated with patients with massive splenomegaly. These risks involve thrombocytopenia that may be difficult to correct secondary to splenic sequestration. Additionally, the surgical anatomy is often distorted secondary to the massive spleen and dissection can be difficult and risky in the presence of abundant enlarged collaterals. These factors can lead to uncontrollable hemorrhage, especially in laparoscopic procedures. With the advent of laparoscopic splenectomy techniques, the size of the spleen in the setting of massive splenomegaly has posed significant challenges in terms of both mobilization and the ability to remove the resected spleen from within the abdominal cavity. Even with the use of in-situ fragmentation techniques, the massively enlarged spleen continues to pose significant challenges.

The concept of preoperative embolization is not a new one. Several early reports demonstrated the feasibility of this technique and its ability to induce devascularization and size reduction as a prelude to open splenectomy. Following a period of decreased utilization, there has been a resurgence in the use of splenic embolization as a preoperative adjunct to reduce splenic size prior to open or (especially) laparoscopic surgery. Numerous subsequent reports have also indicated the relative safety of reduced volume or partial embolization techniques. Some have suggested the use of quantitative goals in reduction in splenic artery flow compared to baseline as a therapeutic goal during splenic artery embolization. In addition to the gradual splenic parenchyma-ischemic effect of partial embolization, some reports indicated a suppressive effect on platelet-associated immunoglobulin G (PA-IgG) after the procedure. These results suggest that a transcatheter splenic arterial embolization not only suppresses the platelet pool in the spleen but may also suppress associated immunologic thrombocytopenia.

When splenic embolization is used as a preoperative adjunct in the urgent setting, complete splenic devascularization may be beneficial. However, because of the risk of postembolic systemic response and the severe pain associated with splenic necrosis, the embolization should be performed immediately before splenectomy, preferably under general anesthesia. Patients who have severe thrombocytopenia should receive platelet transfusions during surgery.

Material used in splenic embolization have included coils and occlusion balloons, autologous clot, Gelfoam, and tissue adhesives. Distal vascular embolization has been performed using polyvinyl alcohol (PVA) microspheres and foam, and silicone particles, among other agents.

In reports describing the use of mechanical occlusion techniques (such as oils), mechanical occlusion of the major splenic arteries can be performed in the proximal, distal, or juxtahilar segments of the splenic artery. Although hilar occlusion is most effective in terms of correction of hematologic complication of hypersplenism, it has a slightly higher rate of complications, such as infarction and infection, whereas more proximal occlusion is associated with a higher rate of therapeutic failure due to abundant collateral circulation.

# F. Conclusions

## *Dionne Skeete*

Laparoscopic splenectomy is a widely performed and well-accepted modality in the operative management for a variety of splenic disorders. This procedure is routinely performed with low morbidity and mortality, and offers the benefits of decreased postoperative analgesia, decreased hospital stay, and faster postoperative recovery as compared to open splenectomy. Despite the technical refinements to the technique since its description in 1991, splenomegaly remains a technical challenge to the laparoscopic technique as it limits the exposure and dissection of the splenic hilum and subsequent removal of the spleen. Patel et al. retrospectively reviewed their experience with laparoscopic splenectomy and found significant differences in patients with splenic size 1000 g or larger (range, 1000 to 4750 g) versus splenic size less than 1000 g (range, 57 to 900 g). Operative times, estimated blood loss, postoperative morbidity, and median postoperative stay were all significantly increased in the patients with splenomegaly. The conversion rate to open splenectomy was also significantly higher at 18% versus 5%.

Preoperative splenic artery embolization (PSAE) has been used with laparoscopic splenectomy to decrease intraoperative blood loss in an effort to decrease the conversion rate and morbidity. Complications include contrast nephropathy, puncture site hemorrhage, postprocedure pain, pancreatitis, and pancreatic necrosis. Avoidance of occlusion of the distal pancreatica magna artery can help decrease the pancreatic complications. Poulin et al. used PSAE in patients with splenic length of 20 to 30 cm and concluded it to be a safe procedure. Postprocedure pain occurred in 46% of the patients, which was readily controlled with patient-controlled analgesia, and there was one case of pancreatitis reported. However, their conversion rate was 17% as compared to 5% in patients with spleens smaller than 20 cm, and 83% of the patients with splenomegaly required transfusion.

Hand-assisted laparoscopic splenectomy has been performed as an alternative treatment in patients with splenomegaly. This technique combines the minimally invasive benefits of laparoscopy with the increased exposure and tactile sensation from the introduction of the surgeon's hand into the operative field. A review of patients undergoing hand-assisted laparoscopic splenectomy with an average splenic weight after morcellation of 1516 g revealed no significant differences in operative times, intraoperative blood loss, hospital length of stay, and complication rates as compared to a group of patients undergoing conventional laparoscopic splenectomy with an average splenic weight of 1031 g. One patient with a splenic weight of 3500 g required conversion to open splenectomy for bleeding, but the authors concluded that the upper limit for splenic size for this approach remains to be determined.

In conclusion, though splenomegaly remains a technical challenge, the literature suggests that hand-assisted laparoscopic splenectomy may provide similar outcomes as compared to conventional laparoscopy, and that preoperative splenic embolization may not be as beneficial. Further studies are needed to compare the two operative techniques and clarify the operative indications for hand-assisted laparoscopic splenectomy. For patients in whom neither laparoscopic approach is feasible, a minimal-access approach such as that described by Casaccia provides an alternative.

# References

Patel A, Parker J, Wallwork B, et al. Massive splenomegaly is associated with significant morbidity after laparoscopic splenectomy. Ann Surg 2003;238:235–240.

Poulin E, Mamazza J, Schlachta M. Splenic artery embolization before laparoscopic splenectomy. Surg Endosc 1998;12:870–875.

# Suggested Readings

Borrazzo EC, Day JM, Morrisey KP, et al. Hand-assisted laparoscopic splenectomy for giant spleens. Surg Endosc 2003;17:918–920.

Brodsky JA, Brody FJ, Walsh RM, Malm JA, Ponsky JL. Laparoscopic splenectomy. Surg Endosc 2002;16(5):851–854.

Casaccia M, Torelli P, Cavaliere D, Santori G, Panaro F, Valente U. Minimal-access splenectomy: a viable alternative to laparoscopic splenectomy in massive splenomegaly. JSLS 2005;9:411–414.

Choy C, Cacchione R, Moon V, Ferzli G. Experience with seven cases of massive splenomegaly. J Laparoendosc Adv Surg Tech A 2004;14(4):197–200.

Donini A, Baccarani U, Terrosu G, et al. Laparoscopic vs open splenectomy in the management of hematologic diseases. Surg Endosc 1999;13(12):1220–1225.

Iwase K, Higaki J, Mikata S, et al. Laparoscopically assisted splenectomy following preoperative splenic artery embolization using contour emboli for myelofibrosis with massive splenomegaly. Surg Laparosc Endosc Percutan Tech 1999;9:197–202.

Iwase K, Higaki J, Yoon HE, et al. Splenic artery embolization using contour emboli before laparoscopic or laparoscopically assisted splenectomy. Surg Laparosc Endosc Percutan Tech 2002;5:331–336.

Kaban GK, Czerniach DR, Cohen R, et al. Hand-assisted laparoscopic splenectomy in the setting of splenomegaly. Surg Endosc 2004;18(9):1340–1343.

Mahon D, Rhodes M. Laparoscopic splenectomy: size matters. Ann R Coll Surg Engl 2003;85(4):248–251.

Ohta M, Nishizaki T, Matsumoto T, et al. Analysis of risk factors for massive intraoperative bleeding during laparoscopic splenectomy. J Hepatobiliary Pancreat Surg 2005;12:433–437.

Rosen M, Brody F, Walsh RM, Ponsky J. Hand-assisted laparoscopic splenectomy vs conventional laparoscopic splenectomy in cases of splenomegaly. Arch Surg 2002;137(12):1348–1352.

Smith L, Luna G, Merg A, McNevin S, Moore M, Bax T. Laparoscopic splenectomy for treatment of splenomegaly. Am J Surg 2004;187:618–620.

Takahashi T, Arima Y, Yokomuro S, et al. Splenic artery embolization before laparoscopic splenectomy in children. Surg Endosc 2005;19:1345–1348.

Targarona EM, Balague C, Cerdan G, et al. Hand-assisted laparoscopic splenectomy (HALS) in cases of splenomegaly: a comparison analysis with conventional laparoscopic splenectomy. Surg Endosc 2002;16(3):426–430.

Targarona EM, Balague C, Trias M. Is the laparoscopic approach reasonable in cases of splenomegaly? Semin Laparosc Surg 2004;11(3):185–190.

Torelli P, Cavaliere D, Casaccia M, et al. Laparoscopic splenectomy for hematological diseases. Surg Endosc 2002;16(6):965–971.

Weiss CA III, Kavic SM, Adrales GL, Park AE. Laparoscopic splenectomy: what barriers remain? Surg Innov 2005;12(1):23–29.

# 32. Insulinoma of Tail of Pancreas

## A. Introduction

Insulinomas are generally benign tumors ideally suited to laparoscopic resection. Surgical management has changed over the years. Small benign tumors of the endocrine pancreas, including insulinomas, can be enucleated if their location is separate from the main pancreatic duct. Those over 2 cm and those close to the main pancreatic duct are generally treated by resection of the distal pancreas. Such a resection may be done as a spleen-preserving operation, or may include splenectomy. This chapter explores options in surgical treatment of a 2-cm insulinoma.

## B. Case

*Carol E.H. Scott-Conner*

A 55-year-old woman developed episodic confusion and was found to be hypoglycemic during one of these episodes. During an attack, at a time when her serum glucose was 35 mg/dL, a serum insulin level of 15 μU/mL (normal less than 6 μU/mL) was measured. Factitious administration of insulin was excluded and a computed tomography (CT) scan showed a 2-cm smooth nodule in the distal third of the pancreas, consistent with benign insulinoma. No other abnormalities were noted. Her physician has excluded other endocrine disorders. She was referred for surgical evaluation.

Her past medical history was significant for rheumatic fever as a child, with only a very mild mitral stenosis as a result. She was asymptomatic, but requires antibiotic prophylaxis before dental procedures. Past surgical history included an appendectomy at age 17, and two cesarean sections. Family history was negative for any endocrine disorders. The patient was active and athletic, and was on no medications. She did not smoke.

On physical examination, she was a slender woman who appeared her stated age. Head, ears, eyes, nose, and throat (HEENT) were normal cephalic and atraumatic (NCAT). A soft holosystolic murmur was audible at the cardiac apex. Respirations are normal. Abdominal exam revealed well-healed McBurney and Pfannenstiel incisions. No masses or tenderness were noted. Rectal and pelvic examinations were normal.

**Which procedure would you recommend—laparoscopic distal pancreatectomy with splenic preservation, laparoscopic distal pancreatectomy with splenectomy, or laparoscopic enucleation?**

# C.  Laparoscopic Distal Pancreatectomy Without Splenectomy

*Basil J. Ammori*

I would recommend laparoscopic distal pancreatectomy with preservation of the spleen.

## Laparoscopic Rather Than Open Distal Pancreatectomy

The former can be accomplished with lower morbidity (mean, 26%) and mortality (mean, 0.5%) and a shorter postoperative hospital stay than those reported after open distal pancreatectomy (morbidity, 31% to 47%; mortality, 0.9% to 4%). The patient carries a low risk for need to convert to open surgery as she is not obese, has had no previous open upper abdominal surgery, does not have a large tumor, and is fit to tolerate a longer operative procedure and pneumoperitoneum. There is no controversy about the application of the laparoscopic approach in patients with benign pancreatic disease, and a patient with a solitary insulinoma is highly likely (90% or more) to have a benign tumor.

## Distal Pancreatectomy Rather Than Enucleation

A lesion of this size (2 cm) is likely to involve or be in very close proximity to the pancreatic duct. Enucleation carries a risk of injury to the pancreatic duct and pancreatic fistula. While laparoscopic ultrasound aids in defining the relationship of the tumor to the pancreatic duct, it is not always available, its interpretation may be inaccurate, and one may not be quite confident that a very close pancreatic duct will not be injured during enucleation. Although distal pancreatectomy also carries a risk of postoperative pancreatic fistula from the stump of the pancreas, it is quite likely that the consequences of pancreatic fistula from enucleation may be graver than those of a distal pancreatectomy and harder to treat. The former is likely to persist longer as the pancreatic tail distal to the fistula site remains intact. While most pancreatic fistulas respond to treatment by observation and percutaneous drainage with or without octreotide (long-acting somatostatin), a fistula arising from the pancreatic stump after distal pancreatectomy may also be readily controlled by endoscopic insertion of a pancreatic duct stent across the ampulla and pancreatic sphincter. Enucleation is quite difficult to accomplish if the tumor is found located on the posterior surface of the gland, and distal pancreatectomy is preferable.

## *Preserve the Spleen Rather Than Performing a Splenectomy*

Preservation of the spleen offers immunologic advantages, as splenectomy is associated with the risk, albeit very small, of postsplenectomy sepsis and reduction of perioperative infectious complications and hospital stay. Preservation of the spleen and splenic vessels during distal pancreatectomy is the standard approach in patients with benign lesions. This is technically easy to accomplish in patients with insulinoma as there are no inflammatory adhesions to the vessels such as those observed in patients with chronic pancreatitis.

The splenic vessels may have to be sacrificed if bleeding that is difficult to control is encountered during a spleen-preserving distal pancreatectomy (DP). The spleen, however, may be preserved as it survives on blood supply from the short gastric vessels, an approach that has been shown to preserve splenic viability and function in more than four fifths of the patients. One fifth of spleens, however, may become ischemic and require subsequent splenectomy, a procedure that could then be accomplished laparoscopically.

## *Surgical Technique*

Under general endotracheal anesthesia, the patient is usually placed in the left lateral position. Some surgeons prefer to place the patient in supine position. Surgery is often accomplished through four ports, and the use of a 30-degree laparoscope is essential for a better visual access to the operative field compared with a 0-degree laparoscope.

Using the ultrasonically activated scalpel (UAS, e.g., Ethicon Endosurgery, Cincinnati, OH) or the Ligasure™ system (Valleylab Inc., Boulder, CO) the splenocolic ligament is divided and the splenic flexure is retracted caudally. The pancreas is exposed by dividing the gastrocolic omentum and any congenital adhesions between the posterior gastric wall and the anterior surface of the pancreas. Care should be exercised to preserve the left gastroepiploic and short gastric vessels. The laparoscopic ultrasound (LapUS) may be employed to localize the lesion (though it is highly likely that the location of a tumor of this size will become readily evident upon exposure of the tail of the pancreas), to aid the decision of whether to proceed to a distal pancreatectomy or enucleation, and to determine the extent of pancreatic resection. The inferior border of the pancreas is then dissected and the pancreas is lifted off the retroperitoneum to expose the splenic vein.

Two approaches to the spleen-preserving distal pancreatectomy may be adopted. A proximal-to-distal approach starts the dissection either at the neck of the gland by exposing the portal vein or at a suitable point along the body or tail of the gland determined by the location of the tumor and extent of the intended pancreatic resection. A careful dissection and division of the small pancreatic venous tributaries using the UAS, Ligasure, or endoclips facilitates separation of the splenic vein and exposure of the splenic artery. A tunnel is created and the pancreas is lifted off, a maneuver that could be aided by the application of a sling for ease of retraction. The pancreas is then transacted with a 30- or 45-mm linear endostapler (blue cartridge). The pancreatic branches of the splenic artery are similarly dissected and divided. Dissection is then continued toward the tail of the gland separating it from the splenic hilum to complete the resection.

The alternative is a distal-to-proximal approach that starts the dissection at the tail of the pancreas by separating it from the hilum of the spleen. The arterial branches of the splenic artery and the venous tributaries to the splenic vein are divided. The division of pancreatic vessels is terminated at a convenient point where the pancreas is then divided with an endostapler.

If preservation of the splenic vessels had to be abandoned for technical reasons such as control of bleeding, the splenic vein may be separated from the body of the gland and divided, exposing the splenic artery. The pancreas is transected and the splenic artery is then divided above the gland. Alternatively, the artery is identified above the body of the gland, dissected and divided before transection of the pancreas. The dissection is continued toward the tail of the gland, and the pancreas is cleared from the hilum of the spleen. The short gastric vessels are preserved allowing perhaps for the spleen to be preserved as it derives its blood supply from the vasa brevia. The spleen, however, should be inspected at the end of surgery as it may become too ischemic to be preserved. Under those circumstances, the short gastric vessels are divided and the spleen is fully mobilized by dividing the lienorenal and lienophrenic ligaments.

The optimal method of handling of the pancreatic stump with view to reduction of postoperative pancreatic fistula formation remains unclear. The large majority of surgeons performing laparoscopic distal pancreatectomy transect the pancreas with staples, and there is no clear evidence to recommend oversewing the pancreatic stump. While there is evidence from open surgery that treatment of the pancreatic stump with tissue glue and the administration of prophylactic perioperative somatostatin or one of its analogues reduce the incidence of postoperative pancreatic fistula, there is no clear evidence from the laparoscopic series to confirm the effectiveness of these measures. Marked reductions of pancreatic fistula rates have been reported after selective ligation of the pancreatic duct in patients undergoing open distal pancreatectomy. In 127 patients undergoing laparoscopic pancreatic resections, Mabrut et al. confirmed by multivariate analysis that selective laparoscopic closure of the pancreatic stump and duct were significant factors affecting the occurrence of postoperative pancreatic-related complications. Selective ligation of the pancreatic duct during laparoscopic DP is therefore recommended whenever feasible.

The operative field is then irrigated with warm saline, and a drain is placed to the pancreatic stump. Some surgeons prefer to examine the drain effluent at 5 to 7 days for amylase concentration before removing the drain. This could be carried out on outpatient basis if the patient was ready for discharge earlier.

The specimen is retrieved in a water-impervious specimen retrieval bag. This is essential to avoid spillage of pancreatic juice into the wound with subsequent necrosis of subcutaneous fat and wound infection.

Surgeons performing laparoscopic pancreatic surgery should keep records of volume of blood lost, need and volume of intraoperative and postoperative blood transfusion, total operating time (from skin incision to skin closure), and any intraoperative or postoperative complications, postoperative hospital stay, and duration and findings of follow-up.

# D. Laparoscopic Distal Pancreatectomy with Spleen Preservation

*David Hazzan, Edward H. Chin, and Barry A. Salky*

Laparoscopic surgery has been applied to an increasing number of indications in recent years. Laparoscopic pancreatic surgery (LPS) has been limited, however, for several reasons: the difficult anatomic location of the pancreas, the relative rarity of surgical pancreatic disorders, the requirements for skillful and experienced laparoscopic surgeons, and the need for advanced technical equipment.

With increased experience and technologic refinements, therapeutic procedures have been developed, including pancreatic pseudocyst drainage, laparoscopic pancreatic necrosectomies, and palliative biliodigestive and gastrointestinal bypasses for unresectable pancreatic malignancies.

Now, more than 10 years since the first reported laparoscopic pancreatic resection by Gagner and Pomp, only 250 additional cases have been published, with very few series exceeding 10 patients.

Insulinoma is the most common endocrine tumor of the pancreas, representing up to 80% of clinically symptomatic endocrine pancreatic tumors. It occurs in all age groups, with a peak incidence during the third to fifth decades, and it is typically <2 cm at presentation. Approximately 90% are solitary, benign, and located predominantly in the body and tail of the pancreas. These favorable features make insulinoma the primary pancreatic neuroendocrine tumor for laparoscopic treatment.

The different options for a solitary insulinoma of the distal pancreas are laparoscopic distal pancreatectomy (LDP) with splenectomy, LDP with spleen preservation, and laparoscopic enucleation.

We have used a laparoscopic spleen-preserving distal pancreatectomy for young patients with body or tail lesions who are not candidates for enucleation (as in the case presented here), most commonly due to tumor proximity to the main pancreatic duct.

Interestingly, Assalia and Gagner reviewed the English-language literature and found a higher incidence of pancreatic leak after enucleation than after distal pancreatectomy for both open and laparoscopic surgery: 30.7% with laparoscopic enucleation and 28.8% with open technique versus 5.1% and 12.5%, respectively. In our experience the incidence of pancreatic fistula is also higher after laparoscopic enucleation than after LDP (28.5% vs. 7.1%).

As with open surgery, splenic preservation in these benign conditions is encouraged whenever technically feasible. In cases of hilar fibrosis and scarring due to past inflammation or abscess formation, or with lesions located very close to the splenic vessels, however, we believe that laparoscopic en bloc pancreaticosplenectomy is the safest technique.

In older patients, no clear long-term benefit is associated with splenic preservation, although a trend toward lower perioperative morbidity has been reported. In our series of LDP ($n = 28$), splenic salvage was attempted in eight (28.6%) and successful in six (75%). One splenectomy was performed for intraoperative bleeding, and a second for splenic devascularization after completion of the pancreatectomy.

Two techniques are described to perform LDP with spleen preservation: LDP with splenic vessel preservation, and LDP with splenic vessel ligation.

Preservation of the splenic vessels requires a longer operating time and laparoscopic expertise. However, after LDP with splenic vessel ligation, the remaining splenic vascular supply is solely from the short gastric vessels. While this is technically a spleen-preserving procedure, immunologic function may be impaired. An intact splenic artery and portal vein have been demonstrated to be critical for splenic clearance of encapsulated organisms. For this reason, we do not recommend this technique over LDP with splenectomy.

## Surgical Technique

The patient is placed in modified lithotomy, with both arms tucked and in the reverse Trendelenburg position. A bolster is placed beneath the left thoracic cage to elevate the left side 20 degrees.

The surgeons stand between the legs, with the first assistant on the patient's left. The video monitor is placed above the head of the patient. Four ports are used. An angled (30 to 45 degrees) scope is recommended.

The body and tail of the pancreas are exposed anteriorly through a window in the gastrocolic ligament, which is created with ultrasonic shears.

The greater curvature of the stomach is retracted with an atraumatic clamp. Laparoscopic ultrasonography is used to localize the lesion, and specifically define the relation with the main pancreatic duct and splenic vessels. At this point, either enucleation or distal pancreatectomy with or without splenectomy is elected.

The posterior peritoneum is incised at the inferior border of the pancreas, which is then dissected to ascertain involvement of the splenic vein or artery. The splenic vein is typically encountered first, and dissected from the posterior aspect of the pancreas. If the tumor is found to be adherent to the splenic vessels, splenic salvage is abandoned.

The posterior peritoneum along the superior border of the pancreas is then incised, and the splenic artery dissected along the adjacent adventitial plane. Once separated from the splenic vessels, the pancreas is transected with a vascular load stapler. The distal pancreas is held with an atraumatic instrument, and the transverse branches of the splenic artery and vein to the pancreas are individually dissected and divided either with clips or ultrasonic shears. The 5-mm Ligasure Lap™ (U.S. Surgical, Norwalk, CT) or the Harmonic Ace (Ethicon Endosurgery, Cincinnati, OH) can be used.

The pancreas is then mobilized from medial to lateral, and the freed specimen placed in an extraction bag. Hemostasis, irrigation, and placement of a closed suction drain complete the procedure.

Nasogastric tubes are removed intraoperatively in all patients, with clear fluids begun on the evening of the operation. Fluid from the closed suction drain is routinely sent to the laboratory for amylase level determination on the third postoperative day. The drain is removed when only serous fluid is obtained, and the amylase level is equal to or less than serum value.

The majority of intraoperative complications are secondary to major bleeding, typically from the splenic artery or vein. Dissection in the proper adventitial plane of these vessels and gentle laparoscopic technique will limit the incidence.

Rapid hemorrhage that cannot be promptly controlled requires urgent conversion to laparotomy. Temporary control can be achieved by direct pressure using a 10-mm instrument while entry to the abdomen is obtained.

If the bleeding source is a transverse pancreatic vessel, and cannot be controlled directly, then more proximal vascular control on the splenic vessel should be obtained, and splenic preservation aborted.

The main postoperative complication after this operation is pancreatic leak and its sequelae. To date, management of the pancreatic remnant following distal pancreatectomy remains a clinically relevant problem in both open and laparoscopic surgery. Ductal ligation, ultrasonic dissection, fibrin glue, synthetic patch and mesh use, pancreaticoenteric anastomosis, and hand-sewn or stapled closure are examples of the numerous attempts made to avoid a fistula. The results are variable, with no clear advantage to one approach.

In our series, pancreatic fistulas developed postoperatively in four patients (11.4% of the total number of patients): two patients of those who were treated with enucleation (28.5%), one patient of those who were treated with distal pancreatectomy and splenectomy (4.5%), and one patient of those who were treated with spleen-preserving distal pancreatectomy (16.5%). Three of the four patients required CT-guided drainage of peripancreatic collections and total parenteral nutrition; all were discharged home on total parenteral nutrition with subsequent spontaneous fistula closure. The fourth patient with a pancreatic fistula did not develop a collection, and had spontaneous closure after 3 weeks.

Our rate of pancreatic fistula using a stapled technique (11.4%) is within the reported range (0% to 30%) of other centers. This large variation stems largely from the inhomogeneous criteria for pancreatic fistula, making comparisons between series confusing if not impossible.

In summary, LDP with spleen preservation for insulinomas located in the body or tail of the pancreas is a safe and effective procedure. The pancreatic fistula rate and overall pancreatic-related complications compare favorably to recent open series.

The successful management of the pancreatic stump remains the challenge of this procedure and is likely independent of the laparoscopic technique.

# E. Conclusions

## Carol E.H. Scott-Conner

In the short time that this book has been in development, laparoscopic surgical opinion has decisively come to favor a single procedure for management of this problem. A tumor of the size described is apt to impinge upon the main pancreatic duct, and enucleation is likely to result in pancreatic fistula. Hence, pancreatic resection becomes the procedure of choice. For a lesion in the body or tail, spleen-preserving distal pancreatectomy is the procedure of choice.

This procedure traces its roots to open surgery for trauma. It was initially described as part of a dedicated attempt to maximize splenic salvage, and to thus minimize the potential infectious complications of the postsplenectomy state.

Successful completion of this procedure, whether open or laparoscopic, requires meticulous attention to control of numerous short,

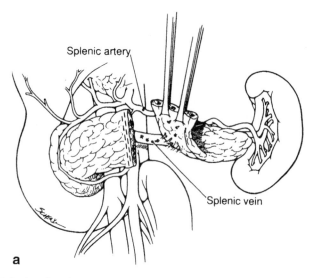

Splenic artery

Splenic vein

a

Fig. 32.1. (continued)

thin-walled tributaries that link the splenic vein to the posterior aspect of the pancreas. A smaller number of arterial branches may also be encountered. These are easily controlled with the ultrasonic shears.

Theoretical advantages of this procedure include preservation of splenic function, but also elimination of a potential space under the left hemidiaphragm (where the spleen normally resides) that might fill with fluid and become infected.

The most common and simplest approach is a proximal to distal (or medial to lateral) dissection that begins by elevating the pancreas at the proposed point of transaction, then separating it from the underlying splenic vessels (Fig. 32.1A). Occasionally, especially for lesions right in the tail, it may be simplest to elevate the tail first and work backward from distal to proximal (Fig. 32.1B). This is particularly true in open surgery, where the surgeon is free to move and change perspective. With the fixed perspective of the laparoscope, this is less natural, and it is more difficult to see under the pancreas unless the laparoscope is moved to a different trocar site.

The laparoscopic approach provides the usual advantages of decreased length of stay and faster return to work. In a case-control comparison, Velanovich demonstrated that major complications including leak rate were similar.

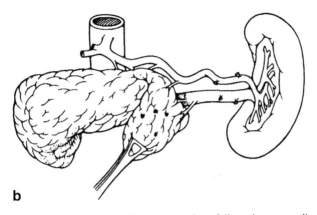

**b**

Fig. 32.1.  (continued) (A) Anatomic representation of dissection proceeding from proximal to distal (medial to lateral). The pancreas has been transected with a stapling device and the distal segment elevated from the underlying splenic artery and splenic vein. Multiple small tributaries must be atraumatically controlled. (B) Anatomic representation of dissection proceeding from distal to proximal. Note that the pancreatic tip must be retracted medially, and that this must be accomplished without obscuring the surgeon's view of the underlying vascular tributaries. (From Scott-Conner CEH, Dawson DL. Operative Anatomy, 2nd ed. Philadelphia: Lippincott Williams & Wilkins, 2003, with permission.)

# References

Assalia A, Gagner M. Laparoscopic pancreatic surgery for islet cell tumors of the pancreas. World J Surg 2004;28:1239–1247.

Gagner M, Pomp A. Laparoscopic pylorus-preserving pancreaticoduodenectomy. Surg Endosc 1994;8:408–410.

Mabrut JY, Fernandez-Cruz L, Azagra JS, et al. Hepatobiliary and Pancreatic Section (HBPS) of the Royal Belgian Society of Surgery, Belgian Group for Endoscopic Surgery (BGES), Club Coelio. Laparoscopic pancreatic resection: results of a multi-center European study of 127 patients. Surgery 2005;137:597–605.

Velanovich V. Case-control comparison of laparoscopic versus open distal pancreatectomy. J Gastrointest Surg 2006;10:95–98.

# Suggested Readings

Ammori BJ, Baghdadi S. Minimally invasive pancreatic surgery—the new frontier? Curr Gastroenterol Rep 2006;8:132–142.

Bilimoria MM, Cormier JN, Mun Y, et al. Pancreatic leak after left pancreatectomy is reduced following main pancreatic duct ligation. Br J Surg 2003;90:190–196.

Ejstrud P, Kristensen B, Hansen JB, et al. Risk and patterns of bacteraemia after splenectomy: a population-based study. Scand J Infect Dis 2000;32:521–525.

Leemans R, Manson W, Snijder JA, et al. Immune response capacity after human splenic autotransplantation: Restoration of response to individual pneumococcal vaccine subtypes. Ann Surg 1999;229:279–285.

Montorsi M, Zago M, Mosca F, et al. Efficacy of octreotide in the prevention of pancreatic fistula after elective pancreatic resections: a prospective, controlled, randomized clinical trial. Surgery 1995;117:26–31.

Ohwada S, Ogawa T, Tanahashi Y, et al. Fibrin glue sandwich prevents pancreatic fistula following distal pancreatectomy. World J Surg 1998;22:494–498.

Park AE, Heniford BT. Therapeutic laparoscopy of the pancreas. Ann Surg 2002;236:149–158.

Patterson EJ, Ganger M, Salky B, et al. Laparoscopic pancreatic resection: single institution experience of 19 cases. J Am Coll Surg 2001;193:281–287.

Shoup M, Brennan MF, McWhite K, et al. The value of splenic preservation with distal pancreatectomy. Arch Surg 2002;137:164–168.

Warshaw AL. Conservation of the spleen with distal pancreatectomy. Arch Surg 1988;123:550–553.

# 33. Preoperative Staging of Pancreatic Adenocarcinoma

## A. Introduction

Surgery offers the primary hope of cure in operable pancreatic cancer. Because of the morbidity associated with surgical resection, accurate preoperative staging to determine operability is of primary importance. New protocols involving neoadjuvant therapy followed by surgery may provide an alternative if resection for cure is deemed not to be feasible. This chapter explores options for preoperative staging of pancreatic adenocarcinoma.

## B. Case

### Eric Pontey

A 60-year-old man consulted his primary care provider because a coworker had noticed that the patient's skin had become yellow and that the patient had lost weight. Upon further questioning, the patient reported a decrease in appetite, general fatigue, and an approximately 2-month history of dark urine. He denied any back pain, shortness of breath, nausea, abdominal pain, bleeding, change in bowel habits, or vomiting.

His past medical history was significant for hypertension. His past surgical history was positive only for a tonsillectomy during childhood. Both parents had chronic obstructive pulmonary disease and adult-onset diabetes. There was no family history of cancer of any kind.

His medications included hydrochlorothiazide and aspirin 80 mg per day. He was allergic to penicillin.

The patient was married with four children, all in good health. He worked as a chemical engineer; his work did not involve chemical exposure. He had a 35-pack-a-year smoking history, but had stopped smoking 4 years earlier. He did not drink any alcoholic beverages. He did drink one cup of coffee per day.

The review of systems was negative except as noted above. On physical examination, he was a slender but well-developed white man in no acute distress. He was obviously jaundiced and had stigmata of recent weight loss.

His temperature was 35.2 °C, pulse 90, and blood pressure 133/76. He was 178 cm tall and weighed 60.5 kg, with a body mass index (BMI) of 19.1.

With the exception of scleral icterus, the head and neck examination was negative. Cardiopulmonary examination was also negative.

On abdominal examination, he was found to have a soft, nontender, nondistended abdomen with normal bowel sounds. No masses were palpable. Rectal examination revealed clay-colored stool, which was guaiac negative. He had a normal prostate, with no masses.

His laboratory results were significant for a hematocrit of 34%, total bilirubin of 26.3, direct bilirubin 18.9, serum glutamic-oxaloacetic transaminase (SGOT) 62, serum glutamate pyruvate transaminase (SGPT) 69, alkaline phosphatase 340, carbohydrate antigen 19-9, 1308 U/mL, and carcinoembryonic antigen 7.3 ng/mL.

A right upper quadrant ultrasound showed a dilated gallbladder without stones, as well as dilated intra- and extrahepatic bile ducts. The common duct measured 18 mm in diameter. The pancreas could not be visualized.

A computed tomography (CT) scan demonstrated a 4-cm mass in the head of the pancreas with biliary and pancreatic ductal dilation. No adenopathy and no evidence of tumor beyond the pancreas were noted. The portal vein and superior mesenteric artery appeared normal. Percutaneous biopsy of the lesion showed adenocarcinoma.

The impression was a carcinoma of the head of the pancreas, apparently operable by radiologic studies.

**How would you proceed? Should this patient undergo preoperative laparoscopic staging?**

# C. Laparoscopic Staging

*Frederick L. Greene and Gamal Mostafa*

The accurate diagnosis and staging of pancreatic cancer is critical to the creation of a treatment plan. Unfortunately, many patients undergo unnecessary laparotomy because of liver, nodal, or peritoneal metastases that were not detected during conventional preoperative testing. The majority of new cases diagnosed in the United States every year present with an advanced stage of the disease. At the time of diagnosis, only 10% of patients have disease confined to the pancreas, 40% exhibit local spread, and 50% demonstrate distant disease.

Surgical resection offers the only chance for long-term survival in these patients, but fewer than 20% of patients are operative candidates because peritoneal, nodal, or hepatic metastases preclude curative resection. Advanced disease eliminates the chance for cure, thereby leaving the surgical palliation of established or impending duodenal or biliary obstruction as the only option. Laparoscopy is both sensitive and specific in the diagnosis and staging of localized or advanced pancreatic cancer and can be completed with minimal morbidity to the patient. This diagnostic and therapeutic tool can provide accurate data for the development of appropriate treatment plans and the completion of palliative care.

The goal of cancer staging is to confirm the diagnosis of malignancy and to differentiate between patients with localized, resectable tumors and those with locally advanced or metastatic disease. Current diagnostic modalities include CT, ultrasound (US), magnetic resonance imaging (MRI), positron emission tomography (PET), and endoscopy. In the workup of patients with pancreatic cancer, all of these modalities may be utilized. In addition, the evaluation of the abdominal cavity with direct laparoscopic visualization and biopsy may mean the difference between managing a patient with unresectable disease nonsurgically and submitting such a patient to an unneeded abdominal procedure.

The goals of laparoscopic evaluation in pancreatic cancer are to assess peripancreatic nodes as well as remote sites that may harbor metastases that have not been identified by preoperative staging. One must perform direct inspection of the pancreas by dividing the gastrocolic and gastrohepatic omental regions and by introducing the laparoscope into the lesser omental bursa. Needle aspiration or biopsy of peripancreatic masses may be accomplished in this manner if the tissue diagnosis has not been obtained previously. Previous episodes of pancreatitis cause increased difficulty in inspection of the lesser sac. Gentle dissection of adhesions usually allows excellent visualization of the body and tail of the pancreas and facilitates laparoscopic-guided biopsy. Tumor ingrowth into the portal venous system may be evaluated using laparoscopic ultrasound (LUS). Using the combination of laparoscopy, laparoscopic intraoperative ultrasound, and CT scans, greater than 90% of unresectable tumors can be identified, thus obviating the morbidity of an exploratory laparotomy. Cytologic investigations of peritoneal washings should be performed if initial laparoscopic evaluation is normal. Neoplastic cells may be obtained from the free peritoneal cavity even when the peritoneum itself is grossly free of metastatic implants. By eliminating nontherapeutic laparotomy and redirecting treatment plans, laparoscopy contributes significantly both to the proper management of patients with pancreatic cancer and to increased efficiency of resource utilization.

Pancreatic cancer has a propensity for early metastasis to the liver and peritoneum. Unfortunately, many patients exhibit local tumor invasion of peripancreatic tissue and metastatic spread by the time symptoms occur and therefore present with unresectable disease. Studies have demonstrated that over 40% of patients may have peritoneal or hepatic metastases despite negative preoperative imaging with US or CT. Most of these implants measure less than 10 mm and many are as small as 1 to 2 mm in diameter. Laparoscopy can play a dominant role in the management of pancreatic cancer and will have a sensitivity and specificity, respectively, of 93% and 100% for detection of these small lesions.

Peritoneal washings for cytologic examination should routinely be obtained during the laparoscopic staging procedure. These washings may be positive in up to 30% of patients with apparently localized disease and therefore indicate an overall poor survival no matter what the resectable nature of the tumor may be. Patients with cancer of the pancreatic body and tail have unexpected peritoneal metastases in up to 50% of cases. Staging laparoscopy is indicated for these patients, who generally present with later symptoms than those with pancreatic head lesions.

Laparoscopic ultrasonography should routinely be applied during evaluation for pancreatic malignancy and resectability. The positive predictive value of LUS in determining local unresectability is approximately 93%, and therefore unnecessary laparotomy may be avoided in as many as 20% of patients. In addition, LUS may provide additional staging information beyond that supplied by laparoscopy alone in as many as 50% to 60% of patients.

The appropriate approach for laparoscopic staging is to attempt to re-create the open dissection and to attempt an evaluation of all appropriate areas surrounding the pancreas. Conlon and his group from Memorial Sloan-Kettering Cancer Center showed that this full evaluation was possible even in patients who had had previous operative exploration for nonpancreatic reasons. In their population, a correct assessment of resectability was made in 76% of patients compared with their previous resection rate of 35%. The possibility of understaging at the time of laparoscopy may be due to liver metastases that are not apparent during visual inspection. Therefore, the use of LUS is recommended to enhance the routine use of laparoscopy.

Patients who undergo laparoscopy for pancreatic evaluation may be managed in the outpatient setting. These patients have minimal morbidity especially if an unnecessary operation is avoided. The combination of routine imaging and laparoscopy plus intraabdominal ultrasound is the most accurate way to identify patients who will benefit from an aggressive surgical approach. In addition, as neoadjuvant regimens are developed for treating pancreatic disease, patients who have marginal resectability may benefit from laparoscopic techniques. These patients may then be treated with preoperative chemotherapy and radiation in order to increase the resectability rates.

# D.  Laparoscopic Ultrasound for Staging Pancreatic Cancer

## *Anand Patel*

If preoperative workup does not preclude resectability, the patient is scheduled for LUS staging. The goal of LUS is to identify occult tumor growth, plan for resection, and avoid morbidity of open exploration by recognizing those patients with unresectable disease. Operative staging consists of peritoneal lavage, laparoscopic examination, and laparoscopic ultrasound to detect metastatic disease to the liver and distant lymph nodes or arterial encasement that would preclude a formal pancreaticoduodenectomy.

Prior to staging or resection, a complete and thorough evaluation of the patient is essential. Patients do not benefit from staging if resection is not a reasonable possibility. Efforts in these patients should be limited to palliation. Many times with long-standing biliary obstruction, an element of liver dysfunction may be present. An evaluation and correction of coagulation parameters is necessary. Vitamin K and fresh frozen plasma can aid the clinician in treating coagulopathy. Ca 19-9 may be of value in following recurrence, but is certainly not diagnostic. Deep venous thrombosis (DVT) prophylaxis is necessary for these patients who are at high risk for DVT.

A proper CT scan is necessary. Often the referring physician obtains a CT scan that is diagnostic but does not aid in surgical evaluation. A proper CT scan must be performed with a "pancreas protocol," which consists of arterial and venous phases, and thin cuts through the pancreas on the best equipment available to the clinician. A 16- or 64-slice CT with axial and coronal cuts greatly enhances evaluation for resectability and planning. This CT scan illustrates the mass with its relationship to surrounding structures, assesses for vascular involvement, identifies lymphadenopathy and liver metastases, and provides clues to unresectability. Drawbacks of CT scan include missing liver lesions less than 1 cm, poor visualization of tumors less than 3 cm, and inability to identify peritoneal implants.

Endoscopic ultrasound (EUS) is a helpful tool to evaluate the pancreas. It is a relatively benign mode of examining the head of the pancreas and provides an avenue for biopsy. It has great capacity to evaluate and plan for resection. The greatest value of EUS is in performing a transduodenal biopsy for tissue diagnosis. Champault found EUS to have 100% sensitivity for staging of small tumors (less than 20 mm), detection of adjacent nodes, and ascertaining the relation between tumor and mesenteric/portal veins. Endoscopic ultrasound can biopsy suspicious nodes distant to the tumor that would preclude resectability. The major drawback of EUS is that it is very user dependent. Endoscopic ultrasound is often performed by gastroenterologists who may overread portal vein involvement and declare a patient unresectable. Surgeons seek criteria for resectability, whereas gastroenterologists seek criteria for unresectability. Portal vein involvement is not necessarily considered unresectable by many pancreatic surgeons. Tseng et al. found that pancreaticoduodenectomy with vascular resection has no impact on survival duration. Properly selected patients with adenocarcinoma of the pancreatic head who required vascular resection had a median survival of approximately 2 years, which does not differ from those who undergo standard pancreaticoduodenectomy and is superior to historical patients believed to have locally advanced disease treated nonoperatively.

Equipment necessary to perform a proper examination includes standard laparoscopic instruments, an ultrasound machine, a laparoscopic ultrasound probe, and sterile saline. A cytopathologist and a surgeon qualified to interpret the ultrasound findings must be available.

The patient is positioned supine with both arms tucked at the side. The patient is properly immobilized to avoid any movement off the bed while extreme positioning is performed. A Betadine scrub is standard in our institution for any patient undergoing an oncologic procedure. Ports and instruments are dipped in Betadine prior to insertion.

We generally use a two-port technique. We have occasionally inserted a third port as needed for manipulation. Preemptive 0.5% Marcaine with epinephrine is used for pain control. A Veress needle is placed in the infraumbilical position. After insufflation, the needle is removed and is replaced by a 10-mm port. A 5-mm port is placed in the right upper quadrant area at approximately the midclavicular line.

Sterile saline, 200cc, is instilled in the perihepatic, periportal, periduodenal, and pelvic areas immediately on entering. At the end of the staging procedure, placing the patient in the Trendelenburg position with right side down recollects the fluid in the right gutter. At least 100cc of fluid recovery is necessary for adequate sampling. Washings are sent for cytology if no contraindications to proceed are found during staging.

The peritoneal surfaces are continuously surveyed throughout the procedure. We begin staging in the pelvis. The patient is placed in the steep Trendelenburg position. This facilitates clearing of the pelvis. The peritoneal surfaces are carefully examined for implants. Bowel is moved as needed for an adequate view. The patient is then repositioned into reverse Trendelenburg. The transverse colon is lifted superiorly and draped over the stomach for examination of the base of the mesentery. This area may hide tumor and metastatic lymphadenopathy. The head of the pancreas is palpated with an instrument to gauge the size and areas of involvement. Our attention then turns toward the liver. The liver surface is inspected at the same time as the ultrasound. The liver is elevated to examine the posterior surfaces and the hepatic hilum.

For ultrasound examination, we use the Entos™ LAP L9-5 probe (Phillips Medical Systems, Andover, MA). It has a flexible linear array scan head. The tip articulates in four directions, allowing examination over most peritoneal surfaces. Ultrasound allows the surgeon to "see" beneath the surface to identify obscure metastatic disease and vascular involvement, and to facilitate biopsy. The ultrasound probe is inserted via the 10-mm port site. The camera is changed to a 5-mm scope, placed through the 5-mm trocar, and is used for direct visualization and guidance.

Ultrasound of the liver is directed by the portal venous system. The portal veins have a hyperechoic lining secondary to the investment of Glisson's capsule. The branches are followed to each segment numerically as designated by the Couinaud/Bismuth classification system. Cautious sequential examination of each segment is performed. Trucut needle biopsy for deep lesions or biopsy forceps for surface tumors are taken as frozen and permanent section biopsies (Figs. 33.1 and 33.2). The position of tumors in relation to portal structures is documented. The biliary tree is examined proximally from the confluence to the distal intrapancreatic portion. Liver metastases are usually well circumscribed and can be hypoechoic, hyperechoic, or isoechoic with a hypoechoic rim. To date, we have identified three patients with biopsy-positive liver lesions found at the time of laparoscopic ultrasound who were not

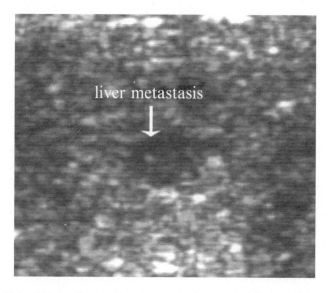

Fig. 33.1. A 7-mm liver metastasis (arrow) found on ultrasound of the liver. This lesion was not apparent on preoperative imaging.

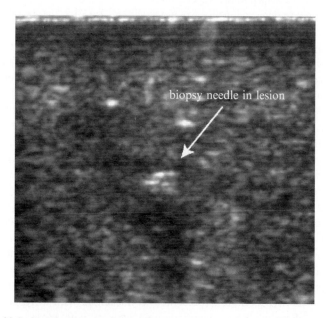

Fig. 33.2. Needle biopsy of the same lesion under ultrasound guidance. The arrow points to the needle.

preoperatively identified. Laparoscopic ultrasound allows for the identification of liver tumors not visible during laparoscopy in up to 33% of patients.

Ultrasound examination of the pancreas begins in the head and uncinate process. The probe is placed directly over the tumor or laterally through a transduodenal or transgastric window. The distal pancreas is optimally viewed through a transgastric acoustic window. Pressure is applied to compress the walls of the stomach to displace intervening air. Tumor characteristics of local invasion and size are visualized. Tumor relation to the portal vein, superior mesenteric vessels, and hepatic artery is essential. Color Doppler is used to assess the patency of the vasculature when tumor encroachment is identified and to distinguish vascular structures from bile or pancreatic ducts. If tumor invasion is suspected, the length and circumference of involvement is noted. The celiac axis, superior mesenteric artery, suprapancreatic, periportal, and paraaortic areas are examined for lymph node involvement. Accessible suspicious-appearing nodes are sampled for histologic evaluation. Peripancreatic lymph nodes are not considered a contraindication to resection, and hence are not biopsied. These nodes are noted and later resected at the time of pancreaticoduodenectomy. Biopsy-proven celiac nodes distant to the pancreas are considered a contraindication.

An ultrasound image of the primary pancreatic cancer typically demonstrates a hypoechoic lesion with poorly defined borders. Sometimes the tumor can demonstrate mixed echogenicity. Dilation of pancreatic and bile ducts is a common finding. The area of dilation is usually free of tumor involvement, as the tumor causing the ductal obstruction is proximal to the dilated segment. Small uncinate process tumors may not demonstrate change in obstructed ducts, whereas pancreatic head lesions often display dilated ductal systems. Patients with chronic pancreatitis may demonstrate diffuse hypoechoic pancreatic parenchyma on ultrasound. This makes it difficult to exam the hypoechoic tumor because of obliteration of the tumor margin. Excessive adipose tissue diminishes ultrasound transmission and may result in suboptimal US images.

Vascular invasion is demonstrated by the loss of an echogenic interface between the tumor and the vessel, and the tumor within the vessel, and increased peripancreatic venous collateralization. The interface of the tumor to vascular structures typically demonstrates hyperechoic delineation due to the adventitial lining of the vessel. An obliterated interface is indicative of vascular invasion (Fig. 33.3). Tumor invasion demonstrates the obliteration of the interface and mass within the confines of the vessel lumen. This can be confirmed by color Doppler.

Benign lymph nodes are usually oval with a hypoechoic rim, or have an isoechoic center and are usually less than 1 cm in size. Loss of nodal architecture may be indicative of metastasis (Fig. 33.4). Pathologic nodes may be of any size but are usually greater than 1 cm, with a hypoechoic center, well circumscribed, and they have a round contour. Exceptions are periportal and suprapancreatic lymph nodes that are oblong and flat. These lymph nodes are often larger than 1 cm.

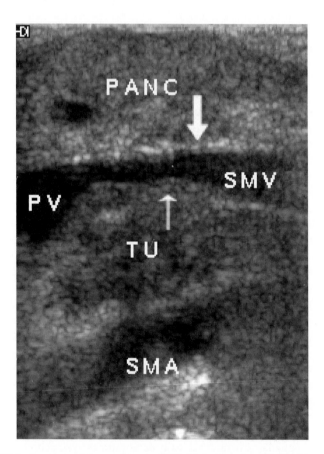

Fig. 33.3. Invasion of the portal vein (PV). Note the adventitial lining on the side opposite the tumor (TU), marked by the thick arrow. The tumor growth has obliterated the wall of the PV, marked by a thin arrow. Superior mesenteric artery (SMA), superior mesenteric vein (SMV), and pancreas (PANC) are visible in this sagittal view over the PV-SMV confluence.

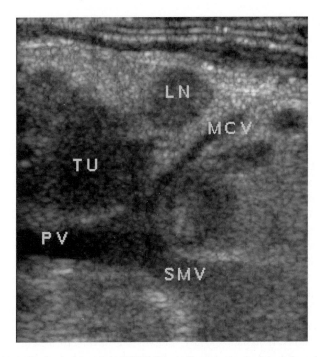

Fig. 33.4. Sagittal view of the PV-SMV confluence. A suspicious lymph node (LN) is visible adjacent to the tumor (TU) and middle colic vein (MCV) insertion on the PV-SMV confluence.

In our laparoscopic staging series, patients with biopsy-proven metastatic lesions were considered unresectable. Different palliative procedures for patients with unresectable disease included laparoscopic gastrojejunostomy, laparoscopic cholecystojejunostomy, laparoscopic choledochojejunostomy, endoscopic enteral stenting, endoscopic biliary stenting, and endoscopic celiac ganglion block. Patients with resectable disease or equivocal findings were brought at a later date to the operating room after all studies were complete. Patients underwent open exploration assessment for resectability. Regional lymphadenopathy or portal vein encroachment was not considered a contraindication to resection.

We compared laparoscopy alone (LA) with LUS to predict resectability at open exploration. Laparoscopy alone had a negative predictive value of 78%, while the negative predictive value of LUS was 90%. Thus negative predictive value means that no disease was found to preclude resectability.

Callery et al. studied the use of staging laparoscopy with and without ultrasound in 50 consecutive patients having only a CT scan for workup. Staging laparoscopy alone demonstrated unresectability in 22% of the cohort. The addition of laparoscopic ultrasound to the staging process demonstrated unresectable disease in another 22% from vascular invasion ($n = 5$), lymph node metastases ($n = 5$), and intraparenchymal tumor ($n = 1$).

Doran et al. studied 190 CT-scan-resectable and 49 CT-scan-unresectable patients with staging laparoscopy and laparoscopic ultrasound; 28 of the CT-resectable patients (15%) were found to have unresectable disease by staging procedures. However, more importantly, four of the CT-unresectable patients (8%) were correctly identified as resectable.

Radiographic studies diagnose pancreatic cancer. However, with only a CT scan, a surgeon is not able to fully assess the extent of disease. Laparoscopic staging is generally accepted as a means for preoperative assessment of pancreatic head cancers. The addition of ultrasound to evaluation is limited by a large learning curve, equipment, and longer operating times. However, laparoscopy alone does not evaluate portal vein involvement, nodal involvement, and small liver metastases. Ultrasound becomes a necessary adjunct to laparoscopic staging. Ultrasound can demonstrate the extent of local spread; characterize and identify liver lesions, lymphadenopathy, and vascular involvement; guide biopsies; and plan for proper resection. By avoiding unnecessary laparotomy, quality of life in these unfortunate patients can be optimized.

# E. Conclusions

## Eiichi Miyasaka

In the United States in 2003, 31,860 new cases of pancreatic cancer were reported and 31,270 deaths occurred due to this disease. The overall prognosis for pancreatic cancer is very poor. Even with a curative resection (pancreaticoduodenectomy, Whipple procedure) with negative margins, the 5-year survival rate is about 21%. Furthermore, despite recent advances in imaging technology including high-resolution CT scan, up to 51% of patients who are deemed to have resectable disease on preoperative noninvasive imaging are found to be unresectable due to metastatic disease at the time of laparotomy. Unnecessary laparotomy compromises the quality of life of patients with these advanced cancers. Because of the limited ability for noninvasive imaging to determine surgical resectability, and the subsequent high percentage of unnecessary laparotomies, some physicians advocate operative imaging prior to proceeding with laparotomy. The two most common imaging modalities are diagnostic laparoscopy and intraoperative ultrasound (IOUS). This section briefly reviews the current literature on these minimally invasive imaging methods.

A review article by Stefanidis et al. provides a good summary of the literature up to 2005 about the role of laparoscopic imaging in the staging of pancreatic neoplasm. Studies in this review found that 15% to 51% of pancreatic neoplasms that are deemed resectable on preoperative noninvasive imaging, including at least high-resolution CT (and may include other modalities such as endoscopic ultrasound, magnetic resonance cholangiopancreatography, and angiography), have findings on laparoscopy or IOUS that preclude curative resection (e.g., peritoneal metastases or invasion of tumor into transverse mesocolon). However, 5% to 16% of patients who were deemed resectable on preoperative imaging were subsequently identified as having unresectable disease on laparotomy. Overall, 10% to 36% of the patients were spared a laparotomy by usage of minimally invasive imaging (combination of laparoscopy, IOUS, and peritoneal cytology).

These numbers indicate that there is a definite role for minimally invasive imaging, but routine prelaparotomy laparoscopy may not be justified, and some authors have looked at which subsets of patients would benefit most from minimally invasive imaging. Morganti et al. found that of 54 patients with pancreatic adenocarcinoma, all patients who were found to have metastatic disease at laparotomy had primary tumor size >3 cm, and concluded that this patient population would benefit most from laparoscopy. Hunerbein et al. looked at CA 19-9 levels and found that at levels >150 U/mL, the positive predictive value of identifying metastatic disease at laparotomy was 88%, and that these patients would benefit most from staging laparoscopy. However, these studies are both retrospective, and, to date, no prospective studies have been done to determine what patient characteristics predict maximum utility of laparoscopy.

Ultrasound is often used as an adjunct to laparoscopy. It is better able to detect nonpalpable small hepatic parenchymal metastases and assess tumor invasion into nearby vascular structures. A review by Camacho et al. reported up to a 98% accuracy in predicting resectability by using laparoscopic ultrasound. In a study by Merchant and Conlon, 90 patients underwent noninvasive imaging, diagnostic laparoscopy, and IOUS. By noninvasive imaging, 65 were considered resectable, 17 unresectable, and eight equivocal. All patients underwent laparoscopy, and it showed 36 patients to be resectable, 41 unresectable, and 13 had equivocal findings. Of these 13 patients with equivocal findings, IOUS identified eight patients as having unresectable disease, and of the five that proceeded to have resection, one was found to be unresectable at laparotomy for involvement of the celiac axis not detected on ultrasound. Intraoperative ultrasound provided added resectability information in 9% of the total number of patients, consistent with reports by other authors of 12% to 14% added benefit.

In conclusion, there is some evidence in the literature supporting the use of laparoscopy prior to proceeding with laparotomy in a certain percentage of patients up to 51%. Laparoscopic ultrasound confers a small increase (~12%) over laparoscopy alone in detecting potentially unresectable disease, though it is unclear whether the increased time, resources, and training needed to obtain its benefits justifies routine use of IOUS in addition to laparoscopy. Certain markers and patient characteristics have been described that may identify patients who would benefit most from minimally invasive imaging, such as tumor >3 cm or CA 19-9 >150 U/mL. However, there is no consensus on whether routine use of laparoscopy or IOUS is indicated in patients with pancreatic cancer who have radiographically resectable disease demonstrated by high-resolution CT scan.

# References

Callery MP, et al. Staging laparoscopy with laparoscopic ultrasonography: optimizing resectability in hepatobiliary and pancreatic malignancy. J Am Coll Surg 1997;185: 33–39.

Camacho D, Reichenbach D, Duerr G, et al. Value of laparoscopy in the staging of pancreatic cancer. J Pancreas (Online) 2005;6(6):552–561.

Champault G. The use of laparoscopic ultrasound in the assessment of pancreatic cancer. Wiad Lek 1997;50(suppl 1):195–203.

Conlon KC, Dougherty E, Klimstra DS, et al. The value of minimal access surgery in the staging of patients with potentially resectable peripancreatic malignancy. Ann Surg 1996;223:134–140.

Doran HE, et al. Laparoscopy and laparoscopic ultrasound in the evaluation of pancreatic and periampullary tumours. Dig Surg 2004;21:305–313.

Hunerbein M, Rau B, Hohenberger P, et al. Value of laparoscopic ultrasound for staging of gastrointestinal tumors. Chirurg 2001;72:914–919.

Merchant NB, Conlon KC. Laparoscopic evaluation in pancreatic cancer. Semin Surg Oncol 1998;15:155–65.

Morganti AG, Brizi MG, Macchia G, et al. The prognostic effect of clinical staging in pancreatic adenocarcinoma. Ann Surg Oncol 2006;12:145–151.

Stefanidis D, Grove KD, Schwesinger WH, et al. The current role of staging laparoscopy for adenocarcinoma of the pancreas: a review. Ann Oncol 2006;17:189–199.

Tseng JF, et al. Pancreaticoduodenectomy with vascular resection: margin status and survival duration. J Gastrointest Surg 2004;8:935–950.

# Suggested Readings

Berber E, Siperstein AE. Laparoscopic ultrasound. Surg Clin North Am 2004;85:1061–1084.

Espat NJ, Brennan MF, Conlon KC. Patients with laparoscopically staged unresectable pancreatic adenocarcinoma do not require subsequent surgical or biliary bypass. J Am Coll Surg 1999;188:649–657.

Jemal A, Murray T, Ward E, et al. Cancer statistics 2005. CA Cancer J Clin 2005;55:10–30.

John TG, Greig JD, Crosbie JL, et al. Superior staging of liver tumors with laparoscopy and laparoscopic ultrasound. Ann Surg 1994;220:711–719.

Koler AJ, Lilly MC, Arregui AE. Suprapancreatic and periportal lymph nodes are normally larger than 1 cm by laparoscopic ultrasound evaluation. Surg Endosc 2004;18:646–649.

Menack MJ, Spitz JD, Arregui ME. Staging of pancreatic and ampullary cancers for resectability using laparoscopy with laparoscopic ultrasound. Surg Endosc 2001;15:129–134.

Minnard EA, Conlon KC, Hoos A, et al. Laparoscopic ultrasound enhances standard laparoscopy in the staging of pancreatic cancer. Ann Surg 1998;228:182–187.

Pratt BL, Greene FL. Role of laparoscopy in the staging of malignant disease. Surg Clin North Am 2000;80:1111–1126.

Van Delden OM, de Wit LT, Bemelman WA, et al. Laparoscopic ultrasonography for abdominal tumor staging; technical aspects and imaging findings. Abdom Imaging 1997;22:125–131.

# 34. Living Related Donor Nephrectomy, Right Side

## A. Introduction

Laparoscopic techniques were first applied to procurement of the left kidney, where the longer vascular pedicle facilitates access. When the left kidney is unsuitable for anatomic reasons, as in the case presented below, the right kidney may be used. Applications of laparoscopic surgery to right donor nephrectomy have been slower in acceptance. This case was chosen to illustrate two possible approaches: an open approach using a small incision, and a hand-assisted laparoscopic surgery (HALS) approach. A purely laparoscopic technique has also been described, but since an incision must be made to retrieve the kidney intact and undamaged, most minimal-access surgeons make the incision at the beginning of the procedure and use a HALS method.

## B. Case

### *Kenneth G. Nepple*

A 27-year-old woman wanted to electively donate a kidney to her older sister, who has end-stage renal disease secondary to diabetic nephropathy from type 1 diabetes. Workup by transplant nephrologist found no medical contraindication to donation.

The donor had no previous medical or surgical problems. She was on no medications and had no allergies. Her mother and father were both alive and in good health. She was married, worked as a medical transcriptionist, and did not smoke or use alcohol. The review of systems was completely negative.

Her physical examination revealed a healthy-appearing female, height 165 cm and weight 65 kg. Her pulse was 72, blood pressure 109/74. The remainder of her physical examination was unremarkable.

Laboratory results included a normal complete blood count (CBC), blood urea nitrogen (BUN) 11, creatinine 0.7, measured creatinine clearance 120, negative urinalysis, and fasting glucose 107. Infectious disease serologies were negative, as was a pregnancy test. Electrocardiogram was normal. Her ABO blood type was compatible with her sister's, and there was a negative donor-recipient crossmatch. Chest x-ray was normal.

Magnetic resonance imaging (MRI), magnetic resonance angiography (MRA), and magnetic resonance urography (MRU) revealed both kidneys to be normal in shape, size, and position. There were nonduplicated, non-obstructed urinary collecting systems bilaterally. There were three left renal arteries. There was a single right renal artery. There were single renal veins bilaterally. Urography revealed no stones and a normal examination.

**What is the best approach to remove the right kidney for donation—open or hand-assisted laparoscopic? What would you advise?**

## C. Donor Nephrectomy via Mini-Incision Technique

*Jason T. Jankowski and Juan R. Sanabria*

The goal in performing any donor nephrectomy, regardless of which technique is used, is to safely procure the donor kidney while exposing the donor to the lowest chance for any morbidity. Factors that must be considered are operative time, surgical blood loss, return of gastrointestinal function, postoperative pain, and return to daily activities. It is also extremely important to consider how the technique used to retrieve the kidney affects graft function. At our institution, we have developed a technique using a minilaparotomy incision to perform open donor nephrectomy. Performed correctly, this technique achieves all of the aforementioned goals.

We have found patient positioning, lighting, and proper retraction to be key elements in performing a mini-incision donor nephrectomy. We place the patient in a standard nephrectomy position (Fig. 34.1A). The patient should be placed on a surgical beanbag at a 60- to 80-degree lateral decubitus position with the iliac crest positioned just below the break in the bed. The bottom leg is flexed to about 75 degrees, with the top leg straight to maintain stability; a pillow is placed between the knees and an axillary roll is positioned in the axilla to prevent compression of the peroneal and axillary nerves, respectively. The lower arm remains extended on a padded armrest and blankets are used to support the extended upper arm so that it remains in a horizontal position. At this point, the bed is flexed to maximize the space between the costal margin and the iliac crest. The skin and abdominal musculature are on tension.

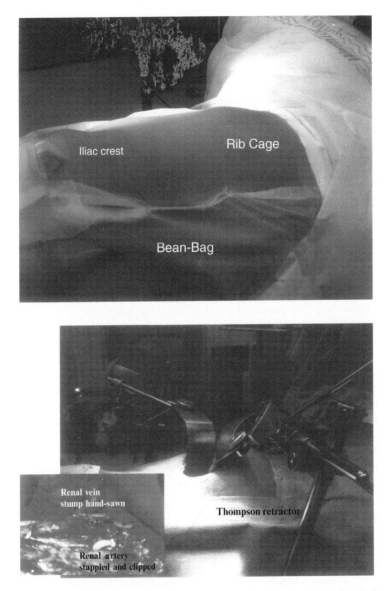

Fig. 34.1. (A) Position of a patient for a donor nephrectomy; the patient is in a lateral decubitus position at 60 to 70 degrees with the surgical bed broken at the level of the iliac crest. (B) The Thompson retractor is in place to maximize exposure through an 8– to 10-cm left subcostal incision. The left renal artery has been stapled and clipped and divided. The renal vein has been divided and hand-sewn with 4–0 Prolene.

The beanbag is placed to suction and the patient is secured to the table. Surgical lights are positioned properly and both a headlight and surgical loupes are worn by the primary surgeon.

A 9-cm (range 8 to 10 cm) anterior subcostal incision is made about two finger-breadths below the costal margin. The incision is carried down through the subcutaneous tissues to the anterior fascia. The muscular plane (external oblique, internal oblique, and transverses muscles and fascia) is divided and the abdominal cavity is entered. A Thompson retractor is positioned (Fig. 34.1B). The colon is then reflected medially by incising the line of Toldt, taking down the hepatocolic ligaments. Gerota's fascia is identified and opened to expose the surface of the kidney. The lateral and posterior attachments are freed and the dissection is carried cephalad to free the upper pole. The lower pole is dissected free until the gonadal vein is identified. The dissection is continued caudal along the medial aspect of the gonadal vein where the ureter is found. The distal ureter is then dissected to the level of the iliac vessels. Attention is turned to the renal hilum. It is easiest to proceed in a cephalad direction along the medial aspect of the gonadal vein until the renal vein is identified. The gonadal vein is divided, the renal vein is circumferentially freed from its adventitial attachments, and the adrenal vein and any associated lumbar branches are identified and divided using silk ties or surgical clips. Prior to beginning dissection of the renal artery, 12.5 g of mannitol and 20 mg of furosemide are administered by the anesthesia team once we have confirmed at least 2 L of crystalloid have been given to the patient. The renal artery, which typically lies posterior to the renal vein, is identified and freed to its origin at the aorta.

When the recipient surgical team is ready, 5000 units of heparin sulfate are administered intravenously and allowed to circulate for 5 minutes. The distal ureter is then clipped with a locking surgical clip at the level of the iliac vessels and divided. The proximal renal artery is then stapled and divided. A Statinsky clamp is placed on the renal vein, which is then divided and the kidney is passed of the field. Fifty milligrams of protamine are then administered by the anesthesia team. The renal vein is oversewn with a running 4-0 Prolene suture and the hilum is inspected for hemostasis. The colon is returned to its normal anatomic position and the fascia is closed in two layers. Subcutaneous catheters are placed to allow continuous infusion of Marcaine by the On-Q system. The skin is closed with a running subcuticular stitch.

In the case of a right nephrectomy, this technique is of a significant advantage to both the donor and the recipient surgeons. Liver retraction is easily achieved with a mechanical retractor with great exposure of the vena cava. This allows removal of the full length of the renal vein.

There is debate in the literature as to whether mini-incision donor nephrectomy matches the low morbidity of a laparoscopic approach. Clearly, the laparoscopic technique has been shown to reduce postoperative complications and hospital stay compared to the traditional flank approach. While some studies have shown laparoscopic donor nephrectomy to be superior to mini-incision donor nephrectomy with regard to donor recovery, hospital stay, and return to work, others have found comparable results. While further studies may provide a more definitive answer, at present, it appears both techniques provide excellent results with relatively low morbidity. We have performed at Case Medical Center (Cleveland, OH) more than 100 consecutive donor nephrectomies during the last year, with equal distribution between laparoscopic and minilaparotomy approaches. We found no differences in any parameter when the two groups were compared.

The effects of these various techniques on graft function have also been debated. Experimental studies by Burgos suggested that the increase in intraabdominal pressure caused by laparoscopic pneumoperitoneum decreases renal blood flow, with a subsequent delay in initial graft function. Warm ischemia time has also been shown to be longer with laparoscopic donor nephrectomy as compared to mini-incision donor nephrectomy. A review of the U.S. United Network for Organ Sharing (UNOS) database showed an increased rate of delayed initial graft function in kidneys that were procured laparoscopically, but no differences in rejection rates and short-term graft survival. Further studies with longer follow-up are needed to assess the impact on long-term graft survival.

Both laparoscopic and mini-incision donor nephrectomy are excellent options for kidney procurement with low morbidity. The mini-incision technique is especially advantageous for those surgeons with limited laparoscopic training and perhaps a better approach for the right-side nephrectomy. It is also an excellent technique for young surgeons well trained in laparoscopy to learn, as they may be required to convert a laparoscopic donor nephrectomy to an open procedure for various technical reasons.

# D.  Hand-Assisted Laparoscopic Donor Nephrectomy

*Kent W. Kercher*

Whether performed laparoscopically or open, live donor nephrectomy for kidney transplantation has traditionally favored utilization of the left kidney in order to maximize vessel length. Relative contraindications to the use of the left kidney include (1) multiple left renal arteries or veins, (2) a small accessory lower pole artery supplying the left ureter, (3) a small right kidney or disproportionately low split renal function of the right kidney, (4) an indeterminate cystic lesion in the right kidney, (5) an extrarenal lesion on the right side requiring concomitant evaluation or treatment, and (6) an extrarenal lesion on the left that could increase operative risk to the donor. Due to differences in adjacent anatomy (inferior vena cava, duodenum, and liver), the need to transect the short right renal vein, as well as relatively limited surgeon experience with right-sided donor nephrectomy, some have argued that the added technical challenges of laparoscopic right donor nephrectomy warrant the use of an open approach.

Since laparoscopic donor nephrectomy was first described in 1997, minimally invasive procurement of live donor kidneys has become the standard of care in most major transplant centers. When compared with the traditional open approach, the laparoscopic technique has resulted in less blood loss, less pain, earlier oral intake, shorter hospital stay, fewer complications, and a faster return to normal activities for live kidney donors. At the same time, multiple centers have documented recipient outcomes and allograft function (as defined by rates of delayed graft function, postoperative creatinine clearance, and long-term graft survival) that are equivalent to those of the open approach. In addition, the introduction of the laparoscopic approach has been shown to increase rates of organ donation, a point that is particularly important in the setting of limited organ resources that are grossly exceeded by the current demand.

Despite these potential advantages, the laparoscopic approach to live kidney procurement is technically challenging. The procedure requires advanced laparoscopic skills in order to allow for the safe dissection, vascular control, and removal of an intact and uninjured solid organ. Disadvantages of purely laparoscopic nephrectomy include the lack of tactile feedback during dissection and retraction of adjacent structures, the potential for trauma to the kidney or adjacent organs by laparoscopic instruments, and difficulty with vascular division and kidney extraction, which may lead to increases in warm ischemia time. Hand-assisted techniques offer solutions to many of these problems while offering most of the potential benefits of a minimally invasive approach.

When compared with purely laparoscopic nephrectomy, multiple studies have demonstrated the hand-assist technique to be similar with respect to postoperative pain and narcotic requirements, time to oral intake, length of stay, and time to convalescence. At the same time, hand-assisted laparoscopic donor nephrectomy (HALDN) facilitates the minimally invasive approach by restoring tactile feedback and allowing for manual manipulation of the kidney. As a result, operative times and warm ischemia times for HALDN are very reasonable and approach those of the standard open operation. We have previously reported (Kercher et al.) that in our institution, the transition from a purely laparoscopic approach to a hand-assisted approach resulted in a 56-minute reduction ($p = .0001$) in mean operative time. This was achieved with no differences in blood loss, length of stay, total charges, or rate of return to normal activity. From a technical standpoint, we have found that the extraction dilemma is eliminated by allowing for kidney removal through the same abdominal incision used for insertion of the hand-assist device.

In our experience, hand-assisted laparoscopic donor nephrectomy is best performed with a midline, periumbilical hand-assist incision and two accessory (12-mm) trocars. On the right side, one additional (5 mm) port is required for retraction of the right lobe of the liver (Figs. 34.2 and 34.3). The hand-assist incision (7 cm) is made at the outset of the

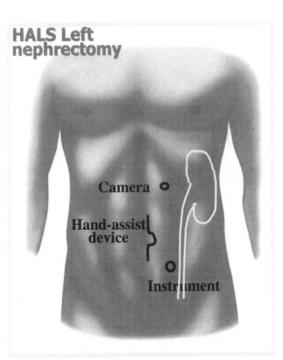

Fig. 34.2. Port placement and site of incision for hand-assisted laparoscopic surgery (HALS) left nephrectomy.

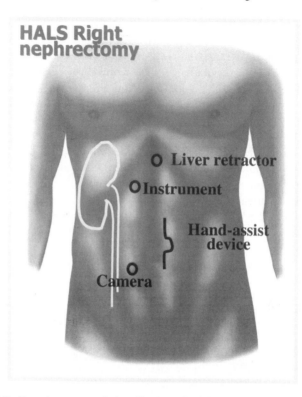

Fig. 34.3. Port placement and site of incision for HALS right nephrectomy.

procedure, and the surgeon's nondominant hand is used primarily for retraction and (occasionally) blunt dissection. For HALS left donor nephrectomy, the camera port and the surgeon's right-hand operating (instrument) port remain constant throughout the case. For right nephrectomy, the division of the short right renal vein and artery require that the hand position and utilization of the camera/instrument ports be altered during the extraction portion of the procedure (which generally takes less than 1 minute). For this maneuver, the camera is placed through the superior port and the articulating linear vascular stapler (2.0 mm/gray load endo–gastrointestinal anastomosis [GIA]) is brought in through the inferior port using the surgeon's left hand. The surgeon's right hand is placed intraperitoneally and elevates the kidney to maximize the length of the vessels during vascular transaction. The artery is divided first (well behind the inferior vena cava to maximize vessel length), followed by the vein (using a second stapler). By brining the stapler in through inferior port, the stapler can be placed perfectly parallel to the inferior vena cava and the right renal vein can be divided flush with the vena cava. The kidney is then rapidly extracted through the base ring of the hand-assist device.

Utilizing the technique described above, we routinely perform HALS right donor nephrectomy when removal of the left kidney is contraindicated. The most common reason for choosing the left kidney is the presence of multiple renal arteries on the left (as in the case presented), particularly if the accessory artery supplies the lower pole, and thrombosis of that vessel in the recipient would therefore jeopardize the blood supply to the left ureter. The other primary indication for using the right kidney is either a size or split renal function discrepancy >20% between the right and left kidney. In this case, the larger or more normal-appearing kidney stays with the donor.

In a recent analysis of 120 hand-assisted laparoscopic donor nephrectomies in our institution, 20 right kidneys were utilized (18%). There were no statistical differences in operative time (192 minutes left vs. 188 minutes right), blood loss (80 mL left vs. 75 mL right), or extraction time (67 seconds left vs. 90 seconds right). Three patients in the left nephrectomy group had major perioperative complications: splenic injury (one), chemical pancreatitis (one), and perioperative blood transfusion (one). There were no major complications in the right donor group. There were no conversions to open surgery and no reoperations in either group. The recipients in both groups were of similar age, same sex, and similar body mass index. For the recipient procedures, there were no significant differences between left and right groups in terms of cold ischemia ($37.6 \pm 115.2$ minutes vs. $34.5 \pm 117.3$ minutes), warm ischemia ($37.7 \pm 11.2$ minutes vs. $36.4 \pm 110.8$ minutes), or estimated blood loss (EBL) (322 vs. 228 cc). No vascular interposition grafts were required for the extension of donor renal vessels, and there were no major intraoperative complications in either group. One recipient (5%) in the right and three patients (2.9%) in the left group had transient graft acute tubular necrosis (ATN). There was one early graft loss in the left laparoscopic donor nephrectomy (LDN) group related to a recipient iliac artery intimal flap dissection. The median discharge serum creatinine was similar (1.75 vs. 2.05 g/dL). One-year graft survival in left and right recipient groups was 98% and 100%, respectively. These same conclusions have been derived from multiple other studies that show no differences in any parameters compared between laparoscopically procured left and right kidneys. These include equivalent operative and cold ischemia times as well as long-term graft survival (>97%).

Hand-assisted laparoscopic right LDN is a safe approach to organ harvest. Despite the perceived difficulty of procuring and implanting a laparoscopically harvested right kidney, this procedure does not appear to result in either increased perioperative donor or recipient morbidity or longer graft ischemia times. In addition, early graft function and long-term graft survival are equivalent for right and left kidneys.

For right donor nephrectomy, the technical considerations of dealing with the adjacent anatomy (inferior vena cava [IVC], duodenum, and liver) as well as the added difficulty of transecting a short renal vein can make the procedure slightly more challenging than left nephrectomy. Compared with pure laparoscopic nephrectomy, the hand-assisted approach reduces operative time and blood loss without increasing total hospital charges or length of stay. This approach also maintains the benefits of a minimally invasive approach in that donor morbidity remains substantially less than with the traditional open procedure. When applied to the procurement of organs for live donor renal transplantation, the use of hand-assisted laparoscopic right donor nephrectomy is well supported and offers the most appropriate solution for both the donor and the recipient in the case described. With proven equivalency in outcomes for the minimally invasive procurement of both right and left donor kidneys, the selection of the most appropriate kidney for donation should be based on the same criteria utilized for the traditional open approach.

# E.  Conclusions

## *Kenneth G. Nepple*

Surgical options for living related renal donation include open nephrectomy, pure LDN, and HALS donor nephrectomy. Since the introduction of laparoscopic donor nephrectomy in 1995, this procedure has become increasingly performed by experienced urologists and general surgeons. Left donor nephrectomy has been more thoroughly studied because the left has been the preferred side for harvest due to the longer left renal vein. The percentage of right donor nephrectomy in series of open nephrectomies (26% to 37%) is greater than in laparoscopic series (0% to 22%). When there is an indication for right-sided donor nephrectomy, there is a debate about the surgical approach.

The indication for harvest of the right kidney most often is anatomic, related to multiple left renal arteries, as in this case. Other reported indications include abnormal right renal artery, retroaortic left renal vein, smaller right kidney, right renal calculus, ureteropelvic junction obstruction, ectopic kidney, right renal cysts, or undiagnosed lesions in the right kidney.

In studies of left donor nephrectomy, mean operating time was longer for LDN and HALS than for open nephrectomy. With experience, laparoscopic operating time decreased. Jacobs et al. reported a shorter operative time for right laparoscopic donor nephrectomy when compared with left LDN. El-Galley et al. reported a shorter time in right LDN compared with right HAL.

Blood loss has been reported to be comparable between the three surgical approaches. When rapid blood loss occurs, open nephrectomy and HALS would seem to have a benefit over LDN in the ability to regain rapid vascular control. There is risk of injury to the liver or vena cava during right donor nephrectomy.

Alston et al. reported that conversion from left laparoscopic to open nephrectomy occurs in 0% to 13% of cases and the indications for conversion may include hemorrhage, endoscopic instrument or stapler malfunction, or the need for improved exposure. Conversion from right laparoscopic to open nephrectomy has been reported to be required in 0% to 11% of cases. Lind et al. reported that ureteral complications are rare, and have not been shown to occur more commonly in LDN (6.5%) compared to open nephrectomy (4.1%). Early experiences with right LDN found increased incidence of renal venous thrombosis and graft loss; however, with changes in surgical technique more recent studies have not found venous thrombosis to be common.

Warm ischemia time is defined as the time from the occlusion of the renal artery to immersion of the kidney in ice slush. El-Galley et al. reported longer warm ischemia time for LDN and HALS when compared with open, for left donor nephrectomy; however, there was no significant difference in serum creatinine of recipients. Right LDN warm ischemia time has been reported to be 3.4 to 4 minutes in several series.

Laparoscopic nephrectomy has been reported to decrease the amount of postoperative pain compared to open nephrectomy, with less need for narcotic pain medication. Hospital stay has been reported to be shorter after left LDN than open donor nephrectomy, and LDN had earlier return to normal physical activities and employment. Buell et al. reported a shorter hospital stay after right LDN than after HALS (48 vs. 65 hours).

Finally, kidney donors may prefer the smaller laparoscopic incisions compared to open nephrectomy. In addition, LDN allows placement of the Pfannenstiel kidney removal incision in a more cosmetic location. However, this has not been objectively studied.

In conclusion, similar technical success has been reported for LDN, HALS, and open nephrectomy with respect to blood loss and long-term recipient outcomes. However, patient preference for shorter hospital stay, less postoperative pain, and improved cosmetic results may lead some patients to prefer the laparoscopic approach. Minimal-access right donor nephrectomy is technically challenging and should be performed only by experienced surgeons.

# References

Alston C, Spaliviero M, Gill I. Laparoscopic donor nephrectomy. Urology 2005;65: 833–839.

Buell J, Edye M, Johnson M, et al. Are concerns over right laparoscopic donor nephrectomy unwarranted? Ann Surg 2001;233:645–51.

Burgos FJ. Influence of laparoscopic live donor nephrectomy in ischemia-reperfusion syndrome and renal function after kidney transplantation: an experimental study. Transplant Proc 2003;35(5):1664–1665.

El-Galley R, Hood N, Young C, et al. Donor nephrectomy: a comparison of techniques and results of open, hand assisted, and full laparoscopic nephrectomy. J Urol 2004;171:40–43.

Jacobs S, Cho E, Foster C, et al. Laparoscopic donor nephrectomy: the University of Maryland 6-year experience. J Urol 2004;171:47–51.

Kercher KW, Heniford BT, Matthews BD, et al. Laparoscopic versus open nephrectomy in 210 consecutive patients: outcomes, cost, and changes in practice patterns. Surg Endosc 2003;17:1889–1895.

Lind M, Hazebroek W, Kirkels W, et al. Laparoscopic versus open nephrectomy: ureteral complications in recipients. Urology 2004;63:36–40.

# Suggested Readings

Abrahams H, Freise C, Kang S, et al. Technique, indications and outcomes of pure laparoscopic right donor nephrectomy. J Urol 2004;171:1793–1796.

Barry J. Editorial: living donor nephrectomy. J Urol 2004;171:61–62.

Buell J, Hanaway M, Potter S, et al. Surgical techniques in right laparoscopic nephrectomy. J Am Coll Surg 2002;195:131–137.

Flowers JL, Jacobs S. Cho E, et al. Comparison of open and laparoscopic live donor nephrectomy. Ann Surg 1997;226:483–489.

Kercher KW, Joels CS, Matthews BD, Lincourt AE, Smith TI, Heniford BT. Hand-assisted surgery improves outcomes for laparoscopic nephrectomy. Am Surg 2003;69:1061–1066.

Khauli RB. A controlled sequential evaluation of laparoscopic donor nephrectomy versus open donor nephrectomy: an update. Transplant Proc 2005;37(2):633–634.

Kok NF. Donor nephrectomy: mini-incision muscle-splitting open approach versus laparoscopy. Transplantation 2006;81(6):881–887.

Lewis GR. A comparison of traditional open, minimal-incision donor nephrectomy and laparoscopic donor nephrectomy. Transplant Int 2004;17(10):589–595.

Lind M, Hazebroek E, Hop W, et al. Right-sided laparoscopic live donor nephrectomy: is reluctance still justified? Transplantation 2002;74:1045–1048.

Neipp M. Living donor nephrectomy: flank incision versus anterior vertical mini-incision. Transplantation 2004;78(9):1356–1361.

Pace KT. Laparoscopic versus open donor nephrectomy. Surg Endosc 2003;17(1):134–142.

Ratner L, Ciseck L, Moore R, et al. Laparoscopic live donor nephrectomy. Transplantation 1995;60:1047–1049.

Ratner LE, Montgomery RA, Maley WR, et al. Laparoscopic live donor nephrectomy: the recipient. Transplantation 2000;69:2319–2323.

Schweitzer EJ, Wilson J, Jacobs S, et al. Increased rates of donation with laparoscopic donor nephrectomy. Ann Surg 2000;3:392–400.

Swartz DE, Cho E, Flowers JL, et al. Laparoscopic right donor nephrectomy: technique and comparison with left donor nephrectomy. Surg Endosc 2001;15:1390–1394.

Troppmann C. Laparoscopic (vs open) live donor nephrectomy: a UNOS database analysis of early graft function and survival. Am J Transplant 2003;3(10):1295–301.

# 35. Adrenal Incidentaloma

## A. Introduction

When a small adrenal mass is found on a computed tomography (CT) scan and biochemical parameters are all normal, the question of observation versus removal arises. When removal required open surgery, a threshold of 6 cm was commonly used to trigger operative removal. As both imaging modalities and laparoscopic techniques have evolved, the question is being reexamined. This chapter uses the case of a 4-cm adrenal mass found incidentally on CT scan to explore these issues.

## B. Case

*Sandy H. Fang*

A 28-year-old man was involved in a rollover motor vehicle accident. His pickup truck was traveling at approximately 65 miles per hours when it slid on ice and rolled over. He was found confused and wandering at the scene. He appeared to be intoxicated. He was brought to the emergency department for evaluation.

He denied any significant illnesses or prior surgeries. He was on no medications. He refused to cooperate with a review of systems. He is currently unemployed. He smoked two packs of cigarettes per day for 13 years and drank six to 12 beers per day.

On physical examination, he was combative and uncooperative. The Glasgow Coma Scale score was 15. He was not able to remember the accident. His pulse was 98, blood pressure was 132/82, weight 98 kg, and height 187 cm. He had multiple superficial lacerations and abrasions on the face and upper extremities. The remainder of his examination was negative. Chest and pelvis x-rays were negative. CT head and cervical spine were negative. Abdomen/pelvis CT scan showed a 4-cm smooth rounded left adrenal mass. All other radiologic studies were negative.

Laboratory tests were as follows: sodium 137 mEq/L, potassium 3.6 mEq/L, blood urea nitrogen (BUN) 15 mg/dL, creatinine 0.8 mg/dL, ethanol 335 mg/dL, complete blood count (CBC) normal, and urine drug screen was positive for amphetamines.

Further workup subsequently revealed total plasma metanephrine 86 pg/mL, plasma metanephrine 53 pg/mL, plasma normetanephrine 33 pg/mL, dehydroepiandrosterone sulfate (DHEAS) 379 ng/mL, serum aldosterone 9.1 ng/dL, 1-mg dexamethasone suppression test plasma cortisol 4.3 μg/dL.

**What would you recommend for the management of this adrenal incidentaloma? Observation or laparoscopic adrenalectomy?**

# C. Observation

## Amal Shibli-Rahhal and Janet Schlechte

The term *adrenal incidentaloma* refers to a clinically inapparent adrenal mass unexpectedly found on imaging for nonadrenal disease. The detection of adrenal incidentalomas has increased significantly in the last 20 years as a result of the widespread use of abdominal imaging modalities. The incidence of incidental adrenal masses increases with age, with a prevalence approaching 7% to 10% in patients 70 years of age or older. The differential diagnosis of an adrenal incidentaloma includes adrenocortical adenoma, pheochromocytoma, adrenocortical carcinoma, and metastatic cancer.

Adrenocortical adenomas form the majority of these lesions, and approximately 70% are nonfunctioning. Functioning adrenal masses produce excess amounts of glucocorticoids, mineralocorticoids, catecholamines, or adrenal androgens. Adrenocortical carcinoma is rare and its incidence in the normal population is estimated at 0.6 to 2 cases per million. Adrenocortical carcinomas can lead to excess hormone secretion, and they generally have a poor prognosis, with a median survival of 18 months. The adrenal glands can also harbor metastases from distant cancers. Lymphomas and carcinoma of the lung and breast are the most common cancers to metastasize to the adrenal glands, followed by melanoma and carcinoma of the kidney, ovaries, and gastrointestinal tract. As a primary malignancy is usually readily apparent when an adrenal incidentaloma is detected, it is rare for metastatic disease to present as an isolated adrenal incidentaloma.

An adrenal incidentaloma does not present a health hazard unless it is malignant or results in hormonal excess. Because the majority of these tumors are benign and nonfunctioning, careful evaluation is needed to select those patients who would benefit from adrenalectomy.

Clinical evaluation starts with a careful medical history and physical examination, looking for signs of a carcinoma or hormone excess. Episodic hypertension, tachycardia, and profuse sweating might suggest a pheochromocytoma, while weight gain, muscle weakness, and bruising might suggest glucocorticoid excess. Hypertension and muscle weakness can also be seen with aldosterone excess, and hirsutism or virilization suggests excess adrenal androgens. Further evaluation should include adrenal imaging and biochemical tests targeted to determine hormone excess.

The likelihood of an adrenal incidentaloma being malignant increases with the size of the tumor. Adrenocortical carcinomas account for 2% of tumors measuring 4 cm or less, 6% of tumors measuring 4.1 to 6 cm, and 25% of tumors larger than 6 cm. A tumor less than 4 cm is usually benign, but the size of the tumor does not reliably predict the presence or absence of malignancy. Benign adrenal adenomas are usually homogeneous and rounded, and have clearly defined margins on CT scan. On the other hand, tumors that have irregular contours or show invasion of surrounding structures are more likely to be malignant. Calcification, hemorrhage, and necrosis are nonspecific findings but are more likely to be seen with malignant lesions. An attenuation coefficient, expressed in Hounsfield units (HU), is another feature on CT scan that is helpful in distinguishing benign from malignant adrenal lesions. Attenuation values are an indirect measure of the intracytoplasmic fat content of the adrenal mass, which is usually high in adenomas. Most adenomas have attenuation values of less than 10 to 20 HU on unenhanced CT. A consensus panel organized by the National Institutes of Health suggested a cutoff value of 10 HU. However, 10% to 40% of adenomas are lipid-poor and show high attenuation values on unenhanced CT. In these cases, delayed enhanced CT imaging is useful since adenomas have a rapid washout of intravenous (IV) contrast. Using a 10- to 15-minute delayed enhanced CT, a washout value of 40% to 50% of the initial enhancement can identify a benign adenoma with a sensitivity of 96% and a specificity of 100%.

Magnetic resonance imaging (MRI) is another imaging modality that is helpful in differentiating benign from malignant adrenal tumors with a diagnostic accuracy that is similar to that of CT. Due to their higher fluid content, malignant masses look denser than adenomas on MRI and appear brighter on T2-weighted images. They also show strong enhancement and delayed washout with paramagnetic contrast due to their low fat content. Chemical-shift MRI is a technique based on the different resonance frequency rates of protons in fat and water. It has been proposed as a method to differentiate malignant adrenal masses from benign adenomas. The high intracytoplasmic lipid content of adenomas results in loss of signal intensity on chemical-shift MRI, while the lipid-poor malignant lesions appear brighter with this technique.

Due to its lower cost and more widespread availability, CT is generally the preferred modality for imaging the adrenal glands.

The results of hormonal testing supplement those of the imaging studies. Subclinical hormonal dysfunction occurs in up to 20% of patients with an adrenal incidentaloma. Subclinical glucocorticoid hypersecretion has been reported in 5% to 47% of cases, subclinical pheochromocytomas in 8% of cases, and subclinical aldosteronomas in 1.6% to 3.8% of cases. The consensus panel organized by the National Institutes of Health recommended an overnight (1-mg) dexamethasone suppression test and determination of fractionated urinary or plasma metanephrines for all patients except those with imaging characteristics of myelolipoma or an adrenal cyst. The test for plasma free metanephrines (normetanephrine and metanephrine) has a sensitivity of 99% and a specificity of 89% and is the test of choice to evaluate for pheochromocytoma. The test for urinary metanephrines has a lower sensitivity but a better specificity (90% and 98%, respectively). The overnight dexamethasone suppression test is performed by administering 1 mg of dexamethasone orally at 11 p.m. followed by measurement of serum cortisol at 8 a.m. the following day. An 8 a.m. serum cortisol level of less than 5 µg/dL excludes the diagnosis of glucocorticoid excess in most cases, but a cutoff of <1.8 µg/dL has been proposed in order to increase the detection of subclinical disease. Serum potassium and a plasma aldosterone concentration/plasma renin activity (PAC/PRA) ratio should be measured in patients with hypertension to screen for primary aldosteronism. A PAC/PRA ratio of more than 30 is highly suggestive of primary aldosteronism.

Benign adrenal adenomas rarely secrete sex hormones. Routine evaluation of testosterone and estradiol is not recommended unless a virilizing or feminizing tumor is clinically suspected or if imaging suggests an adrenocortical carcinoma. Dehydroepiandrosterone sulfate is the most commonly measured hormone in these cases.

Fine-needle aspiration (FNA) may be helpful in the workup of an adrenal incidentaloma in patients with a history of malignancy and an adrenal mass that appears suspicious on imaging. However, because benign findings on FNA do not exclude malignancy, FNA should not be used as a standard procedure during the evaluation of adrenal incidentalomas.

Pheochromocytoma should be excluded before any attempt at FNA is made in order to avoid a potentially life-threatening hypertensive crisis.

Patients whose incidentaloma represents a "silent" pheochromocytoma should undergo adrenalectomy because of their increased risk for a hypertensive crisis. Adrenalectomy is also a reasonable approach for patients with subclinical glucocorticoid overproduction because of their increased risk for insulin resistance and overt Cushing's in the future. However, some debate exists concerning the long-term benefit of adrenalectomy and whether it reverses the metabolic abnormalities in these patients. If adrenalectomy is performed, close follow-up by an endocrinologist is recommended because of the possibility of transient adrenal insufficiency as a result of chronic suppression of the pituitary-adrenal axis. Adrenalectomy is optional for patients with hypertension and an aldosteronoma, since they can be treated medically with aldosterone antagonists.

Nonfunctioning lesions measuring less than 4 cm that exhibit benign features on imaging can be followed conservatively, while lesions larger than 6 cm should be surgically removed. The best therapeutic approach for lesions between 4 and 6 cm is poorly defined. Close follow-up is an acceptable approach for lesions that exhibit benign features on imaging as described above, but adrenalectomy should be strongly considered for lesions that appear suspicious on CT or MRI.

Patients with benign nonfunctioning adenomas should be followed conservatively. Repeat adrenal imaging 6 to 12 months later is recommended. If the lesion remains stable in size, further imaging is not warranted because of the extremely low chance of malignant degeneration. Approximately 20% of patients may develop hormone excess during subsequent follow-up, but this rarely happens with tumors smaller than 3 cm. When hormone excess develops with time, it usually consists of cortisol hypersecretion. Hyperaldosteronism and pheochromocytoma are unlikely to develop during follow-up, once they have been excluded on the initial workup. The current recommendations are to perform the 1-mg dexamethasone suppression test and to measure urinary catecholamines and metabolites at yearly intervals for 3 to 4 years, at which time the risk for tumor hyperfunction plateaus.

In summary, adrenal incidentalomas are being increasingly diagnosed, especially in older patients. Because most of these lesions are benign nonfunctioning adenomas, adrenalectomy is not always necessary and most patients can be followed conservatively. It is, however, important to identify those tumors that present a risk, namely malignant tumors and functioning adenomas and to treat them appropriately.

# D. Laparoscopic Adrenalectomy

## L. Michael Brunt

A patient is referred for evaluation of an incidentally discovered, solitary 4-cm adrenal mass. Two questions should be asked when assessing this patient: (1) Is the mass hyperfunctioning? (2) Is it potentially malignant? If the answer is yes to either question, then adrenalectomy is indicated. The first step in my evaluation of such patients is to perform a careful history and physical examination, specifically looking for a history of hypertension, spells that could be due to a pheochromocytoma, and features of possible increased cortisol production such as obesity or recent weight gain, changes in facial features, diabetes, and osteoporosis. Patients should also be queried about a history of other malignancies because of the potential for adrenal metastasis. Age is another consideration since adrenal adenomas increase in frequency with advancing age and are present in approximately 6.9% of patients older than 70 years of age but in only 0.2% of those under age 30. Adrenocortical carcinomas, on the other hand, peak in incidence in the fourth to sixth decades of life.

The essential biochemical evaluation of this patient should include either plasma fractionated metanephrines or a 24-hour urine for catecholamines and metanephrines to test for pheochromocytoma and an overnight dexamethasone test to exclude subclinical hypercortisolism (1 mg of dexamethasone given at 11 p.m. followed by 8 a.m. plasma cortisol; normals suppress to <3 μg/dL). Approximately 10% of adrenal incidentalomas show evidence of increased hormonal activity on testing, and these are equally divided between pheochromocytomas and subclinical cortisol-producing adenomas (subclinical Cushing's syndrome). Aldosteronomas do not often present as incidentalomas, and it would be unusual for a 4-cm lesion to be aldosterone-producing since most aldosteronomas are less than 1.5 cm in size and aldosterone-producing carcinomas are rare. However, if the patient has a history of either hypertension or hypokalemia, plasma aldosterone and renin levels should be measured to exclude this diagnosis.

Assuming that the biochemical evaluation is negative and this is a nonfunctioning lesion, the question then becomes one of assessing its malignant potential. Most endocrine surgeons agree that nonfunctioning adrenal lesions 4 to 5 cm in size should be removed and lesions smaller than 3.5 to 4 cm are appropriate for observation. These recommendations are based on observations that adrenocortical carcinomas under 5 cm in size are rare although they have been reported. Analysis of reported series indicates that approximately 95% of adrenocortical carcinomas are >4 cm and 95% of adenomas are < 5 cm. In one series, the use of a 4-cm threshold for removal was associated with a 90% sensitivity for detecting adrenocortical carcinomas, although 76% of lesions large than 4 cm that were removed were benign. Therefore, it would appear that a 4-cm size cutoff for adrenalectomy is a reasonable threshold to ensure that an adrenocortical carcinoma is not missed while limiting the number of adrenalectomies done for benign disease. As for the possibility that this lesion could represent an adrenal metastasis, it is important to remember that adrenal metastases usually occur in the setting of other extraadrenal metastatic disease or present as bilateral adrenal masses. The isolated, resectable adrenal metastasis is rare, and so a solitary 4-cm adrenal incidentaloma in the absence of a history of a neoplasm with known adrenal metastatic potential is unlikely to represent a metastatic tumor.

Size alone, however, is not the only feature to be considered in assessing the malignant risk for an adrenal lesion, and the imaging characteristics should also be used to classify these lesions further. Cortical adenomas tend to be smooth, homogeneous, and have low attenuation values (<10 HU) on unenhanced CT. Malignant lesions typically are inhomogeneous and have irregular borders with areas of necrosis, hemorrhage, and calcification and have higher CT attenuation values (>18 HU). However, some overlap in attenuation values between benign and malignant lesions occurs. The appearance on MRI can further characterize lesions that are indeterminate by CT. Adenomas typically have a loss of signal intensity on opposed phase chemical shift imaging due to their high intracellular lipid content, whereas malignant lesions and pheochromocytomas do not show a loss of signal on opposed phase imaging sequences because they have a relatively higher water content. Pheochromocytomas also often have a bright appearance on T2-weighted imaging sequences. Finally, imaging should allow one to identify some adrenal lesions that do not require removal even if >4 cm in size, such as myelolipomas, adrenal cysts, and adrenal hemorrhage.

The role of FNA biopsy in the evaluation of adrenal incidentalomas is very limited. Biopsy does not differentiate benign from malignant primary adrenal tumors and could potentially lead to seeding of tumor or other complications in a patient with a resectable lesion. Biopsy should never be performed unless the patient has first had a pheochromocytoma excluded biochemically. Despite these accepted recommendations, we have seen several patients in recent years who have had an incidentally discovered adrenal lesion biopsied prior to completion of the biochemical workup that is subsequently proven to be a pheochromocytoma. Our personal experience is that adrenal biopsy is rarely informative or alters the management if the patient has a resectable tumor by imaging. Adrenal biopsy should be reserved, therefore, for the patient with *unresectable* primary or metastatic tumor in whom a tissue diagnosis is needed or for the patient who has a suspected infectious or infiltrative process (which is usually bilateral).

The only detail provided in the case scenario presented above is that the patient has a solitary 4-cm adrenal lesion. He is young, and may not be compliant with follow-up due to his substance abuse history. He appears to be a satisfactory risk for surgery. Adrenalectomy would be my recommended treatment. I would use a laparoscopic approach with the expectation of a low risk of complications and a short recovery time. The exceptions to this approach would be if the lesion looked like a myelolipoma or cyst in which case surgery is not indicated, or if the patient is older and has multiple medical comorbidities. In the latter case, provided the lesion has imaging features typical for an adenoma, then careful follow-up with repeat imaging at 4 and 12 months would be most appropriate. For the vast majority of patients who present with this scenario, however, adrenalectomy should be the preferred approach to management.

Finally, it should be emphasized that if the patient has any biochemical evidence of increased production of catecholamines or metabolites, even if the patient has not been hypertensive, preoperative α-adrenergic receptor blockade with phenoxybenzamine is indicated to prevent intraoperative hypertensive exacerbations. Likewise, all patients with subclinical hypercortisolism should receive peri- and postoperative supplemental steroids to avoid adrenal insufficiency.

# E.  Conclusions

## Sandy H. Fang

In the past 20 years, the field of radiology has experienced an explosion of technology with the advent of CT and MRI. The increased utilization of radiologic imaging for screening and diagnosis has inadvertently revealed silent adrenal masses without prior clinical suspicion of adrenal disease; thus, the term *adrenal incidentaloma* has arisen. Definitions vary in the literature. Some exclude those found during staging and workup of cancer. Proper evaluation requires an understanding of the differential diagnosis of adrenal masses, the biochemical workup of hyperfunctioning masses, and identification of malignancy potential—all of which will determine the need for surgical versus medical management.

Autopsy studies reveal that adrenal masses are the most common tumors in humans. Barzon et al. reported that the prevalence of adrenal masses found in a total of 71,206 autopsies was 2.3%, ranging from 1% to 8.7%, with no difference between men and women. The frequency of clinically inapparent adrenal masses detected at autopsy was 0.2% to 1% for patients younger than 30 years of age and increased to 7% to 10% in patients age 70 or older.

Differential diagnosis can be categorized into malignant versus benign masses, hyperfunctioning versus nonfunctioning masses, genetic syndromes, infectious, hemorrhagic, and other etiologies. The differential diagnoses and their distribution in two reported series are depicted in Table 35.1.

Diagnostic evaluation includes a complete history and physical examination, hormone function tests, and possible additional radiologic studies.

History and physical examination may reveal clinical features characteristic of adrenal pathology; however, the signs and symptoms are usually nonspecific. Patients with pheochromocytoma present with hypertension (when severe, they have encephalopathy, proteinuria, or retinopathy) not adequately managed by medical therapy, headache, palpitations, diaphoresis, and anxiety. In addition to hypertension, clinical features of adrenocortical carcinomas include abdominal pain with possible palpation of an abdominal mass, fever, weight loss, weakness, anorexia, nausea, vomiting, severe abdominal gas, and myalgia. The classic symptoms of Cushing syndrome are not commonly associated with adrenal incidentalomas, but hypercortisolism usually presents with more subtle metabolic derangements, such as hypertension, obesity, and diabetes.

An overnight (1-mg) dexamethasone suppression test should be performed to evaluate for hypercortisolism. The morning after dexamethasone is administered, normal individuals suppress serum cortisol levels to less than $5\,\mu g/dL$ ($<138\,nmol/L$), and values greater than $10\,\mu g/dL$ are considered positive. There is a high false-positive rate with this test. A high-dose (8-mg) dexamethasone test may exclude the false positives. The presence of hypertension, hypokalemia, and a PAC/PRA ratio >30 suggests primary aldosteronism. Of note, up to 20% of patients may not have the expected hypokalemia due to restriction of sodium intake, which minimizes potassium losses.

Plasma free metanephrines (normetanephrine >0.6 nmol/d and metanephrine >0.3 nmol/d) is the test of choice for pheochromocytomas.

Table 35.1. Etiology and relative frequency of adrenal incidentalomas.

| Diagnosis | Frequency (%) |
|---|---|
| **Adrenal cortical tumors** | |
| Adenoma | 36–94 |
| Nodular hyperplasia | 7–17 |
| Carcinoma | 1.2–11 |
| **Adrenal medullary tumors** | |
| Pheochromocytoma | 1.5–8 |
| Ganglioneuroma | 0–6 |
| Ganglioneuroblastoma, neuroblastoma, carcinoma | <1 |
| **Other adrenal tumors** | |
| Myelolipoma | 7–15 |
| Lipoma | 0–11 |
| Lymphoma, hemangioma, angiomyolipoma, hamartoma, liposarcoma, myoma, fibroma, neurofibroma, teratoma | <1 |
| Cysts and pseudocysts | 4–22 |
| Hematoma and hemorrhage | 0–4 |
| Infections, granulomatosis | 0–21 |
| Metastases (breast, kidney, lung, ovarian cancer, melanoma, lymphoma, leukemia) | 0–21 |
| Pseudoadrenal masses (stomach, pancreas, kidney, liver, lymph node, vascular lesions, technical artifacts) | 0–10 |

*Source*: Adapted from Barzon et al. and Mansmann et al.

Dehydroepiandrosterone sulfate is a marker of adrenal androgen excess used to identify virilizing and feminizing adrenal tumors.

The current literature proposes that the size and appearance of an adrenal mass on CT and MRI aids in predicting whether the mass is benign or malignant. Grumbach et al. noted that adrenal cortical carcinomas accounted for 2% of tumors less than 4 cm, 6% between 4.1 to 6 cm, and 25% of tumors greater than 6 cm. A benign adrenal adenoma is characterized by a homogeneous mass with a smooth border and an attenuation value of less than 10 HU on unenhanced CT. In contrast, adrenocortical carcinoma demonstrates a larger irregular mass with areas of hemorrhage or tumor necrosis with calcifications in 30% of cases. Concurrently, there may be evidence of metastatic spread to the lymph nodes and other surrounding structures. On MRI, an adrenal adenoma is seen as a signal drop on chemical-shift imaging and intensity similar to that of liver on T2-weighted image, whereas malignancy shows higher signal intensity on T2-weight images.

Other imaging modalities include adrenal scintigraphy and positron emission tomography (PET); however, their use is not standard in the workup of adrenal incidentalomas. Hypersecreting masses and nonhypersecreting adenomas demonstrate radiocholesterol uptake on scintigraphy, whereas primary and secondary adrenal malignancies appear as "cold" nodules. Positron emission tomography may differentiate between benign and malignant masses.

Computed tomography–guided FNA is reserved for the suspicion of metastasis in patients with a prior history of cancer. Lung, breast, stomach, kidney, and ovarian cancer, melanoma, and lymphoma have a predilection to metastasize to the adrenal glands. However, complications of pneumothorax, septicemia, hemorrhage, and seeding of the needle track with metastatic lesions have been reported in 8% to 13% of cases. Of note, benign cytologic diagnosis on FNA does not exclude malignancy because there is a high false-negative rate. In addition, pheochromocytomas should always be excluded prior to performing FNA to avoid the potential of a hypertensive crisis.

The major criteria that determine surgical versus medical management are whether the lesion is functional and whether it is malignant. If the presentation is that of a unilateral incidentaloma, which is confirmed to have glucocorticoid, mineralocorticoid, adrenal sex hormone, or catecholamine excess, then it is classified as functional. Those with pheochromocytomas are at risk for hypertensive crisis, and it has been shown that those with hypercortisolism have future metabolic derangements, for example, insulin resistance or a progression to overt Cushing syndrome. Adrenalectomy is the treatment of choice. Medical management is reserved only for poor surgical candidates; inhibitors of adrenal cortical steroid hormone biosynthesis and aldosterone antagonists are used for Cushing syndrome and aldosterone-secreting tumors, respectively.

In evaluating for malignancy, variables to consider are size, radiologic characteristics, and growth rate. Size is the major determinant of malignancy. About 70% of tumors less than 4 cm are adrenal adenomas and only 2% are cancer. The risk for carcinoma increases to 25% when mass size increases to 6 cm, while adrenal adenomas comprise less than 15%. Thus, 6 cm is designated as the cutoff in which surgical excision is required. If the lesion is less than 4 cm, then observation with follow-up is indicated. There is a gray zone between 4 and 6 cm; either surgical resection or close follow-up is considered acceptable. However, tumor size determined by CT scan is usually less than the diameter reported on histologic examination. Hence, some surgeons use 3 or 5 cm as the cutoff for surgical intervention. In younger patients, some surgeons perform adrenalectomy for masses 3 cm or larger. Adrenalectomy is also considered if the lesion exhibits a rapid growth rate or imaging characteristics not indicative of benign features. Of note, adrenalectomy has no known benefits for patients, who are discovered to have metastasis from a known or unknown primary neoplasm during workup for an adrenal incidentaloma.

Preoperatively, patients with pheochromocytoma should receive $\alpha$-adrenergic blockade with either a calcium channel blocker or phentolamine to avoid a hypertensive crisis during surgery. Patients with subclinical hypercortisolism should receive perioperative glucocorticoids to prevent hypoadrenalism after removal of the functional mass.

The choices for surgical therapy include open versus laparoscopic adrenalectomy. Operative mortality associated with adrenalectomy, in general, is less than 2%. Laparoscopic adrenalectomy has many advantages over the open technique. Patients who undergo a laparoscopic procedure have decreased postoperative pain, decreased time of return to bowel function, shorter hospitalization, and earlier return to work. Contraindications to the laparoscopic approach include malignancy and circumstances in which laparoscopy would be technically difficult.

The recommended follow-up for incidentalomas under observation is a repeat CT or MRI in 3 to 12 months. Radiologic imaging is no longer necessary if the lesion has not increased in size, as concluded by longitudinal studies of up to 10 years. Most adrenal masses remain stable over time, while 3% to 20% enlarge and 3% to 4% decrease in size; 1.7% of patients develop hormone excess, of which cortisol hypersecretion is the most common. The progression to pheochromocytomas, hyperaldosteronism, or malignancy is rare.

# References

Barzon L, Sonino N, Francesco F, et al. Prevalence and natural history of adrenal incidentalomas. Eur J Endocrinol 2003;149:273–285.

Grumbach MM, Biller BMK, Braunstein GD, et al. Management of the clinically inapparent adrenal mass ("incidentaloma"). Ann Intern Med 2003;138:424–429.

Mansmann G, Lau J, Balk E, Rothberg M, Miyachi Y, Bornstein SR. The clinically inapparent adrenal mass: update in diagnosis and management. Endocr Rev 2004;25:309–340.

# Suggested Readings

Angeli A, Osella G, Ali A, et al. Adrenal incidentaloma: an overview of clinical and epide-miological data from the National Italian Study Group. Horm Res 1997;47:279–283.

Angeli A, Terzolo M. Editorial: adrenal incidentaloma—a modern disease with old com-plications. J Clin Endocrinol Metab 2002;87:4869–4871.

Barzon L, Boscaro M. Diagnosis and management of adrenal incidentalomas. J Urol 2000;163:398–407.

Brunt LM, Moley JF. Adrenal incidentaloma. World J Surg 2001;25:905–913.

Hamrahian AH, Ioachimescu AG, Remer EM, et al. Clinical utility of noncontrast com-puted tomography attenuation value (Hounsfield units) to differentiate adrenal adenomas/hyperplasias from nonadenomas: Cleveland Clinic Experience. J Clin Endocrinol Metab 2005;90:871–877.

Mantero F, Terzolo M, Arnaldi G, et al. A survey on adrenal incidentaloma in Italy. J Clin Endocrinol Metab 2000;85:637–644.

Nawar R, Aron D. Adrenal incidentalomas—a continuing management dilemma. Endocr Rel Cancer 2005;12:585–598.

Pocaro AB, Novella G, Ficarra P, et al. Adrenal incidentalomas: surgical treatment in 28 patients and update of the literature. Int Urol Nephrol 2001;32:295–302.

Thompson GB, Young WF Jr. Adrenal incidentaloma. Curr Opin Oncol 2003;15:84–90.

Young WFJ. Management approaches to adrenal incidentalomas: A view from Rochester, Minnesota. Endocrinol Metab Clin North Am 2000;29:159–185.

# 36. Incidental Adrenal Mass with Suspicious Features

## A. Introduction

Laparoscopic adrenalectomy has rapidly superseded open adrenalectomy for most cases of benign adrenal disease. Conversely, open adrenalectomy is preferred when adrenocortical carcinoma is the diagnosis. When the diagnosis is uncertain, but definitely includes adrenocortical cancer, the decision-making process becomes more complex. Chapter 35 discussed options for management of the incidentaloma with benign features. In this chapter, an incidentaloma with some concerning features is presented, and the pros and cons of open versus laparoscopic adrenalectomy are debated.

## B. Case

### Geeta Lal

A 47-year-old woman developed intense interscapular pain 2 weeks after undergoing uneventful laparoscopic cholecystectomy. During the course of her workup a magnetic resonance cholangiopancreatogram (MRCP) was performed to rule out a common bile duct stone. This demonstrated an incidental left adrenal mass. Computed tomography (CT) and magnetic resonance imaging (MRI) scans of the abdomen where then performed (Figs. 36.1 and 36.2) and revealed a 5.4-cm irregularly enhancing left adrenal mass. She had had a basal cell carcinoma excised a few months earlier but otherwise felt well. She denied weight loss, malaise, or fatigue. She had a history of essential hypertension that was controlled on a single medication and had gained 20 pounds over the past 5 years. She denied episodes of headaches, palpitations, and diaphoresis.

Hormonal studies were obtained (see laboratory results, p. 458–459) and demonstrated that the adrenal tumor was nonfunctional. A recent skin exam by her dermatologist did not reveal any new lesions. Recent mammogram and chest x-ray were normal. She denied hematochezia or change in bowel habits.

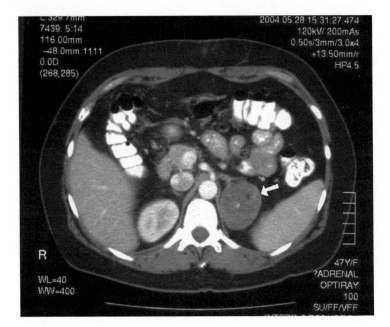

Fig. 36.1. Computed tomography scan showing adrenal mass.

Her past medical history was significant for hypertension and occasional migraine headaches. Her past surgical history included a breast biopsy 22 years earlier (fibroadenoma), tubal ligation 20 years earlier, excision of basal cell carcinoma by a Mohs' procedure 6 months ago, and recent laparoscopic cholecystectomy. There was no family history of thyroid, adrenal, or brain tumors. The patient's only medication was Accupril 30 mg once daily.

Physical examination demonstrated a well-nourished woman appearing her stated age. Vital signs included temperature of 36.9 °C, heart rate 100 and regular, and blood pressure 150/90. Head and neck, chest, and cardiovascular examination were within normal limits. She was not visibly jaundiced. Abdominal examination revealed well-healed trocar sites from recent surgery. There were no masses or tenderness. There were no cutaneous striae. Rectal examination was negative and stool was guaiac negative.

Laboratory results were significant for a normal complete blood count, electrolytes, blood urea nitrogen (BUN), and creatinine. Serum

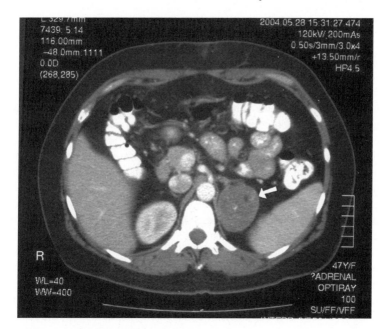

Fig. 36.2. Magnetic resonance imaging scan showing adrenal mass.

metanephrine was 0.36 nmol/L (normal is <0.49), serum normetanephrine 0.42 nmol/L (<0.89), serum aldosterone (upright) 3 ng/dL (3–22), plasma renin activity (upright) 1.8 ng/mL/h (0.5–4), 24-hour urinary cortisol 22 μg (<45), and 24-hour urinary 17-ketosteroids 6.8 mg (normal).

A CT scan showed a 5.4-cm left adrenal mass with heterogeneous enhancement and shotty calcifications (Fig. 36.1). An MRI scan showed a 5-cm adrenal mass containing fat with heterogeneous enhancement (Fig. 36.2).

The impression was a 47-year-old woman with a 5.4-cm nonfunctioning left adrenal mass. The differential diagnosis based on the imaging studies would include an atypical adenoma, myelolipoma, carcinoma, or metastasis.

Adrenalectomy is recommended. The patient is interested in laparoscopic adrenalectomy.

**Which would you recommend—open adrenalectomy or laparoscopic adrenalectomy?**

# C. Open Adrenalectomy

## *James A. Lee and Quan-Yang Duh*

This patient has an adrenal incidentaloma. When faced with an adrenal incidentaloma, one must consider four possibilities: functioning tumor, metastasis, nonfunctioning adenoma, and adrenocortical cancer (ACC). In this case, functional tumors and metastatic disease have effectively been ruled out via age- and risk factor–appropriate cancer screens and biochemical tests. Clearly, the crucial decision is whether this is a nonfunctional adenoma or ACC since the plan of attack is quite different for each. While it is technically feasible to remove very large adrenal lesions laparoscopically, lesions that are suspicious for ACC almost always require an open approach.

There are a number of reasons to suspect ACC in this patient. First and foremost, the size of her tumor suggests the high likelihood of malignancy. Conventional wisdom asserts that the risk of malignancy increases with larger adrenal tumors. Multiple series demonstrate that there is a 35% to 98% chance of malignancy in tumors 5 to 6 cm or greater. At 5.4 cm, the patient's tumor certainly falls into the category of high malignant potential. We also know that cross-sectional imaging can underestimate the size of adrenal lesions by 15%, further increasing this patient's risk. In addition, high signal intensity, irregular borders, invasion, heterogeneity, and calcification on CT or MRI help to distinguish benign from malignant disease. As such, the heterogenous enhancement and shotty calcifications on CT increase the likelihood of cancer. Finally, the acuteness of the patient's pain may be an ominous sign. Unfortunately, the case presentation does not mention if she had left- or right-sided subscapular pain and whether or not she had a common duct stone on MRCP. However, anecdotally, we have found that patients with adrenal incidentaloma who present with acute (not chronic) pain seem to have a higher incidence of malignancy or hemorrhage. Combining these factors, there is a strong likelihood that this is a malignant lesion.

At 0.5 to 2 cases per million, ACC is a rare but highly lethal malignancy. Time and again, retrospective reviews demonstrate that complete surgical resection remains the only potential for cure or meaningful survival. Schulick and Brennan found that the 5-year survival rate of 55% with complete resection plummets to 5% with incomplete resection. As such, it is critical to perform as complete a resection as possible at the first operation. Unfortunately, ACCs are notoriously friable and fracture readily, especially if dissection is carried out in the wrong plane. Tumor rupture is the most important risk factor for recurrence. In addition, ACC fragments readily implant and thrive wherever they land. This is most clearly demonstrated by the literature detailing needle-track seeding after tumor biopsy. Clearly, resection of ACC requires meticulous technique. Furthermore, the surgeon must be prepared to resect surrounding structures such as kidney, spleen, and pancreas if there is invasion. This can be a daunting proposition laparoscopically. Although the magnification afforded by laparoscopic surgery can improve visualization, the lack of tactile feedback and the linear constraints of laparoscopic instruments may limit the surgeon's ability to perform complete resections. Still, surgeons with significant laparoscopic expertise and excellent judgment may choose to start laparoscopically and convert to an open procedure at the first hint of cancer.

Most experts agree that open adrenalectomy is the standard of care for patients with known ACC because this technique minimizes the risks of leaving behind cancer and facilitates removal of involved structures. In essence, open adrenalectomy provides the only chance of meaningful survival for patients. The high likelihood that patients with a tumor greater than 5 to 6 cm will have cancer almost demands an open adrenalectomy. Therefore, for this patient with a 5.4-cm, heterogeneous mass with shotty calcifications, the adrenal lesion should be treated as a cancer until final pathology proves otherwise.

# D. Laparoscopic Adrenalectomy

*Carol E.H. Scott-Conner*

In the proper setting, laparoscopic adrenalectomy may be offered, even when malignancy is part of the differential diagnosis. The case presented is a relatively modest-sized, largely fatty, well-circumscribed lesion. The differential diagnosis includes both benign and malignant lesions. Removal is clearly indicated. The tumor is on the left side, thus dissection should be relatively easy (compared to an equivalent lesion on the right side). An experienced laparoscopist might begin the procedure with careful exposure of the adrenal gland, inspection of the field and a minimal, gentle trial dissection. If, as appears on the MRI scan, the lesion is not adherent to adjacent structures, gentle dissection with extreme care may be successful.

It is important that both patient and laparoscopist understand that the stakes are high. Laparoscopic adrenalectomy is appropriate for benign adenomas and myelolipomas, the two benign lesions included in the radiologic differential diagnosis. The controversy arises with adrenal metastases and adrenocortical carcinoma.

Metastatic lesions are common, but this patient lacks a history of previous malignancy, excluding her basal cell carcinoma (which is unlikely to metastasize). PET-CT scan might yield both additional information about the adrenal mass and help to exclude an occult primary lesion, but would not typically be the next step in workup. Small series of cases attest to the usefulness of laparoscopic adrenalectomy in the setting of metastatic disease.

The real potential for problem arises if the tumor turns out to be an adrenocortical carcinoma. These malignancies are prone to recurrence if dissection in the wrong plane seeds the operative field with tumor cells. Fear of this complication leads many to advocate open adenalectomy in this setting. However, the diagnosis of adrenocortical carcinoma is by no means certain in the present case. In addition, seeding can occur during open as well as laparoscopic surgery. One might argue that the magnification and more precise dissection afforded by laparoscopy would minimize the seeding problem, but this has not been demonstrated.

Thus, in a case such as that presented, where the diagnosis is unknown and the lesion is relatively small and appears well-contained on imaging studies, an experienced laparoscopist might offer laparoscopic adrenalectomy to a suitably informed patient.

# E. Conclusions

*Geeta Lal*

The term *adrenal incidentaloma* is used to denote an adrenal lesion that is identified on imaging studies performed for other reasons and generally excludes tumors discovered on studies performed for evaluation of symptoms of hypersecretion or staging in patients with known cancer. The reported frequency of these lesions identified by CT scan is approximately 0.4% to 4.4% and most (36% to 94%) represent benign, nonfunctioning cortical adenomas. Incidentalomas that are functional, malignant, or potentially malignant are best treated by adrenalectomy. Various series, albeit nonrandomized, have demonstrated that laparoscopic adrenalectomy has been associated with less blood loss, less postoperative pain and narcotic use, shorter hospital stays, and fewer early and late complications. Thus, the procedure has rapidly become the preferred surgical approach for treating benign (both functional and nonfunctional) adrenal lesions. Potentially malignant primary adrenal tumors and adrenal metastases have been traditionally considered to be relative contraindications to the laparoscopic approach. This chapter reviewed the criteria that are useful in assessing the risk of malignancy in adrenal lesions and the results of laparoscopic adrenalectomy for these lesions.

## Risk of Malignancy in Adrenal Lesions

There are no reliable clinical, biochemical, imaging, or cytologic criteria that can be used to predict malignancy preoperatively. Several features, as discussed in the following subsections, need to be considered in deciding the malignant potential of an adrenal lesion.

## Size

Adrenal tumor size has been reported to be the only independent risk factor associated with cancer in several retrospective studies. Although the incidence of primary adrenal cancer in incidentalomas is low (approximately 4% to 5%), the risk increases with tumor size—up to 22% for tumors >4 cm, and to 35% to 98% for tumors >6 cm in size. This has been further substantiated by Sturgeon and Kebebew in their recent comparison of 457 adrenocortical carcinomas identified from the National Cancer Institute Surveillance, Epidemiology, and End Results (SEER) database and 48 benign cortical adenomas treated at their institution. The sensitivity, specificity, and likelihood ratio of tumor size in predicting malignancy for tumors ≥4 cm was 96%, 51%, and 2, respectively, versus 90%, 78%, and 4.1 for tumors ≥6 cm. A recent National Institutes of Health (NIH) state-of-the-science statement recommended that nonfunctioning adrenal incidentalomas ≥6 cm or those with suspicious features on imaging studies be treated by adrenalectomy due to the increased prevalence of malignancy in this group. This is largely based on studies by Copeland, who noted that 92% of 114 adrenocortical carcinomas in the study's series were >6 cm. Ross and Aron also estimated that the risk of malignancy in neoplasms <6 cm in size would be <1/10,000, in the absence of suspicious imaging features. Based on the low risk of malignancy in tumors ≤4 cm in size, observation, with close follow-up is recommended in this group of patients. However, the management of lesions 4 to 6 cm in size with benign imaging features remains controversial; that is, this group of patients can be treated with observation or surgery.

In deciding how to manage these patients, it is important to consider that the size cutoffs are somewhat arbitrary and not absolute because adrenal carcinomas have also been reported in lesions <6 cm, and there are recommendations advocating resection of these tumors at ≥3 cm, ≥4 cm or ≥5 cm. In addition, there are several reports to suggest that imaging studies such as CT scan and MRI can underestimate the size of adrenal masses by 16% to 47% and 20%, respectively. Given the above, and the low morbidity and mortality associated with laparoscopic adrenalectomy, several authors use more aggressive size thresholds, such as 3 cm (rather than 4 cm) for recommending resection in healthy young patients with minimal comorbidities and 5 cm (rather than 6 cm) in older patients with significant comorbidities.

## Imaging Features

Imaging characteristics of incidentalomas have also been used to predict malignancy. Adjacent lymphadenopathy, metastases, or invasion into surrounding organs or blood vessels generally portends malignancy in an adrenal incidentaloma. Other features such as irregular tumor margins, heterogeneity, hemorrhage, necrosis, and hyperdensity (>10 Hounsfield units [HU] on noncontrast CT scans) have also been associated with malignancy, but have also been described in benign lesions. In general, benign adrenal adenomas tend to be homogeneous, encapsulated, and have smooth and regular margins on CT imaging. They also tend to be hypoattenuating lesions (<10 HU). Magnetic resonance imaging has been increasingly used for adrenal imaging, and adrenal metastases have a characteristic high signal intensity on T2-weighted images, whereas adenomas demonstrate low signal intensity. Adrenal to liver signal intensity ratios (on T2-weighted images) have also been investigated, but there is significant overlap among adenomas, metastases, and adrenocortical carcinomas. Radionuclide imaging with NP-59 ($^{131}$I-6β-iodomethyl-19-norcholesterol) has also been used to distinguish between various adrenal lesions, with uptake of NP-59 being reported as 100% predictive of a benign lesion (adenoma). However, this technique has not gained widespread acceptance. More recently, positron emission tomography (PET) scans have been used to identify malignant and metastatic lesions, but these results need further validation.

# Tumor Function

Aldosteronomas are almost always benign and may be safely resected laparoscopically. Approximately 50% of adrenocortical cancers are functional at diagnosis and may secrete cortisol (30%), androgens (20%), estrogens (10%), aldosterone, or a combination of these hormones. Approximately one third of sex-steroid hypersecreting tumors are malignant. Among hormonally active adrenocortical carcinomas, approximately 20% to 30% cause virilization and 10% cause feminization. Thus, the rapid onset of feminization in adult males and virilization at any age should cause heightened suspicious for malignancy. In the absence of other features to suggest adrenocortical cancer, sex-steroid secreting tumors may be approached laparoscopically.

The frequency of malignancy in pheochromocytomas ranges from 2.5% to 26%. However, there are no reliable features to predict malignancy in these tumors. Malignant pheochromocytomas are more likely in extraadrenal tumors, those measuring >6 cm in size, and in those tumors that exclusively secrete dopamine. Often, malignancy is diagnosed when patients develop nodal or locally recurrent disease, or distant metastases during follow-up.

# History of Previous Malignancy

The adrenal is a common site of metastases primarily from tumors of the lung, breast, colon, melanoma, kidney, and lymphoma. In a patient with an adrenal incidentaloma and a history of an extraadrenal malignancy, the tumor represents a metastatic lesion in 32% to 73% of cases. Many studies have documented improved survival with adrenalectomy in the setting of isolated adrenal metastasis. However, this issue, as well as the optimal surgical approach, is still a matter of much debate.

## *Specific Considerations*

### Role of Fine-Needle Aspiration Biopsy

Fine-needle aspiration biopsy (FNAB) under ultrasound or CT guidance has been recommended as a useful tool in distinguishing benign from malignant lesions. It cannot reliably distinguish benign from malignant adrenal lesions and has been associated with complications such as seeding of the biopsy tract with tumor cells and precipitation of a pheochromocytoma crisis. Furthermore, FNAB rarely alters clinical decision making. Thus most authors do not recommend its routine use. Fine-needle aspiration biopsy may be indicated if tumors arising from adjacent tissues are in the differential diagnosis or as part of the diagnostic workup of an adrenal lesion in a patient with a history of malignancy, if the lesion would otherwise be observed.

## Results of Laparoscopic Adrenalectomy for Cancer

The role of laparoscopic adrenalectomy in the management of potential adrenocortical cancers is controversial, mainly due to the paucity of the literature on this subject. Several case reports have described local tumor recurrence, intraabdominal carcinomatosis, and port-site recurrences after adrenalectomy for malignant adrenal tumors that were not appreciated as such either preoperatively or intraoperatively. Sturgeon and Kekebew recently reviewed the outcomes of laparoscopic adrenalectomy for primary and metastatic adrenal lesions based on the published literature. Of a total of 17 patients with primary adrenocortical cancer, only three developed local recurrences and there were no port-site recurrences. One patient developed distant metastasis during a mean follow-up period of 25 months. The three local recurrences were noted in the study by Kebebew et al., representing three of six patients with primary adrenocortical cancer. This 50% recurrence is similar to recurrence rates that were reported for open adrenalectomy (60%); however, the data are difficult to compare because most laparoscopically resected carcinomas were rarely diagnosed preoperatively. The 5-year actuarial survival rates for completely resected adrenocortical carcinoma, as described in the literature, ranges from 32% to 58%.

Of 63 resections performed for metastatic lesions in the same review, there were two local recurrences and two port-site metastases. Fourteen patients developed distant metastases over a mean follow-up of 22 months. Various authors have demonstrated that adrenalectomy for isolated, metachronous adrenal metastasis results in prolonged survival. Luketich and Burt reported an improved median survival of 31 months compared with 8.5 months for chemotherapy alone in their series of open adrenalectomy for non–small cell lung cancer metastases. Kim et al. noted that resection of adrenal metastases ($n = 37$) diagnosed after a disease-free interval of 6 months conferred a survival advantage. Another study by Sarela et al. updated the series with an additional 41 patients and also compared open to laparoscopic metastasectomy. Their results confirmed that a disease-free interval of 6 months was the only significant predictor of improved survival. In their study, actuarial 5-year survival was 29% with a median survival of 28 months. Furthermore, there was no difference in resection margin status or survival between patients treated with open or laparoscopic adrenalectomy. No incisional or port-site recurrences were noted.

Thus, laparoscopic adrenalectomy appears to be safe and effective for locoregional control of solitary metastasis if complete resection is possible and there is no evidence for invasion. Adrenal metastasectomy may be

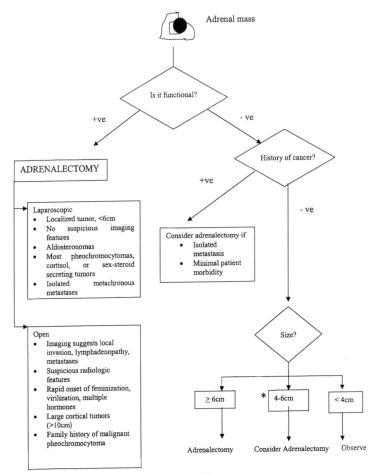

* Refer to discussion in chapter for size threshold

Fig. 36.3. Algorithm for management of incidental adrenal mass.

indicated for diagnosis, curative intent (prolonged survival), or palliation of symptoms. On the other hand, in the absence of further data, open adrenalectomy may be safer for preoperatively known adrenocortical cancers. There is no absolute size criterion for determining which tumors can be resected laparoscopically. Technical considerations and institutional experience usually determine this size threshold. Figure 36.3 is an algorithm for the management of incidentally discovered adrenal lesions.

In conclusion, from the foregoing discussion, it is apparent that there is no single method to reliably distinguish benign from malignant adrenal lesions. Thus, a safe approach is to consider all adrenal masses as potentially malignant and performing laparoscopic resection while keeping the adrenal capsule intact. Laparoscopy can also help determine if the tumor has features of malignancy, which should then lead to conversion to an open adrenalectomy.

# References

Copeland PM. The incidentally discovered adrenal mass. Ann Intern Med 1983;98(6): 940–945.

Kebebew E, Siperstein AE, Clark OH, Duh QY. Results of laparoscopic adrenalectomy for suspected and unsuspected malignant adrenal neoplasms. Arch Surg 2002;137(8):948–951; discussion 952–943.

Kim SH, Brennan MF, Russo P, Burt ME, Coit DG. The role of surgery in the treatment of clinically isolated adrenal metastasis. Cancer 1998;82(2):389–394.

Luketich JD, Burt ME. Does resection of adrenal metastases from non-small cell lung cancer improve survival? Ann Thorac Surg 1996;62(6):1614–1616.

Ross NS, Aron DC. Hormonal evaluation of the patient with an incidentally discovered adrenal mass. N Engl J Med 1990;323(20):1401–1405.

Sarela AI, Murphy I, Coit DG, Conlon KC. Metastasis to the adrenal gland: the emerging role of laparoscopic surgery. Ann Surg Oncol 2003;10(10):1191–1196.

Schulick RD, Brennan MF. Long-term survival after complete resection and repeat resection in patients with adrenocortical carcinoma. Ann Surg Oncol 1999;719–726.

Sturgeon C, Kebebew E. Laparoscopic adrenalectomy for malignancy. Surg Clin North Am 2004;84(3):755–774.

# Suggested Readings

Bardet S, Rohmer V, Murat A, et al. 131I-6 beta-iodomethylnorcholesterol scintigraphy: an assessment of its role in the investigation of adrenocortical incidentalomas. Clin Endocrinol (Oxf) 1996;44(5):587–596.

Barnett CC Jr, Varma DG, El-Naggar AK, et al. Limitations of size as a criterion in the evaluation of adrenal tumors. Surgery 2000;128(6):973–982; discussion 982–973.

Belldegrun A, Hussain S, Seltzer SE, et al. Incidentally discovered mass of the adrenal gland. Surg Gynecol Obstet 1986;163(3):203–208.

Bernini GP, Miccoli P, Moretti A, et al. Sixty adrenal masses of large dimensions: hormonal and morphologic evaluation. Urology 1998;51(6):920–925.

Brunt LM, Moley JF. Adrenal incidentaloma. World J Surg 2001;25(7):905–913.

Cerfolio RJ, Vaughan ED Jr, Brennan TG Jr, Hirvela ER. Accuracy of computed tomography in predicting adrenal tumor size. Surg Gynecol Obstet 1993;176(4):307–309.

Dackiw AP, Lee JE, Gagel RF, Evans DB. Adrenal cortical carcinoma. World J Surg 2001;25(7):914–926.

Doppman JL, Reinig JW, Dwyer AJ, et al. Differentiation of adrenal masses by magnetic resonance imaging. Surgery 1987;102(6):1018–1026.

Dunnick NR, Korobkin M, Francis I. Adrenal radiology: distinguishing benign from malignant adrenal masses. AJR Am J Roentgenol 1996;167(4):861–867.

Francis IR, Gross MD, Shapiro B, Korobkin M, Quint LE. Integrated imaging of adrenal disease. Radiology 1992;184(1):1–13.

Glazer HS, Weyman PJ, Sagel SS, Levitt RG, McClennan BL. Nonfunctioning adrenal masses: incidental discovery on computed tomography. AJR Am J Roentgenol 1982;139(1):81–85.

Graham DJ, McHenry CR. The adrenal incidentaloma: guidelines for evaluation and recommendations for management. Surg Oncol Clin North Am 1998;7(4):749–764.

Gross MD, Shapiro B, Bouffard JA, et al. Distinguishing benign from malignant euadrenal masses. Ann Intern Med 1988;109(8):613–618.

Gross MD, Wilton GP, Shapiro B, et al. Functional and scintigraphic evaluation of the silent adrenal mass. J Nucl Med 1987;28(9):1401–1407.

Guazzoni G, Montorsi F, Bergamaschi F, et al. Effectiveness and safety of laparoscopic adrenalectomy. J Urol 1994;152(5 pt 1):1375–1378.

Herrera MF, Grant CS, van Heerden JA, Sheedy PF, Ilstrup DM. Incidentally discovered adrenal tumors: an institutional perspective. Surgery 1991;110(6):1014–1021.

Hofle G, Gasser RW, Lhotta K, et al. Adrenocortical carcinoma evolving after diagnosis of preclinical Cushing's syndrome in an adrenal incidentaloma. A case report. Horm Res 1998;50(4):237–242.

Kouriefs C, Mokbel K, Choy C. Is MRI more accurate than CT in estimating the real size of adrenal tumours? Eur J Surg Oncol 2001;27(5):487–490.

Lal G, Duh QY. Laparoscopic adrenalectomy—indications and technique. Surg Oncol 2003;12(2):105–123.

Lau H, Lo CY, Lam KY. Surgical implications of underestimation of adrenal tumour size by computed tomography. Br J Surg 1999;86(3):385–387.

Lee MJ, Hahn PF, Papanicolaou N, et al. Benign and malignant adrenal masses: CT distinction with attenuation coefficients, size, and observer analysis. Radiology 1991;179(2):415–418.

Linos DA, Stylopoulos N. How accurate is computed tomography in predicting the real size of adrenal tumors? A retrospective study. Arch Surg 1997;132(7):740–743.

Lombardi CP, Raffaelli M, De Crea C, Bellantone R. Role of laparoscopy in the management of adrenal malignancies. J Surg Oncol 2006;94(2):128–131.

Lumachi F, Borsato S, Tregnaghi A, et al. CT-scan, MRI and image-guided FNA cytology of incidental adrenal masses. Eur J Surg Oncol 2003;29(8):689–692.

McCorkell SJ, Niles NL. Fine-needle aspiration of catecholamine-producing adrenal masses: a possibly fatal mistake. AJR Am J Roentgenol 1985;145(1):113–114.

NIH state-of-the-science statement on management of the clinically inapparent adrenal mass ("incidentaloma"). NIH Consens State Sci Statements 2002;19(2):1–25.

Paivansalo M, Lahde S, Merikanto J, Kallionen M. Computed tomography in primary and secondary adrenal tumours. Acta Radiol 1988;29(5):519–522.

Palazzo FF, Sebag F, Sierra M, Ippolito G, Souteyrand P, Henry JF. Long-term outcome following laparoscopic adrenalectomy for large solid adrenal cortex tumors. World J Surg 2006;30:893–898.

Prinz RA. A comparison of laparoscopic and open adrenalectomies. Arch Surg 1995;130(5):489–492; discussion 492–484.

Shen WT, Lim RC, Siperstein AE, et al. Laparoscopic vs open adrenalectomy for the treatment of primary hyperaldosteronism. Arch Surg 1999;134(6):628–631; discussion 631–622.

Siren JE, Haapiainen RK, Huikuri KT, Sivula AH. Incidentalomas of the adrenal gland: 36 operated patients and review of literature. World J Surg 1993;17(5):634–639.

Staren ED, Prinz RA. Selection of patients with adrenal incidentalomas for operation. Surg Clin North Am 1995;75(3):499–509.

Terzolo M, Ali A, Osella G, Mazza E. Prevalence of adrenal carcinoma among incidentally discovered adrenal masses. A retrospective study from 1989 to 1994. Gruppo Piemontese Incidentalomi Surrenalici. Arch Surg 1997;132(8):914–919.

Thompson GB, Young WF Jr. Adrenal incidentaloma. Curr Opin Oncol 2003;15(1):84–90.

van Erkel AR, van Gils AP, Lequin M, et al. CT and MR distinction of adenomas and non-adenomas of the adrenal gland. J Comput Assist Tomogr 1994;18(3):432–438.

Vassilopoulou-Sellin R, Schultz PN. Adrenocortical carcinoma. Clinical outcome at the end of the 20th century. Cancer 2001;92(5):1113–1121.

Young WF, Jr. Management approaches to adrenal incidentalomas. A view from Rochester, Minnesota. Endocrinol Metab Clin North Am 2000;29(1):159–185, x.

Yun M, Kim W, Alnafisi N, et al. 18F-FDG PET in characterizing adrenal lesions detected on CT or MRI. J Nucl Med 2001;42(12):1795–1799.

# 37. Bilateral Pheochromocytomas

## A. Introduction

Initially, laparoscopic adrenalectomy was applied to very small benign lesions such as aldosteronomas. With increasing experience, larger benign adenomas were tackled (see also Chapters 35 and 36). Because of uncertainties about the effects of pneumoperitoneum on catechol excretion, pheochromocytomas were among the last adrenal tumors to be resected laparoscopically. Questions remain about the best approach when bilateral pheochromocytomas must be removed. This chapter addresses those issues.

## B. Case

### *Howard A. Aubert*

A 24-year-old man presented to the emergency department with sudden onset of severe abdominal pain, which awakened him from sleep at around 2 a.m. He described the pain as 10/10, and localized it to the epigastrium and right upper quadrant. He also complained of nausea, vomiting, diaphoresis, and transient loss of consciousness. His blood pressure was noted to be 220/134. He was treated with intravenous labetalol and nitropaste. A computed tomography (CT) scan of the abdomen was obtained, and bilateral 6- to 7-cm adrenal masses were noted. He was transferred to a tertiary care center for further evaluation and management.

During evaluation at the tertiary care center, the patient stated that he might have had a similar episode of abdominal pain approximately 1 year ago, as well as several less severe spells over the past couple of months. None of these were as bad as the current attack. He denied any significant headache, cardiac palpitations, flushing, diarrhea, or feelings of impending doom. He did complain of intermittent blurred vision that lasted a few seconds and then resolved spontaneously.

His past medical history was significant for viral encephalitis in 1996. His only prior surgery was a repair of a corneal tear in his right eye, sustained in a motor vehicle accident in 2004. His family history was significant for a mother who had bilateral pheochromocytomas resected in 1996. She also had a right eye tumor removed by laser. Her other medical problems include hypothyroidism, insulin resistance, hypertension, and gastroesophageal reflux disease. His father had non–insulin-dependent diabetes mellitus. A sister, aged 21, was healthy. There was no family history of thyroid cancer, hypercalcemia, or other malignancies.

The patient worked in a meat factory. He had smoked half a pack of cigarettes per day for 12 to 13 years, had two to three beers per week, and had used marijuana in the past but denied current usage. He was on no medications and had no allergies.

On physical examination, his vital signs were blood pressure 37/85 and pulse 114 while sitting. Upon standing, his blood pressure was 142/98, pulse 121, and he felt "woozy." He was alert and oriented and in no distress otherwise. His head and neck examination was unremarkable. Specifically, there was no jugular venous distention and his trachea was midline without thyromegaly. There were no masses. His lungs were clear to auscultation bilaterally. His cardiac examination was negative for murmurs, gallops, or rubs.

His abdomen was soft and not distended. It was tender to palpation in the right upper quadrant and right flank. The tenderness increased with deep inspiration. He had normal bowel sounds. The remainder of his examination was negative.

Laboratory results included a hematocrit of 44 with a white cell count of 15.8. Liver function studies included a total bilirubin of 0.5, alanine aminotransferase (ALT) 34, aspartate aminotransferase (AST) 25 U/L, albumin 4.2, alkaline phosphatase 169 U/L, γ-glutamyltransferase (GGT) 169 U/L, and a normal prothrombin time, international normalized ratio (INR), and a normal partial thromboplastin time (PTT). Electrolytes, blood urea nitrogen (BUN), and creatinine were normal. Serum glucose was 66 mg. Amylase and lipase were normal.

Plasma metanephrine levels were normal at 0.24 nmol/L, normetanephrine significantly elevated at 26.9 nmol/L (normal <0.90), calcitonin normal at 2.9 pg/mL, and cortisol 10.3 μg/dL.

A magnetic resonance imaging (MRI) scan of the abdomen demonstrated large bilateral suprarenal masses (Figs. 37.1 to 37.3). There was a bilobed right adrenal mass with lobes measuring 5.4 × 2.7 × 4.7 cm and 2.8 × 2.7 × 2.6 cm. There was also a right aortocaval mass measuring 4.0 × 3.7 × 4.1 cm, as well as an 8-mm mass in the left paraaortic region. These masses showed heterogeneous T1 low signal that did not decrease with the out-phase imaging as well as very high T2 signal, most consistent with pheochromocytoma as well as aortocaval and left paraaortic masses

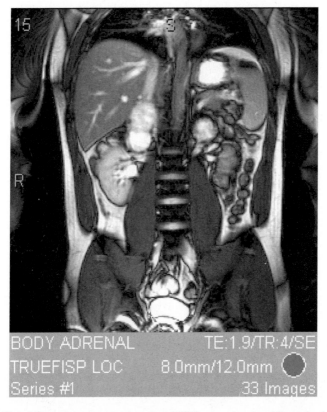

Fig. 37.1. Magnetic resonance imaging (MRI) scan showing bilateral adrenal mass. Note bilobed nature of right adrenal mass.

suggestive of extraadrenal pheochromocytoma. There was also noted to be a low T1, low T2 signal mass in the pancreas (differential diagnosis included islet cell tumor). There were also noted to be large gallbladder stones, with one possibly lodged in the gallbladder neck.

The impression was bilateral pheochromocytomas. He was begun on volume infusions for volume repletion. He was treated with phentolamine and a nitroprusside drip for acute elevations in blood pressure, and with phenoxybenzamine and metyrosine for prevention of catecholamine storm. After adequate control of blood pressure, the patient was started on beta-blockers for extended control. Bilateral adrenalectomy was recommended.

**What route would you recommend—laparoscopic or open?**

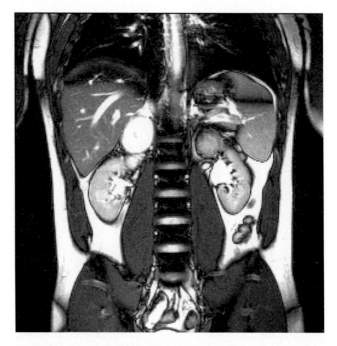

Fig. 37.2. MRI scan showing right paraaortic mass.

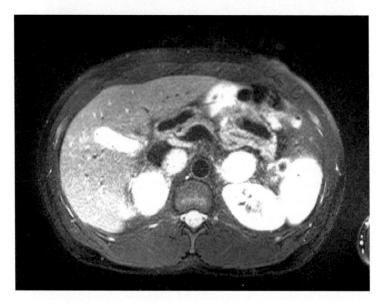

Fig. 37.3. Bilateral pheochromocytomas on MRI.

# C. Bilateral Laparoscopic Adrenalectomy

*Matthew D. Shane and S. Scott Davis, Jr.*

Over the last 10 years, the preferred surgical approach to adrenal disease has undergone a tremendous change. Beginning with the first reported unilateral laparoscopic adrenalectomy by Gagner in 1992, there has been increasing evidence that compared to the open operation, laparoscopic adrenalectomy offers patients shorter hospital stays, less blood loss, and shorter recovery times. Furthermore, despite the use of advanced technologies and equipment, the laparoscopic approach results in decreased overall cost when compared to the open approach. It is for these reasons that the laparoscopic approach is the current gold standard for the surgical management of benign adrenal disease.

Yet do these benefits of laparoscopy apply when a bilateral adrenalectomy is required, or when dealing with complex, hormonally active tumors? Critics would say that longer operative times and the need for intraoperative repositioning of the patient during the bilateral laparoscopic procedure negate any advantages of this approach, and in fact may compromise patient care. Additionally, critics argue that thorough surgical inspection for extraadrenal pheochromocytomas is not possible through the lateral laparoscopic approach. While these concerns may have been valid a decade ago, they have since been refuted by the current published literature. In experienced hands, bilateral laparoscopic adrenalectomy is the preferred approach for bilateral adrenal disease.

As mentioned above, one criticism of the laparoscopic approach is the longer operative times and the need to reposition the patient during the operation. Though operative times are indeed longer in the bilateral laparoscopic approach, they only surpass the open operation by approximately 1 hour in most series. Additionally, as most laparoscopic surgeons in the United States utilize the lateral transperitoneal approach, some of this increased time is simply due to the time needed to reposition and redrape the patient for the bilateral operation. While it is true that repositioning is seldom required in the open approach, with careful attention to airway management and appropriate padding of pressure areas, this represents more of a hassle for the operating room (OR) staff than a true risk to the patient.

More importantly, neither longer operating times nor positioning issues have been shown to have any bearing on patient outcomes after the operation. Retrospective studies of the open versus laparoscopic technique for bilateral adrenal disease demonstrate that the intraoperative blood loss and perioperative hematocrit drop were significantly less in the laparoscopic group. Furthermore, though the bilateral laparoscopic procedure is often akin to two separate procedures performed under a single anesthetic (one side, then the other), the postoperative course is not additive of the two. The length of stay is shorter in the laparoscopic group by an average of 4 days, and the patients return to work a week sooner compared to a similar open group. In short, although the laparoscopic approach may be more demanding for the OR staff and the surgeon, it is better for the patient than an open operation.

Hormonally active tumors of the adrenal gland can be a challenge for both the surgeon and the operating room staff, and bilateral functional tumors can be even more challenging. Yet even in the case of hormonally active tumors, laparoscopy remains the best option for the patient. It is important to remember that for these functional tumors, the bulk of the surgical management actually occurs in the preoperative period. Preoperative imaging with a combination of MRI and $^{123}$I–metaiodobenzylguanidine (MIBG) scintigraphy has demonstrated a sensitivity and positive predictive value for localizing pheochromocytomas of nearly 100%, effectively eliminating the need for intraoperative exploration for other lesions. Preoperative blood pressure control, adrenergic blockade, and the use of experienced anesthesia and surgical staff have allowed pheochromocytomas and other lesions to be successfully managed laparoscopically with the benefits of shorter hospital stays, less postoperative pain, and without increased complication rates for a number of years. With similar attention to preoperative management, even bilateral functioning adrenal masses have been managed definitively laparoscopically with no difference in outcome compared to their nonfunctioning cohorts. It is therefore clear that even in the case of bilateral functional adrenal masses, laparoscopy is superior to the open approach.

Given the superiority of the laparoscopic approach for bilateral adrenalectomy, and that the majority of these procedures are done in the lateral position, the question often arises as to which side should be performed first. In our institution, we prefer to resect the easier side first. While generally this means beginning with resection of the left gland, some patients may benefit from starting with the right side, such as those with chronic pancreatitis or previous operations or infections in the left upper abdomen. The left side is technically easier, with a more consistent position of the adrenal vein (arising from the left renal vein), and with better visualization of the gland itself, due to the need to retract the liver for right-sided lesions. Furthermore, although the overall conversion rate for laparoscopic adrenalectomy is low in experienced hands, there are some data to suggest that intraoperative blood loss and conversion rates may be slightly higher during the resection of right-sided lesions. By starting on the easier side first, in the rare event that a conversion is required, often the incision can be placed on a single flank and not be extended or the patient repositioned to address both glands. Whether the easier side is the right or left, addressing the easier side first will increase the likelihood that the patient have the least morbid operation possible.

Despite its many advantages, laparoscopic bilateral adrenalectomy should not be undertaken by every surgeon. As with any highly specialized surgical procedure, it requires several key factors for success. First and foremost, the operating surgeon must have extensive experience and facility with laparoscopic equipment and techniques, as this is truly an advanced laparoscopic procedure. Similarly, especially in cases of hormonally active tumors, a dedicated and experienced anesthesia staff is a necessity to manage hemodynamic fluctuations, whether the result of positioning or vasoactive factors related to the tumor itself. Dedicated nursing staff familiar with the equipment and troubleshooting is equally important. As long as these criteria are successfully met, in cases of bilateral adrenal disease requiring resection, the laparoscopic approach provides the best care for the patient and should be considered the gold standard.

# D. Open Bilateral Adrenalectomy

## *Carol E.H. Scott-Conner*

I would perform open bilateral adrenalectomy with a thorough abdominal exploration in this patient. There are features on the MRI that suggest extraadrenal involvement, in addition to known bilaterality, gallstones, and an incidental pancreatic mass. Indeed, the presenting symptoms are very suggestive of an attack of acute cholecystitis, with a secondary (albeit very important) diagnosis of pheochromocytoma.

In a complex situation such as this, it is important to triage the order in which the various problems are addressed. I would first proceed with the bilateral adrenalectomies, including a thorough search for other areas of involvement, and then assess patient stability while deciding whether or not to proceed with cholecystectomy and an assessment of the pancreatic mass. Either a bilateral subcostal incision or a midline incision (depending on the angle of the costal margin) would give excellent exposure for all phases of this operation.

If the patient was stable after resection of all hormonally active tissue, I would then proceed with cholecystectomy. Assessing the pancreatic mass would be greatly facilitated by the exposure required for the left adrenalectomy. Further assessment with intraoperative ultrasound and even distal pancreatectomy could be added depending on patient stability and intraoperative findings.

There are several key technical points in performing an open adrenalectomy. On the left side, exposure is best achieved by entry into the lesser sac by widely dividing the gastrocolic omentum. The peritoneum along the inferior aspect of the pancreas is then incised. With the pancreas gently reflected upward, small tumors of the left adrenal gland are easily resected. Larger tumors require reflection of spleen and tail of pancreas medially, a step that would naturally allow careful palpation of the tail of the pancreas and set the stage for subsequent distal pancreatectomy, should that be elected at the end. Gerota's fascia is entered, and the operation proceeds by careful control of adrenal vessels and atraumatic mobilization of the gland.

On the right side, exposure is attained by first mobilizing the hepatic flexure of the colon downward. A generous Kocher maneuver helps by fully exposing the inferior vena cava. The fragile short right adrenal vein must be controlled carefully. If bleeding is encountered, temporary control on the caval side can be achieved by gently grasping the stump with an Allis clamp and running a fine vascular suture under the Allis.

Full exploration of the paraaortic tissues must then be performed. These are exposed by mobilizing the ligament of Treitz and incising the peritoneum. It may be necessary to reflect the colon and small bowel to the right for adequate exposure of the distal aorta and iliacs. Extraadrenal pheochromocytomas (paraganglionomas) are most commonly found at the organ of Zuckerkandl (distal aorta and aortic bifurcation) and superior paraaortic region. The MRI scan gives an excellent delineation of anatomy in this patient and can be used to guide the search.

In summary, I believe that an open approach would provide the best way to remove these pheochromocytomas, allowing assessment of all potential areas of involvement and giving exposure for removal of the gallbladder and even distal pancreas should conditions permit.

# E.  Conclusions

## Howard A. Aubert

Bilateral adrenal pheochromocytoma is usually associated with a familial syndrome, such as Von Hippel–Lindau disease or one of the multiple endocrine neoplastic diseases, as in the current case. Bilateral adrenalectomy has historically been the surgical treatment of choice for familial pheochromocytoma. Currently, the accepted indications to perform an open bilateral adrenalectomy include large tumors, recurrent tumors, suspected malignancy or documented locoregional invasion, or previous adrenal/abdominal surgery, as well as in patients for whom a laparoscopic approach is technically contraindicated. Key aspects of the procedure include the ability to access the adrenal glands without much surgical manipulation, to decrease the amount of catecholamine secretion, and the ability to quickly access and control the adrenal veins.

The open approach for pheochromocytoma is also preferred by some authors due to the possibility of cardiovascular compromise caused by excessive intraoperative catecholamine release, and to allow thorough exploration of retroperitoneal tissues for extraadrenal involvement.

The adrenal glands have a well-defined blood supply, and these tumors are usually small and benign, which makes removal ideally suited to a minimally invasive approach. The difficulty of dissection, the small and flat shape of the gland, and high vascularity and friability increase the risk of damaging the capsule and parenchyma, and can make the procedure very challenging. However, since Gagner et al. performed the first laparoscopic adrenalectomy in 1992, laparoscopic resection has become more popular, and recent studies performed comparing the open and laparoscopic procedures have shown similar outcomes, which advocate that laparoscopic surgery is an adequate alternative to open surgery in treatment of pheochromocytoma. The difficulties are compounded when bilateral tumors must be addressed, because the minimal-access surgeon must reposition from one side to the other.

When performing laparoscopic adrenalectomy, there are several procedural considerations. The options are transperitoneal, retroperitoneal, or bilateral paraspinal. The transperitoneal lateral decubitus approach is considered the favorite for bilateral adrenalectomy, due to the improved working space and gland visualization.

There are some theoretical arguments in favor of helium insufflation. Helium does not cause hypercarbia or acidosis and thus eliminates cardiopulmonary derangements including hypercapnia, respiratory acidosis, increased vascular resistance, decreased cardiac index with elevated oxygen consumption, and increased mean arterial pressure. However, carbon dioxide remains the insufflating gas of choice, and the resulting alterations in cardiopulmonary dynamics are easily managed by an experienced anesthesiologist. There have been no current studies comparing carbon dioxide to helium.

Repositioning patient and trocar sites between sides will require a certain amount of "down" time, which can be minimized by careful planning. In Gagner et al.'s experience, this was reported to be around 20 minutes.

Bjorn et al. performed a study of seven patients treated laparoscopically and nine treated by open resection, which showed that those treated laparoscopically had fewer hypertensive episodes, less need of vasoactive drugs, less postoperative analgesic medication, and decreased hospital stay. Cruz et al. had similar outcomes when performing laparoscopic bilateral adrenalectomy for pheochromocytoma. There was a mean operative time of 330 minutes, blood loss of 440 mL, without need of transfusion, and analgesia of 90 mg, and patients were discharged by postoperative day 4. Mobius found similar results, with decreased blood loss, decreased hospital stay, and decreased need of postoperative analgesia.

The most current trend in the treatment of hereditary forms of bilateral pheochromocytoma has been the introduction of laparoscopic partial adrenalectomy. Although these tumors tend to be bilateral, they are rarely malignant. Partial adrenalectomy eliminates morbidity associated with complete adrenal insufficiency and long-term medical adrenal hormone replacement therapy. McClellan et al. reported mean operative time of 400 minutes, estimated blood loss of 100 cc, postoperative analgesic equivalent to 22 mg morphine, and hospital stay of 4 days. Hartmut et al. found that 2 to 24 months after bilateral laparoscopic partial adrenalectomy, all patients were normotensive, and had normal sodium, potassium, glucose, aldosterone, renin, cortisone serum concentrations, 24-hour excretion of norepinephrine, epinephrine, and vanillylmandelic acid. Abdominal radiologic imaging displayed no remnant or recurrent tumor tissue, and adrenocorticotropic hormone (ACTH) stimulation testing resulted in normal cortisone responses.

In addition to concerns about recurrence, partial adrenalectomy has an additional risk. Because early ligation of the adrenal vein is not feasible, the patient must be extremely well controlled hemodynamically prior to surgery.

Follow-up is recommended at 3 and 6 months after surgery, and then yearly catecholamine determinations and physical examination for at least 5 years. The 5-year survival after removal of benign pheochromocytoma has ranged from 84% to 96%.

In summary, treatment of familial bilateral pheochromocytoma has evolved rapidly since the introduction of the laparoscopic adrenalectomy. Through the teamwork of the entire medical/surgical staff, patients with pheochromocytomas can expect prompt and definitive diagnosis, tumor localization, and preoperative cardiovascular management. With new and improved laparoscopic techniques, most can now also expect less postoperative pain, fewer days of hospital stay, and high success rates similar to those in the past. The future may include greater use of adrenal-sparing surgery; however, more studies with long-term follow-up remain to be conducted.

# References

Bjorn E, Airazat K, Mala T, Pfeffer P, Tonnessen T, Fosse E. Laparoscopic and open surgery for pheochromocytomas. BMC Surg 2001;1:1471–1475.

Cruz L, Sanez A, Benarroch G, Sabater L, Taura P. Total bilateral laparoscopic adrenalectomy in patients with Cushing's syndrome and multiple endocrine neoplasia (IIa). Surg Endosc 1997;11:103–107.

Gagner M, Pomp A, Heniford BT, Pharand D, Lacroix A. Laparoscopic adrenalectomy: lessons learned from 100 consecutive procedures. Ann Surg 1997;226:238–246.

McClellan W, Herring J, Choyke P, Linehan M. Laparoscopic partial adrenalectomy in patients with hereditary forms of pheochromocytoma. J Urol 2000;164:14–17.

Möbius E, Nies C, Rothmund M. Surgical treatment of pheochromocytomas: laparoscopic or conventional? Surg Endosc 1999;13(1):35–39.

# Suggested Readings

Brunt LM, Doherty GM, Norton JA, Soper NJ, Quasebarth MA, Moley JF. Laparoscopic adrenalectomy compared to open adrenalectomy for benign adrenal neoplasms. J Am Coll Surg 1996;183(1):1–10.

Duh Q. Evolving surgical management for patients with pheochromocytoma. J Clin Endocrinol Metab 2001;86:1477–1479.

Gagner M, Breton G, Pharant D, Pomp A. Is laparoscopic adrenalectomy indicated for pheochromocytomas? Surgery 1996;120:1076–1080.

Hasan R, Harold KL, Matthews BD, Kercher KW, Sing RF, Heniford BT. Outcomes for laparoscopic bilateral adrenalectomy. J Laparosc Adv Surg Tech 2002;12(4):233–236.

Hellman P, Linder F, Hennings J, et al. Bilateral adrenalectomy for ectopic Cushing's syndrome- discussions on technique and indication. World J Surg 2006;30(5):909–916.

Heslin MJ, Winzeler AH, Weingarten JO, Diethelm AG, Urist MM, Bland KI. Laparoscopic adrenalectomy and splenectomy are safe and reduce hospital stay and charges. Am Surg 2003;69(5):377–381.

Higashihara E, Baba S, Nakagawa K, et al. Learning curve and conversion to open surgery in cases of laparoscopic adrenalectomy and nephrectomy. J Urol 1998;159(3):650–653.

Horgan S, Sinanan M, Helton WS, Pellegrini CA. Use of laparoscopic techniques improves outcome from adrenalectomy. Am J Surg 1997;173:371–374.

Jaroszewski D, Tessier D, Schlinkert R, et al. Laparoscopic adrenalectomy for pheochromocytoma. Mayo Clin Proc 2003;78:1501–1504.

Kebebew E, Siperstein AE, Duh QY. Laparoscopic adrenalectomy: the optimal surgical approach. J Laparosc Adv Surg Tech 2001;11(6):409–413.

Kim AW, Quiros RM, Maxhimer JB, El-Ganzouri AR, Prinz RA. Outcome of laparoscopic adrenalectomy for pheochromocytomas versus aldosteronomas. Arch Surg 2004;139:526–529.

Korman JE, Ho T. Comparison of laparoscopic and open adrenalectomy. Am Surg 1997;63(10):908–912.

Lumachi F, Tregnaghi A, Zucchetta P, et al. Sensitivity and positive predictive value of CT, MRI and 123I-MIBG scintigraphy in localizing pheochromocytomas: a prospective study. Nucl Med Commun 2006;27(7):583–587.

McClellan W, Keiser, Leinehan M. Pheochromocytoma: evaluation, diagnosis, and treatment. World J Urol 1999;17:35–39.

Mikhail AB, Tolhurst SR, Orvieto MA, et al. Open versus laparoscopic simultaneous bilateral adrenalectomy. Urology 2006;67(4):693–696.

Neuman H, Reincke M, Bender B, Elsner R, Gunter J. Preserved adrenocortical function after laparoscopic bilateral adrenal sparing surgery for hereditary pheochromocytoma. J Clin Endocrinol Metab 1999;84:2601–2610.

Nisiro D, Juries J, Legrans M, Lamy H. Hemodynamic changes during laparoscopic cholecystectomy. Anesth Analg 1992;76:1067–1071.

Pederson L, Lee J. Pheochromocytoma. Current treatment Options Oncol 2003;4:329–337.

Prinz R. A comparison of laparoscopic and open adrenalectomies. Arch Surg 1995;114:1126–1131.

Wells S, Merke D, Cutler G, Norton J, Lacroix A. The role of laparoscopic surgery in adrenal disease. J Clin Endocrinol Metab 1998;83:3041–3042.

# 38. Indirect Inguinal Hernia

## A. Introduction

As techniques for laparoscopic inguinal hernia repair have become standardized, the remaining questions center on indications. The case of a young laborer with a clinically significant indirect inguinal hernia has been chosen to highlight some of these issues. Chapter 39 addresses the issue of which laparoscopic technique to use, if an endoscopic repair is chosen, through a slightly different case scenario.

## B. Case

### *Nate Thepjatri*

A 29-year-old man presented with a 1-month history of right groin pain. He was a construction worker and stated that he noted a bulge in his right groin about 4 weeks earlier. The area became more painful when he stood for prolonged periods of time, and the pain and swelling became worse when he lifted heavy objects at work. The bulge was always reducible, but it had been increasing in size over the prior 2 weeks. The pain was so bothersome he had become unable to work. He did not have any abdominal pain, vomiting, or change in bowel habits.

His past medical and surgical history was negative. He was on no medications and had no allergies. Both parents were alive and well.

His construction job required heavy lifting. He has smoked one pack of cigarettes per day for 10 years. He drinks six beers per week.

On physical examination, he was muscular and well-nourished but not obese. The abdominal exam was negative for masses or tenderness. There was a moderate-sized hernia noted in the right groin, which extended into the scrotum and was easily reducible. The contralateral groin was normal. Testes were normal. The remainder of the exam was negative. Laboratory results were unremarkable.

Impression was a symptomatic right indirect inguinal hernia.

**Would you recommend laparoscopic or open repair?**

# C. Laparoscopic Repair

*Bruce Ramshaw*

The laparoscopic approach for this patient is an ideal option, assuming the surgeon is skilled in the technique. The real dilemma is whether to approach this with a total extraperitoneal (TEP) or transabdominal preperitoneal (TAPP) approach. The TEP approach has the advantage of staying out of the abdominal cavity, avoiding the need to take down the peritoneum and then reperitonealize if a mesh not designed for intraabdominal placement is used. However, a very large scrotal hernia is difficult to reduce using the TEP approach and the reduced hernia contents will likely fill the extraperitoneal space, making mesh placement more difficult. With a TAPP approach, the peritoneum around the internal ring can by incised and the sac left in place, eliminating the need for sac reduction.

Because the size of the hernia on exam was described as moderate and it was easily reducible, I would likely choose a TEP approach. In addition to the advantages over the TAPP approach mentioned above, there are several advantages over an open approach for this patient. First, there is the opportunity to explore the left groin quickly without adding additional incisions. In a review of 1000 laparoscopic inguinal hernia repairs, we noted that 14% of patients had undergone previous contralateral open inguinal hernia repairs and another 12% had undiagnosed contralateral hernias. Taking the patients with bilateral hernias out of this group, almost 50% of patients would potentially benefit from exploration and mesh placement on the contralateral side in a patient with a unilateral inguinal hernia. Exploration of the contralateral groin is especially likely to benefit a young patient who is a physical laborer. In this patient, I would almost always place a mesh on the contralateral side after finding a small indirect defect or a lipoma of the cord.

Another benefit of the laparoscopic approach over an open approach is the decreased pain and faster return to full activity that has been documented in numerous prospective comparative studies. The advantage of the laparoscopic approach in terms of return to activities has been shown to be from 1 day up to several days depending on which study is reviewed. In one of the most thorough evaluations of return to function, Payne et al. showed an 8-day advantage for the laparoscopic approach. The authors evaluated patients with an exercise tolerance test to determine a more objective evaluation of function compared to other studies that usually used patient self-reporting of return to activities.

The potential advantage of decreased recurrence with the laparoscopic approach is debatable. Comparative studies have been inconclusive for the most part. Most of these studies, especially the ones showing increased recurrence rates for the laparoscopic approach, include surgeons with limited laparoscopic experience, but significant experience with the open procedure being studied. Despite this lack of evidence, there are several theoretical advantages for the laparoscopic approach in terms of preventing recurrence. These include using a larger mesh with wider coverage of the myopectineal orifice, including coverage of the femoral and obturator spaces, and mesh placement behind the defect using the intraabdominal pressure holding the mesh in place rather than pushing the mesh away from the defect. Open tension-free repairs, such as the Lichtenstein procedure, where the mesh is placed anterior to the deep muscle layers and coverage includes only the direct and indirect spaces, are susceptible to interstitial hernias between the preperitoneal space and the mesh and to femoral and obturator hernias where the mesh does not provide coverage.

Finally, the incidence of chronic groin pain after inguinal hernia repair has been shown to be significantly less following the laparoscopic approach compared to open alternatives. In Kumar et al.'s study, in which patients responded to a mailed questionnaire, the incidence of chronic pain or discomfort, defined as discomfort when lifting groceries or doing other normal daily activities, was almost twice as high for open (38.3%) compared to laparoscopic (22.5%) hernia repair patients. An open groin incision is not without morbidity. Nerve injuries from dissection or retraction can occur. Other potential causes of chronic pain following open inguinal hernia repair include inadvertent injury from a suture, or nerve irritation due to scarring or the chronic inflammatory reaction to the mesh. The chronic pain associated with open inguinal hernia repair is so prevalent and morbid that some surgeons propose prophylactic division of the nerves to prevent pain resulting in an insensate area of the groin. With appropriate knowledge of the preperitoneal anatomy, limited use of fixation, and use of newer meshes with less chronic foreign body reaction, the incidence of chronic pain after a laparoscopic inguinal hernia repair can be minimized.

In summary, there are numerous reasons to choose a laparoscopic hernia repair for this patient. The opportunity to explore the contralateral groin, less acute pain, quicker return to activity, better mesh placement and coverage of the myopectineal orifice, and lower incidence of chronic pain are all advantages of laparoscopic approach. Of course, these benefits are dependent on the quality and skill of the surgeon in performing this procedure. For a surgeon experienced with laparoscopic inguinal hernia repair, decreased operative times and decreased costs to society can also be achieved in addition to the other benefits mentioned.

# D. Open Repair

*Sathyaprasad C. Burjonrappa*
*and Robert Fitzgibbons, Jr.*

For this patient with an inguinal scrotal hernia, a conventional prosthesis-based tension-free repair (TFR) would be our recommendation. An inguinal scrotal hernia represents a relative contraindication to laparoscopic herniorrhaphy (LIH) especially when it is large. For the purposes of this case scenario, however, we assume that the inguinal scrotal component is not particularly large and that LIH is technically reasonable. The risk of recurrence with a TFR would be between 0.5% and 5%, which is at least as good as for any type of LIH. Most studies that have documented equivalent recurrence rates for LIH and TFR have come from major laparoscopic centers with a keen interest in hernia surgery. A recent randomized control trial conducted in the Veterans Administration (VA) system and reported by Neumayer et al. showed a significantly lower recurrence rate for TFR (4.9%) as compared to LIH (10.1%) in primary unilateral inguinal herniorrhaphies and may be more reflective of the real world.

While certain patient-centered outcomes such as early postoperative pain and resumption of normal activities may be marginally improved with LIH compared to TFR, the risk/benefit ratio still favors TFR in this patient with a unilateral, nonrecurrent inguinal hernia. This is because the slight advantages for the laparoscopic approach must be weighed against potential disadvantages, which include complications related to laparoscopy such as major vascular or bowel injury, possible adhesion formation at trocar sites or where the prosthesis is placed, increased operating room time, increased cost, scarring of the preperitoneal space, and the need for general anesthesia. Other complications that have been reported after LIH include small bowel obstruction, omental infarction, bladder perforation, internal hernia, injury to inferior epigastric or obturator vessels, trocar-site hernia, and intraoperative pneumothorax. These complications are virtually nonexistent with TFR. In a meta-analysis performed by the European Union (EU) Hernia Trialists Group, the incidence of serious adverse events after LIH was 4.7 per 1000 procedures and only 1.1 per 1000 procedures for conventional herniorrhaphy. All of this despite the fact that it is not universally accepted that patient-centered outcomes are actually improved by LIH. For example, in a randomized control study, comparing laparoscopic herniorrhaphy and open TFR performed by Picchio et al., no significant difference was noted in either postoperative analgesic requirement or time to return to unrestricted work.

The overall cost/benefit ratio is an important factor that would further strengthen our recommendations for TFR. That LIH is a more expensive proposition has been unequivocally shown with evidence from meta-analysis by the EU Hernia Trialists Group and the Cochrane Collaboration. Both studies found that longer operating times along with the need for disposable equipment such as trocars and balloon dissectors are the major reasons for the increased cost of LIH. McCormack, Wake et al. conducted a systematic review of comparative studies that included economic evaluations and found that LIH was more costly than TFR in 12 of the 14 studies that met inclusion criteria. The increased immediate cost was estimated to be $520 to $620 per patient. Vale et al. used a Markov cost-effectiveness model to study the subject. They concluded that LIH was not cost-effective.

Another advantage of TFR over LIH is the avoidance of scarring in the preperitoneal space, which results from dissection during LIH. This scar tissue can adversely affect the technical difficulty and complication rate of any subsequent procedure, such as a prostatectomy, performed in that space.

Proponents of LIH for unilateral hernias have touted its ability to diagnose and treat occult contralateral hernias. However, data about the risk of progression and eventual clinical importance of occult hernias are limited, and there is a school of thought that they should not be repaired anyway in deference to the possibility of a postherniorrhaphy pain syndrome in a patient who by definition was asymptomatic.

Our recommendation in this patient would be for a classical Lichtenstein hernia repair. We would perform this repair under local anesthesia with sedation.

We feel that this approach to unilateral hernias is safe, durable, and cost-effective in the real-world setting.

# E.  Conclusions

## *Nate Thepjatri*

The debate continues between open versus laparoscopic approach to repair an inguinal hernia. The two main types of laparoscopic repair are the totally extraperitoneal (TEP), and the transabdominal properitoneal patch (TAPP). In the more common TEP repair, a piece of mesh is placed in the preperitoneal space. In contrast to the TAPP repair, the TEP approach remains completely extraperitoneal. Proponents of each of these laparoscopic techniques argue their respective cases in Chapter 39 of this book.

A review by the Cochrane Database in 2005 identified only one randomized controlled trial comparing these two techniques with an open method. In this study by Schrenk et al., a total of 86 patients were randomized to the Shouldice technique ($n = 34$), TAPP ($n = 28$), or TEP ($n = 24$). There was no statistical difference between the TAPP and TEP in terms of duration of operation, hematoma, length of stay, time to return to usual activity, and recurrence.

In 2005, Schmedt et al. performed a meta-analysis of endoscopic hernia repair versus open repair. A total of 34 randomized controlled trials and 7223 patients were identified. These studies compared both TEP and TAPP with various open hernia techniques. Advantages of laparoscopic repair included lower incidence of wound infection (odds ratio [OR], 0.39; 95% confidence interval [CI] 0.26 to 0.61), lower incidence of hematoma formation (OR, 0.69; 95% CI, 0.54 to 0.90), less nerve injury (OR, 0.46; 95% CI, 0.35 to 0.61), earlier return to work (OR, −1.35; 95% CI, −1.72 to 0.97), and less chronic pain syndromes (OR, 0.56; 95% CI, 0.44 to 0.70). There was no difference in total morbidity; incidence of intestinal, bladder, or vascular lesions; urinary retention; and testicular problems. On the other hand, advantages of the Lichtenstein repair include a shorter operating time (OR, 5.45; 95% CI, 1.18 to 9.73), less seroma (OR, 1.42; 95% CI, 1.13 to 1.79), and fewer recurrences (OR, 2.00; 95% CI, 1.46 to 2.74). One drawback of this analysis was that it included all different types of open repair. Other studies have specifically randomized the laparoscopic versus the Shouldice technique, a method not generally used in United States in the setting described here.

The results from a multicenter VA trial specifically comparing the tension-free open mesh repair to laparoscopic hernia repair were reported by Neumayer et al. in 2004. In this study, 2164 patients with inguinal hernias at 14 VA medical centers were randomly assigned to either an open mesh or laparoscopic mesh repair. A total of 1983 underwent an operation. Two-year follow-up was completed in 1696 (85.5%). The overall recurrence rate was higher in the laparoscopic group (10.1%) versus the open group (4.9%; OR, 2.2; 95% CI, 1.5 to 3.2). In terms of primary hernias, the recurrence rate was higher with laparoscopic repair (10.1% versus 4.0%; adjusted OR, 2.9; 95% CI, 1.8 to 4.5). The recurrence was similar for recurrent hernias (10.0% laparoscopic vs. 14.1%

open; adjusted OR, 0.7; 95% CI, 0.3 to 2). The recurrence rate by either method did not change when there were bilateral hernias.

The complication rate was higher in the laparoscopic group than in the open-surgery group (39.0% vs. 33.4%; adjusted OR, 1.3; 95% CI, 1.1 to 1.6). These complications included injury to the spermatic cord, injury to a vessel, orchitis, and wound infection.

The laparoscopic group had less pain on the day of surgery (difference in mean score on a visual analogue scale, 10.2 mm; 95% CI, 4.8 to 15.6) and at 2 weeks (6.1 mm; 95% CI, 1.7 to 10.5). There was no difference in pain at 3 months. The laparoscopic group returned to normal activity 1 day earlier than the open group (median time 4 days vs. 5 days; adjusted hazard ratio for a shorter time to return to normal activities, 1.2; 95% CI, 1.1 to 1.3).

Surgeon experience was also a factor. Surgeons who performed more than 250 laparoscopic repairs had a recurrence rate of less than 5%, while those performing less than 250 had a rate of greater than 10%. In terms of the open repair, there was no difference in recurrence rate based on surgeon experience.

In conclusion, for primary hernias, existing studies demonstrate that the open repair is better than a laparoscopic approach in terms of recurrence rates and overall safety. Although the pain with laparoscopic repair is less initially, by 3 months there was no difference. If a surgeon chooses to perform a laparoscopic repair, there is a learning curve. It takes about 250 procedures to reduce the recurrence rate by 50%. Laparoscopic hernia repair may have a role in treatment of bilateral or recurrent inguinal hernias.

# References

Kumar S, Wilson RG, Nixon SJ, Macintyre IMC. Chronic pain after laparoscopic and open mesh repair of groin hernia. Br J Surg 2002;89:1479–1479

McCormack K, Wake B, Perez J, et al. Laparoscopic surgery for inguinal hernia repair: systematic review of effectiveness and economic evaluation. Health Technol Assess 2005;9:1–203.

Neumayer L, Giobbie-Hurder A, Jonasson O, et al. Open mesh versus laparoscopic mesh repair of inguinal hernia. N Engl J Med 2004;350:1819–1827.

Payne JH Jr, Grininger LM, Izawa MT, et al. Laparoscopic or open inguinal herniorrhaphy? A randomized prospective trial. Arch Surg 1994;129(9):973–979; discussion 979–981.

Picchio M, Lombardi A, Zolovkins A, Mihelsons M, La Torre G. Tension-free laparo-scopic and open hernia repair: randomized controlled trial of early results. World J Surg 1999;23:1004–1007.

Schmedt CG, Sauerland S, Bittner R. Comparison of endoscopic procedures versus Lich-tenstein and other open mesh techniques for inguinal hernia repair. Surg Endosc 2005;19:188–199.

Schrenk P, Woisetschlager R, Rieger R, et al. Prospective randomized trial comparing postoperative pain and return to physical activity after transabdominal preperito-neal, total preperitoneal or Shouldice technique for inguinal hernia repair. Br J Surg 1997;84(5):728–729.

Vale L, Grant A, McCormack K, Scott NW, EU Hernia Trialists Collaboration. Cost-effectiveness of alternative methods of surgical repair of inguinal hernia. Int J Tech-nol Assess Health Care 2004;20:192–200.

## Suggested Readings

Berndsen F, Arvidsson D, Enander LK, et al. Postoperative convalescence after inguinal hernia surgery: prospective randomized multicenter study of laparoscopic versus Shouldice inguinal hernia repair in 1042 patients. Hernia 2002;6:56–61.

Collaboration EH. Laparoscopic compared with open methods of groin hernia repair: systematic review of randomized controlled trials. Br J Surg 2000;87:860–867.

Grant AM, EU Hernia Trialists Collaboration. Laparoscopic versus open groin hernia repair: meta-analysis of randomized trials based on individual patient data. Hernia 2002;6:2–10.

McCormack K, Scott NW, Go PM, Ross S, Grant AM, EU Hernia Trialists Collaboration. Laparoscopic techniques versus open techniques for inguinal hernia repair. Cochrane Database Syst Rev 2003;1:CD001785.

McCormack K, Scott NW, Go PM, et al., on behalf of the EU Hernia Trialists Collaboration. Laparoscopic techniques versus open techniques for inguinal hernia repair (Cochrane Review). The Cochrane Library 2005;2.

Pokorny H, Klingler A, Scheyer M, Fugger R, Bischof G. Postoperative pain and quality of life after laparoscopic and open inguinal hernia repair: results of a prospective randomized trial. Hernia 2006;10(4):331–337.

Ramshaw B, Frankum C, Young D, et al. 1000 total extraperitoneal (tep) laparoscopic herniorrhaphies: after the learning curve. Published proceedings from the 7th World Congress of Endoscopic Surgery, June 2000.

Wake BL, McCormack K, Fraser C, et al. Transabdominal pre-peritoneal (TAPP) vs totally extraperitoneal (TEP) laparoscopic techniques for inguinal hernia repair. Cochrane Database Syst Rev 2005;1.

# 39. Bilateral Inguinal Hernias

## A. Introduction

The first laparoscopic inguinal hernia repairs were performed using the transabdominal preperitoneal (TAPP) method. As surgeons became more facile in dissection methods, the total extraperitoneal (TEP) repair evolved. Controversy surrounds the choice of method when bilateral hernias require repair. This chapter explores these choices.

## B. Case

*Kent Choi*

A 25-year-old man reported that 3 weeks earlier, while working out at the gym, he noticed pain and then a bulge in his right groin. His physician diagnosed a right inguinal hernia and referred him for repair. The hernia had progressively grown larger, becoming particularly painful after prolonged standing or walking. The patient had always been able to reduce the hernia, with relief of pain.

He was an undergraduate student majoring in premedical studies. He was a nonsmoker and nondrinker. His past medical and surgical history were negative.

On physical examination, he was 180 cm tall and weighed 83 kg. His abdomen was soft without masses, tenderness, or scars. He had a large right inguinal hernia that descended into the scrotum but reduced easily. He also had a palpable left inguinal hernia. The remainder of his examination was negative.

The patient desires laparoscopic repair, and wants to have both hernias fixed at the same setting.

**Would you perform a TAPP or a TEP procedure?**

# C. Bilateral Transabdominal Preperitoneal Repair

## *Leopoldo Sarli*

I would perform a bilateral transabdominal preperitoneal repair. The repair of bilateral inguinal hernias has historically been a persistent problem in hernia surgery. Neither the optimum surgical approach nor the timing of the repair has been clearly defined. In recent years, there has been a trend toward simultaneous hernia repair in view of higher total expenses and more sick leave with sequential unilateral hernia repair. With the spread of laparoscopy, this trend has rapidly accelerated. In fact, while laparoscopic surgery for the repair of inguinal hernia in general surgical practice continues to provoke debate, its role in the simultaneous management of bilateral groin hernias is well established and there are advocates for its routine use in repairing primary hernias. At our center, we have been able to support this view by carrying out a controlled trial in which the laparoscopic TAPP approach to bilateral hernia repair with a single mesh appears to be preferable to the open Lichtenstein tension-free hernioplasty (European Union [EU] Hernia Trialists Collaboration).

The laparoscopic technique that we utilize is a TAPP "bikini" mesh repair. The patient is placed in a supine position with both arms tucked against his body. A Foley bladder catheter is routinely used. After pneumoperitoneum is established, the peritoneal cavity is entered at the umbilicus with a 10-mm trocar and a laparoscope. An additional 12-mm port is placed in both iliac fossae, level with the umbilicus. The inguinal areas are inspected on both sides with their anatomic landmarks. The peritoneum overlying the inguinal regions is transversely separated from the medial umbilical ligament to a point on the iliopubic tract 2 cm lateral to the internal inguinal ring. By blunt dissection, an upper and a lower peritoneal flap are created. The dissection on each side is identical to that of unilateral laparoscopic TAPP repair. Complete visualization of the hernia defects, Cooper's ligaments, transversus abdominis aponeurotic arches, iliopubic tract, and iliac vessels is accomplished with the routine procedure. Both preperitoneal spaces are then joined by continuing the dissection across the midline into the cave of Retzius. A single piece of polypropylene mesh measuring 30 × 10 cm (no splits) is inserted and unfolded to cover spermatic cords, spermatic vessels and all hernial orifices, passing into the cave of Retzius between the bladder and the pubis (Fig. 39.1). The mesh is tacked to the Cooper's ligament and transversalis fascia, using three to five titanium staples at each side.

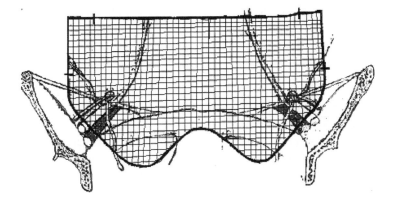

Fig. 39.1. A single piece of polypropylene mesh measuring 30 × 10 cm ("bikini" mesh) is inserted and unfolded to cover spermatic cords, spermatic vessels and all hernial orifices, passing into the space of Retzius between the bladder and the pubis. The mesh is tacked to Cooper's ligament and transversalis fascia, using three to five titanium staples at each side.

The mesh is then fully reperitonealized and the port sites obliterated using titanium clips.

We prefer to utilize a single bikini mesh instead of two individual pieces of mesh (Dean et al.). There are several reasons for this choice. First, this approach covers all hernial orifices and should reduce the risk of medial recurrence as reported in series of laparoscopic and open repairs using two individual pieces of mesh. Second, the positioning of a single bikini mesh, passing into the cave of Retzius between the bladder and the pubis, ensures that, once placed, the prosthesis remains in place and only a few fixing stitches are needed. We maintain that, in this way, besides reducing the operating time, we reduce to a minimum the risk of the long-term postoperative pain often caused by the trapping of nerve endings by the fixing stitches for the prosthesis.

In our experience (Sarli et al.), this technique is seen to have several advantages over the open tension-free technique. The operating time is slightly shorter for the laparoscopic repair than for open repair. This result differs from that usually observed in reports concerning unilateral hernias, in which the duration of the laparoscopic procedure is longer than that of the open procedure. This difference may have occurred because the open procedure for bilateral hernia involves the repetition of the same surgical procedure, first on one side and then on the other, whereas the laparoscopic access is the same for both sides, with a single prosthesis. No patients experienced any major complications; the rate of minor complications was similar in laparoscopic and open procedure patients, although the complication pattern varied between the groups. Seroma and urinary retention were more common after the laparoscopic approach, whereas hematoma and wound infection were more common in the open repair group. Whereas only a few patients undergoing simultaneous open repair of bilateral inguinal hernia were discharged on the first postoperative day, this was possible in a sizable number of patients undergoing the laparoscopic repair.

The most important advantages of the laparoscopic TAPP approach to bilateral hernia over simultaneous open repair are those concerning postoperative pain and the use of medication for pain relief, and this result is in agreement with that of most of the trials comparing laparoscopic hernia repair, unilateral or bilateral, with open techniques. During the first years of our experience, however, right-side shoulder-tip pain occurred only after laparoscopic procedures. The etiology and pathogenic mechanisms of this kind of pain are linked to peritoneal irritation by $CO_2$ and to overstretching of the diaphragmatic muscle fibers owing to the high rate of $CO_2$ insufflation. As we have shown in a previous study, a low insufflation rate significantly reduces both the frequency and the intensity of shoulder-tip pain. Since we began using the precaution of reducing the pneumoperitoneum pressure, we have stopped encountering right-side shoulder-tip pain after bilateral TAPP hernioplasty. We thus advise all those who carry out this type of laparoscopic procedure to reduce carbon dioxide pressure, after the introduction of the trocars, from the initial 13 mm Hg to 9 mm Hg.

It has been suggested that laparoscopic repair is associated with a more rapid return to normal activity and work than is open hernia repair. This difference would appear to be even more marked for bilateral hernias. It has been calculated that the median time to return to work following bilateral laparoscopic hernia repair is 12 to 14 days, which compares favorably to the 28 days reported after simultaneous bilateral open repair.

None of the patients operated on by us returned because of long-term postoperative pain or hernia recurrence. This is encouraging, albeit without any scientific value since we did not carry out a systematic follow-up; also, patients with postoperative pain or hernia recurrence may have turned to other surgeons. In any case, Grant et al. demonstrated in a recent randomized trial that laparoscopic surgery was associated with less long-term numbness and less pain in the groin, and in a Swedish study the recurrence rate after simultaneous laparoscopic surgery was only 2.7% (Berndsen et al.).

For the laparoscopic treatment of bilateral hernia, a proposed alternative to TAPP is TEP. Some studies have compared TEP and TAPP, although none of these compared bilateral hernias specifically. Both repairs allow early return to work and acceptable morbidity rates and low recurrence. A systematic review of the studies comparing TEP and TAPP (McCormack, Wake, Fraser, et al.) concluded that there are insufficient data to allow a conclusion to be drawn as to the relative effectiveness of TEP compared with TAPP. However, there are several reasons why we continue to favor the TAPP technique. Both procedures require a learning curve, but the learning curve for the TEP procedure is longer. Expert laparoscopic surgeons encounter no difficulty in carrying out a transabdominal laparoscopic procedure, whereas the majority of surgeons already skilled in general laparoscopic procedures complain about the technical difficulties of anatomic landmark recognition when they perform the TEP procedure. All in all, we think that TAPP is easier and allows for a better view of the anatomy. This was likely the reason for the longer operating time in TEP patients than in TAPP patients observed in a Brazilian study by Cohen et al. There is yet another reason why we still prefer TAPP hernia repair. In some TEP cases, the procedure has to be converted to TAPP because of large peritoneal tears that cannot be treated by sutures. This conversion is very difficult, because peritoneal closure after TAPP is hard to accomplish owing to the dimension of the peritoneal tear.

We advise the use of TEP, and then only in the hands of a surgeon already skilled in this technique, solely in cases where the transabdominal approach is not suitable, for example on a patient who has undergone previous lower major surgery. However, on a patient affected by bilateral inguinal hernia, with no surgical history or with previous lower minor abdominal operations such as appendectomy, we definitely recommend a transabdominal preperitoneal bikini mesh repair.

For the experienced laparoscopic surgeon, it is easy to perform TAPP, whereas TEP requires a specific learning curve. This is an additional advantage for the TAPP procedure.

# D. Totally Extraperitoneal Hernioplasty

*Jorge Cueto and José A. Vazquez-Frias*

We would perform a totally extraperitoneal repair. In 1991, we watched a live surgery demonstration of a total preperitoneal hernioplasty by Dulucq at the Bordeaux European Association for

Endoscopic Surgery (EAES) Congress of Endoscopic Surgery using primitive instrumentation and technology. It was clear that in time, the well-known advantages of this type of approach (initially described by Cheatle and Henry and popularized by Stoppa and Nyhus) would be applied to endoscopic surgery.

Laparoscopic hernioplasty has not gained wide popularity due to several decisive factors: higher direct costs, a very steep learning curve, and the fact that few surgeons were familiar with the preperitoneal open approach. The completely different surgical anatomic perspective and reduced operating space during TEP repair were thus particularly problematic for many surgeons. In TAPP, though the aforementioned factors apply, the space to work is not as limited as in TEP, and consequently it is less difficult to perform. This is why some surgeons prefer to start with this approach before moving to TEP. In a healthy young man such as the case described here, we would advocate performing bilateral TEP, and we will explain why.

The main indications for a TEP operation are listed in Table 39.1. Bilateral hernias are perhaps the most accepted indication for laparoscopic herniorrhaphy in general and TEP in particular. Recurrent hernias, in particular those initially operated by an anterior conventional approach, form another clear indication for TEP.

In contrast, patients with previous operations such as radical prostatectomy, peritonitis, radiation, and those who have suffered an extensive, infected abdominal/pelvic wound should be operated using a different approach. Although experienced surgeons have reported its feasibility even in this situation, inexperienced surgeons would only experience frustration and complications should they attempt a TEP operation. Likewise, if there is the suspicion of a compromised intestinal loop, a TAPP operation is preferred. A very large, scrotal hernia can be done with either approach, but again the clinical experience of the group and sound surgical criteria must prevail. In these cases, the authors have followed Eduard Phillips's advice of introducing a 3- or a 5-mm laparoscope intraperitoneally to establish the correct diagnosis and then proceed accordingly. This maneuver is also used in those instances where a

Table 39.1. Indications for total extraperitoneal (TEP).

Bilateral hernias
Previous conventional hernia surgery (recurrent hernia)
Scrotal hernia

contralateral hernia is suspected. The TEP method has been shown to be advantageous in single unilateral hernia.

Probably the most important advantage of TEP over TAPP is the fact that it is an abdominal wall procedure. As such, the peritoneum is not entered, and the risk of intraabdominal injury or adhesion formation, considered the main disadvantage of TAPP, is negligible in TEP. Because there is no suture line, staples, or gaps in the peritoneum, the risk of entrapment and small bowel obstruction does not exist.

In the TAPP operation this is an ever-present risk. Suturing the peritoneal incisions in TAPP is not an easy task and the surgeon's position may not be a very comfortable one, which may lead to longer operations and gaps in the suture line. All of this is avoided in TEP. In addition, because TEP avoids direct contact with intestinal loops, ileus does not occur.

Stoppa et al. obtained excellent results applying a similar technique open, and employing a large prosthesis. Some feel that the very low recurrence rate in TEP is due to a more complete dissection than is employed in TAPP, and the use of a larger piece of mesh.

Once the surgical group is comfortable with this approach, the identification of landmarks is straightforward (Cooper's ligament, spermatic cord, the epigastric vessels, etc.). The preperitoneal plane is dissected using both blunt and sharp dissection techniques, and the space of Bogros is entered. A moistened piece of gauze is useful in the dissection particularly in large hernias or reoperations; but even then, bleeding is minimal most of the times.

Endoscopic hernioplasty allows the surgeon to explore the opposite side when other hernias are not diagnosed preoperatively (11.2% in Sayad et al.'s experience) and repair one, if found, without an additional hernia procedure. In this regard, we believe that TEP is a better choice than TAPP, for once the procedure has been finished on one side, it is very simple to extend the dissection to the opposite side through the preperitoneal space already created in the midline. In addition, the dissection done in one side provides a larger operating space for the contralateral repair.

In the repair of large indirect hernias, Stoppa et al. recommended that the sac should be dissected as high as the umbilical level to avoid a recurrence. It may be complicated to achieve this in TAPP, whereas in TEP there is no particular obstacle in doing that. In patients with a large indirect hernia with a weak inguinal floor, our group recommends placing an additional smaller soft mesh under the cord and embracing it, with the edges cut in such a way as to avoid postoperative neuritis. This patient in particular, probably has indirect bilateral hernias, due to his age.

One complication that may occur during the TEP procedure, mainly in patients with previous abdominal/pelvic surgery or in hernia reoperations, is a tear in the peritoneum. In some instances this may lead to a conversion to TAPP. The prevalence of such conversion is between 5% and 10%. Most of the tears can be dealt without the need of a conversion. If the tear is small, a Veress needle can be inserted in the abdominal cavity to vent the pneumoperitoneum. Sutures (interrupted or purse-string type or a preformed loop) can be used as well as clips, and this will usually suffice to control the air leak. If there is a large tear at the beginning of the procedure, a TAPP operation should be done immediately.

Port-site hernias do occur, particularly when 10- to 12-mm trocars are used. This should occur less frequently in the TEP procedure since the peritoneum is not pierced, particularly if the trocars are placed in the midline and sutured properly.

As mentioned before, it is generally recommended that a surgery group should start its experience using the TAPP procedure and then shift to TEP as more experience is obtained. Tutorial guidance is extremely important in the beginning of a surgeon's experience. Review of video presentations is helpful too. Dissecting the preperitoneal space is difficult at first, but it is facilitated by the insertion of disposable balloons, though this adds to the direct costs.

The results obtained with both techniques are similar. The Cochrane review reports that there is only one randomized controlled trial and that review showed no statistical difference between TAPP and TEP when considering operation time, hematomas, hospital stay, recurrence, and time to return to normal activity. That systematic review also reported that eight nonrandomized studies suggest that TAPP is associated with higher rates of port-site hernias and visceral injuries, while there appear to be more conversions associated with TEP.

After a thorough review, McCormack, Wake, Perez, et al. concluded that for unilateral hernias, open repair with mesh is the least costly option but provides fewer quality-adjusted life years (QALYs) than does TEP or TAPP. On average, TEP is estimated to be less costly and more effective. It is likely that for symptomatic bilateral hernias, laparoscopic repair would be more cost-effective as differences in operation time (a key cost driver) may be reduced and differences in convalescence time are more marked (hence QALYs will increase) for laparoscopic compared with open mesh repair. Some surgical groups that routinely perform TEP prefer to carry out the preperitoneal dissection manually with different techniques in an effort to decrease direct costs, but this may lead to longer operating times, and no prospective controlled study has solved this issue.

In summary, laparoscopic hernioplasties are being done more frequently at the present time. Although the results in some series comparing TAPP and TEP are similar, several groups including ours prefer the latter due to the fact that there is less risk and morbidity and fewer recurrences. Bilateral procedures, as in the case of the patient presented here, are particularly suited for this type of approach. The issues of a longer learning curve and higher direct costs are offset by the advantages of a parietal procedure that can be mastered with practice, effort, interest, and patience, as has happened with other endoscopic procedures.

# E.  Conclusions

## *Kent Choi*

Groin hernia management has gone through several revolutions in the last century. It is now widely accepted that mesh repair resulted in a lower recurrence rate. Although there are still some discussions about the merit of open versus laparoscopic repair in simple unilateral groin hernia, the laparoscopic approach has significant advantage in postoperative recovery over traditional open repair in bilateral or recurrent hernias. There are two different approaches in laparoscopic technique—transabdominal preperitoneal (TAPP) and total extraperitoneal (TEP).

There have been multiple publications comparing TAPP and TEP in terms of outcome, complication, and recurrence, but virtually all are retrospective analyses of personal or institutional experiences. There is only one small prospective randomized control trial in the literature. In this trial, Schrenk et al. presented data from 86 patients (34 Shouldice technique, 28 TAPP, and 24 TEP) and reported no difference between TAPP and TEP in terms of length of operation, hematoma, time to return to usual activity, and hernia recurrence. After examining all available data, the Cochrane Group published a comprehensive report that concluded that there are insufficient data to allow conclusions to be drawn about the relative effectiveness of TEP compared with TAPP. Efforts should be made to start and complete adequately powered randomized control trials, which compare the different methods of laparoscopic repair.

The recurrence rate with either technique is relatively low, ranging from less than 1% to 10% in the English-language literature. However, most series have very short follow-up (range, 1 to 28 months). Although no statistical superiority is established, the trending suggested that the total mortality rate is slightly lower with the TEP approach. Surgeon experience plays a major role in the incidence of postoperative morbidity. It appears that it may take 30 to 100 cases to gain sufficient experience in performing laparoscopic hernia repair, although Neumayer et al. suggested that 250 cases were needed.

In conclusion, there is no significant difference or established superiority between TAPP and TEP. Both procedures share the benefits of decreased postoperative pain and shorter recovery time; in both procedures, surgeons can inspect both groins for potential hernia, and avoid going through scar tissue in recurrent cases. Based on current available data, both procedures are effective in managing groin hernia and recurrent groin hernia. Surgeons should choose the procedure according to their training experience and individual patient needs.

# References

Berndsen F, Petersson U, Montgomery A. Endoscopic repair of bilateral inguinal hernias. Short and late outcome. Hernia 2001;5:192–195.

Cohen RV, Alvarez G, Roll S, et al. Transabdominal or totally extraperitoneal laparoscopic hernia repair? Surg Laparosc Endosc 1998;8:264–268.

Deans GT, Wilson MS, Royston CMS, Brough WA. Laparoscopic "bikini mesh" repair of bilateral inguinal hernia. Br J Surg 1995;82:1383–1385.

European Union (EU) Hernia Trialists Collaboration. Laparoscopic compared with open methods of groin hernia repair: systematic review of randomized controlled trials. Br J Surg 2000;87:860–867.

Grant AM, Scott NW, O'Dwyer PJ, MRC Laparoscopic Groin Hernia Trial Group. Five-year follow-up of a randomized trial to assess pain and numbness after laparoscopic or open repair of groin hernia. Br J Surg 2004;91:1570–1574.

McCormack K, Wake BL, Fraser C, Vale L, Perez J, Grant A. Transabdominal preperitoneal (TAPP) versus totally extraperitoneal (TEP) laparoscopic techniques for inguinal repair: a systematic review. Hernia 2005;9:109–114.

McCormack K, Wake B, Perez J, et al. Laparoscopic surgery for inguinal hernia repair: systematic review of effectiveness and economic evaluation. Health Technol Assess 2005;9:1–203.

Neuymayer L, Giobbie-Hurder A, Jonasson O, et al. Open mesh versus laparoscopic mesh repair of inguinal hernia. N Engl J Med 2004;350:1819–1827.

Sarli L, Iusco DR, Sansebastiano G, Costi R. Simultaneous repair of bilateral inguinal hernias: a prospective, randomized study of open, tension-free versus laparoscopic approach. Surg Laparosc Endosc 2001;11:262–267.

Sayad P, Abdo Z, Cachione R, Ferzli G. Incidence of incipient contralateral hernia during laparoscopic hernia repair. Surg Endosc 2000;14:543–545.

Schrenk P, Woisetschlager R, Rieger R, Wayand W. Prospective randomized trial comparing postoperative pain and return to physical activity after transabdominal preperitoneal, total preperitoneal or Shouldice technique for inguinal hernia repair. Br J Surg 1996;83:1563–1566.

Stoppa R, Rives JL, Walamount C, Palot JP, Verhaege PJ, Delattre JF. The use of Dacron in the repair of hernias of the groin. Surg Clin North Am 1984;64:269–285.

# Suggested Readings

Cueto J, Vazquez JA, Weber A. Plastic inguinal laparoscopic transabdominal preperitoneal (TAPP) vs total extraperitoneal (TEP). Ventajas y desventajas. Circ Gen 1998;20(1):36–40.

Cueto J, Vazquez JA, Solis MMA, Valdez GA, et al. Bowel obstruction in the postoperative period of laparoscopic inguinal hernia repair (TAPP). Review of the literature. JSLS 1998;2:277–280.

Felix EL, Michas CA, Conzalez MH Jr. Laparoscopic hernioplasty TAPP vs TEP. Surg Endosc 1995;9:984–989.

Halm JA, Heisterkamp J, Boelhouwer RU, den Hoed PT, Weidema WF. Totally extraperitoneal repair for bilateral inguinal hernia: does mesh configuration matter? Surg Endosc 2005;19:1373–1376.

Kald A, Anderberg B, Smedh K, Karlsson M. Transperitoneal or totally extraperitoneal approach in laparoscopic hernia repair: results of 491 consecutive herniorrhaphies. Surg Laparosc Endosc 1997;7:86–89.

Lau H, Patil NG, WK Yuen. Day-case endoscopic totally extraperitoneal inguinal hernioplasty versus open Lichtenstein hernioplasty for unilateral primary inguinal hernia in males: a randomized trial. Surg Endosc 2006;20:76–81.

Sarli L, Costi R, Sansebastiano G, Trivelli M, Roncoroni L. Prospective randomized trial of low-pressure pneumoperitoneum for reduction of shoulder-tip pain following laparoscopy. Br J Surg 2000;87:1161–1165.

Wake BL, McCormack K, Fraser C, Vale L, Perez J, Grant AM. Transabdominal preperitoneal (TAPP) vs totally extraperitoneal (TEP) laparoscopic techniques for inguinal hernia repair. Cochrane Database Syst Rev 2005;25:CD004703.

# 40. Infantile Hypertrophic Pyloric Stenosis

## A. Introduction

The traditional Ramstedt pyloromyotomy for infantile hypertrophic pyloric stenosis is performed through a very small incision. It has an excellent track record and is associated with rapid recovery and very low complication rate. Thus this procedure seems, at first glance, an unlikely one to be performed laparoscopically. An informal poll of recent graduates of pediatric surgery programs, however, reveals that most preferred the laparoscopic rather than the open approach, as noted later in this chapter. Here we explore the role of minimal-access surgery in this common pediatric surgical procedure, and give tips for both the open and laparoscopic approach.

## B. Case

### Ingrid Lizarraga

A 7-week-old boy developed nonbilious vomiting after every meal. This began 1 week ago. It was initially intermittent, but within the past 3 days it occurred consistently after every feeding. Over the last day it had become projectile. The infant continued to have normal bowel movements, display interest in feeding, and did not appear to be in any pain, although he had become fussy over the last 24 hours. The parents had not noted any fever or abdominal distention.

He was born via uncomplicated spontaneous vaginal delivery at 36 weeks to a 28-year-old primigravida. His birth weight was 3.4 kg and Apgar scores were 9 and 10. He had fed well and had no problems prior to the onset of these symptoms. He had an uncomplicated circumcision at 1 week of age.

The patient's father remembers that his own younger brother had surgery as an infant for a "stomach problem." Both parents were healthy.

On examination, the patient was a crying infant, moderately dehydrated with sunken fontanelles. He had no obvious dysmorphic features.

His heart rate was 152, respiratory rate 36, temperature 37.6 °C, and oxygen saturation 100% on room air. He weighed 4.7 kg and was 55 cm long, putting him at the 40th percentile weight for height.

On gentle palpation of the abdomen, the epigastrium was noted to be slightly distended and a 2- × 3-cm mobile mass was vaguely palpable below the right costal margin. The examination was made difficult by the patient's irritability. Rectal examination was normal.

Laboratory studies included a serum sodium of 146, potassium 2.8, bicarbonate 35, blood urea nitrogen (BUN) 12, and creatinine 0.2. Abdominal ultrasound showed an elongated pylorus with thickening of muscle.

The impression was infantile hypertrophic pyloric stenosis. Pyloromyotomy was recommended. The patient's parents wonder if laparoscopic surgery is feasible for this disorder.

**What would you recommend?**

# C. Open Pyloromyotomy

## Todd A. Ponsky and Anthony Sandler

Although we currently perform >90% of our pyloromyotomies laparoscopically, it is important that surgeons remain facile in the open approach. For this reason, we are writing this case in favor of open pyloromyotomy.

Pyloric stenosis is the most common cause of vomiting in the newborn period that requires surgery. The pathophysiology of pyloric stenosis involves hypertrophy of the musculature of the pyloric channel, the exact etiology of which is unknown. Most children with pyloric stenosis present with projectile, nonbilious vomiting at around 4 weeks of age. Palpating the pyloric olive is diagnostic, but frequently the diagnosis is confirmed by ultrasound or upper gastrointestinal (GI) contrast study. Although pyloric stenosis may resolve spontaneously, it can be associated with significant morbidity and mortality. Thus surgical treatment (pyloromyotomy) is strongly recommended in the United States.

Although recently the laparoscopic approach for the treatment of pyloric stenosis has gained popularity, the traditional open, Fredet-Ramstedt operation remains a safe, tried and true technique. Open pyloromyotomy involves a minilaparotomy through a right upper quadrant, right subcostal or a periumbilical incision. Classically, the pylorus is identified and brought up through the laparotomy incision by eviscerating part of the distal stomach and pylorus. The pyloric muscle is grasped between the index finger and thumb to protect the duodenum and the muscle is sharply incised from the stomach to the pyloric vein of Mayo, just proximal to the duodenum. The muscle fibers are dehisced so that the submucosa freely protrudes through the separated fibers. The entire procedure usually takes 15 to 20 minutes and can usually be performed through a small incision.

In fact, many surgeons who utilize the "omega"-shaped periumbilical incision argue that this open approach may be less invasive and more cosmetic than the laparoscopic approach. This involves a semicircular periumbilical incision that is carried out laterally approximately 1 cm on either side of the umbilicus if needed.

Proponents of the open procedure note that the surgeon loses tactility with the laparoscopic approach, which is important in avoiding a mucosal injury. While some studies suggest that the open approach is a safer technique, others show no difference. St. Peter et al. have proposed that the laparoscopic approach is actually safer.

In a time when the laparoscopic pyloromyotomy is still in its infancy, most pediatric surgeons are still at an early point on the learning curve. Because of this, many academic pediatric surgeons are reluctant to allow a resident to perform pyloromyotomy. This has had a major impact on residency training, because pyloromyotomy has classically been a junior-level resident case.

At our center, over 90% of pyloromyotomies are now performed laparoscopically despite the fact that the authors have never had a perforation or recurrence (inadequate pyloromyotomy) in more than 10 years of performing this procedure open. With the advent of minimally invasive approaches in children, it is important to be familiar with the open approach, and to realize that it does not entail much more pain or morbidity and may even be safer in certain circumstances. For this reason, this approach should remain a valuable option in the treatment of pyloric stenosis.

The operation is performed with attention to the following detailed steps:

1. Place the baby in the supine position.
2. Create a 3- or 4-cm right upper quadrant incision or an "omega" periumbilical incision. This involves a semicircular periumbilical incision that is carried out laterally approximately 1 cm on either side of the umbilicus.
3. Identify the pylorus and deliver the distal stomach and pylorus or pylorus alone up through the incision.

4.  Grasp the pylorus and squeeze it between the index finger and thumb (which will protect the thin-walled duodenum) while incising the muscle with the belly of a scalpel. The incision should be carried from the stomach side of the pylorus to the vein of Mayo on the duodenal side of the pylorus. It is not essential to get every last muscle fiber of the pylorus on the duodenal side, and the pyloric incision can be safely lengthened on the gastric side of the channel.

5.  Spread the fibers with a pyloric spreader or "crack" them with the back of the scalpel handle until the submucosa is clearly seen bulging up between the spread muscle fibers. The muscularis can also be undermined on either side of the pyloromyotomy with the scalpel handle.

6.  Test the myotomy by moving the two split ends of the myotomy parallel to the pylorus but in opposite directions. The two ends should move independently of each other. If not, the myotomy may need to be extended.

7.  Some recommend testing for completion of the pyloromyotomy by submerging the pylorus in saline and insufflating the stomach with 120 cc of air while manually clamping the duodenum. This not only tests for a mucosal injury but also may reveal a persistently tight neck at the proximal end of the pylorus. In this case, the myotomy may need to be extended further toward the stomach.

8.  Following the completion of the myotomy, the fascia should be reapproximated into two layers and the skin closed with a subcuticular stitch.

# D.  Laparoscopic Pyloromyotomy

*John Meehan*

The laparoscopic pyloromyotomy (LP) approach to hypertrophic pyloric stenosis (HPS) is a relatively new method. Introduced in the early 1990s, the technique was performed by only a few surgeons until the late 1990s when smaller equipment finally caught up with pediatric surgical needs. The technique has gained enormous popularity in recent years and has become the preferred method for treating HPS by many surgeons. In fact, an informal account by faculty examiners at the 2006

American Board of Surgery Certifying Oral Board Exam in Pediatric Surgery indicated that all but one examination candidate preferred the laparoscopic approach over the open approach while discussing clinical vignettes.

The operation can be performed with one camera trocar at the umbilicus and two small upper abdominal stab incisions (Fig. 40.1). The camera size is usually 3 mm, although smaller cameras are also available. A standard grasper is used to hold the duodenum through the upper right abdominal stab incision. A pylorotome is brought in through a left upper abdominal stab incision (Fig. 40.2). Before the pylorotomes were commercially manufactured, many surgeons used an arthroscopy knife. This device is an excellent alternative and remains the device that many pediatric surgeons prefer for incising the pyloric serosa.

After the initial longitudinal incision in the pyloric serosa and muscle, the pylorotome is exchanged for a pyloromyotomy spreader and the

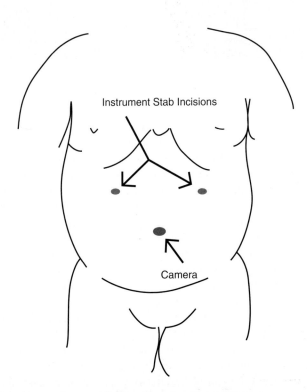

Fig. 40.1.  Trocar placement for laparoscopic pyloromyotomy.

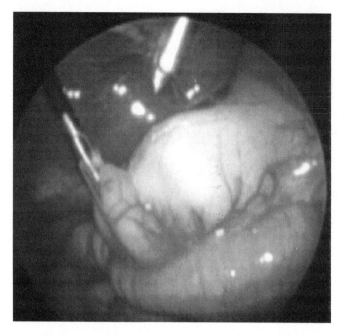

Fig. 40.2. Grasping the pylorus.

muscle fibers are broken down in the standard fashion (Fig. 40.3). These spreaders have evolved over the years, and several options exist. The most recent instrument options bear close resemblance to the Ramstedt pyloric spreader used in open surgery for decades. After the pyloromyotomy is complete, the spreader can act as a grasper, and the superior half of the split pyloric ring is grasped by the grasper and the inferior grasped half by the spreader (Fig. 40.4). The two halves are moved independently to ensure that the ring is adequately broken. Leaks can be tested by having the anesthetist insufflate air into the stomach and visualizing the underlying pyloric mucosa. The umbilical camera port is closed with absorbable suture and the stab wounds require no closure. Postoperatively, patients can be fed as soon as they are sufficiently awake from anesthesia.

As we have seen with other laparoscopic procedures, the laparoscopic pyloromyotomy approach should yield lower wound infection rates. Postoperative pain should also be lower. The cosmesis result is remarkable and the stab incisions are virtually undetectable within a few weeks of the procedure. Length of hospital stay may also decrease, although this would likely need measurements in hours rather than days.

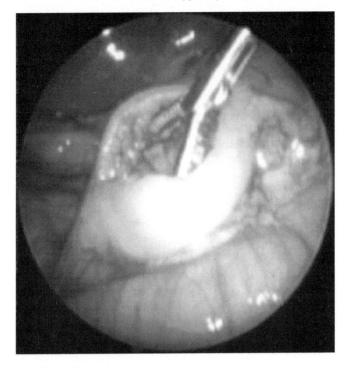

Fig. 40.3. Spreading the myotomy.

The first extramucosal pyloromyotomy was described in 1907 by Fredet and Ramstedt. The first LP series was reported by Alain et al. in 1991. They predicted that LP would likely become a widely used technique. But criticism of the laparoscopic approach was fierce in the first few years after its introduction. Critics argue that the open approach has been time tested, has low complication rates, and most patients can go home within 24 hours. Cosmesis was thought to be the only potential benefit, and perforation rates were projected to be high. Operative times and costs were expected to be prohibitive. None of these criticisms came true.

As expected, the small umbilical incision is well hidden, and the stab incisions are nearly undetectable a few weeks after surgery. But the projected potential downsides of LP never materialized. Multiple retrospective studies have shown that LP is safe and effective with low complication rates and a relatively short learning curve. Yagmurlu published a series of 457 consecutive patients with HPS over a 66-month period. Complications occurred in 4.4% of the open procedures (OPs)

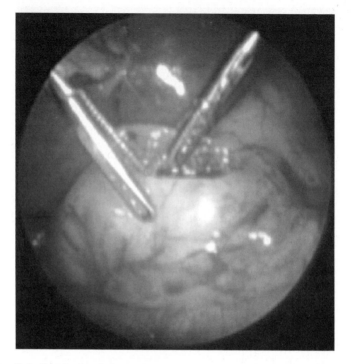

Fig. 40.4. Developing the myotomy.

and in 5.6% of the LPs with more incomplete pyloromyotomies in the LP group and more perforations in the OP group. Kim et al. (2005a) showed an interesting comparison between LP and two different styles of OP—the standard right upper quadrant OP (OP-RUQ) and the umbilical incision (OP-UMB). Once again, a lower perforation rate was seen in the LP group (0 in 51 patients) vs. both open groups (three of 190 in OP-RUQ and three of 49 in OP-UMB). Operative times were the shortest, with the LP group at 25 minutes versus 32 minutes for OP-RUQ and 42 minutes for OP-UMB. This study also addressed the issue of cost. There was a higher cost for the OP-UMB, but no significant difference between the OP-RUQ and LP group, with average costs (including anesthesia) of $2007 for the OP-UMB, $1815 for OP-RUQ, and $1877 for LP. The authors concluded that LP resulted in a shorter operative time with no increase in cost or complications. In another paper, Kim et al. (2005b) showed that the learning curve for LP is relatively short, with the average operative times of about 25 minutes after 30 cases.

In summary, LP is a safe and effective method for treating HPS. Operative times can be shorter with no difference in complication rates and no increase in costs. The cosmetic results for LP are superior to those for OP, and the postoperative scars are nearly invisible a few weeks after surgery. These attributes make LP preferable to OP for the treatment of HPS.

# E. Conclusions

## Ingrid Lizarraga

Infantile hypertrophic pyloric stenosis is among the commonest surgically treated pathologies seen in the neonatal period, with a reported incidence of 1 to 3 per 1000 live births. Ramstedt's pyloromyotomy was first described in 1912, and remains the gold standard of surgical therapy, with minimal morbidity and excellent outcome. The laparoscopic approach was described by Alain et al. in 1991, and has since become widely accepted as an alternative to the traditional procedure. Proponents of laparoscopic pyloromyotomy cite an improved cosmetic appearance and less postoperative discomfort. The literature is rife with studies comparing the two procedures; however, no consensus has emerged on a clearly superior operation. The vast majority of these studies are retrospective and relatively small, with their inherent limitations.

The question was addressed in a meta-analysis by Hall et al., which looked at all English-language papers published between 1996 and December 2002 comparing the two procedures. This study identified eight series, only one of which was a prospective randomized controlled trial. A total of 595 patients were included. The only statistically significant findings were a shorter time to full feeds and shorter length of stay in the laparoscopic group with a mean weighted difference of 8.66 hours and 7.03 hours, respectively. The authors conceded, however, that the differences in feeding protocols among the various institutions made these data heterogeneous and more difficult to interpret. Although mucosal perforations, incomplete pyloromyotomy, and total complications were more frequent in the laparoscopic group, this finding did not reach statistical significance. There was no difference in operating time noted.

This study did not differentiate between pyloric mucosal perforations and duodenal injury. The latter appears to be cited more frequently in relation to laparoscopic pyloromyotomy, and seems to be uniquely related to the use of the grasper in this procedure. A single center retrospective study by Yagmurlu et al. in March 2004 compared 232 laparoscopic and 225 open pyloromyotomies, and found the overall incidence of complications to be similar (5.6% and 4.4%, respectively). However, the spectrum of complications differed between the two procedures. Gastric mucosal perforation was seen in 3.6% of open cases compared to 0.4% of laparoscopic cases, and this was statistically significant. Alternatively, the only two duodenal injuries occurred during laparoscopic pyloromyotomies. A 2.2% incidence of incomplete pyloromyotomy requiring reoperation was noted for laparoscopy only, a finding that also reached statistical significance. The authors theorized that a less aggressive pyloromyotomy was more typical of the minimally invasive approach, thus explaining the lower rate of mucosal perforation and higher rate of incomplete pyloromyotomy. Notably, in this series, the operating time was found to be significantly longer for the open procedure with a mean time of 24.3 versus 29 minutes. It is questionable whether this difference is truly significant either clinically or economically.

A shorter operating time for laparoscopic pyloromyotomy has been reported elsewhere. A recent study by Kim et al. (2005a) of 290 patients comparing laparoscopic to open surgery via a right upper quadrant or umbilical approach found the operating time to be significantly less for laparoscopy. Again, the complication rate and outcome was comparable for all three. They also found operating room charges to be similar for open right upper quadrant and laparoscopic surgery. This finding has varied from center to center, with other papers reporting lower operating costs for open surgery.

Even proponents of the minimally invasive approach admit that there is a definite learning curve associated with this procedure compared to the traditional operation, as with all advanced laparoscopic surgery. Both Kim et al. (2005b) and Ford et al. found that operating times and complication rates were significantly higher in their first 20 patients. Campbell et al. also made the observation that as laparoscopic pyloromyotomy became more popular, there was a decrease in the operative experience of general surgery residents in favor of pediatric surgery fellows at their institution. This may be important to teaching programs, considering that many general surgeons in community hospitals do treat pyloric stenosis.

In experienced hands, laparoscopic pyloromyotomy appears to be as safe as open surgery with comparable or shorter operating times. The wide variation in outcomes reported may reflect the apparent learning curve, and this is important to consider since traditionally this procedure is associated with very low morbidity. An awareness of the potential complications peculiar to the laparoscopic approach is imperative. At this time there does not appear to be a clear advantage of one procedure over the other, and the issue will only be resolved with a large prospective randomized controlled study.

# References

Alain JL, Grousseau D, Terrier G. Extramucosal pyloromyotomy by laparoscopy. Surg Endosc 1991;5:174–175.

Campbell BT, McLean K, Barnhart D, Drongowski R, Hirschl R. A comparison of laparoscopic and open pyloromyotomy at a teaching hospital. J Pediatr Surg 2002;37(7):1068–1071.

Ford WD, Crameri JA, Holland AJ. The learning curve for laparoscopic pyloromyotomy. J Pediatr Surg 1997;32(4):552–554.

Hall NJ, Van Der Zee J, Tan HL, et al. Meta-analysis of laparoscopic versus open pyloromyotomy. Ann Surg 2004;240(5):774–778.

Kim SS, Lau ST, Lee SL, et al. Pyloromyotomy: a comparison of laparoscopic, circumumbilical, and right upper quadrant operative techniques. J Am Coll Surg 2005a;201(1):66–70.

Kim SS, Lau ST, Lee SL et al. The learning curve associated with laparoscopic pyloromyotomy. J Laparoendosc Adv Surg Tech [A] 2005b;15(5):474–477.

St. Peter SD, et al. Open versus laparoscopic pyloromyotomy for pyloric stenosis: a prospective, randomized trial. Ann Surg 2006;244:363–370.

Yagmurlu A, Barnhart DC, Vernon A, et al. Comparison of the incidence of complications in open and laparoscopic pyloromyotomy: a concurrent single institution series. J Pediatr Surg, 2004;39(3):292–296.

# Suggested Readings

Adibe OO, et al. Comparison of outcomes after laparoscopic and open pyloromyotomy at a high-volume pediatric teaching hospital. J Pediatr Surg 2006;41:1676–1678.

Fredet P, Lesne E. Stenose du pylore chez le nourrisson. Resultat anatomique de la pyloromyotomie sur un cas traite et gueri depruis 3 mois. Bull Mem Soc Nat Chir 1908;54:1050.

Hall NJ, et al. Retrospective comparison of open versus laparoscopic pyloromyotomy. Br J Surg 2004;91:1325–1329.

Meehan JJ. Pediatric minimally invasive surgery: general considerations; Pediatric laparoscopy: specific surgical procedures. In: Scott-Conner CEH, ed. The SAGES Manual: Fundamentals of Laparoscopy, Thoracoscopy, and GI Endoscopy, 2nd ed. New York: Springer-Verlag, 2006:491–509.

# 41. Variceal Bleeding

## A. Introduction

Endoscopic management of variceal hemorrhage has revolutionized the emergency treatment of this lethal complication of portal hypertension. In conjunction with other maneuvers, such as the transjugular intrahepatic portosystemic shunt (TIPS), these therapies allow the patient to be stabilized and buy time for evaluation for possible liver transplantation. This chapter explores two common methods of obtaining endoscopic hemostasis: variceal injection sclerotherapy and endoscopic variceal banding.

## B. Case

### Anne T. Mancino

A 44-year-old man presented with a 2- to 3-day history of black, tarry stools. On the day of admission, he had three to four episodes of vomiting dark, clotted blood followed by several cups of fresh blood. He had not had any hematochezia. He had been drinking one-fourth to one-half pint of whiskey every day for at least the last several days. He complained of nausea, but had not had any abdominal pain.

His past medical history was significant for chronic hepatitis C, cirrhosis, alcohol abuse, and hemorrhoids. He had had a variceal hemorrhage in 2002, at which time grade 2 esophageal varices and a small prepyloric ulcer were noted on endoscopy. He had a previous right inguinal hernia repair.

He lived with his mother, and had never married. In addition to chronic daily alcohol consumption, he had a history of occasional marijuana and prior intravenous heroin and cocaine abuse. He smoked half a pack of cigarettes per day for the past 30 years.

His medications included furosemide 20 mg per day, propranolol HCl 10 mg b.i.d., omeprazole 20 mg daily, and potassium chloride 10 mEq daily. He had no allergies. The review of systems was otherwise negative.

On physical examination, his height was 168 cm and his weight was 71 kg. His pulse was 101 and his blood pressure 129/83. He was alert and oriented. He was noticeably icteric. His abdomen was soft with mild tenderness, no hepatosplenomegaly, and minimal ascites. Rectal examination revealed melena, no masses, and hemorrhoids.

Laboratory results were significant for a hemoglobin of 10.6 and hematocrit of 32.8, white blood count (WBC) of 3.9, and platelets 56,000. Other results was as follows: sodium 141, potassium 3.4, chloride 106, glucose 101, blood urea nitrogen (BUN) 5, and creatinine 0.7. His protime was 16.6 seconds (international normalized ratio [INR] 1.3), and his partial thromboplastin time (PTT) was 28.1 seconds. Aspartate aminotransferase (AST [SGOT]) was 224 U/L, alanine aminotransferase (ALT [SGPT]) was 74 U/L, total bilirubin 3.1 mg/dL, direct bilirubin 1.4 mg/dL, alkaline phosphatase 165 U/L, γ-glutamyltransferase (GGT) 492 U/L, albumin 3 g/dL, amylase 271 U/L, and lipase 62 U/L.

He was admitted to the intensive care unit (ICU) and begun on continuous infusions of proton pump inhibitors and octreotide.

Esophagogastroduodenoscopy was performed. No stigmata of recent bleeding were noted to the third portion of the duodenum. He was noted to have a single column of grade 2 to 3 esophageal varices (Fig. 41.1). He also had mild portal hypertensive gastropathy.

**Would you perform injection sclerotherapy or variceal banding on this patient?**

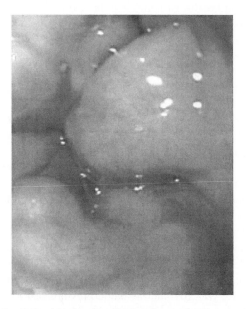

Fig. 41.1. Endoscopic view showing single column of varices.

# C.  Endoscopic Sclerotherapy

*Choichi Sugawa*

Endoscopic sclerotherapy (ES) and variceal banding (VB) are currently accepted as primary treatment modalities for bleeding esophageal varices. When variceal hemorrhage is found to be the cause of bleeding by initial diagnostic endoscopy, the patient is best served if the endoscopist proceeds to definitive control of bleeding with ES or endoscopic band ligation (EBL). This patient is a suitable candidate for endoscopic sclerotherapy.

Sclerotherapy controls acute variceal bleeding in 75% to 95% of patients. Most clinical reports show that ES reduces recurrent bleeding from esophageal varices. There have been a few controlled studies indicating that when compared with medical therapy, ES of esophageal varices improves overall survival.

Several prospective randomized controlled trials have compared EBL with ES. In all studies, EBL and ES were equally effective in controlling active bleeding, but complications were significantly lower with EBL in all studies. Rebleeding rates and mortality rates in EBL were lower in some studies. Currently, we use band ligation as the first-line endoscopic therapy for acute variceal bleeding.

Endoscopic sclerotherapy is still performed routinely in some institutions. In addition, there may be instances in which either EBL is not possible or ES is the more feasible and effective treatment. There are three identifiable occasions when EBL is not technically possible: (1) equipment for EBL is not available, (2) the band ligation device cannot pass beyond the cricopharyngeal sphincter, and (3) varices are too small to be suctioned into the banding apparatus.

In case of massive bleeding, we usually intubate the patient to prevent aspiration, which is relatively common in these patients. Endoscopic band ligation is difficult to perform in this situation. The endoscope is removed and the ligation device is attached to the tip of the endoscope, thus making it difficult to reinsert and examine the actively bleeding varices. In patients with torrential bleeding, ES is possible when bleeding varices are diagnosed at the initial examination.

Endoscopic sclerotherapy can complement band ligation for complete eradication of varices. Endoscopic band ligation is less effective in smaller varices and in repeat endoscopic therapy. In these situations fibrosis caused by previous banding or sclerotherapy renders suction of residual varices difficult. Following a course of initial band ligation, small residual varices were treated by ES. Lo et al. (2000) reported that this approach reduced the rates of both recurrent varices and recurrent bleeding during a median follow-up period of 2 years.

Prophylactic ES in patients who have not yet experienced variceal hemorrhage is controversial. There are both positive and negative reports on this. Advantages of sclerotherapy are largely offset by the morbidity associated with the treatment except polidocanol. Currently, we do not perform prophylactic ES.

Geography and operator preference determine the choice of sclerosant. In the United States, three effective sclerosing agents are available (Table 41.1).

The reported complication rate of ES varies depending on the injection methods and sclerosants used. In the United Kingdom, Japan, North America, and South Africa, sodium tetradecyl sulfate and ethanolamine oleate are widely employed, whereas a mixture of 1 to 20 mg/mL of polidocanol with 0.05 mL of ethanol is used most frequently in continental Europe. In the clinical setting, Kitano et al. reported that ethanolamine oleate was more effective than sodium tetradecyl sulfate with respect to rebleeding and complication of esophageal ulcers. We first developed a canine experimental model of esophageal varices in 1978. At that time, 5% sodium morrhuate was used as sclerosant. To evaluate possible value of this sclerotherapy for treating achalasia, we injected 2 cc of 5% sodium morrhuate into the distal esophagus of a normal dog. We found that injection to the esophageal wall caused perforation of the injection site and ultimate death of the dog. Clinically, we used 1% sodium tetradecyl sulfate and found the rebleeding rate was quite high. We changed the sclerosing agent to a thrombogenic sclerosant cocktail, with better results. After ethanolamine oleate became available in the United States, we have been using ethanolamine oleate as sclerosant with good results.

Table 41.1.  Sclerosing agents available in the United States.

| Sodium morrhuate | |
| --- | --- |
| Sodium tetradecyl sulfate | • 0.75–1.5% solution, or<br>• 1% in combination with 33% ethanol and 0.3% normal saline |
| Ethanolamine oleate | • Used extensively in Europe and Japan<br>• Most expensive agent<br>• Author's sclerosant of choice |

Cyanoacrylate has also been used for the control of gastric variceal hemorrhage. Cyanoacrylate works by polymerization on exposure to moisture when injected into varices. This polymer produces vessel occlusion by variceal embolization. Either isobutyl-2 or $N$-butyl-cyanoacrylate is mixed with lipiodol and injected directly into the varices, producing a virtual acrylic cast of the varices. It appears to be quite effective, but major concerns include the lack of a licensed, deliverable agent and the potential for damage to the endoscope.

Liver function remains the most important prognostic indicator and appears independent of treatment or prophylaxis of bleeding. If the condition of the liver improves, endoscopic therapy will be effective—either EBL or ES. Some patients with advanced liver disease may require liver transplantation after stabilization with endoscopic treatment of varices.

# D.  Endoscopic Band Ligation

*Gregory Van Stiegmann*

The patient presented in this chapter has known cirrhosis and portal hypertension resulting from chronic hepatitis and alcohol abuse. Physical examination and laboratory data indicate he is a Child-Pugh class B patient. Child-Pugh class reflects hepatic functional reserve and correlates with survival. His first variceal bleed in 2002 was apparently treated with a low dose of propranolol in an attempt to prevent recurrent bleeding. He now has another upper gastrointestinal bleed. Patients with one documented bleed from esophageal varices have up to a 70% chance of rebleeding if untreated. The risk of rebleeding is highest during the first week after a documented variceal bleed.

The management described, including fluid resuscitation, proton pump inhibitor therapy, octreotide drip, and blood transfusion if needed, is appropriate. Patients with known cirrhosis and possible bleeding from varices should also be treated with prophylactic antibiotic therapy. If variceal bleeding is confirmed, antibiotic treatment should be continued for 5 to 7 days, which results in a lower incidence of short-term variceal rebleeding when compared with patients who do not receive antibiotic treatment. A fluoroquinolone drug, given first intravenously and then orally, is appropriate.

The patient is slightly tachycardic but has normal blood pressure. Endoscopy should be done within 24 hours in patients with upper gastrointestinal hemorrhage who are stable on admission. Those who have hemodynamic instability on admission benefit by undergoing endoscopy as soon as hemodynamic stability has been achieved. This patient was found to have mild portal hypertensive gastropathy and a single column of varices on initial endoscopy. No other potential source of bleeding was identified. Although the varices found in this patient do not appear impressive (in size or quantity), it is important to recognize that immediately following a bleeding episode, in spite of the presence of stable vital signs, many patients are relatively volume depleted. The true size and extent of varices may become apparent only at a subsequent endoscopy. Mild or moderate portal hypertensive gastropathy is seldom a cause of major bleeding.

Injection sclerotherapy (ES), EBL, and vasoactive pharmacologic therapy are the commonly employed treatments for patients with an acute bleeding episode. Patients with acute bleeding from esophageal varices are best treated with a combination of pharmacologic and endoscopic methods. Drug therapy (octreotide) should be started as soon as possible after admission and continued for several days after endoscopic treatment in order to maximize its value. There is little difference in short-term (3 to 5 days) control of acute variceal bleeding between pharmacologic treatment alone and ES alone; however, there is a higher incidence of complications with the latter. Endoscopic band ligation has advantages over sclerotherapy, both in efficacy for controlling acute bleeding and in safety.

Endoscopic band ligation is the preferred endoscopic treatment for patients with an acute variceal bleed. It is done with a device attached to the endoscope that allows the varix to be aspirated into the device and ligated with a small elastic band (Fig. 41.2). Treatment of active bleeding is similar for both endoscopic methods. If a discrete bleeding site is identified, ES or EBL should be done below and above the site in an attempt to thrombose the varix. In this situation, EBL can also be used directly at the bleeding site, usually with prompt cessation of hemorrhage. If a defined site of bleeding is not found, but no other lesions are present that could account for the bleeding, all varices in the distal esophagus and proximal stomach should be treated. Either endoscopic method controls acute variceal bleeding in 80% to 90% of patients. Endoscopic band ligation is superior for controlling spurting bleeding as compared with oozing.

After bleeding is controlled and the patient is discharged from the hospital, repeat endoscopic treatments aimed at preventing rebleeding by obliterating varices are performed at 7- to 14-day intervals. Endoscopic band ligation is the preferred endoscopic treatment for eradication of

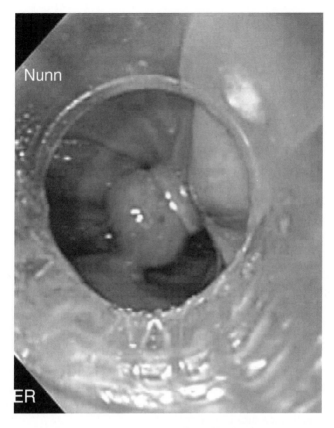

Fig. 41.2. Endoscopic view showing varix ligated by band.

varices and usually requires a total of three or four outpatient treatments. Once varices are eradicated, patients should have repeat endoscopy at 6-month intervals to detect and treat any varices that recur.

Recurrent variceal bleeding after initial endoscopic control occurs in up to 40% of patients and is less common after EBL than after ES. Most patients who rebleed do so prior to eradication of their varices. Repeat endoscopic treatment is indicated for patients who experience one or two episodes of recurrent variceal hemorrhage. Most patients who experience a third episode of variceal bleeding during the course of endoscopic treatment should be considered for alternate treatments such as transjugular intrahepatic shunt or operative shunt insertion.

Outcomes for patients with acute bleeding from esophageal varices have improved substantially in recent decades. Mortality for a first variceal bleed is now approximately 20% as compared with 40% to 60% as recently as 20 to 30 years ago. Elective endoscopic therapy (EBL) to obliterate varices is more effective in preventing recurrent variceal bleeding than long-term pharmacologic therapy using beta-blockade. Long-term treatment using a combination of beta-blockade and EBL appears to offer an additional advantage if the patient is compliant with drug regimen and can tolerate the drug side effects.

# E.  Conclusions

## Anne T. Mancino

Bleeding from esophageal varices is a serious, life-threatening complication of portal hypertension. In patients with cirrhosis, mortality of up to 50% has been reported after the index hemorrhage, with 30% mortality associated with subsequent bleeding episodes. Improvements in both prophylaxis and treatment methods for bleeding have improved these results significantly. Prophylactic treatment with nonselective beta-blockers such as propranolol or nadolol has been shown to prevent or delay the first episode of bleeding. For this reason it is important to identify which patients with cirrhosis have varices and to institute prophylactic measures as is appropriate.

The most recent American Society of Gastrointestinal Endoscopists (ASGE) guidelines recommend screening esophagogastroduodenoscopy (EGD) in all patients with established cirrhosis, especially in patients with Childs B and C disease, and in those patients with signs of portal hypertension such as a platelet count $< 140,000/mm^3$. Patients with no varices on initial EGD should be rescreened every 3 years. If small varices are found, a repeat EGD is indicated in 1 to 2 years. Prophylaxis should be considered in patients with varices at high risk for bleeding. Characteristics of high-risk varices include large varices and the presence of red wale markings, cherry red spots, and hematocystic spots. If high-risk varices are identified, the patient should be started on beta-blocker given in doses that lower the heart rate by 25%. Beta-blockade has been shown to reduce hepatic vein pressure gradient, prevent or delay the onset of variceal bleeding, and slow the growth of varices. Endoscopic variceal ligation (EBL) can be used for prophylaxis and has been shown to significantly reduce the rate of initial variceal hemorrhage and overall mortality. Current recommendations are that EBL should be reserved for patients with contraindications for use of beta-blockers or whose hepatic vein pressure gradient is not reduced by >20%. Endoscopic sclerotherapy is not recommended for primary prophylaxis, as studies showed an increased mortality in treated groups.

Endoscopic sclerotherapy is an effective treatment for active bleeding, and it has been shown to prevent repeat bleeding as well. Sclerotherapy involves the injection of sclerosant either into the varices or in paravariceal tissues. Agents used include sodium tetradecyl sulfate, sodium morrhuate, ethanolamine oleate, polidocanol, and ethanol in varying doses and treatment intervals. Complications of ES include retrosternal pain, dysphagia, bleeding, and fever. More serious events such as perforation, mediastinitis, bronchoesophageal fistula, pleural effusion, and acute respiratory distress syndrome (ARDS) have also been reported.

Endoscopic variceal band ligation (EBL) has been successfully used both for control of active variceal bleeding and for obliteration of other varices for secondary prophylaxis. It involves tenting up the varix and placing small rubber bands on the varices in a manner similar to hemorrhoidal banding. Newer applicators have been developed to allow placement of multiple bands without removing the scope between bandings. Multiple randomized prospective trials have compared EBL with ES, and a meta-analysis by Laine and Cook confirmed that EBL is superior to ES in all of the major outcomes. It eradicates varices more rapidly, has less recurrent bleeding, and has fewer complications such as ulceration and stricture formation.

Although variceal ligation is the preferred method for treating variceal bleeding, there is an increased rate of recurrence of varices in comparison to sclerosis, as ligation does not address the deeper collaterals. The addition of sclerotherapy to EBL has been shown to decrease the probability of variceal recurrence. But a meta-analysis of studies combining the two methods for treatment of bleeding and secondary prophylaxis showed no significant improvement in rebleeding, time to obliteration, or survival. The addition of sclerotherapy, however, did result in an increased incidence of esophageal strictures. The current recommendation is to add ES only when EBL is not effective in treatment of initial bleeding.

Endoscopic clipping of varices is a newer method that has been proposed as an alternative treatment for bleeding varices. The clipping device was originally developed to treat bleeding gastric ulcers. The device targets vessels with minimal damage to surrounding tissue, and may be advantageous over bands in tissue that is scarred or less compliant.

In a randomized trial, Yol et al. compared the two methods and demonstrated that the clips had a high initial hemostasis rate, decreased risk of rebleeding, and fewer sessions needed for eradication. Their study reported an increased risk of iatrogenic tear of varices, but reclipping of the varices easily controlled the resultant bleeding. Although there are some early indications that clipping might be as good a method or even better for control of bleeding, it has had only limited use in the United States and is currently not recommended over EBL.

In conclusion, patients with cirrhosis and portal hypertension should have screening EGD, and prophylaxis should be instituted if high-risk varices are identified. Beta-blockade should be the initial therapy, and EBL should be used for primary prophylaxis only if beta-blockers are contraindicated. Follow-up EGD schedule is based on findings at the initial EGD.

In patients with current or prior bleeding, EBL is the recommended treatment and is superior to ES; ES should be added to EBL only if bleeding is not controlled. After the initial treatment, EBL should be repeated every 2 to 4 weeks until varices are eradicated. Beta-blockers should be considered as adjuvant treatment. Follow-up EGD should be performed every 6 to 12 months and EBL performed for any recurrent varices.

# References

Kitano S, Iso Y, Koyanagi N, et al. Ethanolamine oleate is superior to polidocanol (Athoxysklerol) for endoscopic injection sclerotherapy of esophageal varices: a prospective randomized trial. Hepatogastroenterology 1987;34:19–23.

Laine L, Cook D. Endoscopic ligation compared with sclerotherapy for treatment of esophageal variceal bleeding. A meta-analysis. Ann Intern Med 1999;123;280–287.

Yol S, Belviranli M, Toprak S, Kartal A. Endoscopic clipping vs band ligation in the management of bleeding esophageal varices. Surg Endosc 2003;17:38–42.

# Suggested Readings

ASGE Guideline. The role of endoscopy in the management of variceal hemorrhage, updated July 2005. Gastrointest Endosc 2005;62:651–655.

Banares RAA, Rincon D, Alonso S, et al. Endoscopic treatment versus endoscopic plus pharmacologic treatment for acute variceal bleeding: a meta-analysis. Hepatology 2002;35(3):609–615.

Carbonell N, Pauwels A, Serfaty L, Fourdan O, Levy VG, Poupon R. Improved survival after variceal bleeding in patients with cirrhosis over the past two decades. Hepatology 2004;40:652–659.

Chalasani N, Kahi C, Francois F, et al. Improved patient survival after acute variceal bleeding: a multicenter, cohort study. Am J Gastroenterol 2003;98(3):653–659.

Cheng Y-S, Pan S, Lien G-S, et al. Adjuvant sclerotherapy after ligation for the treatment of esophageal varices: a prospective, randomized long-term study. Gastroenterol Endosc 2001;53:566–571.

D'Amico G, Pagliaro L, Bosch J. Pharmacologic treatment of portal hypertension: an evidence based approach. Semin Liver Dis 1999;19:475–505.

D'Amico G, Pagliaro L, Bosch J. The treatment of portal hypertension: a meta-analytic review. Hepatology 1995;22:332–355.

Fardy JM, Laupacis A. A meta-analysis of prophylactic endoscopic sclerotherapy for esophageal varices. Am J Gastroenterol 1994;89:1938–1948.

Garrett KO, Reilly JJ, Schade RR, et al. Bleeding esophageal varices treatment by sclerotherapy and liver transplantation. Surgery 1988;104:819–823.

Hayashi T, Yonezawa M, Kuwabara T. The study on stanch clip for the treatment by endoscopy. Gastroenterol Endosc 1975;17:92–101.

Hou M-C, Chen W-C, Lin H-C, Lee F-Y, Chang F-Y, Lee S-D. A new "sandwich" method of combined endoscopic variceal ligation and sclerotherapy versus ligation alone in the treatment of esophageal variceal bleeding: a randomized trial. Gastrointest Endosc 2001;53:572–578.

Hou MC, Lin HC, Kuo BI, Chen CH, Lee FY, Lee SD. Comparison of endoscopic variceal injection sclerotherapy and ligation for the treatment of esophageal variceal hemorrhage: a prospective randomized trial. Hepatology 1995;21(6):1517–1522.

Hou MC, Lin HC, Liu TT, et al. Antibiotic prophylaxis after endoscopic therapy prevents rebleeding in acute variceal hemorrhage: a randomized trial. Hepatology 2004;39(3):746–753.

Infante-Rivard C, Esnaola S, Villeneuve J-P. Role of endoscopic variceal sclerotherapy in the long-term management of variceal bleeding: a meta-analysis. Gastroenterology 1989;96:1087–1092.

Kamath PS. Esophageal variceal bleeding: primary prophylaxis. Clin Gastroenterol Hepatol 2005;3:90–93.

Karsan HA, Morton SC, Shekelle PG, et al. Combination endoscopic band ligation and sclerotherapy compared with endoscopic band ligation alone for the secondary prophylaxis of esophageal variceal hemorrhage: a meta-analysis. Dig Dis Sci 2005;50:399–406.

Khuroo MS, Khuroo NS, Farahat KL, Khuroo YS, Sofi AA, Dahab ST. Meta-analysis: endoscopic variceal ligation for primary prophylaxis of oesophageal variceal bleeding. Aliment Pharmacol Ther 2005;21:347–361.

Krige JE, Shaw JM, Bornman PC. The evolving role of endoscopic treatment for bleeding esophageal varices. World J Surg 2005;29:966–973.

Laine L, El-Newihi HM, Migikovsky B, et al. Endoscopic ligation compared with sclerotherapy for treatment of bleeding esophageal varices. Ann Intern Med 1993;119:1–7.

Lay C-S, Tsai Y-T, Teg C-Y, et al. Endoscopic variceal ligation in prophylaxis of first variceal bleeding in Cirrhotic patients with high risk esophageal varices. Hepatology 1997;25:1346–1350.

Lo GH, Lai KH, Cheng JS, et al. Emergency banding ligation versus sclerotherapy for the control of active bleeding from esophageal varices. Hepatology 1997;25:1101–1105.

Lo GH, Lai KH, Cheng JS, et al. The additive effect of sclerotherapy to patients receiving repeated endoscopic variceal ligation: a prospective randomized trial. Hepatology 1998;28:391–395.

Lo GH, Lai KH, Cheng JS, et al. Endoscopic variceal ligation plus nadolol and sucralfate compared with ligation alone for the prevention of variceal rebleeding: a prospective, randomized trial. Hepatology 2000;32(3):461–465.

Lyons SD, Sugawa C, Geller EF, Vandenberg DM. Comparison of 1% sodium tetradecyl sulfate to a thrombogenic sclerosant cocktail for endoscopic sclerotherapy. Am Surg 1988;54:81–84.

Merkel C, Marin R, Angeli P, et al. A placebo controlled clinical trial of nadolol in the prophylaxis of growth of small esophageal varices in cirrhosis. Gastroenterology 2004;127:476–484.

Nakamura R, Bucci LA, Sugawa C, et al. Sclerotherapy of bleeding esophageal varices using a thrombogenic cocktail. Am Surg 1991;57:226–230.

Stiegmann GV. Variceal banding. In: Scott-Conner CEH, ed. The SAGES Manual: Fundamentals of Laparoscopy, Thoracoscopy, and GI Endoscopy. New York: Springer-Verlag, 2006:583–586.

Stiegmann GV, Goff JS, Michaletz-Onody PA, et al. Endoscopic sclerotherapy as compared with endoscopic variceal ligation for bleeding esophageal varices. N Engl J Med 1992;326:1527–1532.

Sugawa C, Okumura Y, Lucas CE, Walt AJ. Endoscopic sclerosis of experimental esophageal varices in dogs. Gastrointest Endosc 1978;24:114–116.

Sugawa C. Sclerotherapy of variceal bleeding. In: Scott-Conner CEG, ed. The SAGES Manual: Fundamentals of Laparoscopy, Thoracoscopy, and GI Endoscopy. New York: Springer-Verlag, 2006:587–594.

# 42. Laparoscopic or Endoscopic Management of Gastroesophageal Reflux Disease

## A. Introduction

There are now several endoscopic alternatives to standard fundoplication for the management of gastroesophageal reflux. This chapter explores two of these, endoscopic suturing and the Stretta procedure, in contrast to laparoscopic fundoplication, the proven surgical procedure. Earlier chapters in this manual have discussed other aspects of laparoscopic fundoplication and issues related to medical versus surgical management.

## B. Case

### *José E. Torres*

A 53-year-old man was referred for evaluation for surgical management of gastroesophageal reflux disease. He had a 3-month history of epigastric and substernal chest pain that worsened after greasy meals and when he lay down. His symptoms have not improved with the cessation of drinking caffeine and eating high-fat meals, and with the loss of 20 pounds. He did not want to stay on medications and was interested in surgical options.

His past medical history was significant for asthma and hypertension, both under medical control. He had not undergone surgery previously. His mother was alive with heartburn, hypertension, and diabetes. His father had died from a cerebrovascular accident at age 82. He had a brother who had undergone surgery for a hiatus hernia, with excellent results.

His medications included Prilosec and atenolol. He had no known allergies. The review of symptoms was negative except as noted above.

On physical examination, he was a well-developed, well-nourished white male. His abdomen was soft without masses, scars, or tenderness. Rectal exam was negative and stool was guaiac negative. Laboratory results were unremarkable.

Upper gastrointestinal series showed a 2-cm sliding hiatal hernia. Upper gastrointestinal endoscopy had not shown esophagitis or Barrett's metaplasia. Esophageal manometry was negative for achalasia. Ambulatory pH monitor revealed the pH to be less than 4.0 for 12% of the study time.

He is interested in repair and wonders if endoscopic repair, which he has read about on the Internet, is feasible.

**What would you recommend?**

# C. Laparoscopic Nissen Fundoplication

*Rob Schuster and Sherry M. Wren*

We would recommend laparoscopic Nissen fundoplication, which is the gold standard against which other methods must be judged.

Since 1936, when Rudolph Nissen first wrapped the fundus of the stomach around the lower esophagus to buttress an anastomotic line and postoperatively noticed resolution of heartburn, many other treatments for gastroesophageal reflux disease (GERD) have been introduced, modified, examined, and possibly abandoned. These include medical, surgical, and endoluminal therapies. The surgical approaches have included thoracotomy, laparotomy, thoracoscopy, and laparoscopy. The most recent development is the potential role of endoluminal therapies to treat GERD. Although more minimally invasive novel therapies seem attractive, long-term results have yet to be evaluated and compared with the procedure that has been studied the most extensively: the laparoscopic Nissen fundoplication.

Nissen first described wrapping the anterior and posterior walls of the stomach fundus around the esophagus after mobilization of the lower 5 to 8 cm of the esophagus. This antireflux barrier formed the basis of the repair, and multiple groups reported results. Polk and Zeppa described 994 GERD patients treated with Nissen fundoplication, of whom 96% were symptom-free at 2.5 years. However, several groups such as Woodward et al. noted a 24% postoperative dysphagia rate and gas bloat syndrome in 54% of patients postoperatively. This led to the development of the "short floppy" fundoplication by DeMeester. This consisted of a 1-cm fundoplication over a 60-French esophageal bougie and complete mobilization of the fundus with division of the short gastric vessels. At 10 years, 91% of DeMeester's patients were symptom-free with a dysphagia rate of 3%.

The minimally invasive era for GERD began in the early 1990s, with the first reported laparoscopic Nissen fundoplication performed by Bernard Dallemagne and colleagues. Since then, several reports comparing the open versus the laparoscopic Nissen fundoplication have documented improvements in postoperative pain, respiratory status, disability, and hospital stay in the laparoscopic group. Based on these results, laparoscopic Nissen fundoplication has become the procedure of choice for GERD.

Excellent results that have withstood the test of time are available for laparoscopic Nissen fundoplication. Peters et al. prospectively followed 100 patients with typical GERD symptoms for 21 months after laparoscopic Nissen fundoplication. The GERD symptoms were relieved in 96% of patients, and 95% discontinued medications after the procedure. Bammer et al. provided data on 171 patients after laparoscopic Nissen fundoplication and followed them for 6.4 years. Overall satisfaction was achieved in 96.5% of patients and nearly all were free of symptoms at follow-up. Carlson and Frantzides performed a meta-analysis of 10,735 patients and found that greater than 90% of patients achieved symptomatic success.

These studies show that laparoscopic Nissen fundoplication has been extremely successful in achieving not only symptomatic relief but equally important an overall improved quality of life, which also is a significant advantage to this approach. The Department of Veterans' Affairs (VA) Cooperative Study enrolled patients to antireflux surgery or medical therapy and found the surgery group had significantly better outcome (Spechler et al.). In addition, the Nordic study randomized 310 patients to antireflux surgery or omeprazole therapy. At 3- and 5-year follow-up, Lundell et al. reported that symptomatic relief and quality-of-life scores were significantly improved in the surgery group. Eubanks et al., in a larger series with 640 patients after laparoscopic Nissen fundoplication, noted that 80% of patients had normalization of reflux by pH monitoring and 93% were satisfied with improvement of their reflux symptoms. Finally, Holzman et al., in a recent study of Tennessee Medicaid patients, evaluated the costs of GERD patients treated with medication or surgery. Although the utilization of medical resources was increased in the perioperative period for the surgery group, most patients had a reduction in their medication use that may over the long term decrease overall health care usage.

Although proponents of medical and endoluminal therapies cite safety and efficacy, a basic understanding of the pathophysiology of GERD will show that these options are bound to fail over time. The competency of the antireflux barrier forms the basis of GERD and treatment. Lower esophageal sphincter (LES) pressure, presence of a hiatal hernia, and a short intraabdominal segment of the esophagus all contribute to GERD. Medical treatments do not address these issues, and endoluminal treatments have not been shown to provide this antireflux barrier over time. On the other hand, antireflux surgery, most notably laparoscopic Nissen fundoplication, is the only option that permanently corrects all the factors involved in the pathophysiology of GERD.

Endoscopic treatment for GERD most commonly involves endoscopic suturing, polymer injection, or radiofrequency scar formation at the gastroesophageal junction (GEJ). Filipi et al. reported that at 6-month follow-up after endoscopic suturing for GERD in 64 patients, there was no difference in LES pressure after the procedure, no change in esophageal acid exposure, and 62% of patients were still taking medication. The Enteryx solution is an inert polymer solution injected at the GEJ to create a mechanical barrier to prevent reflux. Johnson et al. studied 85 GERD patients injected with Enteryx at the GEJ. At 6-month follow-up, 26% of patients were still taking proton pump inhibitors (PPIs) and 22% of patients required repeat treatments. On October 14, 2005, the Food and Drug Administration (FDA) recalled Enteryx due to several reports of transmural injection and serious adverse events, including death.

Radiofrequency delivery at the gastroesophageal junction, the Stretta procedure, has been evaluated with modest results. Triadafilopoulos et al. prospectively evaluated 118 patients with GERD who underwent the Stretta procedure. Although improvements at 12 months were noted for GERD symptoms, 30% still required PPIs, esophageal acid exposure was still abnormal in the majority of patients, and there was no improvement in the incidence of esophagitis. Of note, there was an 8.6% complication rate. Richards and colleagues prospectively evaluated 140 GERD patients who underwent either the Stretta procedure or laparoscopic fundoplication. In the patients who underwent the Stretta procedure, only 36% had normalization of their acid exposure time and no change in the mean LES pressure. When compared with laparoscopic fundoplication group, 58% of patients were off their PPIs after the Stretta procedure versus 97% after fundoplication. Partial or no response was noted in 42% of patients after the Stretta procedure compared to only 3% after laparoscopic fundoplication, indicating the superiority of the surgical procedure.

These studies reinforce the improvement not only of GERD symptoms after laparoscopic Nissen fundoplication, but also satisfaction, quality of life, and possible decreased health care resource utilization. These have not been addressed by current endoluminal therapy options. However, as technologic improvements and long-term follow-up become available, these less invasive alternatives may become a more accepted treatment for GERD. In the meantime, laparoscopic Nissen fundoplication remains the gold standard for anatomic correction of GERD.

# D. Endoscopic Suturing

*Bruce V. MacFadyen, Jr.*

I would recommend endoscopic suturing.

Gastroesophageal reflux disease is a common problem in the United States, where 50% of the population has symptoms of heartburn and bloating each month, and 10% have symptoms every day. Diagnostic studies to identify GERD should include upper endoscopy, 24-hour pH monitoring of the acid and bilirubin content of the upper and lower esophagus, cine esophagram, and esophageal motility and manometry. The first line of management should be to maximize medical therapy including using 20 mg of a PPI medication 1 hour before breakfast and dinner along with a histamine receptor H2 blocker at bedtime. Lifestyle modifications should include instituting a low-fat diet, eliminating caffeine, nicotine, and alcohol from the diet; and elevating the head of the bed by 4 to 6 inches.

Although these changes may relieve the symptoms of GERD in 75% to 90%, symptom recurrence in 3 to 4 months is high (40% to 50%) if the PPI is discontinued. An additional 25% have progression of their disease, producing complications such as esophageal stricture, erosive esophagitis, Barrett's esophagus, and a short esophagus. The underlying etiology of GERD is often related to an anatomic problem involving a combination of a defective LES, a hiatal hernia, and alteration in the angle of His at the esophagogastric junction. None of these are altered by medical therapy. Laparoscopic Nissen fundoplication procedure *does* re-create an effective LES mechanism and restores a normal angle of His at the gastroesophageal junction. This operation is successful in eliminating GERD in 93% to 97% of the cases with a type 1 hiatal hernia and is effective for 10 to 15 years.

In the patient presented above, the adequacy of the medical therapy is not clear, and the type 1 hiatal hernia is small (2 cm). However, the percent of time that the acid reflux pH is <4% in a 24-hour period in this

Table 42.1. Endoluminal therapies for gastroesophageal reflux disease (GERD).

| Mechanical | Radiofrequency | Injection* |
|---|---|---|
| NDO Plicator™ | Stretta™ | Enteryx™ |
| EndoCinch Suturing System™ | | Gatekeeper Reflux Repair System™ |
| Sew–Right Device™ | | PMMA Plexiglas Submucosal Injection |
| Endoscopic Suturing Device (ESD)™ | | |

*None FDA approved at the time of this writing.

patient is moderately severe. The acid reflux time is graded as follows: grade 1, normal, <4%; grade 2, mild, 4% to 8%; grade 3, moderately severe, 8% to 12%; and grade 4, severe, >12%. A pH study should also measure acid and bilirubin content in the upper and lower esophagus, as it has been observed that acid and bilirubin in the refluxate have been associated with Barrett's esophagus. Additionally, obesity has been reported to have an increasing effect on GERD symptoms when the body mass index (BMI) is greater than 30.

The question is whether the laparoscopic Nissen fundoplication should be performed in all cases when medical therapy has failed or is there an intermediate therapy before surgery is performed. Over the past 5 years, gastroesophageal endoluminal therapies have been developed as a bridge between medical therapy and surgery. These therapies can be categorized into three types: mechanical, injection, and radiofrequency (Table 42.1) and they can be used in all cases. The exclusion criteria are listed in (Table 42.2). In the mechanical category, the NDO Plicator/endoscope is introduced orally over a Savory guidewire into the stomach and is retroflexed. The esophagogastric junction is plicated with two to three polypropylene full-thickness sutures along the lesser curvature starting 1 cm below the Z line to create a fundoplication in the gastric cardia. Pleskow et al. reported a 12-month prospective multicenter trial in which

Table 42.2. Exclusion criteria for endoluminal therapy.

- Dysphagia
- Esophagitis greater than grade 2
- Body mass index >40
- Gastroesophageal reflux disease refractory to proton pump inhibitor
- Hiatal hernia >2 cm

68% of the patients discontinued PPI medication. The majority of the group had a significant decrease in distal acid exposure and 30% had a normal 24-hour pH study. The most common complications included a sore throat (41%) and 20% had postprocedure abdominal pain. The EndoCinch™ and the Sew-Right™ devices are similar technologies based on an endoscopic sewing machine technology developed in 1986.

The EndoCinch™ device is advanced into the esophagus. A suturing/suction capsule is placed on the esophageal mucosa and a needle is advanced through the mucosa and submucosa 1 cm below the Z line. Two to three additional sutures are similarly applied. In a sham study by Schwartz, distal acid exposure was similar to that in patients treated by PPI medication alone. Thus far this device has had limited clinical benefit.

In the injection therapy category, a 12-month injection therapy trial with Enteryx (composed of ethylene vinyl alcohol, tantalum powder, and dimethyl sulfoxide) was reported by Johnson et al., in which they noted that 88% of patients were able to discontinue PPI therapy and 39% had a normal 24-hour pH study, but there was no change in the LES pressure. However, this injectable solution has been associated with several complications, including death, and has been withdrawn from the market. The Gatekeeper system (polyacrylonitrile hydrogel) and the polymethylmethacrylate (PMMA) injection technique are not used clinically as there are limited data as to the effectiveness of these esophageal submucosal injections.

The use of radiofrequency in the distal esophagus above and below the Z line has been reported using the Stretta procedure (p. 534). This flexible catheter with radially placed electrodes is advanced over a guidewire introduced via a flexible upper endoscope. The electrodes are inserted into the muscle of the esophagus and cardia of the stomach above and below the squamocolumnar junction, and radiofrequency energy is applied. A 3-year study by Lufti et al. demonstrated a significant decrease from 7.8% to 5.1% in distal acid exposure in 40%, an improvement of the DeMeester score from 40.2 to 29.5, and 64% were able to eliminate or significantly reduce PPI medication at 3 years.

Endoluminal therapies are early in their development. They have their limitations, which include the fact that the hiatal hernia is not repaired, the LES is neither returned to its normal position nor fixed to intraabdominal structures, and sutures may not be placed full thickness or reach the deep layer of muscle. The patient presented here does not appear to be well controlled on PPI medication and hence further therapy is needed to control the GERD. I would recommend endoluminal therapy.

My preference is the NDO Plicator because the technique produces a full-thickness fundoplication at the level of the gastroesophageal junction. Early results have been favorable, and this procedure is particularly useful in a patient who may have respiratory or cardiac risk factors. In addition, it is less invasive, and if it is not successful, the patient can proceed to laparoscopic Nissen fundoplication. The risks of the procedure are low and technically it can be performed in a short time (20 to 30 minutes) as an outpatient.

# E. Stretta Procedure

*Richard Nguyen and William Richards*

We would offer this patient a Stretta procedure, which was approved by the FDA in April 2000. It can be offered as therapy before more invasive surgical procedures for selected patients with GERD. Although a new addition to treatment options, it appears to be a safe and effective technology for the treatment of GERD, with documented clinical trial data supporting its efficacy, safety, and patient satisfaction. Our argument for incorporation of Stretta involves informed consent because most patients who are amenable to Stretta treatment could also be treated with escalation of medical therapy or laparoscopic fundoplication. We believe that the patient presented needs additional evaluation and medical treatment.

The Stretta incorporates constant tissue temperature monitoring and automated modulation of radiofrequency (RF) power output to control tissue heating of the needle electrodes, which are inserted into the gastroesophageal junction (Figs. 42.1 to 42.3). The RF power is automatically modulated to achieve a target temperature of 85 °C, but not exceed 100 °C. The technical aspects of this procedure are described in detail in Mellinger and MacFadyen. Collagen contraction occurs when temperatures reach 65 °C, resulting in collagen shrinkage and an increase in wall thickness of the LES. Studies in human and animal subjects have shown that RF treatment reduces the frequency of inappropriate transient lower esophageal sphincter relaxations (TLESRs), increases postprandial LES pressure, and increases the gastric yield pressure. The randomized sham verses Stretta trial demonstrated that the Stretta-treated patients had a significant improvement in their GERD symptoms while there was no effect in the sham treated patients.

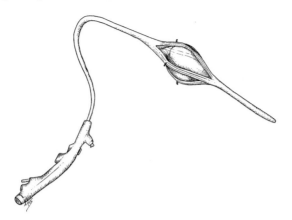

Fig. 42.1. Stretta balloon catheter device. (From Scott-Conner CEH, ed. The SAGES Manual: Fundamentals of Laparoscopy, Thoracoscopy, and GI Endoscopy, 2nd ed. New York: Springer-Verlag 2006.).

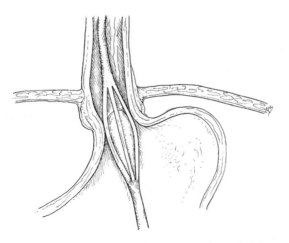

Fig. 42.2.  Catheter positioned appropriately at gastroesophageal junction.(From Scott-Conner CEH, ed. The SAGES Manual: Fundamentals of Laparoscopy, Thoracoscopy, and GI Endoscopy, 2nd ed. New York: Springer-Verlag 2006.).

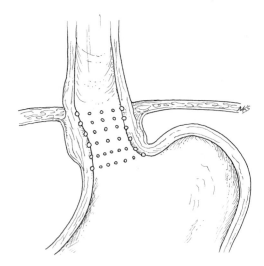

Fig. 42.3. Desired pattern of radiofrequency lesions. (From Scott-Conner CEH, ed. The SAGES Manual: Fundamentals of Laparoscopy, Thoracoscopy, and GI Endoscopy, 2nd ed. New York: Springer-Verlag 2006.).

Ideal candidates for Stretta are those who

- suffer from frequent heartburn or regurgitation that requires PPI use to control;
- have adequate esophageal peristalsis;
- have a 24-hour pH study demonstrating pathologic acid reflux (total acid exposure time >4%, or a DeMeester composite score >14.7); or
- have nonerosive reflux disease or grade I or II esophagitis by Savary-Miller criteria, or have higher grades of esophagitis healed by drug therapy.

Patients who are not considered candidates for Stretta are those who

- have a more than 3-cm-long hiatal hernia detected endoscopically;
- have significant dysphagia;
- have grade III or IV esophagitis by Savary-Miller criteria;
- have inadequate esophageal peristalsis or incomplete LES relaxation in response to swallow;
- have gastroesophageal reflux (GER)-induced asthma or recurrent aspiration pneumonia; or
- have Barrett's esophagus.

In the patient presented here, several aspects of the history, physical exam, and diagnostic workup are missing that would help the surgeon and patient determine the best course of action. It is unusual in our experience not to see improvement in heartburn symptoms with use of a PPI, and thus this history throws a red flag up for the surgeon about to treat him. Patients who initially respond well to alleviation of heartburn symptoms with PPI use generally respond well to Stretta or laparoscopic fundoplication (LF). We would as a first course of action escalate his PPI to twice-daily dosing and make sure that he takes the medications prior to meals, because the PPIs work best to reduce meal-stimulated acid production. We would also switch him from Prilosec to another PPI to identify if he has a better response to the different formulation. He continues to smoke, and with his asthma history we are concerned about his pulmonary function. Adult-onset asthma frequently can be associated with significant GER, and a dual-probe pH study to evaluate the extent of reflux into the proximal esophagus would be helpful in determining the degree to which GERD is exacerbating his asthma. Neither medical therapy nor Stretta has been shown to be effective in patients with GER-induced asthma and would be a relative contraindication for both medical and Stretta therapy in this patient if he has significant proximal esophageal acid exposure. We would insist that he immediately cease smoking and we would not proceed to Stretta or surgery until he has been smoke free for 3 months. A chest radiograph and arterial blood gas determination prior to surgery is indicated with his smoking and asthma history.

His weight, height, waist circumference, and BMI are not reported, and this information is one of the fundamental determinants of therapy. Obesity is a major factor in GERD and must be addressed. Weight loss alone may significantly reduce his symptoms; however, many of these patients have failed many weight loss diets and have BMIs greater than 35. Although such patients come to us for alleviation of symptomatic GERD, their real surgical problem is morbid obesity, hypertension, and the potential for early cardiovascular death. This patient has a strong family history of diabetes, hypertension, and cardiovascular pathology, and probably has the metabolic syndrome of central obesity, dyslipidemia, hypertension, and insulin resistance. We would obtain a fasting glucose and lipid profile and measure his waist circumference. He may be unaware that he is at very high risk for cardiovascular death, and these factors must be addressed prior to treatment of non–life-threatening GERD. Moreover, performance of a laparoscopic fundoplication in a morbidly obese patient would be prone to failure from the elevated intraabdominal pressure, and would make subsequent bariatric surgery exceedingly difficult.

Setting these considerations aside, and assuming that the patient had complied with medical management as noted above, Stretta is an ideal choice for this patient. Technically this procedure is as easy to perform in a patient with a BMI of 60 as it is in a patient with a BMI of 21. Moreover, it does not cause any scarring on the serosa of the stomach or in the periesophageal tissues of the mediastinum. Thus, should an obese patient subsequently decide to undergo bariatric surgery, he will be able to undergo the procedure without the negative aspect of intraabdominal adhesions at the GEJ, which would subsequently significantly complicate the surgery.

We also use the esophageal manometry to make decisions about the continuation of medical therapy or choice of fundoplication or Stretta. If there is a critically low LES pressure, that is, <5 mm Hg, then long term we believe the patient will fail Stretta and medical therapy. However, most patients have TLERs as the primary mechanism of GER, and thus Stretta is an acceptable treatment for these patients. We generally do not bother with upper GI series unless we are evaluating patients with paraesophageal hiatal hernias. We find that our own endoscopic evaluation is much superior to radiologic evaluation. We are surprised that the endoscopy did not reveal a sliding hiatal hernia, so we would personally repeat the endoscopy so that we could further evaluate the patient as to the best course of action. Surgeons need to perform their own endoscopy so that surgery can be planned and that the anatomy can be fully appreciated by the surgeon.

Long-term follow-up with radiofrequency treatment in patients with GERD is emerging. The precise role of this endoscopic therapy for GERD requires further study and long-term follow-up. However, among the available endoscopic procedures, the Stretta procedure appears to be modestly effective, is technically easy to perform, and after 6 years of treatment in more than 10,000 patients has emerged as a safe therapy with complications reported in only 0.02%. We certainly would entertain the use of Stretta in this patient after a more complete workup and medical treatment.

# E. Conclusions

*José E. Torres*

Gastroesophageal reflux disease is the mechanical failure of the antireflux mechanism at the LES caused by a defective LES, failed esophageal peristalsis, or a gastric emptying disorder. This abnormality allows the abnormal reflux of gastric contents into the esophagus. Complications of this disease range from heartburn to esophageal mucosal damage, which may lead to Barrett's esophagus, a premalignant lesion.

The treatment of this disease includes behavior modification, medications that reduce acid production and improve esophageal motility, and surgical therapy via a laparoscopic or open Nissen fundoplication. Approximately 20% of the individuals affected use nonprescription medications for the treatment of this disorder. Patients inflicted with this disease continually seek medical advice for further medical or surgical treatment.

Recent advances in endoscopy have produced three minimally invasive procedures for the treatment of GERD: endoscopic full-thickness suturing of the gastroesophageal mucosa; the application of controlled RF energy to the LES—the Stretta procedure; and the injection of a biopolymer into the LES—the Enteryx procedure.

The first procedure uses an endoscopic suturing device that allows the user to place a suture through the muscularis propria at the gastroesophageal junction. The EndoCinch™ system allows one to place a dual-channel endoscope into the esophagus and place a series of sutures into the muscularis propria by using a vacuum to draw tissue into the suturing device, allowing a suture to be deployed in a figure-of-eight fashion. The knot is then secured with a knot pusher and the process is repeated several more times until the desired effect is achieved.

Patients in initial studies who did not have dysphagia, a BMI greater than 40, grade two esophagitis, GERD refractory to proton pump inhibitors, or a hiatal hernia >2 cm reported subjective improvement in heartburn symptoms 6 months after the procedure. Objective measures such as LES pressure and acid exposure in the esophagus were modest. There was a decrease in the amount of medication requirements in 62% of the patients. The complications were self-limited and included one suture perforation, abdominal pain, vomiting, and pharyngitis, and the requirement of repeat procedures to complete the placation. Subsequent follow-up studies revealed that the effect of the procedure was not permanent. Most patients were on antisecretory medications within 2 years of the placation or underwent a Nissen fundoplication.

Initial studies demonstrate that endoscopic suturing is relatively safe and may become a viable therapeutic option in the treatment algorithm of GERD. Continued research and development is directed at developing full-thickness plicators with the ability to place sutures more accurately and retroflex the endoscope.

The second endoscopic procedure entails the delivery of RF energy to the LES—the Stretta procedure. In this procedure the LES is identified endoscopically, a balloon catheter with four small metallic prongs (Fig. 42.1) is passed orally and positioned at the LES. The metallic prongs are embedded into the esophageal wall (Fig. 42.2). Radiofrequency energy is applied to create thermal lesions, while water cooling protects the mucosa from injury. This process is repeated multiple times (Fig. 42.3) to create a ring of lesions.

Several hypotheses have been developed to explain the mechanism of action, including the shortening of collagen molecules, macrophage, and fibroblast responses, all of which may tighten the GEJ. The Stretta procedure improves the symptoms of GERD, decreases esophageal acid exposure, and significantly decreases the need for antisecretory drugs; the FDA reported a complication rate of less than 0.6%.

The third endoscopic procedure utilizes the injection of a biocompatible polymer into the muscularis of the LES under fluoroscopic control—the Enteryx procedure. It initially gained FDA approval, and small studies revealed improvement of symptoms and decreased use of PPIs. But 24-hour pH studies have shown only modest improvement, and several deaths attributed to injection of the polymer into extraesophageal tissue have been reported. As noted previously, this procedure is no longer available in the U.S.

Although patients report symptomatic relief with these novel procedures, physiologic evidence suggesting improvement of GERD in patients is lacking. At this time, no long-term clinical studies have been performed to evaluate these procedures. Additionally, these endoscopic procedures are limited by current contraindications:

1. Severe esophagitis or Barrett's esophagus
2. Morbid obesity
3. Prior antireflux surgery
4. Hiatal hernias greater than 2 cm
5. Severe dysphagia

In the early 1990s the laparoscopic Nissen fundoplication was described and added to the armamentarium for treatment of GERD. The results for open and laparoscopic fundoplication have been shown to be identical. Laparoscopic fundoplication has been demonstrated to lead to rapid recuperation and significant success rates in the vast majority of patients with low rates of morbidity and mortality when performed by an experienced surgeon. Similar to other laparoscopic procedures, laparoscopic Nissen fundoplication has several advantages over its open counterpart:

• Minimal postoperative discomfort
• Reduced duration of hospitalization

- Shortened recovery time
- Earlier return to work

Minimally invasive surgery is considered the first-line treatment for achalasia, and laparoscopic fundoplication is considered more readily and at an earlier stage in the management of GERD, with high levels of patient satisfaction and physiologic improvement at 5 years, including a statistically significant increase in LES pressure and a significant drop in duration of acid reflux in 24 hours. Ganderath et al. reported a conversion rate of 0.4%, and a morbidity rate of 7%, including a 4.8% laparoscopic redoprocedure rate due to failure of the primary intervention. No mortalities were reported. The few studies that have compared medical therapy to surgical treatment (see Chapter 10) have demonstrated that quality of life (QOL) scores in patients undergoing laparoscopic Nissen fundoplication were superior to those in patients undergoing medical treatment, and that the majority of patients are happy with their outcomes. Thus, if the patient presented here should fail improved medical or endoscopic therapy, a laparoscopic Nissen fundoplication would become the procedure of choice.

# References

Bammer T, Hinder RA, Klaus A, Klingler PJ. Five- to eight-year outcome of the first laparoscopic Nissen fundoplications. J Gastrointest Surg 2001;5:42–48.

Carlson MA, Frantzides CT. Complications and results of primary minimally invasive antireflux procedures: a review of 10,735 reported cases. J Am Coll Surg 2001;193:428–439.

Dallemagne B, Weerts JM, Jenaes C. Laparoscopic Nissen fundoplication: preliminary report. Surg Laparosc Endosc 1991;1:138–143.

Eubanks TR, Omelanczuk P, Richards C, et al. Outcomes of laparoscopic antireflux procedures. Am J Surg 2000;179:391–395.

Filipi CJ, Lehman GA, Rothstein RI, et al. Transoral, flexible endoscopic suturing for treatment of GERD: a multicenter trial. Gastrointest Endosc 2001;53:416–422.

Ganderath FA, Kamotz T, Schweiger UM, et al. Long-term results of laparoscopic antireflux surgery: Surgical outcomes and analysis of failure after 500 laparoscopic antireflux procedures. Surg Endosc 2002;16:753–757.

Holzman MD, Mitchel EF, Ray WA, Smalley WE. Use of healthcare resources among medically and surgically treated patients with gastroesophageal reflux disease: a population-based study. J Am Coll Surg 2001;192:17–24.

Johnson DA, Aisenberg J, Deviere J, et al. Enteryx solution, a minimally invasive injectable treatment for GERD: analysis of X-ray findings over 12 months. Dig Dis Week 2003;abstract 107493.

Lufti RE, Torwuati A, Kaiser J, Holzman M, Richards WO. Three year's experience with the Stretta procedure. Did it really make a difference? Surg Endosc 2005;19:289–295.

Lundell L, Miettinen P, Myrvold HE, et al. Continued (5–year) followup of a randomized clinical study comparing antireflux surgery and omeprazole in gastroesophageal reflux disease. J Am Coll Surg 2001;192:172–181.

Mellinger JD, MacFadyen BV Jr. Endoluminal approaches to gastroesophageal reflux disease. In: Scott-Conner CEH, ed. The SAGES Manual: Fundamentals of Laparoscopy, Thoracoscopy, and GI Endoscopy, 2nd ed. New York: Springer-Verlag 2006:602–607.

Peters JH, DeMeester TR, Crookes P, et al. The treatment of gastroesophageal reflux disease with laparoscopic Nissen fundoplication: prospective evaluation of 100 patients with "typical" symptoms. Ann Surg 1998;228:40–50.

Pleskow D, Rothstein R, Lo S, et al. Endoscopic full-thickness plication for the treatment of GERD: 12 month follow-up for the North American open-label trial. Gastrointest Endosc 2005;61(6):643–649.

Polk HC, Zeppa R. Hiatal hernia and esophagitis. A survey of indications for operation and technique and results of fundoplication. Ann Surg 1971;173:775–781.

Richards WO, Scholz S, Khaitan L, Sharp KW. Initial experience with the Stretta procedure for the treatment of gastroesophageal reflux disease. J Laparoendosc Adv Surg Tech [A] 2001;11:267.

Schwartz MP. A blinded, randomized, sham-controlled trial of endoscopic gastroplication for the treatment of gastro-esophageal reflux disease (GERD): Preliminary results. Dig Dis Week 2005;abstract 496.

Speckler SJ et al. Longterm outcomes in medical and surgical therapies for gastroesophageal reflux disease: followup of a randomized controlled trial. JAMA 2001;285(18):2331–2338.

Triadafilopoulos G, DiBaise JK, Nostrant TT, Stollman NH. The Stretta procedure for the treatment of GERD: 6 and 12 month follow-up of the U.S. open label trial. Gastrointest Endosc 2002;55:149.

Woodward ER, Thomas HF, McAlhany JC. Comparison of crural repair and Nissen fundoplication in the treatment of esophageal hiatus hernia with peptic esophagitis. Ann Surg 1971;173:782–792.

# Suggested Readings

Corley DA, Katz P, Wo JM, Stefan A. Improvement of gastroesophageal reflux symptoms after radiofrequency energy: a randomized, sham-controlled trial. Gastroenterology 2003;125:668.

Demeester TR, Bonavina L, Albertucci M. Nissen fundoplication for gastroesophageal reflux disease. Evaluation of primary repair in 100 consecutive patients. Ann Surg 1986;204:9–20.

Fernando HC, Schauer PR, Rosenblatt M, et al. Quality of life after antireflux surgery compared with nonoperative management for severe gastroesophageal reflux disease. J Am Coll Surg 2002;194:23–27.

Houston H, Khaitan L, Holzman M, Richards WO. First year experience of patients under-
    going the Stretta procedure. Surg Endosc 2003;17:401.

Hunter JG, Trus TL, Branum GD, Waring JP, Wood WC. A physiologic approach
    to laparoscopic fundoplication for gastroesophageal reflux disease. Ann Surg
    1996;223(6):673–687.

Johnson DA, Ganz R, Ainsberg J, et al. Endoscopic implantation of Enteryx for the treat-
    ment of GERD: 12 month results of a prospective multicenter trial. Am J Gastroen-
    terol 2003;98(9):1921–1930.

Lundell L. Surgery of gastroesophageal reflux disease: a competitive or complementary
    procedure? Dig Dis 2004;22(2):161–170.

Richards WO, Houston HL, Torquati A, et al. Paradigm shift in the management of gastro-
    esophageal reflux disease. Ann Surg 2003;237:638–649.

Savarino V, Dulbecco P. Optimizing symptom relief and preventing complications in adults
    with gastro-oesophageal reflux disease. Digestion 2004;69(1):9–16.

Torquati, A, Houston, HL, Kaiser, J, et al. Long-term follow-up study of the Stretta
    procedure for the treatment of gastroesophageal reflux disease. Surg Endosc
    2004;18:1475–1479.

Triadafilopoulos G, Dibaise JK, Nostrant TT, et al. Radiofrequency energy delivery to
    the gastroesophageal junction for the treatment of GERD. Gastrointest Endosc
    2001;53:407.

Trus TL, Laycock WS, Waring JP, Branum GD, Hunter JG. Improvement in quality of life
    measures after laparoscopic antireflux surgery. Ann Surg 1999;229:331–336.

Utley DS, Kim M, Vierra MA, Triadafilopoulos G. Augmentation of lower esophageal
    sphincter pressure and gastric yield pressure after radiofrequency energy delivery to
    the gastroesophageal junction: a porcine model. Gastrointest Endosc 2000;52:81.

Wolfsen HC, Richards WO. The Stretta procedure for the treatment of GERD: a registry of
    558 patients. J Laparoendosc Adv Surg Tech [A] 2002;12:395.

# 43. Screening Colonoscopy: Endoscopic or Virtual

## A. Introduction

With improvements in computed tomography (CT) scan resolution, virtual colonoscopy using reconstructed CT images has emerged as a potential alternative to endoscopy. This chapter explores the role of this alternative to traditional colonoscopic examination.

## B. Case

*Nora A. Royer*

A 55-year-old man presented for a routine physical examination. He had no complaints, and had not had a full physical exam in the previous 10 years.

His past medical history was significant for hypertension, hypothyroidism, and depression. His past surgical history consisted of a right ankle repair after trauma and a total thyroidectomy (benign follicular adenoma). His mother had colon cancer at age 78. There was no other family history of cancer.

His medications included metoprolol 25 mg PO b.i.d., hydrochlorothiazide 25 mg PO daily, levothyroxine 150 µg PO daily, and Prozac 40 mg PO daily.

He worked as a manager at a local store. He had smoked one pack of cigarettes per day for 5 years, and quit 30 years ago. He had occasional alcohol consumption totaling two to three glasses of wine per month. He ate a healthy diet and biked approximately 100 miles per week. The review of symptoms was negative.

Physical examination revealed a well-developed male with a body mass index (BMI) of 24.6. His blood pressure was 118/76, and heart rate 64. Abdominal examination demonstrated no masses or tenderness. Rectal examination revealed a smooth prostate, no masses, and guaiac-negative stool. The remainder of the physical examination was negative, except for well-healed surgical scars on the medial right ankle and the lower neck.

As part of his health maintenance, colonoscopy was recommended. **Would you recommend conventional or virtual (CT) colonoscopy?**

# C. Conventional Colonoscopy

*Tracey D. Arnell*

We would recommend that this patient undergo conventional colonoscopy. There is no debate at this time about whether screening for colon cancer should be performed. Colorectal cancer is the second most common cancer in the United States and it is estimated that 1 in 18 people will develop colorectal cancer during their lifetime, of which 60% will be diagnosed with disease beyond the colon. In patients who present with symptomatic disease, at least 75% have regional or distant metastasis. Screening colonoscopy offers the opportunity for identification of all neoplastic growths, including adenomatous polyps. Approximately 15% to 20% of polyps have the potential to become invasive, following a polyp-to-cancer pathway; therefore, removal of adenomatous polyps prevents the development of cancer. Despite the consensus that screening should be performed as part of general health maintenance, less than 30% of Americans are compliant. There are many reasons for this including patient fear, embarrassment, and failure of primary care physicians to refer patients. Virtual colonoscopy, or CT colonography (CTC), has been proposed as a more acceptable means of screening to patients and an opportunity to increase the availability of whole colon screening. Unfortunately, presently both CTC and fiberoptic colonoscopy (FOC) require a bowel preparation and there has been minimal difference noted in terms of patient discomfort between the two. More importantly, the accuracy, reproducibility. and treatment plan for patients found to have lesions on CTC must be understood.

To address the question of accuracy, Mulhall et al. performed a large meta-analysis of studies comparing FOC and CTC. The per patient sensitivity varied from 21% to 96% for CTC, although it did improve with increasing polyp size (48% for <6 mm, 70% for 6 to 9 mm, 85% for >9 mm). Included in this meta-analysis was one of the largest prospective series of tandem colonoscopies by Cotton et al., in which CTC was only 55% accurate in identifying polyps > 10 mm in size. It should be noted that these studies involved expert radiologists and should represent the best outcomes. Fiberoptic colonoscopy is overall more sensitive and consistent with sensitivities of 74%, 87%, and 98% for polyps <6 mm, 6 to 10 mm, and >10 mm, respectively. There are many reasons for the wide variability in accuracy of CTC including differences in equipment, software, technique, and interpretation. There is no universal protocol; therefore, the quality of CTC at an individual institution cannot be predicted.

Assuming that the physician caring for the patient in this scenario knows the accuracy of CTC at his or her institution, the next question is, Is this patient a reasonable candidate for a CTC? Since lesions seen on CTC cannot be biopsied or removed, the ideal candidate should have a low likelihood of having a need for a polypectomy or biopsy. The National Polyp Study found that 53.8% of patients undergoing colonoscopy had a polyp of which 37.5% were neoplastic. Traditionally, advanced polyps are those >10 mm, or with villous or dysplastic changes. In this series 10.5% of patients had an advanced neoplasm, but 12% of these were considered advanced based on histology alone and were <10 mm in size. If the National Polyp Study had been performed using CTC, 53.8% of patients would have required FOC assuming the screening accuracy was equal. If only those lesions >10 mm in size were referred, 12% of villous or dysplastic lesions would not have been removed. This patient has a first-degree relative with colon cancer, placing him in an above-average risk category. Therefore, the potential for finding significant lesions that require therapeutic intervention via an FOC is even higher.

Ideally, the best situation in which to perform CT colonography is in a patient with a low risk of having a neoplastic finding by an experienced radiologist with advanced colonography software confirmed to have accuracy and sensitivity. This patient does not fit the former characterization and most centers do not know if they fit the latter.

## D.  Virtual Colonoscopy

*Srinath C. Yeshwant and Ronald M. Summers*

We would advocate virtual colonoscopy. Virtual colonoscopy (VC), also known as CT colonography (CTC), is a minimally invasive technique that uses two-dimensional (2D) and three-dimensional (3D) images of the colon acquired from thin-section CT images to scan for colonic polyps and cancer. The rapid evolution of this technology over the last decade has been a source of considerable interest among radiologists, gastroenterologists, and patients as it may provide a faster, safer, and more tolerable means for detecting colorectal neoplasia than optical colonoscopy.

There are several benefits to using virtual colonoscopy as a screening method. These include its ability to screen segments of the colon that lie beyond an occluding lesion and to function as an alternate examination for patients for whom colonoscopy was incomplete or could not be performed. However, the results from several recent multiinstitutional clinical studies that have attempted to clarify the clinical value of virtual colonoscopy for polyp detection are not consistent. In one trial, the sensitivity for adenomas 10 mm and larger was equivalent for virtual colonoscopy and for optical colonoscopy (93.8% and 87.5%, respectively). Halligan et al. reported that meta-analysis revealed virtual colonoscopy to have a sensitivity of 95.9% for cancers. Conversely, Cotton et al. reported a virtual colonoscopy sensitivity for adenomas 10 mm and larger of only 55% with two missed cancers. Poor sensitivity has been attributed to inadequate training of the image interpreters or outdated scanning technology. Despite these conflicting results, it is believed that virtual colonoscopy may provide a reliable alternative for colon cancer screening.

Attention to technique is important. Patient preparation, scanning protocol, and interpretation all must be optimized. Patients examined by virtual colonoscopy must undergo a bowel preparation prior to scanning. The first requirement of this preparation is a thorough cleansing of the colon, a step that improves visualization of the bowel mucosa and minimizes the potential for false positives due to residual fecal matter. Cleansing can be achieved by administration of one of a variety of bowel preparation regimes that use cathartics such as Phospho-Soda, magnesium citrate, or polyethylene glycol.

Some investigators have recently incorporated fecal tagging into the bowel preparation to facilitate the identification of residual fecal material during interpretation. This process involves the ingestion of an oral contrast agent prior to imaging. The contrast material mixes with fecal matter and appears on the CT scans as bright white regions due to its high attenuation. Using subtraction software, the oral contrast can be eliminated from the images, along with any stool it has mixed with, leaving the colon wall intact for inspection.

The second fundamental requirement of bowel preparation for virtual colonoscopy is adequate distention of the colon immediately prior to and during examination. This step is necessary since a well-distended colon allows for better detection of abnormalities on the CT and VC images and minimizes the chances of misinterpreting normal structures in the colon, such as haustral folds, for false-positive lesions. Insufflation is typically achieved by pumping either room air or carbon dioxide ($CO_2$) into the colon through a small flexible rectal catheter. Air is used by many institutions because it is inexpensive and readily available. $CO_2$, however, is believed to reduce abdominal cramping since it is better absorbed by the colon. Examiners may also select between a basic manual pump and an electronic pump that automatically provides an influx of gas to keep pressure inside the colon constant during the exam. The use of spasmolytics such as glucagon and buscopan (the latter available outside the U.S.) has been somewhat controversial.

Scanning protocols have continued to improve. Over the last decade, advances in CT imaging technology have benefited virtual colonoscopy. For example, multidetector CT scanners have led to reduced radiation exposure, decreased scan time, and improved image resolution. Current standards require that patients be scanned during a single breath hold in a helical CT scanner (with four or more detectors), a slice width of at most 3 mm, and a reconstruction interval of at most 2 mm. Scans of the patient are routinely obtained in both supine and prone positions to optimize colon distention, compensate for changes in residual fluid, and identify mobile residual fecal material.

One concern regarding virtual colonoscopy is the risk associated with patient exposure to the radiation. The dose per examination has been reported as 8.3 mSv. However, there have been a number of attempts to reduce this amount by altering x-ray tube output, scanning pitch, and collimation. These studies have suggested that the sensitivity of virtual colonoscopy remains high despite the application of dose-reducing techniques that have lowered x-ray exposure to less than 3 mSv.

Once the patient has been scanned, the resulting images must be interpreted. Image processing and interpretation are generally performed using commercially available virtual colonoscopy software. These software packages construct digital volumetric models of the colon from a series of CT images and provide a diagnostic interface that allows readers to view the colon on both 2D and 3D views.

There are two methods for interpreting virtual colonoscopy data: a primary axial 2D image review with 3D images for problem solving or a primary 3D image review. In a primary 2D interpretation, the supine colon is evaluated by scrolling through the axial images while examining the colon wall for abnormalities from the rectum to the cecum. When an abnormality is detected, the coronal, sagittal, and 3D endoluminal views can be used to assist with its identification as a polyp, fold, or fecal matter. The prone images are also examined to increase diagnostic confidence. Optical and 3D endoluminal virtual colonoscopic images of the same 1.4 cm polyp are shown in Figs. 43.1 and 43.2.

Interpretation by a primary 3D read involves an assessment of the volumetric reconstruction of the colon. This digital model is evaluated by performing a virtual "fly-through" of the colon lumen (the "endoluminal" or 3D view) in both antegrade and retrograde directions to detect polyps. The 2D slice views are readily available to confirm the presence of a polyp after its initial detection on the endoluminal view.

Comparisons between primary 2D and 3D methods have revealed advantages and disadvantages to both. A 2D interpretation, for instance, allows the entire colon to be examined in a single pass since polyps cannot be hidden by folds from this perspective. A 3D interpretation, on the other hand, can require antegrade and retrograde passes on both supine and prone images to ensure the visualization of all abnormalities in the

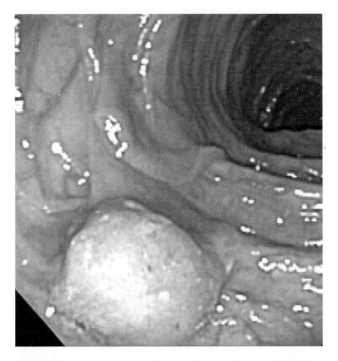

Fig. 43.1. Optical image of a 1.4-cm polyp in the transverse colon of a 64-year-old woman.

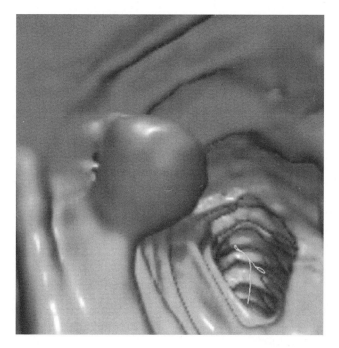

Fig. 43.2. Three-dimensional virtual colonoscopy image of same polyp. A portion of the colon centerline is shown in the lower right corner.

colon. This difference has a significant effect on interpretation times as indicated by a recent study by Macari et al. that showed a mean 2D reading time of 16 minutes versus 40 minutes for primary 3D reading with similar sensitivities for both. This difference, however, may be reduced with the application of better 3D visualization and automated polyp detection software.

A strong defense for the use of a primary 3D read has been reported in a study by Pickhardt et al. This study suggests that interpretation on an endoluminal view increases polyp conspicuity and therefore increases the sensitivity of the examination. In addition, the mean reading time using this method was found to be significantly shorter than previous reports.

A current focus of virtual colonoscopy research involves improving the consistency and sensitivity of this technique using computer-aided polyp detection (CAD) systems. A CAD system is essentially a software package that automatically identifies the colon lumen and wall, locates and segments candidate polyps, and uses a feature-based classification scheme to distinguish true polyps from false detections. The CAD system can then mark the location of each polyp on the primary axial CT images or on a 3D volumetric reconstruction of the colon. A recent multiinstitutional trial of virtual colonoscopy using CAD showed that performance of the CAD system was comparable to that of optical colonoscopy for patients having polyps ≥8 mm. This result indicates the strong potential for CAD to be a valuable addition to virtual colonoscopy interpretation methods.

At its present stage of development, virtual colonoscopy has an established role for detecting mass lesions and for evaluating the colon proximal to an occluding lesion or when colonoscopy is incomplete. Further research must be conducted to optimize colon preparation, confirm accuracy for detecting polyps, and assess clinical implementation of computer-assisted diagnosis.

*Acknowledgments*:    This work was supported by the intramural research program of the National Institutes of Health Clinical Center.

# E.  Conclusions

## *Nora A. Royer*

Colorectal cancer is one of the most common cancers to afflict adults in the United States today. The lifetime incidence is approximately 5% with a 3.7 per 1000 per year incidence by age 80. It is the third most common cancer and leading cause of cancer death in both men and women. The mortality for those afflicted is between 1 in 3 and 1 in 4. Over 90% of the cases occur in those over 50 years of age. The known risk factors for colon cancer include a family history of colon cancer in a first-degree relative, hereditary nonpolyposis colon cancer, familial adenomatous polyposis, prior colorectal cancer or dysplastic polyps in another region of colon, inflammatory bowel disease, and possibly exposure to radiation.

Colon cancer is considered one of the more ideal cancers for screening because the progression of the disease usually follows a predictable timeline of advancement and can be treated and removed if caught early in this progression. Colon cancer generally progresses over a period of approximately 10 years from a small, less than 5 mm, polyp to a larger polyp greater than 1.0 cm, to a larger dysplastic polyp, and finally to a frank cancer. Screening examinations for colon cancer have been geared toward identifying early lesions that could be removed before progression of disease. Traditional screening progressed from the use of Hemoccult cards to look for blood in the stool, lower gastrointestinal examination with barium to look for narrowing or masses in the lumen, flexible sigmoidoscopy to examine the left colon, where a greater percentage of lesions occur on statistical studies, to colonoscopy, which examines the entire colon.

Colonoscopy is the current preferred screening examination for colon cancer. It offers a view of the entire colon and the advantage of being able to intervene and remove or biopsy suspicious lesions as well as mark areas of suspicion with tattooing to ease in identification of lesions in the operating room should removal become necessary in the future. It requires highly trained examiners and is not acceptable to all patients, due to fear and expense. A finite rate of complications including perforation add to these concerns, and hence there has been great interest recently in less invasive ways of viewing the colon. Much has been touted recently in the popular media about CT colonography, also known as virtual colonoscopy.

Optical colonoscopy, where a scope is advanced to the cecum and the colon is visualized while the scope is withdrawn, has been the gold standard to date for the detection of polyps and colorectal cancers. The "miss rates" for optical colonoscopy has been between 0% to 6% in various studies using a technique of back-to-back colonoscopy, meaning the technique acts as its own gold standard in these studies.

There have been numerous studies published recently comparing optical to virtual colonoscopy. Cotton et al., in a nonrandomized comparison of the two modalities, demonstrated a sensitivity of 100% for polyps greater than 10 mm and 99% for polyps greater than 6 mm using traditional colonoscopy; the sensitivities for virtual colonoscopy were 39% for lesions greater than 6 mm and 55% for those greater than 10 mm. The sensitivities for the less than 6 mm polyps were greatly colored in this study by the most experienced center, where the sensitivity for detection was 82%, while the aggregate for all others was 24%. The technique used in this study was 2D technology and CT scanners with a slice width varying between 2.5 and 5 mm with reconstruction increments of 1 to 1.5 mm. There was a 20% referral rate to traditional colonoscopy in the virtual colonoscopy group.

Rockey et al. compared air contrast barium enema, virtual colonoscopy, and optical colonoscopy and found that traditional methods had a sensitivity for lesion detection of 98% and 99% for polyps greater than 10 mm and 6 mm, respectively, while virtual methods had detection rates of 59% and 51% for 10-mm and 6-mm lesions. Mulhall et al., in a meta-analysis of studies for virtual colonoscopy, found that a total of 33 studies covering 6393 patients demonstrated a sensitivity for polyp detection of 48% for lesions less than 6 mm in size, 70% for lesions greater than 6 mm in size, and 85% for lesions greater than 9 mm in size.

Many of these studies also used patient satisfaction questionnaires to determine which method patients preferred. The bowel preparation regimen in these studies was often the same, as the patients underwent both studies on the same day. Virtual studies still needed to use air insufflation of the bowel to assist with visualization. Patient satisfaction across all of the studies noted was lower for virtual colonoscopy, likely related to the fact that no sedation is given for the virtual colonoscopy procedure, so the patient is aware of and recalls the discomfort associated with air insufflation and the presence of a rectal tube.

Pickhardt et al. have provided the main study noting that virtual colonoscopy was better at lesion detection than traditional colonoscopy. Their research was carried out by the military using various military hospitals. The sensitivities for detection of lesions was 87.5%, 91.5%, and 92.3% for lesions greater than 10 mm, 8 mm, and 6 mm, respectively, for optical colonoscopy; 93.8%, 93.9%, and 88.7% for lesions greater than 10 mm, 8 mm, and 6 mm, respectively, for virtual colonoscopy. This is the only study that demonstrated that virtual colonoscopy was better at polyp detection than traditional colonoscopy. The technology used was different than the majority of other studies in that they used very thin slice machines and were able to use software that allows 3D reconstruction with a "fly-through" of the colon. This technology is not widely available in all hospitals at this time. An issue of bias is also possible in these results, in that the authors considered colonoscopy as a variable, meaning that they considered virtual colonoscopy as a gold standard rather than assuming that traditional colonoscopy was the standard. All of the studies noted that the sensitivity of lesion detection went up greatly with operator experience in reading this type of study. The best results come from centers where the author of the study was a pioneer in the field of virtual colonoscopy.

Although optical colonoscopy is not perfect in that lesions on folds and near the rectum can be missed, it does offer the advantage of being able to screen and intervene using only one test. Patient satisfaction is lower with virtual testing at this time, as patients must undergo the same bowel preparation and are aware during the entire examination. The current literature supports the use of virtual colonoscopy as a research tool at this time, but there are not sufficient data to support its use as a screening examination. The sensitivity of detection using the most widely available technology for slice width and reconstruction do not have a high enough level to ensure that even high-risk individuals will not have a false-negative screening examination. In the future, as slice width and 3D reconstruction software is perfected and as the possibility of stool subtraction oral contrast agents are expanded, virtual colonoscopy may become an appropriate screening tool for some individuals.

# References

Cotton PB, Durkalski VL, Benoit PC, et al. Computed tomographic colonography (virtual colonoscopy)—a multicenter comparison with standard colonoscopy for detection of colorectal neoplasia. JAMA 2004;291:1713–1719.

Halligan S, Altman DG, Taylor SA, et al. CT colonography in the detection of colorectal polyps and cancer: systematic review, meta-analysis, and proposed minimum data set for study level reporting. Radiology 2005;237:893–904.

Macari M, Milano A, Lavelle M, Berman P, Megibow AJ. Comparison of time-efficient CT colonography with two- and three- dimensional colonic evaluation for detecting colorectal polyps. AJR Am J Roentgenol 2000;174:1543–1549.

Mulhall BP, Veerappan GR, Jackson JL. Meta-Analysis: Computed tomographic colonography. Ann Intern Med 2005;142:635–650.

Pickhardt PJ, Choi JR, Hwang I, et al. Computed tomographic virtual colonoscopy to screen for colorectal neoplasia in asymptomatic adults. N Engl J Med 2003;349:2191–2200.

Rockey DC, Paulson E, Niedzwiecki D, et al. Analysis of air contrast barium enema, computed tomographic colonography, and colonoscopy: prospective comparison. Lancet 2005;365:305–311.

# Suggested Readings

Callstrom MR, Johnson CD, Fletcher JG, et al. CT colonography without cathartic preparation: feasibility study. Radiology 2001;219:693–698.

Fenlon HM, Barish MA, Clarke PD, Ferrucci JT. Virtual colonoscopy in occlusive colon carcinoma: preoperative evaluation of the proximal colon. Radiology 1998;209P:689.

Hixson LJ, Fennerty MB, Samplinger RE, Garewal HS. Prospective blinded trial of the colonoscopic miss-rate of large colorectal polyps. Gastrointestinal Endoscopy 1991;37:125–7.

Iannaccone R, Laghi A, Catalano C, et al. Detection of colorectal lesions: lower-dose multi-detector row helical CT colonography compared with conventional colonoscopy. Radiology 2003;229:775–781.

Johnson CD, Toledano AY, Herman BA, et al. Computerized tomographic colonography: performance evaluation in a retrospective multicenter setting. Gastroenterology 2003;125:688–695.

Lefere PA, Gryspeerdt SS, Dewyspelaere J, Baekelandt M, Van Holsbeeck BG. Dietary fecal tagging as a cleansing method before CT colonography: initial results polyp detection and patient acceptance. Radiology 2002;224:393–403.

Lieberman DA, Weiss DG, Bond JH, Ahnen DJ, Garewal H, Chejec G. Use of colonoscopy to screen asymptomatic adults for colorectal cancer. N Engl J Med 2000;83:162–169.

Macari M, Berman P, Dicker M, Milano A, Megibow AJ. Usefulness of CT colonography in patients with incomplete colonoscopy. AJR Am J Roentgenol 1999;173:561–564.

Pickhardt PJ, Choi JR, Hwang I, Schindler WR. Nonadenomatous polyps at CT colonography: prevalence, size distribution, and detection rates. Radiology 2004;232:784–790.

Pickhardt PJ, Nugent PA et al. Location of adenomas missed by optical colonoscopy. Ann Intern Med 2004;141:352–359.

Rex DK, Cutler CS, Lemmet GT, Rahmani EY, et al. Colonoscopic miss rates of adenomas determined by back-to-back colonoscopies. Gastroenterology 1997;112:24–28.

Summers RM, Yao J, Pickhardt PJ, et al. Computed tomographic virtual colonoscopy computer-aided polyp detection in a screening population. Gastroenterology 2005;129:1832–1844.

van Gelder RE, Venema HW, Serlie IW, et al. CT colonography at different radiation dose levels: feasibility of dose reduction. Radiology 2002;224:25–33.

Zalis ME, Hahn PF. Digital subtraction bowel cleansing in CT colonography. AJR Am J Roentgenol 2001;176:646–648.

# 44. Sessile Right Colon Polyp

## A. Introduction

As techniques for laparoscopic right colon resection have become standardized, it has emerged as an attractive alternative to sequential polypectomies for extirpation of the benign, but large, sessile colon polyp. This chapter uses the example of a sessile polyp in the cecum to explore these alternatives.

## B. Case

*Chad R. Laurich*

A 62-year-old man underwent screening colonoscopy after his wife was diagnosed with colon cancer. A large sessile cecal polyp was identified. Biopsy revealed a benign tubular adenoma. He denied any abdominal symptoms, including nausea, vomiting, bright red blood per rectum, abdominal pain, change in bowel habits, or change in weight or appetite.

His past medical history was significant for gastroesophageal reflux disease, peptic ulcer disease, non–insulin-dependent diabetes mellitus, hyperlipidemia, and depression. His past surgical history included a right inguinal hernia repair in 1994, carpal tunnel surgery on the left wrist in 1988, and a tonsillectomy during childhood. His father died at age 78 from laryngeal and lung cancer, and his mother was alive and healthy at 83, His two siblings were alive and healthy. No one in his family had developed colon cancer.

He worked as a dentist and lived with his wife. He had never smoked or used alcohol. The review of symptoms was negative, except as noted above.

On physical examination, he was a well-developed and well-nourished white male. Temperature was 36.0 °C, pulse 66, blood pressure 128/82, respirations 16, height 172 cm, and weight 94.6 kg. Examination of his head and neck, heart, and lungs were all normal.

Abdominal examination revealed a soft, nontender, nondistended abdomen. Bowel sounds were normal. No masses were palpable. There was a well-healed right inguinal incision. No hernias were noted. Rectal examination was negative and stool was guaiac negative.

Laboratory examination included a hemoglobin of 12.5 and hematocrit of 36.

**Would you recommend serial colonoscopic excisions or laparoscopic segmental colectomy for this benign tubular adenoma?**

# C. Serial Colonoscopic Polypectomies

*Kenneth A. Forde*

The question of whether a sessile lesion of the colon discovered endoscopically should be removed at colonoscopy or by colon resection (laparoscopic, laparoscopically assisted, or open) is of interest not only to the patient but also to the endoscopist (gastroenterologist or surgeon) as well as the surgeon.

The advantages of endoscopic resection are many. Inpatient hospital stay is not usually required, the procedure is performed with minimal or no conscious sedation, there is usually little interruption in the patient's activities, and the potential complications of general anesthesia and colon resection are avoided.

However, not every patient with a sessile lesion that is benign on biopsy is a candidate for the endoscopic approach. The biopsy sample may be inadequate and not representative of the entire lesion. Sessile polyps of the cecum larger than 1 cm in diameter are more commonly villous (as opposed to tubular) adenomas, which, as a group, have a greater malignant potential. Any evidence suggesting malignancy would deter me from choosing endoscopic excision, except for a large particle biopsy. This is especially relevant in the patient under discussion, who is anemic with a sessile right colon lesion.

When a sessile lesion with the gross appearance of a benign adenoma is visualized in the cecum colonoscopy, its general appearance, size, and configuration help in deciding which approach one should consider. Size is often inaccurately estimated. I have used the open biopsy 7-mm forceps placed immediately over the lesion to estimate its dimensions. The larger a villous adenoma, the greater the likelihood of malignant change but this should not be a total deterrent to endoscopic excision since many totally benign villous adenomas may attain enormous size in the right colon (as they often do in the rectum).

The lesion is described in our patient as a sessile polyp that on biopsy is a *tubular* adenoma. If it has a smooth surface and does not have villous features, I would be more aggressive with the endoscopic approach. If such a lesion is soft, not ulcerated, and glides over the deeper tissues of the bowel wall, even if villous, even if of larger size (3 cm or more), and even if in the more capacious cecum it occupies much of the circumference of the bowel wall, it might yet be feasible and appropriate to remove it at endoscopy.

If such a lesion is well demarcated from the surrounding bowel mucosa, does not have pseudopod-like extensions or satellite nodules, and its margins do not straddle more than two mucosal folds, I would certainly proceed endoscopically.

I remain hesitant about submucosal injection of saline solution to form a cushion against transmural burn during snare-cautery excision because (1) it is not universally protective; and (2) if there is malignant infiltration in the lesion, one could theoretically cause dissemination of malignant cells into lymphatic channels.

The cecal wall is deceptively thin, especially when distended by air insufflation during endoscopic manipulation. Unlike the rectum, with its thicker wall and even to some extent the left colon, the use of cautery may penetrate deeper in the cecal wall than is initially apparent to the endoscopist, and the risk of immediate or delayed perforation is thus increased.

If a sessile adenoma, tubular or villous, is found in a patient with known inflammatory disease involving the colon, I would not attempt total colonoscopic removal for fear that the inflamed bowel might not heal well and that bleeding or perforation might ensue. If the disease is ulcerative colitis of many years' duration, the presence of the adenoma may be an indication for colectomy (total) rather than polypectomy.

With respect to specifics of technique, I prefer to encircle the entire lesion, if feasible, or excise it in two or three fragments with snare and cautery. If further resection is necessary, one should be concerned about applying further cautery to the same area, and it is more prudent to defer further excision to a later date. Generally, I try to excise overhanging areas first and then move further centrally on the lesion. If it is clear that further endoscopic excision will be required in the future, I do not return in less than 4 to 6 weeks because earlier application of cautery might be through an area of granulation tissue, which is apt to be quite vascular and bleed significantly.

When I remove a large villous adenoma in fragments, I carefully "mock up" the segments, placing them back together in their proper position. This orients the specimen for the pathologist so that if malignant tissue is identified histologically, analysis for invasion will be easier in case consideration of resection becomes necessary.

I plan ahead for retrieval of large fragments, whether by basket, grasper, snare, or other device. If the lesion has been demonstrated by previous endoscopic or radiologic study and appears large, I find that the use of a double-channel colonoscope may facilitate specimen collection since one channel may be used for the snare and the other for retrieval instruments. Sometimes fragments of an excised lesion are temporarily lost at the site. Instilling a small amount of water in the area allows the specimen to be more readily found because it will fall into the dependent portion of the lumen and thus be seen in the "puddle." At times it may be necessary to change the patient's position to accomplish this.

Even if all fragments of a sessile polyp removed at a particular endoscopic session are histologically benign, the endoscopist must realize that residual neoplastic tissue will continue to grow and may become malignant in the interval between endoscopic sessions. The lesion has to be reevaluated critically at each endoscopic encounter in case a change in strategy (for example, resection) becomes indicated.

It is unnecessary to tattoo the polypectomy site when it is in the cecum, because resection, if indicated, conventionally involves this area (ileocolectomy).

When all visible tissue has been removed, close endoscopic follow-up is necessary, since any remaining microscopic foci of neoplasia may continue to grow. I usually reexamine patients twice in the first year following excision of a sessile lesion before resuming a longer-term follow-up (3 to 5 years). If the entire sessile lesion has been removed at the initial session and the pathologist is able to identify normal tissue at the margin of resection, a longer follow-up interval is satisfactory, depending on the risk category.

Patients in categories of higher risk for colon cancer—previous personal history or family history, history of previous adenoma (tubular or villous)—should make us less aggressive about performing endoscopic sessile polypectomy for fear of inadequately treating a cancer.

In patients with known coagulopathy, special care needs to be taken to replace the missing factors before embarking on endoscopic polypectomy. Since many treatments may be anticipated, one may opt for resection as a one time risk in selected patients.

As can be concluded from the above discussion, the primary risks of endoscopic resection of sessile colonic lesions are bleeding, perforation, and delay in the diagnosis of cancer, a risk that is greater than for pedunculated polyps. These risks may be reduced through thorough preprocedure evaluation, careful endoscopic examination, safe excision, and close follow-up.

In the future, endoscopic ultrasound may prove useful in assessing the depth of a neoplastic lesion, and safer methods of thermal ablation such as argon plasma coagulation may assist in reducing recurrence or persistence of some sessile lesions after endoscopic polypectomy.

# D. Laparoscopic Right Colon Resection

## Steven A. Lee-Kong and Daniel L. Feingold

The purpose of intervention in this case is to completely remove all neoplastic tissue in the cecum. If the colonoscopic biopsy is representative of the entire lesion and the neoplasm is only a tubular adenoma, complete removal of the lesion will disrupt the adenoma-carcinoma sequence, preventing potential future malignant transformation and will also prevent the lesion from causing symptoms in the future. In addition, given the inherent sampling error of colonoscopic biopsies and the possibility of a large adenoma harboring occult invasive adenocarcinoma, complete removal of the lesion facilitates histopathologic analysis that may very well influence treatment if a malignancy is discovered.

When considering possible therapeutic interventions in this case, it is important to consider the association between adenoma size and occult malignancy. In a landmark study, Muto et al. investigated the malignant potential of adenomas, and reported that of nearly 2500 colorectal adenomas, 1.3% of polyps smaller than 1 cm, 9.5% of polyps between 1 and 2 cm, and 46% of polyps larger than 2 cm harbored invasive cancer. The National Polyp Study further substantiated this association by demonstrating a correlation between colorectal adenoma size and the presence of high-grade dysplasia.

Based on the clinical details presented, there are two options for treatment in this case: serial colonoscopic excisions and colectomy. Attempting to completely remove a large, sessile neoplasm via a colonoscope is inherently risky in the thin-walled cecum. These lesions often have a carpet-like appearance with indiscrete borders and may be partially obscured by folds (in this case by the ileocecal valve), making complete endoscopic removal difficult. Given the risk of perforation, colonoscopic excision of a sessile, cecal adenoma is often performed piecemeal and usually requires multiple procedures. It is important to recognize and consider the need for short-interval endoscopic follow-up in these patients. Attempts at colonoscopic excision may utilize advanced techniques such as endoscopic mucosal resection, whereby a submucosal injection of dilute epinephrine is used to elevate a sessile polyp off of the muscularis propria to facilitate snare polypectomy. Although the colonoscopic approach in expert hands may be feasible in certain situations, the more appropriate alternative in the present case, in our opinion, is to perform a colon resection.

Once the decision is made to recommend colectomy, one must consider the extent of resection to be performed. In this scenario, there is no compelling reason to perform a limited resection by way of ileocecectomy; rather, a formal right colectomy is indicated. Central to this issue is the likelihood of demonstrating invasive cancer within the specimen. Although an estimate of the size of the adenoma is not offered in this case (it is only described as "large and sessile"), given the association between the size of an adenoma and the risk of occult cancer reviewed previously, a formal oncologic operation should be performed. Even though a tubular adenoma is considered to have less malignant potential as compared to a villous adenoma, formal colectomy is warranted. In the event that pathologic review demonstrates a cancer in the specimen, this approach will ensure oncologic adequacy in terms of margins and nodal catch. If any question remains regarding the proposed extent of resection, it may be helpful to keep in mind that the additional colon mobilization and length of colon resected in a right colectomy as compared to an ileocecectomy add negligible risk of morbidity to the operation and do not impact functional outcomes whatsoever.

In terms of the surgical approach in this case, a laparoscopic right colectomy is preferred over a comparable open operation. The patient in this case has no contraindications to laparoscopic colectomy. Specifically, he has an American Society of Anesthesiologists (ASA) score of 2 and a body mass index (BMI) of 32 and has had no prior abdominal surgery. In addition, the lesion is well localized by the fact that the polyp is in the cecum. The anatomic landmarks of the appendiceal orifice, cecal strap, and ileocecal valve are used to confidently localize mucosal lesions in the cecum and ascending colon during colonoscopy and usually obviate the need for further localization (i.e., tattooing). Clearly, adequate preoperative localization is required prior to undertaking laparoscopic-assisted colectomy. These kinds of considerations facilitate the laparoscopic approach in this particular case. The caveat remains, however, that laparoscopic colectomy is technically challenging and should be performed only by surgeons proficient in this technique who have adequate experience dealing with colonic neoplasms.

# E.  Conclusions

## *Chad R. Laurich*

Colon polyps are categorized as pedunculated if there is a mucosal stalk between the polyp and the colon wall or sessile if the base of the polyp is attached to the colon wall. Polyps are commonly removed endoscopically by forceps or snare excision. Pedunculated polyps readily lend themselves to excision. Sessile polyps, especially large ones (over 2 cm), often require piecemeal excision with close colonoscopic follow-up every 3 to 6 months initially. In a study by Walsh and colleagues evaluating patients after colonoscopic excision of large sessile polyps, 28% persisted or recurred requiring re-resection, but overall 88% of the endoscopically managed patients were ultimately cured, with a low 3% total complication rate. Thus endoscopic resection of sessile polyps, even larger adenomas, can be both safe and effective when performed by experienced colonoscopists, and when patients are carefully followed.

When a large sessile polyp cannot be safely or completely resected endoscopically, however, laparoscopic segmental colectomy has been shown to be an excellent alternative, with the added advantages of decreased operative morbidity and pain, shorter length of stay, quicker return to work, and improved cosmesis over open techniques. In their series of laparoscopic segmental colectomies, Lo and Law demonstrated low intraoperative complications (4.5%), low total complications (15.6%), and no mortalities. Gracia and colleagues further demonstrated that patients undergoing laparoscopic colectomy for polyps versus other reasons had lower morbidity, less need for conversion, and shorter operative time, suggesting laparoscopic colectomy may be particularly suited for the treatment of polyps.

The treatment of choice for the removal of colon polyps, including sessile polyps, is endoscopic resection. When a sessile polyp is particularly large or in a difficult anatomic position, safe and complete resection can be carried out by segmental laparoscopic colectomy with significant advantages over open techniques.

# References

Gracia E, Targarona EM, Garriga J, Pujol J, Trias M. Laparoscopic treatment of colorectal polyps. Gastroenterol Hepatol 2000;23(5):224–227.

Lo SH, Law WL. Laparoscopic colorectal resection for polyps not suitable for colonoscopic removal. Surg Endosc 2005;19:1252–1255.

Muto T, Bussey HJ, Morson BC. The evolution of cancer of the colon and rectum. Cancer 1975;36:2251–2270.

Walsh RM, Ackroyd FW, Shellito PC. Endoscopic resection of large sessile colorectal polyps. Gastrointest Endosc 1992;38:303.

# Suggested Readings

Church JM. Experience in the endoscopic management of large colonic polyps. ANZ J Surg 2003;73:988–995.

Conio M, Repici A, Demarquay JF, Blanchi S, Dumas R, Filiberti R. EMR of large sessile colorectal polyps. Gastrointest Endosc 2004;60:234–241.

Feingold DL, Addona T, Forde KA, et al. Safety and reliability of tattooing colorectal neoplasms prior to laparoscopic resection. J Gastrointest Surg 2004;8:543–546.

Heldwein W, Dollhopf M, Rosch T, et al. The Munich Polypectomy study: prospective analysis of complications and risk factors in 4000 colonic snare polypectomies. Endoscopy 2005;37:1116–1122.

Higaki S, Hashimoto S, Harada K, et al. Long-term follow-up of large flat colorectal tumors resected endoscopically. Endoscopy 2003;35:845–849.

Lohnert MS, Wittmer A, Doniec JM. Endoscopic removal of large colorectal polyps. Zentralbl Chir 2004;129:291–295.

Nivatvongs S, Snover DC, Fang DT. Piecemeal snare excision of large sessile colon and rectal polyps: is it adequate? Gastrointest Endosc 1984;30(1):18–20.

O'Brien MJ, Winawer SJ, Zauber AG, et al. The National Polyp Study. Patient and polyp characteristics associated with high-grade dysplasia in colorectal adenomas. Gastroenterology 1990;98:371–379.

Pokala N, Delaney CP, Kiran RP, Brady K, Senagore AJ. Outcome of laparoscopic colectomy for polyps not suitable for endoscopic resection. Surg Endosc 2006;21(3):400–403.

Prohn P, Weber J, Bonner C. Laparoscopic-assisted coloscopic polypectomy. Dis Colon Rectum 2001;44:746–748.

Senagore AJ, Delaney CP, Brady KM, Fazio VW. Standardized approach to laparoscopic right colectomy: outcomes in 70 consecutive cases. J Am Coll Surg 2004;199:675–679.

Stergiou N, Riphaus A, Lange P, Menke D, Kockerling F, Wehrmann T. Endoscopic snare resection of large colonic polyps: how far can we go? Int J Colorectal Dis 2003;18(2):131–135.

Thaler K, Dinnewitzer A, Mascha E, et al. Long-term outcome and health-related quality of life after laparoscopic and open colectomy for benign disease. Surg Endosc 2003;17:1404–1408.

Young-Fadok TM, Radice E, Nelson H, Harmsen WS. Benefits of laparoscopic-assisted colectomy for colon polyps: a case-matched series. Mayo Clin Proc 2000;75(4):344–348.

# 45. Rectal Villous Adenoma

## A. Introduction

Villous adenomas are benign lesions that, if untreated, may progress to colon carcinoma. They tend to be sessile and may carpet a region of colon or rectum. Complete resection is necessary and may be accomplished endoscopically, surgically, or by endoscopic mucosal resection. This chapter uses a case of a distal rectal villous adenoma to explore alternatives in transanal management. A related topic, serial polypectomies, was discussed in Chapter 44, as applied to a sessile polyp of the cecum. In a way, these transanal excisions might be considered an example of natural orifice surgery, an area under active development at present.

## B. Case

*Chad R. Laurich*

A 57-year-old woman complained of a 4-month history of bright red blood per rectum and blood mixed with stool. She had not noted any other change in bowel habits and ascribed the bleeding to her hemorrhoids. A friend saw an article in a health magazine about the warning signs of cancer and urged her to seek medical attention. She normally had one to two firm bowel movements per day with no constipation, diarrhea, change in caliber, or abdominal pain. She had not experienced nausea, vomiting, or loss of appetite. She had not lost weight.

Her past medical history was significant for hypertension, hypothyroidism, ovarian carcinoma (stage IIC, treated by resection and chemotherapy 9 years earlier, currently no evidence of disease), renal insufficiency with a creatinine up to 1.8, and a history of anemia. She had been told that she had hemorrhoids about 10 years earlier. Her surgical history was significant for a total abdominal hysterectomy and bilateral salpingo-oophorectomy in 1999, as noted above. Her mother had colon cancer. There was no other family history of cancer.

The patient's medications are hydrochlorothiazide and thyroid hormone replacement therapy. She had no known drug allergies.

She was single and had not worked since her ovarian cancer treatment. She was a nonsmoker and did not drink alcoholic beverages. She walked 1 to 2 miles per day. The review of systems was negative, except as noted above.

On physical examination, she was a well-developed, well-nourished female in no acute distress. Vital signs included a temperature of 36.7 °C, pulse 82, and blood pressure 136/89. She was 170 cm tall and weighed 76 kg. Her head and neck and cardiopulmonary examinations were negative.

Abdominal examination revealed a soft, nontender abdomen with a lower midline scar (well healed without evidence of hernia). There were no masses or tenderness. No hernias were found.

Inspection of the anus revealed external hemorrhoids. Digital rectal examination revealed a suggestion of a soft mass at fingertip. Stool was streaked with mucus and blood and was guaiac positive.

Laboratory investigations were remarkable for a hematocrit of 35%, a blood urea nitrogen (BUN) of 31, and creatinine 1.7. The remainder of her labs were normal. Chest x-ray was negative.

Colonoscopy revealed a 3.5-cm sessile polyp in the rectum, 5 cm from the anal verge. The remainder of the examination was negative. Biopsy of the polyp revealed a villous adenoma without high-grade dysplasia or invasive carcinoma.

The impression was a rectal villous adenoma. She has been told that endoscopic polypectomy is inadvisable, and wishes to avoid open surgery.
**What would you recommend?**

# C. Transanal Endoscopic Microsurgery

*John H. Marks*

When approaching a patient with a rectal polyp, as in this case, surgeon must first decide whether they agree with the original description of the lesion: is it truly benign, and is the location as reported? Then the surgeon must focus on determining the optimal procedure for removing the polyp. In general, the treatment options include endoscopic polypectomy, transanal excision, or transabdominal resection with or without sphincter preservation (low anterior resection versus abdominoperineal resection). At our center we emphasize the role of local excision (either endoscopic or transanal) and use a decision tree for choosing the best approach for rectal polyp removal.

The surgeon evaluating a rectal polyp that has been deemed unresectable endoscopically must be wary of the possibility of an inadequately biopsied cancer as well as the exact location of the mass. Accurate characterization of the polyp and its malignant potential together with its location critically inform the surgeon's operative approach. Measurements of polyp level, even in the rectum, are notoriously inconsistent, and the significance of polyp location for the surgeon planning an excision is different than for the gastroenterologist. Both of these points highlight the essential necessity of evaluating the patient oneself.

This physical exam includes a digital rectal examination in a patient who is prepped with an enema, and some form of endoscopic evaluation. Flexible sigmoidoscopy allows a better ability in the office to determine the exact morphology and extent of the tumor. Attention must be paid to the mucosa around the obvious polyp so one does not miss a carpet-like extension of the villous adenoma around the raised polyp. This method also facilitates visually inspecting the polyp, looking for signs of invasion. A sense of firmness and ulceration should raise the suspicion of an underlying cancer. However, another possibility is reactive induration and ulceration secondary to an endoscopic biopsy. Often this exam is augmented by a rigid sigmoidoscopy, which facilitates identifying precisely in what quadrant in the rectum the lesion lies, as this can be difficult to determine with a flexible sigmoidoscope.

On endoscopic and digital rectal examination, attention must be focused on the fine points that will impact the surgical approach. In abdominal surgery the important descriptor for a rectal lesion is the inferior margin of the border. This is proper, as the challenge is to perform the anastomosis in the low rectum, and the question is whether one will be able to reach there through the pelvis. In transanal surgery the level of the tumor relative to the anal sphincter is important to ensure that the sphincter is not damaged. However, the more central point of information is the cephalad extent of the mass, as the surgeon must be able to reach the apex of the tumor transanally to ensure an adequate margin of resection. Particular attention should be paid to the morphology of the lesion, its size, the distal and cephalad extent of the tumor, ulceration, and mobility. If questions exist regarding the possibility of an underlying cancer, it should be re-biopsied in the office with endoscopic biopsy forceps, even if previous endoscopic biopsies have been benign. If one has the strong clinical impression that the polypoid mass is an underlying cancer, repetitive biopsies must be performed. Sometimes it is necessary to use large rigid biopsy forceps in the operating room or endoscopy suite with the patient under anesthesia to obtain a better tissue sample to confirm the diagnosis so that an invasive cancer is not mistakenly violated transanally. If questions remain, endoscopic ultrasound (EUS) may also be used. Again, previous biopsies make results difficult to interpret reliably.

A second factor that must be clearly considered and documented, especially in women, is the patient's fecal continence status and bowel habits. A history of frequency, control, and ability to defer both solid liquid stool and flatus should be obtained. In addition, any history of previous anorectal surgery, vaginal delivery, episiotomy, or tear at the time of delivery should be noted. On clinical examination the status of the perineal body, anal wink (which confirms the sensory and motor innervation of S2-4), and voluntary contraction on the examining index finger at the time of digital rectal examination are simple easy methods to identify problems and perform initial continence evaluation. Any irregularities found should be so noted and can be evaluated as deemed necessary.

Assuming there are no contraindicating factors and the lesion is indeed as described, the next question is how it should be treated. The primary goal of the surgeon's approach is to effectively remove the pathology with a low level of local recurrence and minimal patient morbidity. If necessary a low anterior resection (LAR) is a reasonable option, but clearly for a benign polyp if one can avoid an abdominal operation, this is to the patient's great benefit. For the purpose of this discussion, we will focus on the options of colonoscopic polypectomy versus transanal excision. From a theoretical standpoint, endoscopic polypectomy, if it can be accomplished effectively, is clearly the least invasive for the patient. For a patient referred by the gastroenterologist, already one endoscopist has decided the polyp cannot be removed endoscopically, but this should not override your clinical judgment. View the lesion with an open mind regarding your comfort level endoscopically and what you are willing to undertake. Lipof et al. recently demonstrated that 32% of patients referred for colectomy by a gastroenterologist were able to avoid abdominal surgery after a repeat colonoscopy by the surgeon.

The location of the tumor has impact on the treatment options. Anteriorly based polyps, especially in a woman where deep coagulation could end in a thermal injury to the rectum, vagina, or extend into the pouch of Douglas and the peritoneal cavity, must be handled much more carefully. With a posteriorly based lesion one need not be as concerned about using thermal coagulation, as the mesorectum will serve to seal a small burn without great problems, as been demonstrated in the electrocoagulation fulguration of cancers. It is important that the patient undergo complete bowel prep, in the event that a more extensive procedure is necessary. The tools available to the endoscopist include saline injection underneath the polyp to raise it to perform a polypectomy, which may be augmented with a laser to address areas of the polyp that cannot be adequately treated by snare. The approach will be, by definition, a piecemeal snare polypectomy. In general it requires multiple returns to the endoscopy suite at 3- to 6-month intervals. The operative consideration in these patients has to be that less is more. A persistent benign polyp with no evidence of dysplasia is far preferable to an endoscopic perforation requiring emergent surgery. The caveat is that there is a high incidence of persistent/recurrent polyps in this scenario. There is little downside other than patient inconvenience because of the multiple endoscopic polypectomies, as long as there is no evidence of dysplasia or invasive neoplasia. Patient compliance with follow-up must be considered in weighing this treatment approach. In addition, if more unfavorable pathology is encountered over time, which is a significant possibility, surgeons must be willing to alter their approach and then must move to a more definitive approach, meaning a transanal or abdominal operation.

My preference for removal of a large polyp such as the one described in this case is transanal excision because it is an en bloc resection that allows good visualization and evaluation of the lesion's margins, and low local recurrence rates (Fig. 45.1). As stated earlier, the challenge of operating transanally is comfortably reaching the cephalad margins of the tumor. Transanal endoscopic microsurgery (TEM) offers advantages over conventional transanal excision of improved visualization and greater control of resection.

Transanal endoscopic microsurgery or transanal endoscopic microsurgery was first described by Dr. Gerhardt Buess in Germany in 1983. The basic equipment involves a 4-cm-diameter operating microscope (Figs. 45.2 and 45.3) that is inserted into the rectum with the patient under general anesthesia. It allows for gentle insufflation and distention of the rectum. The visualization of pathology with binocular stereoscopic vision is clearly superior to the view afforded transanally, especially as one approaches the cephalad margin and it is much easier to clearly evaluate the surrounding normal mucosa and perform a controlled resection. The surgeon is only able to operate on the bottom 180 degrees of the operating lumen, which highlights the necessity for careful preoperative evaluation.

For posterior lesions the patient is placed in the lithotomy position, for an anterior lesion the patient is placed in the prone position, and for right- or left-sided lesions the patient is placed in the right lateral or left lateral decubitus position, respectively. Once the patient is positioned

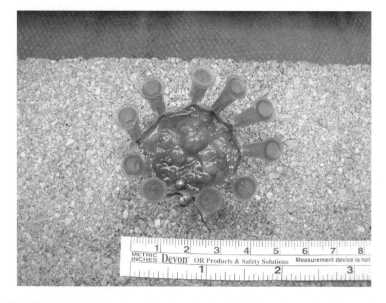

Fig. 45.1. Transanal endoscopic microsurgery (TEM) specimen pinned on cork. Note that complete excision with a rim of normal mucosa has been accomplished, and that the specimen is oriented for the pathology.

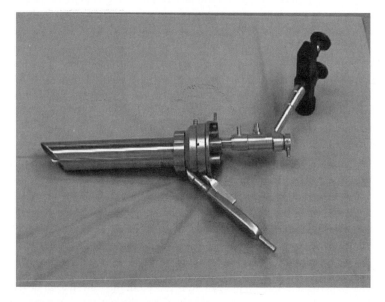

Fig. 45.2. Operating endoscope used for TEM.

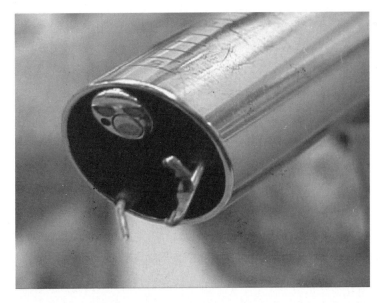

Fig. 45.3. View of the end of the scope, showing optical and operating channels in use.

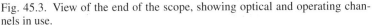

and under anesthesia, digital rectal examination is performed to confirm the location of the tumor. The rectum is gently prepped and draped and the anus is gently dilated. The 4-cm obturator is inserted into the rectum and positioned with the faceplate in place to ensure that adequate visualization of the lesion and reaching it are possible. The tubing is then passed off the field, which allows for insufflation into the lumen of carbon dioxide and monitoring the intrarectal pressure, irrigating the operative scope and aspirating excess liquid.

With the TEM equipment in place, a left-handed grasper is inserted to retract the lesion, and then for a benign polyp, a 5-mm to 1-cm rim of normal mucosa around the polyp is marked or "tattooed" with electrocautery circumferentially around the lesion (Fig. 45.4). This is essential to identifying what will be resected. Without this marking, once the resection is started, even with only a small amount of blood, smoke, and char on the field, it is often difficult to determine the exact area of desired resection. After this is accomplished, we find it very helpful to inject 1% lidocaine with 100,000 to 200,000 units of epinephrine solution in the submucosal plane. This elevates the level in which the surgeon will be working and then makes it easier to stay out of the deeper muscular layer.

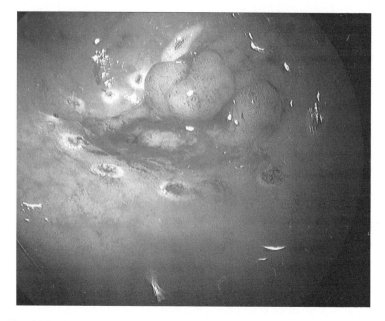

Fig. 45.4.  Mucosa tattooed prior to TEM.

One starts inferiorly connecting the dots, and the dissection is taken submucosally using the normal mucosa as a handle. Great care is taken not to handle the adenoma itself, as generally it is quite friable and will start to bleed. Working in a small field, such as one encounters when working endoluminally, becomes a major impediment to the operation. Do not be surprised in some patients to find adipose tissue in the submucosal plane. Likewise it is not uncommon to inadvertently venture into the muscularis propria and even through the full thickness of the muscularis, which is often much thinner than you would expect in the distal rectum. Early on in the dissection it is often helpful to place a marking stitch inferiorly, which can be used both as a handle as well as to orient the specimen once it is removed. Depending on the morphology of the polyp, one can work from inferior to superior in the submucosal plane or connect all the dots circumferentially and then work underneath from inferior to superior to excise the polyp. If all the markings are not connected originally, be careful as you come to the cephalad margin of the lesion. It is quite common to dissect much more proximally than one had intended. While this is not a problem per se, and often this mobilization helps with closure, it is better to be aware that one is doing this intentionally rather than doing it inadvertently.

Once the specimen is removed, instruments are washed with a dilute Betadine solution, as is the operative field, and then the gloves are changed. This minimizes the possibility of inadvertently seeding viable cells into the open wound. The defect is generally bisected with a 4-cm stitch of 2-0 PDS. The anastomosis is then carried out using a running 2-0 PDS suture starting from the right side and continuing laterally over to the left side. Generally it takes two to three stitches to successfully close the defect. Once the defect is closed in its entirety, it is a good idea to inspect the anastomosis and check for any gaps in the closure. Often the running stitch simply needs to be tightened with an additional clip placed on the tightened suture in order to complete the closure, or simple interrupted stitches can be utilized.

Postoperatively patients receive perioperative antibiotics for 24 hours. A Foley catheter is left in place for the first operative night, and depending on patients' medical comorbidities, they are generally started on liquids later that evening or the following morning. It is impossible to effectively constipate these patients, and the risk of a large hard bulky stool disrupting the anastomosis outweighs any other considerations. For that reason, patients are generally started the following day on a half to one ounce of milk of magnesia, which is continued for 1 week postoperatively. Patients are instructed to titrate it up or down in order to avoid active diarrhea yet keep the stools loose. Patients are discharged with narcotics for pain, but these patients have very little in the way of actual pain.

The onset of pain and mucoid discharge between 3 and 10 days postoperatively generally heralds a wound disruption. In general these are managed conservatively by an oral antibiotic regimen. This is a common occurrence and in our TEM experience, occurring in 26% of patients. Likewise in follow-up in these patients, it is not uncommon to find a small area of granulation tissue. It should be biopsied aggressively to rule out the possibility of a recurrence. These areas can then be fulgurated to effectively eradicate them.

The specimen itself is prepared on a cork board with the edges rolled out and pinned to assist the pathologist in evaluating margin involvement (Fig. 45.1). If the margins are negative and there is no invasive carcinoma in situ or high-grade dysplasia, the patients are generally followed at 6-month intervals endoscopically with flexible sigmoidoscopy in the office at 6, 18, and 24 months, and a colonoscopy is done at 12 months postoperatively. This schedule should be adequate, as 80% of local recurrence occurs in the first 24 months. If all these assessments remain negative, then patients are placed in a normal surveillance program for colorectal polyps.

# D. Conventional Transanal Excision

*John H. Marks*

If one does not have TEM equipment available, the procedure can also be performed transanally under direct visualization.

The preparation and postoperative follow-up are exactly the same as cited above, but the intraoperative details vary somewhat. A Pratt speculum or a Sawyer hemicircumferential retractor is best used to gain good visualization in the rectum. Generally the patients are operated on in a prone jackknife position for lesions other than those directly posteriorly. Those patients are best operated on in an extended lithotomy position. Again, the operation is started by using the electrocautery to mark circumferentially around the polyp with a 5-mm to 1-cm margin. The inferior margin is often marked with a stitch both to help handle the polyps and to orient the specimen at the conclusion of the operation. It is a good idea to avoid grasping the polyp itself, as that will cause fragmentation of the lesion as well as significant bleeding, which will obscure the operative field. An effort should be made to avoid grasping or putting a stitch above the polyp. This only serves to pull the normal mucosa from above over the area where you need to be working, in a fashion similar to a window shade. If there is a concern that there will retraction of the mucosa as the specimen is finally removed, stitches can be placed in a cephalad area to the right and left of the lesion, and place hemostats, which will serve to provide access to the proximal mucosa. Similar strategies regarding epinephrine solution and dissection are utilized. In general, closures are undertaken using interrupted 3-0 Vicryl stitches, which are placed serially and tied when all have been placed to avoid misaligning the closure.

The significant concept to highlight as one approaches a rectal polyp is eradicating the adenomatous tissue. If one elects to start this approach endoscopically and is not having success, or if there is a question of dysplasia or invasive neoplasia, there must be a very low threshold to then recommend a definitive transanal resection. In the case presented a transanal excision is a viable and straightforward option. The discussion becomes more complex when dealing with larger polyps and those with high-grade dysplasia that have a higher likelihood of housing an invasive neoplasia. In addition, lesions more proximal, while still reachable by TEM resection, become more challenging transanally. These issues must be factored into the surgeon endoscopist's decision of how best to remove a rectal polyp.

# E. Conclusions

*Chad R. Laurich*

Adenomas are dysplastic by definition and thus have malignant potential. They are classified as tubular, villous, or tubulovillous based on the glandular architecture and are graded as low or high dysplasia. The histologic features and size largely determine malignant potential. Villous histology and larger size (>1 cm in diameter) are independent risk factors for high-grade dysplasia and colorectal cancer formation. As up to 35% of rectal villous adenomas may contain malignancy, complete resection is necessary.

A variety of methods have been described to remove rectal villous adenomas. Colonoscopic excision has been a common approach and has been shown to be both safe and effective. Larger tumors often have to be removed in piecemeal fashion, however, decreasing the effectiveness of the pathologic examination. Ongoing surveillance is also necessary, as rates of retained tissue or recurrence have been reported to range from 3% to 28%.

Transanal excision is another described method of removing rectal villous adenomas that allows for a more complete resection and histologic analysis of the tumor at the initial intervention. It is also a one-step procedure that does not require specialized instrumentation. In their 2004 study, Featherstone and colleagues reported a residual tumor rate of 2.1% with no significant preoperative morbidity and no mortality. Other series have reported recurrence rates up to 36% with significant complications in 19%. Pigot and colleagues suggested that this high variability in published results may be due to variable completeness of tumor excision because of difficulties in dissection. Their 2003 study describes a tractable cutaneomucous flap procedure they developed to lower the rectal tumor to the anal verge where dissection is easier, resulting in a 3.6% recurrence rate with a 4% complication rate.

Excellent results have been achieved with TEM. The procedure produces a complete specimen for thorough pathologic examination and has been extended to stage T1 rectal tumors with curative intent. Meng and colleagues reported their series in 2004 in which they had no recurrences and no significant complications or mortality. Other series have reported recurrence rates of 6%, with significant complications up to 10.3%. When compared directly to other methods, TEM shows significantly decreased recurrence rates, with complication rates that trended lower but did not reach significance. Although the results with TEM are excellent, the equipment is expensive and may be used relatively infrequently in many institutions, which creates barriers to widespread use.

While colonoscopic polypectomies, transanal excision, and TEM have all been shown to be safe and effective, they do have their specific advantages and disadvantages. Colonoscopic excision is technically familiar for most practitioners and inexpensive, but requires close ongoing surveillance, and piecemeal excision results in poor pathologic examination. Transanal excision allows for more complete resection, but has a high variability in published results. Transanal endoscopic microsurgery has excellent results, but cost and practicality hamper its widespread use.

# References

Featherstone JM, Grabham JA, Fozard JB. Per-anal excision of large, rectal, villous adenomas. Dis Colon Rectum 2004;47(1):86–89.

Lipof T, Bartus C, Sardella W, Johnson K, Vignati P, Cohen J. Preoperative colonoscopy decreases the need for laparoscopic management of colonic polyps. Dis Colon Rectum 2005;48:1076–1080.

Meng WC, Lau PY, Yip AW. Treatment of early rectal tumours by transanal endoscopic microsurgery in Hong Kong: prospective study. Hong Kong Med J 2004;10(4): 239–243.

Pigot F, Bouchard D, Mortaji M, et al. Local excision of large rectal villous adenomas: long-term results. Dis Colon Rectum 2003;46(10):1345–1350.

# Suggested Readings

Bardan E, Bat L, Melzer E, Shemesh E, Bar-Meir S. Colonoscopic resection of large colonic polyps—a prospective study. Isr J Med Sci 1997;33:777–780.

Buess G, Hutterer F, Theiss J, Bobel M, Isselhard W, Pichlmaier H. A system for a trananal endoscopic rectum operation. Surg Gynecol Obstet 1988;166:393–396.

Church JM. Experience in the endoscopic management of large colonic polyps. ANZ J Surg 2003;73:988–995.

Dell'Abate P, Iosca A, Galimberti A, Piccolo P, Soliani P, Foggi E. Endoscopic treatment of colorectal benign-appearing lesions 3 cm or larger: techniques and outcome. Dis Colon Rectum 2001;44:112–118.

Doniec JM, Lohnert MS, Schniewind B, Bokelmann F, Kremer B, Grimm H. Endoscopic removal of large colorectal polyps: prevention of unnecessary surgery? Dis Colon Rectum 2003;46(3):340–348.

Iishi H, Tatsuta M, Iseki K, et al. Endoscopic piecemeal resection with submucosal saline injection of large sessile colorectal polyps. Gastrointest Endosc 2000;51:697–700.

Marks JH, Marchionni C, Marks GJ. Transanal endoscopic microsurgery in the treatment of select rectal cancers or tumors suspicious for cancer. Surg Endosc 2003;17:1114–1117.

Middleton PF, Sutherland LM, Maddern GJ. Transanal endoscopic microsurgery: a systematic review. Dis Colon Rectum 2005;48(2):270–284.

O'Brien MJ, Winawer SJ, Zauber AG, et al. The National Polyp Study. Patient and polyp characteristics associated with high-grade dysplasia in colorectal adenomas. Gastroenterology 1996;98:371–379.

Salvati EP, Rubin RJ, Eisenstat TE, Siemons GO, Mangione JS. Electrocoagulation of selected carcinoma of the rectum. Surg Gynecol Obstet 1988;166:393–396.

Stergiou N, Riphaus A, Lange P, Menke D, Kockerling F, Wehrmann T. Endoscopic snare resection of large colonic polyps: how far can we go? Int J Colorectal Dis 2003;18(2):131–135.

Walsh RM, Ackroyd FW, Shellito PC. Endoscopic resection of large sessile colorectal polyps. Gastrointest Endosc 1992;38:303.

# 46. Thoracoscopic Sympathectomy for Hyperhidrosis: A Lagniappe

## A. Introduction

The *Oxford English Dictionary* defines *lagniappe* as "something given as a bonus or gratuity, extra reward." This brief chapter discusses thoracoscopic sympathectomy, the only nongastrointestinal subject included in this manual. The editor offers it as a lagniappe. As such, it is briefer than the previous chapters, and opposing viewpoints are not given.

## B. Case

*Kalpaj R. Parekh*

A 24-year-old woman presented with severe lifestyle-limiting palmar hyperhidrosis. She had undergone multiple, unsuccessful medical therapies. These therapies included topical aluminum chloride and repeated injections of botulinum toxin. The sweating was so excessive that it interfered with day-to-day activities such as typing on a computer, playing the clarinet, and, most importantly, social interactions. She was otherwise healthy and had no medical problems.

Family history was significant for a paternal uncle with hyperhidrosis. Physical examination was negative with the exception of wet palms, with dripping sweat, bilaterally. She was referred for thoracic sympathectomy for management of her refractory hyperhidrosis.

## C. Thoracoscopic Sympathectomy

*Kalpaj R. Parekh*

Historically, several techniques have been described to perform thoracic sympathectomy. The anterior approach was initially used by Jonnesco, Leriche, and Royle in the 1930s. The posterior approach was described by Adson and Brown in 1929, while Telford described the anterior cervical approach in 1935.

Hughes, a British surgeon, was the first to describe endoscopic thoracic sympathectomy in 1942. Since then, advances in the endoscopic video technology have been applied, and video assisted thoracoscopy (VATS) thoracic sympathectomy has become the current standard of care in the treatment of primary hyperhidrosis.

Primary hyperhidrosis is a disorder of unknown etiology that is characterized by excessive perspiration. It most commonly affects the palms, the axillae, and, to a lesser extent, the face and trunk. The main drawback that it imposes on patients is a psychosocial burden, which affects their professional and personal life and their daily activities. Medical treatment in the form of topical aluminium chloride, iontophoresis, anticholinergics, and botulinum toxin injection has been less than satisfactory and provides only transient relief. Thoracic sympathectomy leads to complete resolution of the upper extremity hyperhidrosis and is now the treatment of choice for this pathophysiologic condition.

The sympathetic chain ganglia lie in the retropleural region over the head of the ribs at their articulation with the transverse process of the vertebral body (Fig. 46.1). The inferior cervical and T1 ganglia fuse to

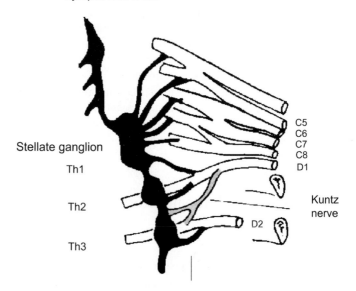

Fig. 46.1. Anatomy of the thoracic sympathetic chain.

form the stellate ganglion. The T1 root mainly supplies the head and neck region, whereas most of the innervation to the hand originates in the T2 ganglion and partly from the T3 ganglia. The axillary region is supplied by the T4 and T5 ganglia of the sympathetic chain. The nerve of Kuntz arises from the postganglionic fibers of T2 and T3, which bypass the stellate ganglion and carry sympathetic fibers to the inferior portion of the brachial plexus.

For VATS thoracic sympathectomy, the patient is usually intubated with a double-lumen endotracheal tube. The thoracic cavity is approached via an incision in the midaxillary line. Two additional 3- to 5-mm ports are placed in the second and third intercostals space and the lung is collapsed (Fig. 46.2). Carbon dioxide insufflation can be used to improve visualization; however, intrathoracic pressures above 15 mm Hg are associated with hemodynamic instability and should be used with extreme caution. The sympathetic chain is then identified running over the rib heads, and the overlying pleura is excised (Fig. 46.3).

The method and extent of nerve ablation is a subject of controversy and varies from institution to institution. Sympathetic nerve ablation has been achieved in a number of ways. Electrocauterization of the chain using a two-hole approach was described by Tan and Nam in 1998, while transection of the sympathetic trunk was described with good results by

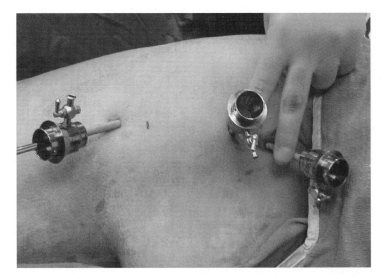

Fig. 46.2. Port sites used for VATS sympathectomy.

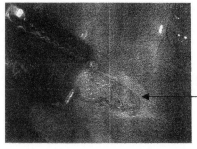

Mediastinal Pleura

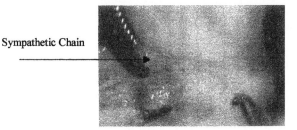

Sympathetic Chain

Fig. 46.3. (A,B) Dissection of the sympathetic chair after dividing the mediastinal pleura.

Rex and colleagues in the same year. Other techniques, such as division of the rami communicantes and resection of a segment of nerve, have also been described. Finally, some authors have advocated clipping the thoracic sympathetic chain without division; this has the advantage of being reversible if the rare symptoms of compensatory hyperhidrosis become unbearable. We prefer to resect the chain.

The next important question is the extent of ablation. Several authors have suggested that limiting the extent of sympathectomy may reduce the occurrence of compensatory sweating. Generally for palmar hyperhidrosis, just excision of T2 is indicated, while for axillary hyperhidrosis most surgeons will take T2 along with T3 and frequently the T4 ganglion as well.

Pneumothorax is the most common early complication and is seen in up to 75% of patients. Most patients are simply observed; chest tube drainage is rarely required. Other complications that have been reported include subcutaneous emphysema, injury to the subclavian artery, and chylothorax. Gossot et al. reported a 5.3% incidence of significant (300 to 600 mL) intraoperative bleeding.

Rebound sweating is a temporary occurrence in 31% of patients. Horner syndrome is seen in less than 1% of patients.

The commonest long-term complication is compensatory sweating. The incidence of compensatory sweating varies considerably in the literature and is reported to be as high as 89%. However, only 35% of the patients were severely affected by it. The severity was higher in patients who T2-4 ablation for axillary hyperhidrosis compared to patients who had only T2 ablation for palmar hyperhidrosis.

Another long-term complication is gustatory sweating, and the reason for this is still obscure. The incidence varies from 38% to 50% in the literature and is particularly related to spicy foods or foods with acidity like oranges or apples.

In conclusion, VATS thoracic sympathectomy is a safe and effective treatment for hyperhidrosis when performed by an experienced team for the right indication. This approach has less morbidity than open techniques, though compensatory sweating and gustatory sweating are frequent complications. The newer modality of clipping offers the option of reversibility in the face of unbearable side effects. However, the extent and technique of ablation needs to be studied in large multicenter randomized trials.

# References

Adson A, Brown GE. The Treatment of Raynaud's Disease by Resection of the Upper Thoracic and Lumbar Sympathetic Ganglia and Trunks. Surg Gynecol Obstet 1929;48:577.

Gossot D, Kabiri H, Caliandro R, Debrosse D, Girard P, Grunenwald D. Early complications of thoracic endoscopic sympathectomy: a prospective study of 940 procedures. Ann Thorac Surg 2001;71(4):1116.

Hughes J. Endothoracic sympathectomy. Proc R Soc Med 1942;35:585.

Rex LO, Drott C, Claes G, Gothberg G, Dalman P. The Boras experience of endoscopic thoracic sympathicotomy for palmar, axillary, facial hyperhidrosis and facial blushing. Eur J Surg Suppl 1998;(580):23.

Tan V, Nam H. Results of thoracoscopic sympathectomy for 96 cases of palmar hyperhidrosis. Ann Thorac Cardiovasc Surg 1998;4(5):244.

Telford E. The Technique of Sympathectomy. Br J Surg 1935;77:1043–1045.

# Suggested Readings

Asking B, Svartholm E. Degeneration activity: a transient effect following sympathectomy for hyperhidrosis. Eur J Surg Suppl 1994;(572):41.

Baumgartner FJ, Toh Y. Severe hyperhidrosis: clinical features and current thoracoscopic surgical management. Ann Thorac Surg 2003;76(6):1878.

Gossot D, Toledo L, Fritsch S, Celerier M. Thoracoscopic sympathectomy for upper limb hyperhidrosis: looking for the right operation. Ann Thorac Surg 1997;64(4):975.

Herbst F, Plas EG, Fugger R, Fritsch A. Endoscopic thoracic sympathectomy for primary hyperhidrosis of the upper limbs. A critical analysis and long-term results of 480 operations. Ann Surg 1994;220(1):86.

Kao MC. Complications in patients with palmar hyperhidrosis treated with transthoracic endoscopic sympathectomy. Neurosurgery 1998;42(4):951.

Krasna MJ, Demmy TL, McKenna RJ, Mack MJ. Thoracoscopic sympathectomy: the U.S. experience. Eur J Surg Suppl 1998;(580):19.

Licht PB, Pilegaard HK. Severity of compensatory sweating after thoracoscopic sympathectomy. Ann Thorac Surg 2004;78(2):427.

Lin CC, Mo LR, Lee LS, Ng SM, Hwang MH. Thoracoscopic T2-sympathetic block by clipping—a better and reversible operation for treatment of hyperhidrosis palmaris: experience with 326 cases. Eur J Surg Suppl 1998;(580):13.

Ojimba TA, Cameron AE. Drawbacks of endoscopic thoracic sympathectomy. Br J Surg 2004;91(3):264.

Sung SW, Kim YT, Kim JH. Ultra-thin needle thoracoscopic surgery for hyperhidrosis with excellent cosmetic effects. Eur J Cardiothorac Surg 2000;17(6):691.

# Index